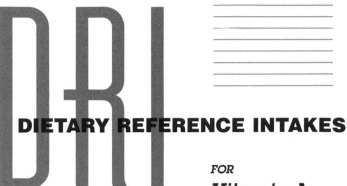

DIETARY REFERENCE INTAKES

FOR

Vitamin A, Vitamin K, Arsenic, Boron, Chromium, Copper, Iodine, Iron, Manganese, Molybdenum, Nickel, Silicon, Vanadium, and Zinc

A Report of the
Panel on Micronutrients,
Subcommittees on Upper Reference Levels of Nutrients and of
Interpretation and Uses of Dietary Reference Intakes, and the
Standing Committee on the Scientific Evaluation of
Dietary Reference Intakes

Food and Nutrition Board
Institute of Medicine

NATIONAL ACADEMY PRESS
Washington, D.C.

NATIONAL ACADEMY PRESS • 2101 Constitution Avenue, N.W. • Washington, DC 20418

NOTICE: The project that is the subject of this report was approved by the Governing Board of the National Research Council, whose members are drawn from the councils of the National Academy of Sciences, the National Academy of Engineering, and the Institute of Medicine. The members of the committee responsible for the report were chosen for their special competences and with regard for appropriate balance.

This project was funded by the U.S. Department of Health and Human Services Office of Disease Prevention and Health Promotion, Contract No. 282-96-0033, T03; the National Institutes of Health Office of Dietary Supplements; the Centers for Disease Control and Prevention, National Center for Chronic Disease Prevention and Health Promotion, Division of Nutrition and Physical Activity; Health Canada; the Institute of Medicine; the Dietary Reference Intakes Private Foundation Fund, including the Dannon Institute and the International Life Sciences Institute; and the Dietary Reference Intakes Corporate Donors' Fund. Contributors to the Fund to date include Daiichi Fine Chemicals, Inc., Kemin Foods, L.C., M&M/Mars, Mead Johnson Nutritionals, Nabisco Foods Group, Natural Source Vitamin E Association, Roche Vitamins Inc., U.S. Borax, and Weider Nutritional Group. The opinions or conclusions expressed herein do not necessarily reflect those of the funders.

Library of Congress Cataloging-in-Publication Data

Dietary reference intakes for vitamin A, vitamin K, arsenic, boron, chromium, copper, iodine, iron, manganese, molybdenum, nickel, silicon, vanadium, and zinc : a report of the Panel on Micronutrients ... [et al.], Standing Committee on the Scientific Evaluation of Dietary Reference Intakes, Food and Nutrition Board, Institute of Medicine.
    p. cm.
Includes bibliographical references and index.
ISBN 0-309-07279-4 (pbk.)—ISBN 0-309-07290-5 (hc.)
    1. Trace elements in nutrition. 2. Vitamin A in human nutrition. 3. Vitamin K. 4. Reference Values (Medicine) I. Institute of Medicine (U.S.). Panel on Micronutrients.

QP534 .D54 2002
612.3'924--dc21   2001052139

This report is available for sale from the National Academy Press, 2101 Constitution Avenue, N.W., Box 285, Washington, DC 20055; call (800) 624-6242 or (202) 334-3313 (in the Washington metropolitan area), or visit the NAP's on-line bookstore at **http://www.nap.edu**.

For more information about the Institute of Medicine or the Food and Nutrition Board, visit the IOM home page at **http://www.iom.edu**.

Printed in the United States of America

The serpent has been a symbol of long life, healing, and knowledge among almost all cultures and religions since the beginning of recorded history. The image adopted as a logotype by the Institute of Medicine is based on a relief carving from ancient Greece, now held by the Staatliche Museen in Berlin.

"Knowing is not enough; we must apply.
Willing is not enough; we must do."
—Goethe

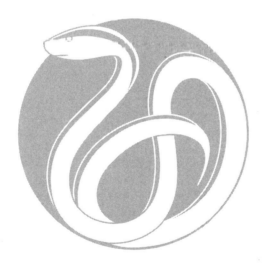

INSTITUTE OF MEDICINE

Shaping the Future for Health

THE NATIONAL ACADEMIES

National Academy of Sciences
National Academy of Engineering
Institute of Medicine
National Research Council

The **National Academy of Sciences** is a private, nonprofit, self-perpetuating society of distinguished scholars engaged in scientific and engineering research, dedicated to the furtherance of science and technology and to their use for the general welfare. Upon the authority of the charter granted to it by the Congress in 1863, the Academy has a mandate that requires it to advise the federal government on scientific and technical matters. Dr. Bruce M. Alberts is president of the National Academy of Sciences.

The **National Academy of Engineering** was established in 1964, under the charter of the National Academy of Sciences, as a parallel organization of outstanding engineers. It is autonomous in its administration and in the selection of its members, sharing with the National Academy of Sciences the responsibility for advising the federal government. The National Academy of Engineering also sponsors engineering programs aimed at meeting national needs, encourages education and research, and recognizes the superior achievements of engineers. Dr. Wm. A. Wulf is president of the National Academy of Engineering.

The **Institute of Medicine** was established in 1970 by the National Academy of Sciences to secure the services of eminent members of appropriate professions in the examination of policy matters pertaining to the health of the public. The Institute acts under the responsibility given to the National Academy of Sciences by its congressional charter to be an adviser to the federal government and, upon its own initiative, to identify issues of medical care, research, and education. Dr. Kenneth I. Shine is president of the Institute of Medicine.

The **National Research Council** was organized by the National Academy of Sciences in 1916 to associate the broad community of science and technology with the Academy's purposes of furthering knowledge and advising the federal government. Functioning in accordance with general policies determined by the Academy, the Council has become the principal operating agency of both the National Academy of Sciences and the National Academy of Engineering in providing services to the government, the public, and the scientific and engineering communities. The Council is administered jointly by both Academies and the Institute of Medicine. Dr. Bruce M. Alberts and Dr. Wm. A. Wulf are chairman and vice chairman, respectively, of the National Research Council.

PANEL ON MICRONUTRIENTS

ROBERT RUSSELL (*Chair*), Jean Mayer U.S. Department of Agriculture Human Nutrition Research Center on Aging, Tufts University, Boston, Massachusetts

JOHN L. BEARD, Department of Nutrition, The Pennsylvania State University, University Park

ROBERT J. COUSINS, Center for Nutritional Sciences, University of Florida, Gainesville

JOHN T. DUNN, University of Virginia Health System, Charlottesville

GUYLAINE FERLAND, Department of Nutrition, University of Montreal, Quebec, Canada

K. MICHAEL HAMBIDGE, Department of Pediatrics, University of Colorado Health Sciences Center, Denver

SEAN LYNCH, Veterans Administration Medical Center, Hampton, Virginia

JAMES G. PENLAND, U.S. Department of Agriculture Human Nutrition Research Center, Grand Forks, North Dakota

A. CATHARINE ROSS, Department of Nutrition, The Pennsylvania State University, University Park

BARBARA J. STOEKER, Department of Nutritional Sciences, Oklahoma State University, Stillwater

JOHN W. SUTTIE, Department of Biochemistry, University of Wisconsin, Madison

JUDITH R. TURNLUND, U.S. Department of Agriculture Western Human Nutrition Research Center, Davis, California

KEITH P. WEST, Center for Human Nutrition, Johns Hopkins School of Hygiene and Public Health, Baltimore, Maryland

STANLEY H. ZLOTKIN, Departments of Pediatrics and Nutritional Sciences, The Hospital for Sick Children and The University of Toronto, Ontario, Canada

Consultants

LEWIS BRAVERMAN, School of Medicine, Harvard University, Boston, Massachusetts

FRANCOISE DELANGE, Department of Pediatrics, Hôpital Saint-Pierre, Brussels, Belgium

Staff

PAULA R. TRUMBO, Study Director

ALICE L. VOROSMARTI, Research Associate

MICHELE RAMSEY, Senior Project Assistant

v

SUBCOMMITTEE ON UPPER REFERENCE LEVELS OF NUTRIENTS

IAN C. MUNRO *(Chair)*, CanTox, Inc., Mississauga, Ontario, Canada

GEORGE C. BECKING, Phoenix OHC, Kingston, Ontario, Canada

RENATE D. KIMBROUGH, Institute for Evaluating Health Risks, Washington, D.C.

RITA B. MESSING, Division of Environmental Health, Minnesota Department of Health, St. Paul

SANFORD A. MILLER, Graduate School of Biomedical Sciences, University of Texas Health Sciences Center, San Antonio

HARRIS PASTIDES, School of Public Health, University of South Carolina, Columbia

JOSEPH V. RODRICKS, The Life Sciences Consultancy LLC, Washington, D.C.

IRWIN H. ROSENBERG, Clinical Nutrition Division, the Jean Mayer U.S. Department of Agriculture Human Nutrition Research Center on Aging, Tufts University and New England Medical Center, Boston, Massachusetts

STEVE L. TAYLOR, Department of Food Science and Technology and Food Processing Center, University of Nebraska, Lincoln

JOHN A. THOMAS, Retired, University of Texas Health Science Center at San Antonio

GARY M. WILLIAMS, Department of Pathology, New York Medical College, Valhalla

Staff

SANDRA SCHLICKER, Study Director

ELISABETH A. REESE, Research Associate

MICHELE RAMSEY, Senior Project Assistant

SUBCOMMITTEE ON INTERPRETATION AND USES OF DIETARY REFERENCE INTAKES

SUZANNE MURPHY *(Chair)*, Cancer Research Center of Hawaii, University of Hawaii, Honolulu

LENORE ARAB, University of North Carolina School of Public Health, Chapel Hill

SUSAN I. BARR, University of British Columbia, Vancouver

SUSAN T. BORRA, International Food Information Council, Washington, D.C.

ALICIA CARRIQUIRY, Iowa State University, Ames

BARBARA L. DEVANEY, Mathematica Policy Research, Princeton, New Jersey

JOHANNA T. DWYER, Frances Stern Nutrition Center, New England Medical Center and Tufts University, Boston, Massachusetts

JEAN-PIERRE HABICHT, Cornell University, Ithaca, New York

HARRIET V. KUHNLEIN, Centre for Indigenous Peoples' Nutrition and Environment, McGill University, Ste. Anne de Bellevue, Quebec, Canada

Staff

MARY POOS, Study Director
ALICE L. VOROSMARTI, Research Associate
SHELLEY GOLDBERG, Senior Project Assistant

PAULA TRUMBO, Senior Program Officer
ALICE L. VOROSMARTI, Research Associate
KIMBERLY FREITAG, Research Assistant
MICHELE RAMSEY, Senior Project Assistant
GAIL E. SPEARS, Administrative Assistant

Preface

This report is one in a series that presents a comprehensive set of reference values for nutrient intakes for healthy U.S. and Canadian populations. It is a product of the Food and Nutrition Board of the Institute of Medicine (IOM) working in cooperation with Canadian scientists.

The report establishes a set of reference values for vitamin A, vitamin K, chromium, copper, iodine, iron, manganese, molybdenum, and zinc to replace previously published Recommended Dietary Allowances (RDAs) and Recommended Nutrient Intakes (RNIs) for the United States and Canada. The report also examines data about arsenic, boron, nickel, silicon, and vanadium. Although all reference values are based on data, available data often were scanty or drawn from studies that had limitations in addressing the various questions that confronted the Panel. Thus, although governed by reasoning, informed judgments often were required in setting reference values. The reasoning used is described for each nutrient in Chapters 4 through 13.

Close attention was given to the evidence relating intake of micronutrients to reduction of the risk of chronic disease, and the daily amounts needed to maintain normal status based on biochemical indicators and daily body losses. In addition, a major task of the Panel on Micronutrients, Subcommittee on Upper Reference Levels of Nutrients (UL Subcommittee), and the Standing Committee on the Scientific Evaluation of Dietary Reference Intakes (DRI Committee) was to analyze the evidence on beneficial and adverse effects of arsenic, boron, nickel, silicon, and vanadium—in the context of setting Dietary Reference Intakes (DRIs).

Another major task of the report was to outline a research agenda to provide a basis for future public policy decisions related to recommended intakes of these micronutrients and ways to achieve those intakes. Many of the questions that were raised about requirements for and recommended intakes of micronutrients were not answered fully because of inadequacies in the published database. Apart from studies of overt deficiency diseases, there is a dearth of studies that address specific effects of inadequate micronutrient intakes on health status. For most of the micronutrients, there is no direct information that permits estimating the amounts required by children, adolescents, the elderly, and pregnant and lactating women. For four of the micronutrients, data were sparse for setting Tolerable Upper Intake Levels (ULs), precluding reliable estimates of how much can be ingested safely. For some of these micronutrients, there are questions about how much is contained in the foods North Americans eat.

Readers are urged to recognize that the establishment of DRIs is an iterative process that is expected to evolve as its conceptual framework is applied to new nutrients and food components. With more experience, the proposed models for establishing reference intakes of nutrients and food components that play a role in health will be refined. Also, as new information or new methods of analysis are adopted, these reference values undoubtedly will be reassessed.

Thus, because the project is ongoing, many comments were solicited and have been received on the reports that have been previously published. Refinements that have resulted from this iterative process have been included in the general information regarding approaches used (Chapters 1 through 3) and in the discussion of uses of DRIs (Chapter 14 in this report).

The Subcommittee on the Interpretation and Uses of Dietary Reference Intakes (Uses Subcommittee), formed subsequent to the release of the first two reports, has been primarily responsible for chapter 14, which addresses major issues conceptually included since the beginning of the DRI process that relate to the anticipated uses and applications of reference values as developed further by the Uses Subcommittee.

This report reflects the work of the Food and Nutrition Board's DRI Committee, its expert Panel on Micronutrients, and the UL and Uses Subcommittees. We gratefully acknowledge the support of the government of Canada and Canadian scientists in this initiative that represents a pioneering first step in the standardization of nutrient reference intakes at least within a major part of one continent. A brief description of the overall project of the DRI Committee and of the panel's task is given in Appendix A. We hope that the critical, comprehensive analyses of available information and knowledge gaps contained in this initial series of reports will assist the private sector, foundations, universities, government laboratories, and other institutions with the development of a productive research agenda for the next decade.

The DRI Committee, the Panel on Micronutrients, the UL and Uses Subcommittees, and the Food and Nutrition Board wish to extend sincere thanks to the many experts who assisted with this report by giving presentations, providing written materials, participating in discussions, analyzing data, and other means. Many, but far from all, of these individuals are named in Appendix B. Special thanks go to George Beaton and the staff at the National Center for Health Statistics, the Food Surveys Research Group of the Agricultural Research Service, ENVIRON Corporation, Health Technomics, and the Department of Statistics at Iowa State University for extensive analyses of survey data.

The respective chairs and members of the Panel on Micronutrients and subcommittees have performed their work under great time pressure. Their dedication made the completion of this report possible. All gave of their time willingly and without financial reward; the public and the science and practice of nutrition are among the major beneficiaries.

The DRI Committee and the Food and Nutrition Board wish to acknowledge, in particular, the commitment shown by Robert Russell, Chair of the Panel on Micronutrients, who guided this difficult project through challenging and innovative paths. His ability to keep the effort and various biases moving in a positive direction is very much appreciated. Thanks are also due to the DRI Committee members, Lindsay Allen and William Rand, who served as in-depth internal reviewers for this report.

Special thanks also are expressed to the staff of the Food and Nutrition Board and foremost to Paula Trumbo, who was the study director for the panel and without whose assistance, both intellectual and managerial, this report would neither have been as polished nor as timely in its release. It is, of course the Food and Nutrition Board staff who get much of the work completed and so the panel, committees, and the Food and Nutrition Board wish to thank Allison Yates, Director of the Food and Nutrition Board, for her and her staff's constant assistance. Thus, we also recognize and appreciate the contributions of Sandra Schlicker, Mary Poos, Elisabeth Reese, Alice Vorosmarti, Gail Spears, and Michele Ramsey and thank Pat Stephens for editing the manuscript, Jacqueline Dupont for technical review, and Claudia Carl for assistance with publication.

Vernon Young
Chair, Standing Committee on the Scientific
    Evaluation of Dietary Reference Intakes

Cutberto Garza
Chair, Food and Nutrition Board

Reviewers

This report has been reviewed in draft form by individuals chosen for their diverse perspectives and technical expertise, in accordance with procedures approved by the NRC's Report Review Committee. The purpose of this independent review is to provide candid and critical comments that will assist the institution in making its published report as sound as possible and to ensure that the report meets institutional standards for objectivity, evidence, and responsiveness to the study charge. The review comments and draft manuscript remain confidential to protect the integrity of the deliberative process. We wish to thank the following individuals for their review of this report:

Sarah L. Booth, Tufts University
James D. Cook, Kansas University Medical Center
Mark L. Failla, University of North Carolina
Jeanne Freeland-Graves, University of Texas
James K. Friel, Memorial University of Newfoundland
Walter Mertz, Rockville, Maryland
Phylis B. Moser-Veillon, University of Maryland
Robert S. Parker, Cornell University
John B. Stanbury, Massachusetts General Hospital
Clive E. West, Wageningen Agricultural University

Although the reviewers listed above have provided many constructive comments and suggestions, they were not asked to endorse the conclusions or recommendations nor did they see the final draft of the report before its release. The review of this report was overseen by Kurt J. Isselbacher, Massachusetts General Hospital and Ronald W. Estabrook, University of Texas Southwestern Medical Center at Dallas. Appointed by the National Research Council and Institute of Medicine, they were responsible for making certain that an independent examination of this report was carried out in accordance with institutional procedures and that all review comments were carefully considered. Responsibility for the final content of this report rests entirely with the authoring committees and the institution.

Contents

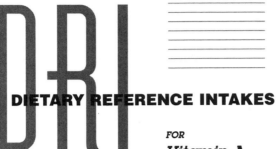

DIETARY REFERENCE INTAKES

FOR

Vitamin A,
Vitamin K,
Arsenic, Boron,
Chromium,
Copper,
Iodine, Iron,
Manganese,
Molybdenum,
Nickel, Silicon,
Vanadium,
and Zinc

Summary

This report provides quantitative references intakes for vitamin A, vitamin K, boron, chromium, copper, iodine, iron, manganese, molybdenum, nickel, vanadium, and zinc. No recommendations are provided for arsenic and silicon. This is one volume in a series of reports that presents dietary reference values for the intake of nutrients by Americans and Canadians. The development of Dietary Reference Intakes (DRIs) expands and replaces the series of Recommended Dietary Allowances (RDAs) in the United States and Recommended Nutrient Intakes (RNIs) in Canada. A major impetus for the expansion of this review is the growing recognition of the many uses to which RDAs and RNIs have been applied and the growing awareness that many of these uses require the application of statistically valid methods that depend on reference values other than RDAs and RNIs. This report includes a review of the roles that micronutrients are known to play in traditional deficiency diseases and evaluates possible roles in chronic diseases.

The overall project is a comprehensive effort undertaken by the Standing Committee on the Scientific Evaluation of Dietary Reference Intakes (the DRI Committee) of the Food and Nutrition Board, Institute of Medicine, The National Academies, with active involvement of Health Canada. (See Appendix A for a description of the overall process and its origins.) This study was requested by the U.S. Federal Advisory Steering Committee for Dietary Reference Intakes in collaboration with Health Canada.

1

Major new approaches and findings in this report include the following:

• The establishment of new estimates for the conversion of provitamin A carotenoids to vitamin A: 1 μg retinol activity equivalent (μg RAE) is equal to 1 μg all-*trans*-retinol, 12 μg β-carotene, and 24 μg α-carotene or β-cryptoxanthin. This recognizes that 50 percent less bioconversion of carotenoids to vitamin A occurs than was previously thought, a change that means twice as much provitamin A-rich carotenoids contained in green leafy vegetables and certain fruits are required to provide a given amount of vitamin A activity. Given possible future changes in equivalency, weight of carotenoids should be given in food tables.
• The establishment of RDAs for copper and molybdenum.
• The establishment of Tolerable Upper Intake Levels (ULs) for vitamin A, boron, copper, iodine, iron, manganese, molybdenum, nickel, vanadium, and zinc.
• Research recommendations for information needed to advance understanding of human micronutrient requirements and the adverse effects associated with intake of higher amounts.

WHAT ARE DIETARY REFERENCE INTAKES?

Dietary Reference Intakes (DRIs) are reference values that are quantitative estimates of nutrient intakes to be used for planning and assessing diets for apparently healthy people. They include not only Recommended Dietary Allowances (RDAs) but also three other types of reference values (see Box S-1). Although the reference values arc based on data, the data were often scanty or drawn from studies that had limitations in addressing the question. Thus, scientific judgment was required for evaluating the evidence and in setting the reference values, and that process is delineated for each nutrient in Chapters 4 through 13.

Recommended Dietary Allowances

The process for setting the RDA depends on being able to set an *Estimated Average Requirement* (EAR). Before the EAR is set, a specific criterion of adequacy is selected on the basis of a careful review of the literature. In the selection of the criterion, reduction of disease risk is considered along with many other health parameters.

Box S-1 Dietary Reference Intakes

Recommended Dietary Allowance (RDA): *the average daily dietary nutrient intake level sufficient to meet the nutrient requirement of nearly all (97 to 98 percent) healthy individuals in a particular life stage and gender group.*

Adequate Intake (AI): *the recommended average daily intake level based on observed or experimentally determined approximations or estimates of nutrient intake by a group (or groups) of apparently healthy people that are assumed to be adequate—used when an RDA cannot be determined.*

Tolerable Upper Intake Level (UL): *the highest average daily nutrient intake level that is likely to pose no risk of adverse health effects to almost all individuals in the general population. As intake increases above the UL, the potential risk of adverse effects may increase.*

Estimated Average Requirement (EAR): *the average daily nutrient intake level estimated to meet the requirement of half the healthy individuals in a particular life stage and gender group.*

If the standard deviation (SD) of the EAR is available and the requirement for the nutrient is symmetrically distributed, the RDA is set at two SDs above the EAR:

$$RDA = EAR + 2\ SD_{EAR}.$$

If data about variability in requirements are insufficient to calculate an SD, a coefficient of variation (CV) for the EAR of 10 percent is assumed, unless available data indicate a greater variation in requirements.

If 10 percent is assumed to be the CV, then twice that amount when added to the EAR is defined as equal to the RDA. The resulting equation for the RDA is then

$$RDA = 1.2 \times EAR.$$

This level of intake statistically represents 97.5 percent of the requirements of the population. If the distribution of the nutrient requirement is known to be skewed for a population, as with iron, other approaches are used to find the ninety-seventh to ninety-eighth percentile to set the RDA.

The RDA for a nutrient is a value to be used as a goal for dietary intake for the healthy individual. As discussed in Chapter 14, the RDA is not intended to be used to assess the diets of either individuals or groups or to plan diets for groups. Only if intakes have been observed for a large number of days (i.e., usual intake) and are at or above the RDA, or if observed intakes for fewer days are well above the RDA, should one have a high level of confidence that the intake is adequate (see Box S-2). The EAR is also used as the basis to address diets of groups.

Adequate Intakes

The *Adequate Intake* (AI) is set instead of an RDA if sufficient scientific evidence is not available to calculate an EAR. The main intended use of the AI is as a goal for the nutrient intake of individuals. For example, the AI for young infants, for whom human milk is the recommended sole source of food for most nutrients up through the first 4 to 6 months of age, is based on the daily mean nutrient intake supplied by human milk for apparently healthy, full-term infants receiving human milk. The goal may be different for infants consuming infant formula for which the bioavailability of a nutrient may be different from that in human milk, such as iron, which is high in infant formula due to its lower bioavailability than that found in human milk.

Comparison of Recommended Dietary Allowances and Adequate Intakes

Although both the RDA and AI are to be used as a goal for intake by individuals, the RDA differs from the AI. Intake of the RDA for a nutrient is expected to meet the needs of 97 to 98 percent of the apparently healthy individuals in a life stage and gender group (see Figure S-1). However, because no distribution of requirements is known for nutrients with an AI, it is not possible to know what percentage of individuals are covered by the AI. The AI for a nutrient is expected to exceed the RDA for that nutrient, and thus it should cover the needs of more than 97 to 98 percent of the individuals. The degree to which an AI exceeds the RDA is likely to differ among nutrients and population groups.

For people who have diseases that increase specific nutrient requirements or who have other special health needs, the RDA and

Box S-2 Uses of Dietary Reference Intakes for Healthy Individuals and Groups

Type of Use	For the Individual[a]	For a Group[b]
Assessment	**EAR:** use to examine the probability that usual intake is inadequate.	**EAR:** use to estimate the prevalence of inadequate intakes within a group.
	RDA: usual intake at or above this level has a low probability of inadequacy.	**RDA:** do not use to assess intakes of groups.
	AI[c]**:** usual intake at or above this level has a low probability of inadequacy.	**AI**[c]**:** mean usual intake at or above this level implies a low prevalence of inadequate intakes.
	UL: usual intake above this level may place an individual at risk of adverse effects from excessive nutrient intake.	**UL:** use to estimate the percentage of the population at potential risk of adverse effects from excess nutrient intake.
Planning	**RDA:** aim for this intake.	**EAR:** use to plan an intake distribution with a low prevalence of inadequate intakes.
	AI[c]**:** aim for this intake.	**AI**[c]**:** use to plan mean intakes.
	UL: use as a guide to limit intake; chronic intake of higher amounts may increase the potential risk of adverse effects.	**UL:** use to plan intake distributions with a low prevalence of intakes potentially at risk of adverse effects.

RDA = Recommended Dietary Allowance
EAR = Estimated Average Requirement
AI = Adequate Intake
UL = Tolerable Upper Level

[a] Evaluation of true status requires clinical, biochemical, and anthropometric data.
[b] Requires statistically valid approximation of distribution of usual intakes.
[c] For the nutrients in this report, AIs are set for infants for all nutrients, and for other age groups for vitamin K, chromium, and manganese. The AI may be used as a guide for infants as it reflects the average intake from human milk.

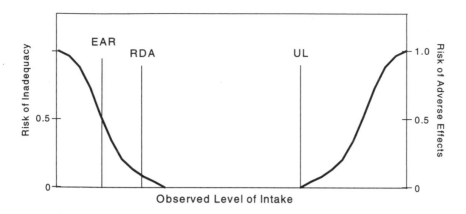

FIGURE S-1 Dietary reference intakes. This figure shows that the Estimated Average Requirement (EAR) is the intake at which the risk of inadequacy is 0.5 (50 percent) to an individual. The Recommended Dietary Allowance (RDA) is the intake at which the risk of inadequacy is very small—only 0.02 to 0.03 (2 to 3 percent). The Adequate Intake (AI) does not bear a consistent relationship to the EAR or the RDA because it is set without being able to estimate the average requirement. It is assumed that the AI is at or above the RDA if one could be calculated. At intakes between the RDA and the Tolerable Upper Intake Level (UL), the risks of inadequacy and of excess are both close to 0. At intakes above the UL, the potential risk of adverse effects may increase.

AI each may serve as the basis for adjusting individual recommendations. Qualified health professionals should adapt the recommended intake to cover higher or lower needs.

Tables S-1 through S-9 provide the recommended intake levels, whether RDAs or AIs, for vitamin A, vitamin K, chromium, copper, iodine, iron, manganese, molybdenum, and zinc by life stage and gender group. For most of these micronutrients, AIs rather than RDAs are proposed for infants to age 1 year. EARs and RDAs, however, are proposed for iron and zinc for infants 7 to 12 months of age because the level of iron and zinc in human milk does not meet the needs of the older infants and because factorial data are available to estimate the average requirement. Neither AIs nor RDAs were proposed for arsenic, boron, nickel, silicon, or vanadium.

Tolerable Upper Intake Levels

The *Tolerable Upper Intake Level* (UL) is the highest level of daily nutrient intake that is likely to pose no risk of adverse health effects for almost all individuals in the general population (see Table S-10). As intake increases above the UL, the potential risk of adverse effects may increase. The term "tolerable intake" was chosen to avoid implying a possible beneficial effect. Instead, the term is intended to connote a level of intake that can, with high probability, be tolerated biologically. The UL is not intended to be a recommended level of intake. There is no established benefit for apparently healthy individuals if they consume nutrient intakes above the RDA or AI.

ULs are useful because of the increased interest in and availability of fortified foods and the increased use of dietary supplements. ULs are based on total intake of a nutrient from food, water, and supplements if adverse effects have been associated with total intake. However, if adverse effects have been associated with intake from supplements or food fortificants only, the UL is based on nutrient intake from one or both of those sources only, rather than on total intake. The UL applies to chronic daily use.

For vitamin K, arsenic, chromium, and silicon, there are insufficient data for developing a UL. This does not mean that there is no potential for adverse effects resulting from high intake; for example, arsenic is a human poison at high intakes. However, at levels below what is known to be toxic, little data are available. Where data about adverse effects are extremely limited, extra caution may be warranted.

APPROACH FOR SETTING DIETARY REFERENCE INTAKES

The scientific data used to develop Dietary Reference Intakes (DRIs) have come from observational and experimental studies. Studies published in peer-reviewed journals were the principal source of data. Life stage and gender were considered to the extent possible, but the data did not provide a basis for proposing different requirements for men and for nonpregnant and nonlactating women in different age groups for many of the micronutrients. Two of the categories of reference values—the Estimated Average Requirement (EAR) and Recommended Dietary Allowance (RDA)—are defined by specific criteria of nutrient adequacy; the third, the Tolerable Upper Intake Level (UL), is defined by a specific endpoint of adverse effect, when one is available. In all cases, data were examined closely to determine whether a functional endpoint could

TABLE S-1 Criteria and Dietary Reference Intake Values for
Vitamin A by Life Stage Group

Life Stage Group	Criterion
0 through 6 mo	Average vitamin A intake from human milk
7 through 12 mo	Extrapolation from 0 through 6 mo AI
1 through 3 y	Extrapolation from adult EAR
4 through 8 y	Extrapolation from adult EAR
9 through 13 y	Extrapolation from adult EAR
14 through 18 y	Extrapolation from adult EAR
> 18 y	Adequate liver vitamin A stores
Pregnancy	
14 through 18 y	Adolescent female EAR plus estimated daily accumulation by fetus
19 through 50 y	Adult female EAR plus estimated daily accumulation by fetus
Lactation	
14 through 18 y	Adolescent female EAR plus average amount of vitamin A secreted in human milk
19 through 50 y	Adult female EAR plus average amount of vitamin A secreted in human milk

[a] EAR = Estimated Average Requirement. The intake that meets the estimated nutrient needs of half of the individuals in a group.

[b] RDA = Recommended Dietary Allowance. The intake that meets the nutrient need of almost all (97–98 percent) of individuals in a group.

[c] AI = Adequate Intake. The observed average or experimentally determined intake by a

be used as a criterion of adequacy. The quality of studies was examined by considering study design; methods used for measuring intake and indicators of adequacy; and biases, interactions, and confounding factors.

Although the reference values are based on data, the data were often scanty or drawn from studies that had limitations in addressing the various questions that confronted the panel. Therefore, many of the questions raised about the requirements for and recommended intakes of these micronutrients cannot be answered fully because of inadequacies in the present database. Apart from studies of overt deficiency diseases, there is a dearth of studies that address specific effects of inadequate intakes on specific indicators of health status, and a research agenda is proposed (see Chapter 15). The

EAR (µg RAE/d)[a]		RDA (µg RAE/d)[b]		
Male	Female	Male	Female	AI (µg/d)[c]
				400
				500
210	210	300	300	
275	275	400	400	
445	420	600	600	
630	485	900	700	
625	500	900	700	
	530		750	
	550		770	
	885		1,200	
	900		1,300	

defined population or subgroup that appears to sustain a defined nutritional status, such as growth rate, normal circulating nutrient values, or other functional indicators of health. The AI is used if sufficient scientific evidence is not available to derive an EAR. For healthy infants receiving human milk, the AI is the mean intake. **The AI is not equivalent to an RDA.**

reasoning used to establish the values is described for each nutrient in Chapters 4 through 13. While the various recommendations are provided as single rounded numbers for practical considerations, it is acknowledged these values imply a precision not fully justified by the underlying data in the case of currently available human studies.

The scientific evidence related to the prevention of chronic degenerative disease was judged to be too nonspecific to be used as the basis for setting any of the recommended levels of intake for all these nutrients. For all of the micronutrients, the EAR is higher than the amount needed to prevent overt deficiency diseases in essentially all individuals in the life stage group and is based on limited data indicating laboratory evidence of sufficiency. The indicators used in deriving the EARs, and thus the RDAs, are described below.

TABLE S-2 Criteria and Dietary Reference Intake Values for Vitamin K by Life Stage Group

Life Stage Group	Criterion
0 through 6 mo	Average vitamin K intake from human milk
7 through 12 mo	Extrapolation from 0 through 6 mo AI
1 through 3 y	Median intake of vitamin K from the Third National Health and Nutrition Examination Survey (NHANES III)
4 through 8 y	Median intake of vitamin K from NHANES III
9 through 13 y	Median intake of vitamin K from NHANES III
14 through 18 y	Median intake of vitamin K from NHANES III
> 18 y	Median intake of vitamin K from NHANES III
Pregnancy	
14 through 18 y	Adolescent female median intake
19 through 50 y	Adult female median intake
Lactation	
14 through 18 y	Adolescent female median intake
19 through 50 y	Adult female median intake

[a] AI = Adequate Intake. The observed average or experimentally determined intake by a defined population or subgroup that appears to sustain a defined nutritional status, such as growth rate, normal circulating nutrient values, or other functional indicators of health. The AI is used if sufficient scientific evidence is not available to derive an

NUTRIENT FUNCTIONS AND THE INDICATORS USED TO ESTIMATE REQUIREMENTS

Vitamin A functions to maintain normal reproduction, vision, and immune function. A deficiency of vitamin A, although uncommon in North America, can result initially in abnormal dark adaptation (night blindness) followed by xerophthalmia. The method used to set an Estimated Average Requirement (EAR) for vitamin A is based on a computational analysis to assure adequate body stores of vitamin A. The Recommended Dietary Allowance (RDA) for adults for vitamin A is set at 900 µg RAE/day for men and 700 µg RAE/day for women. One µg retinol activity equivalent (µg RAE) is equal to 1 µg all-*trans*-retinol, 12 µg β-carotene, and 24 µg α-carotene or β-cryptoxanthin.

Vitamin K functions as a coenzyme in the synthesis of the biologically active form of a number of proteins involved in blood coagulation and bone metabolism. Because of the lack of data to set an

AI (μg/d)[a]	
Male	Female
2.0	2.0
2.5	2.5
30	30
55	55
60	60
75	75
120	90
	75
	90
	75
	90

Estimated Average Requirement (EAR). For healthy infants receiving human milk, the AI is the mean intake. **The AI is not equivalent to a Recommended Dietary Allowance (RDA).**

EAR, an Adequate Intake (AI) is set based on representative dietary intake data from healthy individuals from the Third Nutrition and Health Examination Survey (NHANES III). The AI for adults is 120 and 90 μg/day, for men and women, respectively.

Chromium potentiates the action of insulin in vivo and in vitro. There was not sufficient evidence to set an EAR for chromium. Therefore, an AI was set based on estimated intakes of chromium derived from the average amount of chromium/1,000 kcal of balanced diets and average energy intake from NHANES III. The AI is 35 μg/day for young men and 25 μg/day for young women.

Copper functions to catalyze the activity of many copper metalloenzymes that act as oxidases to achieve the reduction of molecular oxygen. Frank copper deficiency in humans is rare; the deficiency symptoms include normocytic and hypochromic anemia, leukopenia, and neutropenia. The method used to set an EAR for copper is based on the changes in a combination of biochemical indicators

TABLE S-3 Criteria and Dietary Reference Intake Values for Chromium by Life Stage Group

Life Stage Group	Criterion
0 through 6 mo	Average chromium intake from human milk
7 through 12 mo	Average chromium intake from human milk and complementary foods
1 through 3 y	Extrapolation from adult AI
4 through 8 y	Extrapolation from adult AI
9 through 13 y	Extrapolation from adult AI
14 through 18 y	Extrapolation from adult AI
19 through 50 y	Average chromium intake based on the chromium content of foods/1,000 kcal and average energy intake[b]
≥ 51 y	Average chromium intake based on the chromium content of foods/1,000 kcal and average energy intake[b]
Pregnancy	
14 through 18 y	Extrapolation from adolescent AI based on body weight
19 through 50 y	Extrapolation from adult woman AI based on body weight
Lactation	
14 through 18 y	Adolescent female intake plus average amount of chromium secreted in human milk
19 through 50 y	Adult female intake plus average amount of chromium secreted in human milk

[a] AI = Adequate Intake. The observed average or experimentally determined intake by a defined population or subgroup that appears to sustain a defined nutritional status, such as growth rate, normal circulating nutrient values, or other functional indicators of health. AI is used if sufficient scientific evidence is not available to derive an Estimated Average Requirement (EAR). For healthy infants receiving human milk, AI is the

resulting from varied levels of copper intake. The RDA for copper is 900 µg/day for men and women. There were insufficient data to set a different EAR and RDA for each gender.

Iodine is an important component of the thyroid hormones that are involved with the regulation of metabolism. Severe iodine deficiency can result in impaired cognitive development in children and goiter in adults. The method used to set an EAR for iodine is iodine accumulation and turnover. The adult RDA for iodine is 150 µg/day. There were insufficient data to set a different EAR and RDA for each gender.

Iron functions as a component of hemoglobin, myoglobin, cytochromes, and enzymes. Iron deficiency anemia is the most common

AI (μg/d)[a]		
Male	Female	
0.2	0.2	
5.5	5.5	
11	11	
15	15	
25	21	
35	24	
35	25	
30	20	
	29	
	30	
	44	
	45	

mean intake. **The AI is not equivalent to a Recommended Dietary Allowance (RDA).**
[b] The average chromium content in well balanced diets was determined to be 13.4 μg/ 1,000 kcal and the average energy intake for adults was obtained from the Third National Health and Nutrition Examination Survey.

nutritional deficiency in the world, resulting in fatigue and impaired cognitive development and productivity. The required amount of absorbed iron is estimated based on factorial modeling. The EAR is determined by dividing the required amount of absorbed iron by the fractional absorption of dietary iron, estimated to be 18 percent for adults for the typical North American diet. The RDA for men and premenopausal women is 8 and 18 mg/day, respectively. The RDA for pregnant women is 27 mg/day.

Manganese is involved in the formation of bone and in amino acid, lipid, and carbohydrate metabolism. There were insufficient data to set an EAR for manganese. An AI was set based on median intakes reported from the U.S. Food and Drug Administration Total Diet

TABLE S-4 Criteria and Dietary Reference Intake Values for Copper by Life Stage Group

Life Stage Group	Criterion
0 through 6 mo	Average copper intake from human milk
7 through 12 mo	Average copper intake from human milk and complementary foods
1 through 3 y	Extrapolation from adult EAR
4 through 8 y	Extrapolation from adult EAR
9 through 13 y	Extrapolation from adult EAR
14 through 18 y	Extrapolation from adult EAR
19 through 50 y	Plasma copper, serum ceruloplasmin, and platelet copper concentrations and erythrocyte superoxide dismutase activity
≥ 51 y	Extrapolation from 19 through 50 y
Pregnancy	
14 through 18 y	Adolescent female EAR plus fetal accumulation of copper
19 through 50 y	Adult female EAR plus fetal accumulation of copper
Lactation	
14 through 18 y	Adolescent female EAR plus average amount of copper secreted in human milk
19 through 50 y	Adult female EAR plus average amount of copper secreted in human milk

a EAR = Estimated Average Requirement. The intake that meets the estimated nutrient needs of half of the individuals in a group.
b RDA = Recommended Dietary Allowance. The intake that meets the nutrient need of almost all (97–98 percent) of individuals in a group.
c AI = Adequate Intake. The observed average or experimentally determined intake by a

Study. The AI for adult men and women is 2.3 and 1.8 mg/day, respectively.

Molybdenum functions as a cofactor for several enzymes in a form called molybdopterin. An inborn error of metabolism that leads to a deficiency of sulfite oxidase is due to the lack of molybdopterin, which results in neurological dysfunction and mental retardation. Molybdenum balance data were used to set an EAR. The RDA for adults for molybdenum is 45 μg/day for men and women. There were insufficient data to set a different EAR and RDA for each gender.

EAR (μg/d)[a]		RDA (μg/d)[b]		AI (μg/d)[c]
Male	Female	Male	Female	
				200
				220
260	260	340	340	
340	340	440	440	
540	540	700	700	
685	685	890	890	
700	700	900	900	
700	700	900	900	
	785		1,000	
	800		1,000	
	985		1,300	
	1,000		1,300	

defined population or subgroup that appears to sustain a defined nutritional status, such as growth rate, normal circulating nutrient values, or other functional indicators of health. The AI is used if sufficient scientific evidence is not available to derive an EAR. For healthy infants receiving human milk, the AI is the mean intake. **The AI is not equivalent to an RDA.**

Zinc functions through the catalysis of various enzymes, the maintenance of the structural integrity of proteins, and the regulation of gene expression. Overt human zinc deficiency is rare, and the symptoms of a mild deficiency are diverse due to zinc's ubiquitous involvement in metabolic processes. Factorial analysis of zinc losses and requirements for growth, as well as fractional absorption, were used to set an EAR. The RDA for zinc is set at 11 mg/day for men and 8 mg/day for women.

TABLE S-5 Criteria and Dietary Reference Intake Values for Iodine by Life Stage Group

Life Stage Group	Criterion
0 through 6 mo	Average iodine intake from human milk
7 through 12 mo	Extrapolation from 0 through 6 mo AI
1 through 3 y	Balance data on children
4 through 8 y	Balance data on children
9 through 13 y	Extrapolation from adult EAR
14 through 18 y	Extrapolation from adult EAR
19 through 50 y	Iodine turnover
≥ 51 y	Extrapolation of iodine turnover studies from 19 through 50 y
Pregnancy	
14 through 18 y	Balance data during pregnancy
19 through 50 y	Balance data during pregnancy
Lactation	
14 through 18 y	Adolescent female average requirement plus average amount of iodine secreted in human milk
19 through 50 y	Adult female average requirement plus average amount of iodine secreted in human milk

[a] EAR = Estimated Average Requirement. The intake that meets the estimated nutrient needs of half of the individuals in a group.
[b] RDA = Recommended Dietary Allowance. The intake that meets the nutrient need of almost all (97–98 percent) of individuals in a group.
[c] AI = Adequate Intake. The observed average or experimentally determined intake by a

CRITERIA AND PROPOSED VALUES FOR TOLERABLE UPPER INTAKE LEVELS

A risk assessment model is used to derive Tolerable Upper Intake Levels (ULs). The model consists of a systematic series of scientific considerations and judgments. The hallmark of the risk assessment model is the requirement to be explicit in all of the evaluations and judgments made.

The adult ULs for vitamin A (3,000 µg/day), boron (20 mg/day), copper (10,000 µg/day), iodine (1,100 µg/day), iron (45 mg/day), manganese (11 mg/day), molybdenum (2,000 µg/day), nickel (1.0

EAR (µg/d)[a]		RDA (µg/d)[b]		AI (µg/d)[c]
Male	Female	Male	Female	
				110
				130
65	65	90	90	
65	65	90	90	
73	73	120	120	
95	95	150	150	
95	95	150	150	
95	95	150	150	
	160		220	
	160		220	
	209		290	
	209		290	

defined population or subgroup that appears to sustain a defined nutritional status, such as growth rate, normal circulating nutrient values, or other functional indicators of health. The AI is used if sufficient scientific evidence is not available to derive an EAR. For healthy infants receiving human milk, the AI is the mean intake. **The AI is not equivalent to an RDA.**

mg/day), vanadium (1.8 mg/day), and zinc (40 mg/day), as shown in Table S-10, were set to protect the most sensitive individuals in the general population (such as those who might be below the reference adult weight).

Members of the general, apparently healthy population should be advised not to routinely exceed the UL. However, intake above the UL may be appropriate for investigation within well-controlled clinical trials to ascertain if such intakes are of benefit to health for specific reasons. Clinical trials of doses above the UL should not be discouraged, as it is expected that participation in these trials will require informed consent that will include discussion of the possi-

TABLE S-6 Criteria and Dietary Reference Intake Values for Iron by Life Stage Group

Life Stage Group	Criterion
0 through 6 mo	Average iron intake from human milk
7 through 12 mo	Factorial modeling
1 through 3 y	Factorial modeling
4 through 8 y	Factorial modeling
9 through 13 y	Factorial modeling
14 through 18 y	Factorial modeling
19 through 30 y	Factorial modeling
31 through 50 y	Factorial modeling
51 through 70 y	Factorial modeling
> 70 y	Extrapolation of factorial analysis from 51 through 70 y
Pregnancy	
14 through 18 y	Factorial modeling
19 through 50 y	Factorial modeling
Lactation	
14 through 18 y	Adolescent female EAR minus menstrual losses plus average amount of iron secreted in human milk
19 through 50 y	Adult female EAR minus menstrual losses plus average amount of iron secreted in human milk

[a] EAR = Estimated Average Requirement. The intake that meets the estimated nutrient needs of half of the individuals in a group.

[b] RDA = Recommended Dietary Allowance. The intake that meets the nutrient need of almost all (97–98 percent) of individuals in a group.

[c] AI = Adequate Intake. The observed average or experimentally determined intake by a

bility of adverse effects and will employ appropriate safety monitoring of trial subjects.

The ULs for vitamin A, boron, copper, iodine, iron, manganese, molybdenum, nickel, and zinc are based on adverse effects of intake from diet, fortified foods, and/or supplements. ULs could not be established for vitamin K, arsenic, chromium, and silicon because of lack of suitable data, a lack that indicates the need for additional research. The absence of data does not necessarily signify that people can tolerate chronic intakes of these substances at high levels, particularly elements such as arsenic which are known to cause serious adverse effects at very high levels of intake. Like all chemical agents, nutrients and other food components can produce adverse effects

EAR (mg/d)[a]		RDA (mg/d)[b]		AI (mg/d)[c]
Male	Female	Male	Female	
				0.27
6.9	6.9	11	11	
3.0	3.0	7	7	
4.1	4.1	10	10	
5.9	5.7	8	8	
7.7	7.9	11	15	
6	8.1	8	18	
6	8.1	8	18	
6	5	8	8	
6	5	8	8	
	23		27	
	22		27	
	7		10	
	6.5		9	

dcfined population or subgroup that appears to sustain a defined nutritional status, such as growth rate, normal circulating nutrient values, or other functional indicators of health. The AI is used if sufficient scientific evidence is not available to derive an EAR. For healthy infants receiving human milk, the AI is the mean intake. **The AI is not equivalent to an RDA.**

if intakes are excessive. Therefore, when data are extremely limited, extra caution may be warranted.

USING DIETARY REFERENCE INTAKES TO ASSESS NUTRIENT INTAKES OF GROUPS

Suggested uses of Dietary Reference Intakes (DRIs) appear in Box S-2. The transition from using previously published Recommended Dietary Allowances (RDAs) and Reference Nutrient Intakes (RNIs) to using each of the DRIs appropriately will require time and effort by health professionals and others.

For statistical reasons that are addressed in the report *Dietary*

TABLE S-7 Criteria and Dietary Reference Intake Values for Manganese by Life Stage Group

Life Stage Group	Criterion
0 through 6 mo	Average manganese intake from human milk
7 through 12 mo	Extrapolation from adult AI
1 through 3 y	Median manganese intake from the Food and Drug Administration's (FDA) Total Diet Study
4 through 8 y	Median manganese intake from FDA Total Diet Study
9 through 13 y	Median manganese intake from FDA Total Diet Study
14 through 18 y	Median manganese intake from FDA Total Diet Study
≥ 19 y	Median manganese intake from FDA Total Diet Study
Pregnancy	
14 through 18 y	Extrapolation of adolescent female AI based on body weight
19 through 50 y	Extrapolation of adult female AI based on body weight
Lactation	
14 through 18 y	Median manganese intake from FDA Total Diet Study
19 through 50 y	Median manganese intake from FDA Total Diet Study

a AI = Adequate Intake. The observed average or experimentally determined intake by a defined population or subgroup that appears to sustain a defined nutritional status, such as growth rate, normal circulating nutrient values, or other functional indicators of health. The AI is used if sufficient scientific evidence is not available to derive an

Reference Intakes: Applications in Dietary Assessment (IOM, 2000) and briefly in Chapter 14, the Estimated Average Requirement (EAR) is the appropriate reference intake to use in assessing the nutrient intake of groups, whereas the RDA is not appropriate. When assessing nutrient intakes of groups, it is important to consider the variation in intake in the same individuals from day to day, as well as underreporting. With these considerations, the prevalence of inadequacy for a given nutrient may be estimated by using national survey data and determining the percent of the population below the EAR. Assuming a normal distribution of requirements, the percent of surveyed individuals whose intake is less than the EAR equals the percent of individuals whose diets are considered inadequate based on the criteria of inadequacy chosen to determine the requirement. For example, intake data from the Continuing Survey of Food Intakes by Individuals and the Third National Health and Nutrition Examination Survey, which collected 24-hour diet recalls for 1 or 2 days, indicate that:

AI $(mg/d)^a$		
Male	Female	
0.003	0.003	
0.6	0.6	
1.2	1.2	
1.5	1.5	
1.9	1.6	
2.2	1.6	
2.3	1.8	
	2.0	
	2.0	
	2.6	
	2.6	

Estimated Average Requirement (EAR). For healthy infants receiving human milk, the AI is the mean intake. **The AI is not equivalent to a Recommended Dietary Allowance (RDA).**

- Between 10 and 25 percent of children 1 to 3 years of age consume dietary vitamin A or its precursors at a level less than the EAR. The percent of adults consuming intakes of vitamin A below the EAR is higher than for children. The EAR is based on a criterion of adequate vitamin A stores in the liver (> 20 µg vitamin A/g liver); thus, these data suggest that a considerable number of people have liver vitamin A stores that are less than desirable. It should be recognized that this does not represent a clinical deficiency state, such as dark adaptation, which is not commonly seen in North Americans.
- Between 5 and 10 percent of adolescent girls consume dietary iron at a level less than the EAR. The criterion chosen for the EAR for this age group was based on iron loss and accretion, using an upper limit of absorption that provides minimal iron stores.
- The prevalence of iron intakes less than the EAR ranges from 15 to 20 percent for premenopausal women which corresponds with a 13 to 16 percent prevalence of low iron status (based on serum ferritin concentration).

TABLE S-8 Criteria and Dietary Reference Intake Values for Molybdenum by Life Stage Group

Life Stage Group	Criterion
0 through 6 mo	Average molybdenum intake from human milk
7 through 12 mo	Extrapolation from 0 through 6 mo
1 through 3 y	Extrapolation from adult EAR
4 through 8 y	Extrapolation from adult EAR
9 through 13 y	Extrapolation from adult EAR
14 through 18 y	Extrapolation from adult EAR
19 through 30 y	Balance data
≥ 31 y	Extrapolation of balance data from 19 through 30 y
Pregnancy	
14 through 18 y	Extrapolation of adolescent female EAR based on body weight
19 through 50 y	Extrapolation of adult female EAR based on body weight
Lactation	
14 through 18 y	Adolescent female EAR plus average amount of molybdenum secreted in human milk
19 through 50 y	Adult female EAR plus average amount of molybdenum secreted in human milk

[a] EAR = Estimated Average Requirement. The intake that meets the estimated nutrient needs of half of the individuals in a group.
[b] RDA = Recommended Dietary Allowance. The intake that meets the nutrient need of almost all (97–98 percent) of individuals in a group.
[c] AI = Adequate Intake. The observed average or experimentally determined intake by a

• A high percentage of pregnant women consume dietary iron at a level less than the EAR; this corresponds with a high prevalence of low hemoglobin concentration (anemia).

CONSIDERATION OF THE RISK OF CHRONIC DEGENERATIVE DISEASE

Close attention was given to the evidence relating intake of all the micronutrients to reduction of the risk of chronic disease. Data linking intake of vitamin K and chromium with the risk of chronic disease in North America were available but insufficient to set Estimated Average Requirements (EARs).

EAR (µg/d)[a]		RDA (µg/d)[b]		AI (µg/d)[c]
Male	Female	Male	Female	
				2
				3
13	13	17	17	
17	17	22	22	
26	26	34	34	
33	33	43	43	
34	34	45	45	
34	34	45	45	
	40		50	
	40		50	
	35		50	
	36		50	

defined population or subgroup that appears to sustain a defined nutritional status, such as growth rate, normal circulating nutrient values, or other functional indicators of health. The AI is used if sufficient scientific evidence is not available to derive an EAR. For healthy infants receiving human milk, the AI is the mean intake. **The AI is not equivalent to an RDA.**

Bone Health and Osteoporosis

The notion that vitamin K may have a role in osteoporosis was first suggested with reports of lower circulating phylloquinone concentrations in osteoporotic patients having suffered a spinal crush fracture or fracture of the femur. A potential role of vitamin K in bone metabolism has been investigated by studying the vitamin K-dependent bone protein, osteocalcin, and its under-γ-carboxylated form. Increases in undercarboxylated osteocalcin have been associated with an increased risk of hip fracture. These associations should be interpreted with caution because most studies did not control for confounding factors such as other nutrients known to influence

TABLE S-10 Tolerable Upper Intake Levels (UL)[a], by Life Stage Group

Life Stage Group	Preformed Vitamin A (µg/d)	Boron (mg/d)	Copper (µg/d)	Iodine (µg/d)
0 through 6 mo	600	ND[b]	ND	ND
7 through 12 mo	600	ND	ND	ND
1 through 3 y	600	3	1,000	200
4 through 8 y	900	6	3,000	300
9 through 13 y	1,700	11	5,000	600
14 through 18 y	2,800	17	8,000	900
≥ 19 y	3,000	20	10,000	1,100
Pregnancy				
14 through 18 y	2,800	17	8,000	900
19 through 50 y	3,000	20	10,000	1,100
Lactation				
14 through 18 y	2,800	17	8,000	900
19 through 50 y	3,000	20	10,000	1,100

NOTE: Because of the lack of suitable data, ULs could not be established for vitamin K or chromium. In the absence of ULs, extra caution may be warranted in consuming levels of these nutrients above recommended intakes. Although a UL was not determined for arsenic, there is no justification for adding arsenic to food or supplements. In addition, although silicon has not been shown to cause adverse effects in humans, there is no justification for adding silicon to supplements.

[a] The highest level of daily nutrient intake that is likely to pose no risk of adverse health effects to almost all individuals in the general population. As intake increases above the

RESEARCH RECOMMENDATIONS

Five major types of information gaps were noted: a lack of data demonstrating a specific role of some of these micronutrients in human health; a dearth of studies designed specifically to estimate average requirements in presumably healthy humans; a lack of data on the micronutrient needs of infants, children, adolescents, the elderly, and pregnant women; a lack of studies to determine the role of these micronutrients in reducing the risk of certain chronic diseases; and a lack of studies designed to detect adverse effects of chronic high intakes of these many of these micronutrients.

Highest priority is thus given to studies that address the following research topics:

Iron (mg/d)	Manganese (mg/d)	Molybdenum (μg/d)	Nickel (μg/d)	Vanadium (mg/d)^c	Zinc (mg/d)
40	ND	ND	ND	ND	4
40	ND	ND	ND	ND	5
40	2	300	200	ND	7
40	3	600	300	ND	12
40	6	1,100	600	ND	23
45	9	1,700	1,000	ND	34
45	11	2,000	1,000	1.8	40
45	9	1,700	1,000	ND	34
45	11	2,000	1,000	ND	40
45	9	1,700	1,000	ND	34
45	11	2,000	1,000	ND	40

UL, the risk of adverse effects increases. Unless specified otherwise, the UL represents total nutrient intake from food, water, and supplements.

^{b} ND = not determinable due to lack of data of adverse effects in this age group and concern about lack of ability to handle excess amounts. Source of intake should be from food only to prevent high levels of intake.

^{c} Although vanadium in food has not been shown to cause adverse effects in humans, there is no justification for adding vanadium to food, and vanadium supplements should be used with caution. The UL is based on adverse effects in laboratory animals and this data could be used to set a UL for adults, but not for children or adolescents.

- studies to identify and further understand the functional (e.g., cognitive function, regulation of insulin, bone health, and immune function) and biochemical endpoints that reflect sufficient and insufficient body stores of vitamin A, vitamin K, arsenic, boron, chromium, copper, iodine, iron, manganese, molybdenum, nickel, silicon, vanadium, and zinc;
- studies to further identify and quantify the effects of interactions between micronutrients and interactions between micronutrients and other food components, the food matrix, food processing, and life stage on micronutrient (vitamin A, vitamin K, chromium, copper, iron, and zinc) bioavailability and therefore dietary requirement;

• studies to further investigate the role of arsenic, boron, nickel, silicon, and vanadium in human health; and

• studies to investigate the influence of non-nutritional factors (e.g., body mass index, glucose intolerance, infection) on the biochemical indicators for micronutrients currently measured by U.S. and Canadian nutritional surveys, such as for iron and vitamin A.

1

Introduction to Dietary Reference Intakes

Dietary Reference Intakes (DRIs) comprise a set of nutrient-based reference values, each of which has special uses. The development of DRIs expands on the periodic reports, *Recommended Dietary Allowances*, which have been published since 1941 by the National Academy of Sciences and the *Recommended Nutrient Intakes* of Canada. This comprehensive effort is being undertaken by the Standing Committee on the Scientific Evaluation of Dietary Reference Intakes of the Food and Nutrition Board, Institute of Medicine, National Academies, with the active involvement of Health Canada. See Appendix A for a description of the overall process and its origins.

WHAT ARE DIETARY REFERENCE INTAKES?

The reference values, collectively called the Dietary Reference Intakes (DRIs), include the Estimated Average Requirement (EAR), Recommended Dietary Allowance (RDA), Adequate Intake (AI), and Tolerable Upper Intake Level (UL).

A requirement is defined as the lowest continuing intake level of a nutrient that will maintain a defined level of nutriture in an individual. The chosen criterion of nutritional adequacy is identified in each chapter; note that the criterion may differ for individuals at different life stages. Hence, particular attention is given throughout this report to the choice and justification of the criterion used to establish requirement values.

This approach differs somewhat from that used by the World Health Organization, Food and Agriculture Organization, and International Atomic Energy Agency (WHO/FAO/IAEA) Expert Consultation on *Trace Elements in Human Nutrition and Health* (WHO, 1996). That publication uses the term *basal requirement* to indicate the level of intake needed to prevent pathologically relevant and clinically detectable signs of a dietary inadequacy. The term *normative requirement* indicates the level of intake sufficient to maintain a desirable body store or reserve. In developing RDAs and AIs, emphasis is placed instead on the reasons underlying the choice of the criterion of nutritional adequacy used to establish the requirement. They have not been designated as basal or normative.

Unless otherwise stated, all values given for EARs, RDAs, and AIs represent the quantity of the nutrient or food component to be supplied by foods from a diet similar to those consumed in Canada and the United States. If the food source of a nutrient is very different (as in diets of some ethnic groups) or if the source is supplements, adjustments may have to be made for differences in nutrient bioavailability. When this is an issue, it is discussed for the specific nutrient in the section "Special Considerations".

RDAs and AIs are levels of intake recommended for individuals. They should reduce the risk of developing a condition that is associated with the nutrient in question and that has a negative functional outcome. The DRIs apply to the apparently healthy general population. Meeting the recommended intakes for the nutrients would not necessarily provide enough for individuals who are already malnourished, nor would they be adequate for certain disease states marked by increased nutritional requirements. Qualified medical and nutrition personnel must tailor recommendations for individuals who are known to have diseases that greatly increase nutritional requirements or who are at risk for developing adverse effects associated with higher intakes. Although the RDA or AI may serve as the basis for such guidance, qualified personnel should make necessary adaptations for specific situations

CATEGORIES OF DIETARY REFERENCE INTAKES

Each type of Dietary Reference Intake (DRI) refers to average daily nutrient intake of individuals over time. In most cases, the amount taken from day to day may vary substantially without ill effect.

Recommended Dietary Allowance

The *Recommended Dietary Allowance* (RDA) is the average daily dietary intake level that is sufficient to meet the nutrient require-

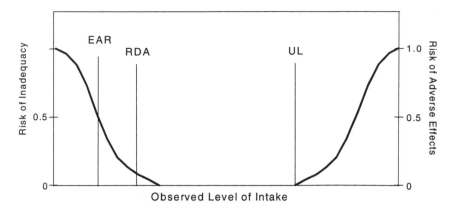

FIGURE 1-1 Dietary reference intakes. This figure shows that the Estimated Average Requirement (EAR) is the intake at which the risk of inadequacy is 0.5 (50 percent) to an individual. The Recommended Dietary Allowance (RDA) is the intake at which the risk of inadequacy is very small—only 0.02 to 0.03 (2 to 3 percent). The Adequate Intake (AI) does not bear a consistent relationship to the EAR or the RDA because it is set without being able to estimate the requirement. At intakes between the RDA and the Tolerable Upper Intake Level (UL), the risks of inadequacy and of excess are both close to 0. At intakes above the UL, the risk of adverse effects may increase.

ment of nearly all (97 to 98 percent) healthy individuals in a particular life stage and gender group (see Figure 1-1). The RDA is intended to be used as a goal for daily intake by individuals. The process for setting the RDA is described below; it usually depends on being able to set an Estimated Average Requirement (EAR). That is, if an EAR cannot be set, no RDA will be set.

Estimated Average Requirement[1]

The *Estimated Average Requirement* (EAR) is the daily intake value that is estimated to meet the requirement, as defined by the specified indicator or criterion of adequacy, in half of the apparently healthy individuals in a life stage or gender group (see Figure 1-1). A normal or symmetrical distribution (median and mean are simi-

---

[1] The definition of EAR implies a median as opposed to a mean, or average. The median and average would be the same if the distribution of requirements followed a symmetrical distribution and would diverge as a distribution became skewed.

lar) is usually assumed for nutrient requirements. At this level of intake, the other half of a specified group would not have its nutritional needs met. The general method used to set the EAR is the same for all the nutrients. The specific approaches, which are provided in Chapters 4 through 12, differ because of the different types of data available. For many of the nutrients, there are few direct data on the requirements of children. Thus, EARs and RDAs for children are based on extrapolations from adult values. The method is described in Chapter 2.

Method for Setting the RDA when Nutrient Requirements Are Normally Distributed

If the requirement for the nutrient is normally distributed, and the standard deviation (SD) of the EAR is available, the RDA is defined as equal to the EAR plus 2 SDs of the EAR:

$$RDA = EAR + 2\ SD_{EAR}.$$

If data about variability in requirements are insufficient to calculate an SD, a coefficient of variation (CV_{EAR}) of 10 percent will be ordinarily assumed and used to estimate the SD:

$$CV_{EAR} = SD_{EAR}/EAR$$

and

$$SD = (EAR \times CV_{EAR});$$

the resulting equation for the RDA is

$$RDA = EAR + 2\ (0.1 \times EAR)$$

or

$$RDA = 1.2 \times EAR.$$

The assumption of a 10 percent CV is based on extensive data on the variation in basal metabolic rate (FAO/WHO/UNA, 1985; Garby and Lammert, 1984), which contributes about two-thirds of the daily energy needs of many individuals residing in Canada and the United States (Elia, 1992) and on the similar CV of 12.5 percent estimated for the protein requirements in adults (FAO/WHO/

UNA, 1985). If data are not available for estimation of a standard deviation, then a CV of 10 percent is assumed depending on the information that is available.

Method for Setting the RDA when Nutrient Requirements Are Not Normally Distributed

When factorial modeling is used to estimate the distribution of requirements from the distributions of the individual components of requirement (e.g., losses, accretion), it is necessary to add the individual distributions. For normal component distributions, this is straightforward since the resultant distribution is also normal, with a mean that is the sum of component means and a variance (the square of the SD) that is the sum of the individual variances. The ninety-seven and one half percentile is then estimated as the mean value plus two SDs.

If the requirement of a nutrient is not normally distributed but can be transformed to normality, its EAR and RDA can be estimated by transforming the data, calculating a fiftieth and a ninety-seventh and one-half percentile, and transforming these percentiles back into the original units. In this case, the difference between the EAR and the RDA cannot be used to obtain an estimate of the CV because skewing is usually present.

If normality cannot be assumed for all of the components of requirement, then Monte Carlo simulation is used for the summation of the components. This approach involves simulation of a large population of individuals (e.g., 100,000) each with his or her own requirement for a particular nutrient. To accomplish this, the component parts of nutrient needs (the factorial components) are treated as coming from independent random distributions.

Using iron as an example (see Chapter 9), for basal iron loss, a distribution of expected losses was generated. For each individual in the simulated population, a randomly selected iron loss value was drawn from that distribution of iron losses. This is done for each component of iron need and then these components were summed for each individual yielding the simulated iron needs. The total requirement is then calculated for each individual and the median and the ninety-seven and one-half percentile calculated directly.

Information about the distribution of values for the requirement components is modeled on the basis of known physiology. Monte Carlo approaches may be used in the simulation of the distribution of components; or, where large data sets exist for similar populations (such as growth rates in infants), estimates of relative variability may be transferred to the component in the simulated population (Gentle, 1998). At each step, the goal is to achieve distribution values for the component that not only reflect known physiology or known direct observations, but also values that can be transformed into a distribution that can be modeled and used in selecting random members to contribute to the final requirement distribution. When the final distribution representing the convolution of components has been derived, then the median and ninety-seven and one-half percentile of the distribution can be directly estimated. It is recognized that in its simplest form, the Monte Carlo approach ignores possible correlation among components. In the case of iron, however, expected correlation is built into the modeling of the requirement where components are linked to a common variable, such as growth rate, so that not all sources of correlation are neglected.

Other Uses of the EAR

The EAR may also be used in the assessment of the intake of groups (IOM, 2000) or, together with an estimate of the variance of intake, be used in planning for the intake of groups (Beaton, 1994) (see Chapter 14).

Adequate Intake

If sufficient scientific evidence is not available to calculate an EAR, a reference intake called an *Adequate Intake* (AI) is provided instead of an RDA. The AI is a value based on experimentally derived intake levels or approximations of observed mean nutrient intakes by a group (or groups) of healthy people. In the judgment of the Standing Committee on the Scientific Evaluation of Dietary Reference Intakes, the AI for children and adults is expected to meet or exceed the amount needed to maintain a defined nutritional state or criterion of adequacy in essentially all members of a specific healthy population. Examples of defined nutritional states include normal growth, maintenance of normal circulating nutrient values, or other aspects of nutritional well-being or general health.

The AI is set when data are considered to be insufficient or inadequate to establish an EAR on which an RDA would be based. For example, for young infants for whom human milk is the recommended sole source of food for most nutrients for the first 4 to 6 months, the AI is based on the daily mean nutrient intake supplied by human milk for healthy, full-term infants who are exclusively fed human milk. For adults, the AI may be based on data from a single experiment, on estimated dietary intakes in apparently healthy population groups (e.g., vitamin K, chromium, or manganese), or on a review of data from different approaches that considered alone do not permit a reasonably confident estimate of an EAR.

Similarities Between the AI and the RDA

Both the AI and RDA are to be used as a goal for individual intake. In general, the values are intended to cover the needs of nearly all persons in a life stage group. (For infants, the AI is the mean intake when infants in the age group are consuming human milk. Larger infants may have greater needs, which they meet by consuming more milk.) As with RDAs, AIs for children and adolescents may be extrapolated from adult values if no other usable data are available.

Differences Between the AI and the RDA

There is much less certainty about the AI value than about the RDA value. Because AIs depend on a greater degree of judgment than is applied in estimating the EAR and subsequently the RDA, the AI may deviate significantly from and be numerically higher than the RDA. For this reason, AIs must be used with greater care than is the case for RDAs. Also, the RDA is usually calculated from the EAR by using a formula that takes into account the expected variation in the requirement for the nutrient (see previous section, "Estimated Average Requirement").

Tolerable Upper Intake Level

The *Tolerable Upper Intake Level* (UL) is the highest level of daily nutrient intake that is likely to pose no risk of adverse health effects for almost all individuals in the specified life stage group (see Figure 1-1). As intake increases above the UL, the potential risk of adverse effects may increase. The term *tolerable intake* was chosen to avoid implying a possible beneficial effect. Instead, the term is intended to connote a level of intake that can, with high probability, be tolerated biologically. The UL is not intended to be a recommended level of intake, and there is no established benefit for healthy individuals if they consume a nutrient in amounts exceeding the recommended intake (the RDA or AI).

The UL is based on an evaluation conducted by using the methodology for risk assessment of nutrients (see Chapter 3). The need for setting ULs grew out of the increased fortification of foods with nutrients and the use of dietary supplements by more people and in larger doses. The UL applies to chronic daily use. As in the case of applying AIs, professionals should avoid very rigid application of ULs and first assess the characteristics of the individual and group of concern, such as source of nutrient, physiological state of the individual, length of sustained high intakes, and so forth.

For some nutrients such as vitamin K, arsenic, chromium, and silicon, data are not sufficient for developing a UL. This indicates the need for caution in consuming amounts greater than the recommended intakes; it does not mean that high intakes pose no risk of adverse effects.

The safety of routine, long-term intake above the UL is not well documented. Although members of the general population should be advised not to routinely exceed the UL, intake above the UL may be appropriate for investigation within well-controlled clinical trials. Clinical trials of doses above the UL should not be discouraged as long as subjects participating in these trials have signed informed consent documents regarding possible toxicity and as long as these trials employ appropriate safe monitoring of trial subjects.

Determination of Adequacy

In the derivation of the EAR or AI, close attention has been paid to the determination of the most appropriate indicators of adequacy. A key question is, Adequate for what? In many cases, a continuum of benefits may be ascribed to various levels of intake of the same nutrient. One criterion may be deemed the most appropriate to determine the risk that an individual will become deficient in the nutrient whereas another may relate to reducing the risk of chronic degenerative disease, such as diabetes mellitus or osteoporosis.

Each EAR and AI is described in terms of the selected criterion. The potential role of the nutrient in the reduction of disease risk was considered in developing the EARs. With the acquisition of additional data relating intake to chronic disease or disability, the choice of the criterion for setting the EAR may change.

PARAMETERS FOR DIETARY REFERENCE INTAKES

Life Stage Groups

The life stage groups described below were chosen by keeping in mind all the nutrients to be reviewed, not only those included in this report. Additional subdivisions within these groups may be added in later reports. If data are too sparse to distinguish differences in requirements by life stage or gender group, the analysis may be presented for a larger grouping.

Infancy

Infancy covers the period from birth through 12 months of age and is divided into two 6-month intervals. The first 6-month interval was not subdivided further because intake is relatively constant during this time. That is, as infants grow they ingest more food; however, on a body weight basis their intake remains the same. During the second 6 months of life, growth velocity slows, and thus total daily nutrient needs on a body weight basis may be less than those during the first 6 months of life.

For a particular nutrient, the average intake by full-term infants who are born to healthy, well-nourished mothers and exclusively fed human milk has been adopted as the primary basis for deriving the Adequate Intake (AI) for most nutrients during the first 6 months of life. The value used is thus not an Estimated Average Requirement (EAR); the extent to which intake of human milk may result in exceeding the actual requirements of the infant is not known, and ethics of experimentation preclude testing the levels known to be potentially inadequate. Therefore, the AI is not an EAR in which only half of the group would be expected to have their needs met.

Using the infant fed human milk as a model is in keeping with the basis for estimating nutrient allowances of infants developed in the last Recommended Dietary Allowances (RDA) (NRC, 1989) and Recommended Nutrient Intakes (RNI) (Health Canada, 1990) reports. It also supports the recommendation that exclusive human milk feeding is the preferred method of feeding for normal full-term infants for the first 4 to 6 months of life. This recommendation has also been made by the Canadian Paediatric Society (Health Canada, 1990), the American Academy of Pediatrics (AAP, 1997) and in the Food and Nutrition Board report *Nutrition During Lactation* (IOM, 1991).

In general, for this report special consideration was not given to possible variations in physiological need during the first month after birth or to the variations in intake of nutrients from human milk that result from differences in milk volume and nutrient concentration during early lactation. Specific Dietary Reference Intakes (DRIs) to meet the needs of formula-fed infants are not proposed in this report. The previously published RDAs and RNIs for infants have led to much misinterpretation of the adequacy of human milk because of a lack of understanding about their derivation for young infants. Although they were based on human milk composition and volume of intake, the previous RDA and RNI values allowed for lower bioavailability of nutrients from nonhuman milk.

Ages 0 through 6 Months. To derive the AI value for infants ages 0 through 6 months, the mean intake of a nutrient was calculated on the basis of the average concentration of the nutrient from 2 through 6 months of lactation with use of consensus values from several reported studies (Atkinson et al., 1995), and an average volume of milk intake of 0.78 L/day as reported from studies of full-term infants by test weighing, a procedure in which the infant is weighed before and after each feeding (Butte et al., 1984; Chandra, 1984; Hofvander et al., 1982; Neville et al., 1988). Because there is variation in both of these measures, the computed value represents the mean. It is expected that infants will consume increased volumes of human milk as they grow.

Ages 7 through 12 Months. Except for iron and zinc, which have relatively high requirements, there is no evidence for markedly different nutrient needs during the period of infants' growth acceleration and gradual weaning to a mixed diet of human milk and solid foods from ages 7 through 12 months. The basis of the AI values derived for this age category was the sum of the specific nutrient provided by 0.6 L/day of human milk, which is the average volume of milk reported from studies in this age category (Heinig et al., 1993), and that provided by the usual intakes of complementary weaning foods consumed by infants in this age category (Specker et al., 1997). This approach is in keeping with the current recommendations of the Canadian Paediatric Society (Health Canada, 1990), the American Academy of Pediatrics (AAP, 1997), and *Nutrition During Lactation* (IOM, 1991) for continued feeding of human milk to infants through 9 to 12 months of age with appropriate introduction of solid foods.

One problem encountered in trying to derive intake data in infants was the lack of available data on total nutrient intake from a combination of human milk and solid foods in the second 6 months of life. Most intake survey data do not identify the milk source, but the published values indicate that cow milk and cow milk formula were most likely consumed.

Toddlers: Ages 1 through 3 Years

The greater velocity of growth in height during ages 1 through 3 years compared with ages 4 through 5 years provides a biological basis for dividing this period of life. Because children in the United States and Canada from age 4 years onwards begin to enter the public school system, ending this life stage prior to age 4 years seemed appropriate. Data are sparse for indicators of nutrient adequacy on which to derive DRIs for these early years of life. In some cases, DRIs for this age group were derived from data extrapolated from studies of infants or of adults aged 19 years and older.

Early Childhood: Ages 4 through 8 Years

Because major biological changes in velocity of growth and changing endocrine status occur during ages 4 through 8 or 9 years (the latter depending on onset of puberty in each gender), the category of 4 through 8 years is appropriate. For many nutrients, a reasonable amount of data is available on nutrient intake and various criteria for adequacy (such as nutrient balance measured in young children ages 5 through 7 years) that can be used as the basis for the EARs and AIs for this life stage group.

Puberty/Adolescence: Ages 9 through 13 Years and 14 through 18 Years

Because current data support younger ages for pubertal development, it was determined that the adolescent age group should begin at 9 years. The mean age of onset of breast development (Tanner Stage 2) for white females in the United States is 10.0 ± 1.8 (standard deviation) years; this is a physical marker for the beginning of increased estrogen secretion (Herman-Giddens et al., 1997). In African-American females, onset of breast development is earlier (mean 8.9 years ± 1.9). The reason for the observed racial differences in the age at which girls enter puberty is unknown. The onset of the growth spurt in girls begins before the onset of breast development (Tanner, 1990). The age group of 9 through 13 years allows for this early growth spurt of females.

For males, the mean age of initiation of testicular development is 10.5 to 11 years, and their growth spurt begins 2 years later (Tanner, 1990). Thus, to begin the second age category at 14 years and to have different EARs and AIs for females and males for some nutrients at this age seems biologically appropriate. All children continue to grow to some extent until as late as age 20 years; therefore, having these two age categories span the period 9 through 18 years of age seems justified.

Young Adulthood and Middle Ages: Ages 19 through 30 Years and 31 through 50 Years

The recognition of the possible value of higher nutrient intakes during early adulthood on achieving optimal genetic potential for peak bone mass was the reason for dividing adulthood into ages 19 through 30 years and 31 through 50 years. Moreover, mean energy expenditure decreases during this 30-year period, and needs for nutrients related to energy metabolism may also decrease. For some nutrients, the DRIs may be the same for the two age groups. However, for other nutrients, especially those related to energy metabolism, EARs (and RDAs) are likely to differ for these two age groups.

Adulthood and Older Adults: Ages 51 through 70 Years and Over 70 Years

The age period of 51 through 70 years spans active work years for most adults. After age 70 years, people of the same age increasingly display variability in physiological functioning and physical activity. A comparison of people over age 70 years who are the same chronological age may demonstrate as much as a 15- to 20-year age-related difference in level of reserve capacity and functioning. This is demonstrated by age-related declines in nutrient absorption and renal function. Because of the high variability in functional capacity of older adults, the EARs and AIs for this age group may reflect a greater variability in requirements for the older age categories. This variability may be most applicable to nutrients for which requirements are related to energy expenditure.

Pregnancy and Lactation

Recommendations for pregnancy and lactation may be subdivided because of the many physiological changes and changes in nutrient needs that occur during these life stages. In setting EARs and AIs for these life stages, however, consideration is given to adaptations to increased nutrient demand, such as increased absorption and greater conservation of many nutrients. Moreover, nutrients may undergo net losses due to physiological mechanisms regardless of the nutrient intake. Thus, for some nutrients, there may not be a basis for EAR values that are different during these life stages than they are for other women of comparable age.

Reference Weights and Heights

The reference weights and heights selected for children and adults are shown in Table 1-1. The values are based on anthropometric data collected from 1988–1994 as part of the Third National Health and Nutrition Examination Survey (NHANES III) in the United States. When extrapolation to a different age group was conducted, these reference weights were used, except for iron which used weights with known coefficients of variation that were required for factorial modeling.

Using NHANES III data, the median heights for the life stage and gender groups through age 30 years were identified, and the median weights for these heights were based on reported median Body Mass Index (BMI) for the same individuals. Since there is no evidence that weight should change as adults age if activity is maintained, the reference weights for adults ages 19 through 30 years are applied to all adult age groups.

The most recent nationally representative data available for Canadians (from the 1970–1972 Nutrition Canada Survey [Demirjian, 1980]) were reviewed. In general, median heights of children from

TABLE 1-1 Reference Heights and Weights for Children and Adults in the United States[a]

Gender	Age	Median Body Mass Index (kg/m^2)	Reference Height, cm (in)	Reference Weight[b] kg (lb)
Male, female	2–6 mo	–	64 (25)	7 (16)
	7–11 mo	–	72 (28)	9 (20)
	1–3 y	–	91 (36)	13 (29)
	4–8 y	15.8	118 (46)	22 (48)
Male	9–13 y	18.5	147 (58)	40 (88)
	14–18 y	21.3	174 (68)	64 (142)
	19–30 y	24.4	176 (69)	76 (166)
Female	9–13 y	18.3	148 (58)	40 (88)
	14–18 y	21.3	163 (64)	57 (125)
	19–30 y	22.8	163 (64)	61 (133)

[a] Adapted from the Third National Health and Nutrition Examination Survey (NHANES III), 1988–1994.
[b] Calculated from body mass index and height for ages 4 through 8 years and older.

1 year of age in the United States were greater by 3 to 8 cm (1 to 3 inches) than those of children of the same age in Canada measured two decades earlier (Demirjian, 1980). This difference could be partly explained by approximations necessary to compare the two data sets but more likely by a continuation of the secular trend of increased heights for age noted in the Nutrition Canada Survey when it compared data from that survey with an earlier (1953) national Canadian survey (Pett and Ogilvie, 1956).

Similarly, median weights beyond age 1 year derived from the recent survey in the United States (NHANES III) were also greater than those obtained from the older Canadian survey (Demirjian, 1980). Differences were greatest during adolescence, ranging from 10 to 17 percent higher. The differences probably reflect the secular trend of earlier onset of puberty (Herman-Giddens et al., 1997), rather than differences in populations. Calculations of BMI for young adults (e.g., a median of 22.6 for Canadian women compared with 22.8 for U.S. women) resulted in similar values, thus indicating greater concordance between the two surveys by adulthood.

The reference weights chosen for this report were based on the most recent data set available from either country, with recognition that earlier surveys in Canada indicated shorter stature and lower weights during adolescence than did surveys in the United States.

Reference weights are used primarily when setting the EAR or Tolerable Upper Intake Level for children or when relating the nutrient needs of adults to body weight. For the 4- to 8-year-old age group, a small 4-year-old child can be assumed to require less than the EAR and that a large 8-year-old child will require more than the EAR. However, the RDA or AI should meet the needs of both.

SUMMARY

Dietary Reference Intakes (DRIs) is a generic term for a set of nutrient reference values that includes the Estimated Average Requirement, Recommended Dietary Allowance, Adequate Intake, and Tolerable Upper Intake Level. These reference values are being developed for life stage and gender groups in a joint U.S. and Canadian activity. This report, which is one volume in a series, covers the DRIs for vitamins A and K, arsenic, boron, chromium, copper, iodine, iron, manganese, molybdenum, nickel, silicon, vanadium, and zinc.

REFERENCES

AAP (American Academy of Pediatrics). 1997. Breastfeeding and the use of human milk. *Pediatrics* 100:1035–1039.

Atkinson SA, Alston-Mills BP, Lonnerdal B, Neville MC, Thompson MP. 1995. Major minerals and ionic constituents of human and bovine milk. In: Jensen RJ, ed. *Handbook of Milk Composition.* California: Academic Press. Pp. 593–619.

Beaton GH. 1994. Criteria of an adequate diet. In: Shils ME, Olson JA, Shike M, eds. *Modern Nutrition in Health and Disease,* 8th ed. Philadelphia: Lea & Febiger. Pp. 1491–1505.

Butte NF, Garza C, Smith EO, Nichols BL. 1984. Human milk intake and growth in exclusively breast-fed infants. *J Pediatr* 104:187–195.

Chandra RK. 1984. Physical growth of exclusively breast-fed infants. *Nutr Res* 2:275–276.

Demirjian A. 1980. *Anthropometry Report. Height, Weight, and Body Dimensions: A Report from Nutrition Canada.* Ottawa: Minister of National Health and Welfare, Health and Promotion Directorate, Health Services and Promotion Branch.

Elia M. 1992. Energy expenditure and the whole body. In: Kinney JM, Tucker HN, eds. *Energy Metabolism: Tissue Determinants and Cellular Corollaries.* New York: Raven Press. Pp. 19–59.

FAO/WHO/UNA (Food and Agriculture Organization of the United Nations/World Health Organization/United Nations Association). 1985. *Energy and Protein Requirements Report of a Joint FAO/WHO/UNA Expert Consultation.* Technical Report Series, No. 724. Geneva: WHO.

Garby L, Lammert O. 1984. Within-subjects between-days-and-weeks variation in energy expenditure at rest. *Hum Nutr Clin Nutr* 38:395–397.

Gentle JE. 1998. *Random Number Generation and Monte Carlo Methods.* New York: Springer-Verlag.

Health Canada. 1990. *Nutrition Recommendations. The Report of the Scientific Review Committee 1990.* Ottawa: Canadian Government Publishing Centre.

Heinig MJ, Nommsen LA, Peerson JM, Lonnerdal B, Dewey KG. 1993. Energy and protein intakes of breast-fed and formula-fed infants during the first year of life and their association with growth velocity: The DARLING Study. *Am J Clin Nutr* 58:152–161.

Herman-Giddens ME, Slora EJ, Wasserman RC, Bourdony CJ, Bhapkar MV, Koch GG, Hasemeier CM. 1997. Secondary sexual characteristics and menses in young girls seen in office practice: A study from the Pediatric Research in Office Settings network. *Pediatrics* 99:505–512.

Hofvander Y, Hagman U, Hillervik C, Sjolin S. 1982. The amount of milk consumed by 1–3 months old breast- or bottle-fed infants. *Acta Paediatr Scand* 71:953–958.

IOM (Institute of Medicine). 1991. *Nutrition During Lactation.* Washington, DC: National Academy Press.

IOM 2000. *Dietary Reference Intakes: Applications in Dietary Assessment.* Washington, DC: National Academy Press.

Neville MC, Keller R, Seacat J, Lutes V, Neifert M, Casey C, Allen J, Archer P. 1988. Studies in human lactation: Milk volumes in lactating women during the onset of lactation and full lactation. *Am J Clin Nutr* 48:1375–1386.

NRC (National Research Council). 1989. *Recommended Dietary Allowances,* 10th ed. Washington, DC: National Academy Press.

Pett LB, Ogilvie GH. 1956. The Canadian Weight-Height Survey. *Hum Biol* 28:177–188.

Specker BL, Beck A, Kalkwarf H, Ho M. 1997. Randomized trial of varying mineral intake on total body bone mineral accretion during the first year of life. *Pediatrics* 99:E12.

Tanner JM. 1990. *Growth at Adolescence.* Oxford: Oxford University Press.

WHO (World Health Organization). 1996. *Trace Elements in Human Nutrition and Health.* Geneva: WHO.

2

Overview and Methods

This report focuses on fourteen micronutrients—vitamin A, vitamin K, arsenic, boron, chromium, copper, iodine, iron, manganese, molybdenum, nickel, silicon, vanadium, and zinc. These micronutrients fall into two categories: (1) those known to have a beneficial role in human health and (2) those that lack sufficient evidence of their specific role in human health and lacking a reproducibly observed human indicator in response to their absence in the diet.

The micronutrients that have a beneficial role in human health include vitamin A, vitamin K, chromium, copper, iodine, iron, manganese, molybdenum, and zinc. Vitamin A is required for normal vision, gene expression, cellular differentiation, morphogenesis, growth, and immune function. Vitamin K plays an essential role in the coagulation of blood. Chromium improves the efficiency of insulin in individuals with impaired glucose tolerance. Copper is associated with many metalloenzymes and is necessary for proper development of connective tissue, myelin, and melanin. Iodine prevents dwarfism, cretinism, and goiter. Iron, via hemoglobin and myoglobin, is necessary for the movement of oxygen from the air to the various tissues and the prevention of anemia. Manganese is associated with a number of metalloenzymes and is involved with the formation of bone and the metabolism of amino acids, lipids, and carbohydrates. Molybdenum is a cofactor of several enzymes, and a deficiency of these enzymes can result in neurological abnormalities and death. Zinc is associated with catalytic activity of more than 200 enzymes and regulatory proteins, including transcription factors.

The micronutrients reviewed that lack a demonstrated role in human health include arsenic, boron, nickel, silicon, and vanadium. Arsenic has been shown to have a role in methionine metabolism in rats, and a deprivation of arsenic has been associated with impaired growth in various animals. Embryonic defects have been demonstrated in boron-depleted trout. Abnormal metabolism of vitamin D and estrogen has been proposed as a related function for boron in humans. Nickel has been demonstrated to be essential for animals, and its deprivation in rats can result in retarded growth. Silicon is involved with the formation of bone and collagen in animals. Vanadium has been shown to mimic insulin and stimulate cell proliferation and differentiation in animals.

METHODOLOGICAL CONSIDERATIONS

Types of Data Used

The scientific data for developing the Dietary Reference Intakes (DRIs) have essentially come from observational and experimental studies in humans. Observational studies include single-case and case-series reports and cross sectional, cohort, and case-control studies. Experimental studies include randomized and nonrandomized therapeutic or prevention trials and controlled dose-response, balance, turnover, and depletion-repletion physiological studies. Results from animal experiments are generally not applicable to the establishment of DRIs, but selected animal studies are considered in the absence of human data.

Animal Models

Basic research using experimental animals affords considerable advantage in terms of control of nutrient exposures, environmental factors, and even genetics. In contrast, the relevance to free-living humans may be unclear. In addition, dose levels and routes of administration that are practical in animal experiments may differ greatly from those relevant to humans. Nevertheless, animal feeding experiments were sometimes included in the evidence reviewed to determine the ability to specify DRIs.

Human Feeding Studies

Controlled feeding studies, usually in a confined setting such as a metabolic ward, can yield valuable information on the relationship between nutrient consumption and health-related biomarkers.

Much of the understanding of human nutrient requirements to prevent deficiencies is based on studies of this type. Studies in which the subjects are confined allow for close control of both intake and activities. Complete collections of nutrient losses through urine and feces are possible, as are recurring sampling of biological materials such as blood. Nutrient balance studies measure nutrient status in relation to intake. Depletion-repletion studies, by contrast, measure nutrient status while subjects are maintained on diets containing marginally low or deficient levels of a nutrient; then the deficit is corrected with measured amounts of that nutrient. Unfortunately, these two types of studies have several limitations: typically they are limited in time to a few days or weeks, and so longer-term outcomes cannot be measured with the same level of accuracy. In addition, subjects may be confined, and findings are therefore not always generalizable to free-living individuals. Finally, the time and expense involved in such studies usually limit the number of subjects and the number of doses or intake levels that can be tested.

In spite of these limitations, feeding studies play an important role in understanding nutrient needs and metabolism. Such data were considered in the DRI process and were given particular attention in the absence of reliable data to directly relate nutrient intake to disease risk.

Observational Studies

In comparison to human feeding studies, observational epidemiological studies are frequently of direct relevance to free-living humans, but they lack the controlled setting. Hence they are useful in establishing evidence of an association between the consumption of a nutrient and disease risk but are limited in their ability to ascribe a causal relationship. A judgment of causality may be supported by a consistency of association among studies in diverse populations, and it may be strengthened by the use of laboratory-based tools to measure exposures and confounding factors, rather than other means of data collection, such as personal interviews. In recent years, rapid advances in laboratory technology have made possible the increased use of biomarkers of exposure, susceptibility, and disease outcome in "molecular" epidemiological research. For example, one area of great potential in advancing current knowledge of the effects of diet on health is the study of genetic markers of disease susceptibility (especially polymorphisms in genes encoding metabolizing enzymes) in relation to dietary exposures. This development is expected to provide more accurate assessments of the risk associated with different levels of intake of both nutrients and nonnutritive food constituents.

While analytic epidemiological studies (studies that relate exposure to disease outcomes in individuals) have provided convincing evidence of an associative relationship between selected nondietary exposures and disease risk, there are a number of other factors that limit study reliability in research relating nutrient intakes to disease risk. First, the variation in nutrient intake may be rather limited in populations selected for study. This feature alone may yield modest relative risk trends across intake categories in the population, even if the nutrient is an important factor in explaining large disease rate variations among populations.

A second factor, one that gives rise to particular concerns about confounding, is the human diet's complex mixture of foods and nutrients that includes many substances that may be highly correlated. Third, many cohort and case-control studies have relied on self-reports of diet, typically food records, 24-hour recalls, or diet history questionnaires. Repeated application of such instruments to the same individuals show considerable variation in nutrient consumption estimates from one time period to another with correlations often in the 0.3 to 0.7 range (e.g., Willett et al., 1985). In addition, there may be systematic bias in nutrient consumption estimates from self-report as the reporting of food intakes and portion sizes may depend on individual characteristics such as body mass, ethnicity, and age. For example, total energy consumption may tend to be substantially underreported (30 to 50 percent) among obese persons, with little or no underreporting among lean persons (Heitmann and Lissner, 1995). Such systematic bias, in conjunction with random measurement error and limited intake range, has the potential to greatly impact analytic epidemiological studies based on self-reported dietary habits. Note that cohort studies using objective (biomarker) measures of nutrient intake may have an important advantage in the avoidance of systematic bias, though important sources of bias (e.g., confounding) may remain.

Randomized Clinical Trials

By randomly allocating subjects to the (nutrient) exposure of interest, clinical trials eliminate the confounding that may be introduced in observational studies by self-selection. The unique strength of randomized trials is that, if the sample is large enough, the study groups will be similar with respect not only to those confounding variables known to the investigators, but also to any unknown factors that might be related to risk of the disease. Thus, randomized trials achieve a degree of control of confounding that is simply not possible with any observational design strategy, and thus they allow for the testing of small effects that are beyond the ability of observational studies to detect reliably.

Although randomized controlled trials represent the accepted standard for studies of nutrient consumption in relation to human health, they too possess important limitations. Specifically, persons agreeing to be randomized may be a select subset of the population of interest, thus limiting the generalization of trial results. For practical reasons, only a small number of nutrients or nutrient combinations at a single intake level are generally studied in a randomized trial (although a few intervention trials to compare specific dietary patterns have been initiated in recent years). In addition, the follow-up period will typically be short relative to the preceding time period of nutrient consumption that may be relevant to the health outcomes under study, particularly if chronic disease endpoints are sought. Also, dietary intervention or supplementation trials tend to be costly and logistically difficult, and the maintenance of intervention adherence can be a particular challenge.

Because of the many complexities in conducting studies among free-living human populations and the attendant potential for bias and confounding, it is the totality of the evidence from both observational and intervention studies, appropriately weighted, that must form the basis for conclusions about causal relationships between particular exposures and disease outcomes.

Weighing the Evidence

As a principle, only studies published in peer-reviewed journals have been used in this report. However, studies published in other scientific journals or readily available reports were considered if they appeared to provide important information not documented elsewhere. To the extent possible, original scientific studies have been used to derive the DRIs. On the basis of a thorough review of the scientific literature, clinical, functional, and biochemical indicators of nutritional adequacy and excess were identified for each nutrient.

The quality of the study was considered in weighing the evidence. The characteristics examined included the study design and the representativeness of the study population; the validity, reliability, and precision of the methods used for measuring intake and indicators of adequacy or excess; the control of biases and confounding factors; and the power of the study to demonstrate a given difference or correlation. Publications solely expressing opinions were not used in setting DRIs. The assessment acknowledged the inherent reliability of each type of study design as described above, and it applied standard criteria concerning the strength and dose-response and temporal pattern of estimated nutrient-disease or adverse effect associations, the consistency of associations among studies of various types, and the specificity and biological plausibility of the suggested relationships (Hill, 1971). For example, biological plausibility would not be sufficient in the presence of a weak association and lack of evidence that exposure preceded the effect.

Data were examined to determine whether similar estimates of the requirement resulted from the use of different indicators and different types of studies. For a single nutrient, the criterion for setting the Estimated Average Requirement (EAR) may differ from one life stage group to another because the critical function or the risk of disease may be different. When no or very poor data were available for a given life stage group, extrapolation was made from the EAR or Adequate Intake (AI) set for another group; explicit and logical assumptions on relative requirements were made. Because EARs can be used for multiple purposes, they were established whenever sufficient supporting data were available.

Data Limitations

Although the reference values are based on data, the data were often scanty or drawn from studies that had limitations in addressing the various questions that confronted the Panel. Therefore, many of the questions raised about the requirements for and recommended intakes of these nutrients cannot be answered fully because of inadequacies in the present database. Apart from studies of overt deficiency diseases, there is a dearth of studies that address specific effects of inadequate intakes on specific indicators of health status, and thus a research agenda is proposed (see Chapter 15). For many of these nutrients, estimated requirements are based on factorial, balance, and biochemical indicator data because there is little information relating health status indicators to functional sufficiency or insufficiency.

Thus, after careful review and analysis of the evidence, including examination of the extent of congruent findings, scientific judgment was used to determine the basis for establishing the values. The reasoning used is described for each nutrient in Chapters 4 through 13.

Method for Determining the Adequate Intake for Infants

The AI for young infants is generally taken to be the average intake by full-term infants who are born to healthy, well-nourished mothers and who are exclusively fed human milk. The extent to which intake of a nutrient from human milk may exceed the actual requirements of infants is not known, and ethics of experimentation preclude testing the levels known to be potentially inadequate. Using the infant exclusively fed human milk as a model is in keeping with the basis for earlier recommendations for intake (e.g., Health Canada, 1990; IOM, 1991). It also supports the recommendation that exclusive intake of human milk is the preferred method of feeding for normal full-term infants for the first 4 to 6 months of life. This recommendation has been made by the Canadian Paediatric Society (Health Canada, 1990), the American Academy of Pediatrics (AAP, 1997), the Institute of Medicine (IOM, 1991), and many other expert groups, even though most U.S. babies no longer receive human milk by age 6 months.

In general, this report does not cover possible variations in physiological need during the first month after birth or the variations in intake of nutrients from human milk that result from differences in milk volume and nutrient concentration during early lactation.

In keeping with the decision made by the Standing Committee on the Scientific Evaluation of Dietary Reference Intakes, specific DRIs to meet the needs of formula-fed infants have not been proposed in this report. The use of formula introduces a large number of complex issues, one of which is the bioavailability of different forms of the nutrient in different formula types.

Ages 0 through 6 Months

To derive the AI for infants ages 0 through 6 months, the mean intake of a nutrient was calculated based on (1) the average concentration of the nutrient from 2 to 6 months of lactation using consensus values from several reported studies, if possible, and (2) an average volume of milk intake of 0.78 L/day. This volume was reported from studies that used test weighing of full-term infants. In this procedure, the infant is weighed before and after each feeding (Butte et al., 1984; Chandra, 1984; Hofvander et al., 1982; Neville et al., 1988). Because there is variation in both the composition of milk and the volume consumed, the computed value represents the mean. It is expected that infants will consume increased volumes of human milk during growth spurts.

Ages 7 through 12 Months

Except for iron and zinc, during the period of infant growth and gradual weaning to a mixed diet of human milk and solid foods from ages 7 through 12 months, there is no evidence for markedly different nutrient needs. The AI can be derived for this age group by calculating the sum of (1) the content of the nutrient provided by 0.6 L/day of human milk, which is the average volume of milk reported from studies of infants receiving human milk in this age category (Heinig et al., 1993) and (2) that provided by the usual intakes of complementary weaning foods consumed by infants in this age category. Such an approach is in keeping with the current recommendations of the Canadian Paediatric Society (Health Canada, 1990), the American Academy of Pediatrics (AAP, 1997), and the Institute of Medicine (IOM, 1991) for continued feeding of infants with human milk through 9 to 12 months of age with appropriate introduction of solid foods. The amounts of vitamin A, copper, iron, and zinc consumed from complementary foods were determined by using Third National Health and Nutrition Examination Survey data, and they are discussed in the nutrient chapters.

For some of the nutrients, two other approaches were considered as well: (1) extrapolation downward from the EAR for young adults by adjusting for metabolic or total body size and growth and adding a factor for variability and (2) extrapolation upward from the AI for infants ages 0 through 6 months by using the same type of adjustment. Both of these methods are described below. The results of the methods are compared in the process of setting the AI.

Human milk does not provide sufficient levels of iron and zinc for proper growth and development of the older infant. Because factorial data were available for iron and zinc in the older infants, an EAR for iron and zinc has been established for infants ages 7 through 12 months.

Method for Extrapolating Data from Adults to Infants and Children

Setting the EAR or AI for Children

For vitamin A, chromium, copper, iodine, and molybdenum, data were not available to set the EAR and Recommended Dietary Allowance (RDA) or an AI for children ages 1 year and older and adolescents. Therefore, the EAR or AI has been extrapolated down by using a consistent basic method. The method relies on at least four assumptions:

1. Maintenance needs for vitamin A, chromium, copper, iodine, and molybdenum, expressed with respect to metabolic body weight ([kilogram of body weight]$^{0.75}$), are the same for adults and children. Scaling requirements to the 0.75 power of body mass adjusts for metabolic differences demonstrated to be related to body weight, as described by Kleiber (1947) and explored further by West et al. (1997). By this scaling, a child weighing 22 kg would require 42 percent of what an adult weighing 70 kg would require—a higher percentage than that represented by actual weight. If there is a lack of evidence demonstrating an association between metabolic rate and nutrient requirement, needs are estimated directly proportional to total body weight.

2. The EAR for adults is an estimate of maintenance needs.

3. The percentage of extra vitamin A, chromium, copper, and molybdenum needed for growth is similar to the percentage of extra protein needed for growth.

4. On average, total needs do not differ substantially for males and females until age 14, when reference weights differ.

The formula for the extrapolation is

$$EAR_{child} = EAR_{adult} \times F,$$

where $F = (Weight_{child}/Weight_{adult})^{0.75} \times (1 + growth\ factor)$. Reference weights from Table 1-1 are used. If the EAR differs for men and women, the reference weight used for adults differs in the equation by gender; otherwise, the average for men and women is used. The approximate proportional increase in protein requirements for growth (FAO/WHO/UNA, 1985) is used as an estimate of the growth factor as shown in Table 2-1. If only an AI has been set for adults, it is substituted for the EAR in the above formula, and an AI is calculated; no RDA will be set.

Setting the RDA for Children

To account for variability in requirements because of growth rates and other factors, a 10 percent coefficient of variation (CV) for the requirement is assumed for children just as for adults unless data are available to support another value, as described in Chapter 1.

TABLE 2-1 Estimated Growth Factor, by Age Group

Age Group	Growth Factor
7 mo–3 y	0.30
4–8 y	0.15
9–13 y	0.15
14–18 y	
Males	0.15
Females	0.0

SOURCE: Proportional increase in protein requirements for growth from FAO/WHO/UNA (1985) used to estimate the growth factor.

Setting the Tolerable Upper Intake Level for Children

When data are not available to set the Tolerable Upper Intake Level (UL) for children, the UL for adults is extrapolated down using the reference body weights in Table 1-1:

$$UL_{child} = UL_{adult} \times Weight_{adult}/Weight_{child}.$$

Method for Extrapolating Data from Young to Older Infants

Using the metabolic weight ratio method to extrapolate data from young to older infants involves metabolic scaling but does not include an adjustment for growth because it is based on a value for a growing infant. To extrapolate from the AI for infants ages 0 through 6 months to an AI for infants ages 7 through 12 months, the following formula is used:

$$AI_{7-12\,mo} = AI_{0-6\,mo} \times F,$$

where $F = (Weight_{7-12\,mo}/Weight_{0-6\,mo})^{0.75}$.

Methods for Determining Increased Needs for Pregnancy

It is known that the placenta actively transports certain nutrients from the mother to the fetus against a concentration gradient (Hytten and Leitch, 1971). However, for many nutrients, experimental data that could be used to set an EAR and RDA or an AI for pregnancy are lacking. In these cases, the potential increased need for these nutrients during pregnancy is based on theoretical considerations, including obligatory fetal transfer, if data are available, and on increased maternal needs related to increases in energy or protein metabolism, as applicable. For chromium, manganese, and molybdenum, the AI or EAR is determined by extrapolating up according to the additional weight gained during pregnancy. Carmichael et al. (1997) reported that the median weight gain of 7,002 women who had good pregnancy outcomes was 16 kg. No consistent relationship between maternal age and weight gain was observed in six studies of U.S. women (IOM, 1990). Therefore, 16 kg is added to the reference weight for nonpregnant adolescent girls and women for extrapolation.

Methods for Determining Increased Needs for Lactation

It is assumed that the total nutrient requirement for lactating women equals the requirement for nonpregnant, nonlactating women of similar age plus an increment to cover the amount needed for milk production. To allow for inefficiencies in the use of certain nutrients, the increment may be greater than the amount of the nutrient contained in the milk produced. Details are provided in each nutrient chapter.

ESTIMATES OF NUTRIENT INTAKE

Reliable and valid methods of food composition analysis are crucial in determining the intake of a nutrient needed to meet a requirement. For nutrients such as chromium, analytic methods to determine the content of the nutrient in food have serious limitations.

Methodological Considerations

The quality of nutrient intake data varies widely across studies. The most valid intake data are those collected from the metabolic study protocols in which all food is provided by the researchers, amounts consumed are measured accurately, and the nutrient composition of the food is determined by reliable and valid laboratory analyses. Such protocols are usually possible with only a few subjects. Thus, in many studies, intake data are self-reported (e.g., through 24-hour recalls of food intake, diet records, or food frequency questionnaires).

Potential sources of error in self-reported intake data include over- or underreporting of portion sizes and frequency of intake, omission of foods, and inaccuracies related to the use of food composition tables (IOM, 2000; Lichtman et al., 1992; Mertz et al., 1991). In addition, because a high percentage of the food consumed in the United States and Canada is not prepared from scratch in the home, errors can occur due to a lack of information on how a food was manufactured, prepared, and served. Therefore, the values reported by nationwide surveys or studies that rely on self-report are often inaccurate and possibly biased, with a greater tendency to underestimate actual intake (IOM, 2000).

Adjusting for Day-to-Day Variation

Because of day-to-day variation in dietary intakes, the distribution of 1-day (or 2-day) intakes for a group is wider than the distribution of usual intakes even though the mean of the intakes may be the same (for further elaboration, see Chapter 14). To reduce this problem, statistical adjustments have been developed (NRC, 1986; Nusser et al., 1996) that require at least 2 days of dietary data from a representative subsample of the population of interest. However, no accepted method is available to adjust for the underreporting of intake, which may average as much as 20 percent for energy (Mertz et al., 1991).

DIETARY INTAKES IN THE UNITED STATES AND CANADA

Sources of Dietary Intake Data

The major sources of current dietary intake data for the U.S. population are the Third National Health and Nutrition Examination Survey (NHANES III), which was conducted from 1988 to 1994 by the U.S. Department of Health and Human Services, and the Continuing Survey of Food Intakes by Individuals (CSFII), which was conducted by the U.S. Department of Agriculture (USDA) from 1994 to 1996. NHANES III examined 30,000 subjects aged 2 months and older. A single 24-hour diet recall was collected for all subjects. A second recall was collected for a 5 percent nonrandom subsample to allow adjustment of intake estimates for day-to-day variation. The 1994 to 1996 CSFII collected two nonconsecutive 24-hour recalls from approximately 16,000 subjects of all ages. Both surveys used the food composition database developed by USDA to calculate nutrient intakes (Perloff et al., 1990) and were adjusted by the method of Nusser et al. (1996). For boron, which is not included in the USDA food composition database, the Boron Nutrient Database (Rainey et al., 1999) was used to calculate boron intakes from these surveys. National survey data for Canada are not currently available, but data have been collected in Québec and Nova Scotia. The extent to which these data are applicable nationwide is not known.

The Food and Drug Administration (FDA) Total Diet Study was used for estimating the intakes for many of the micronutrients reviewed that were not covered by NHANES III and CFSII. The FDA Total Diet Study utilized a number of FDA Market Basket Surveys collected between the third quarter of 1991 and the first quarter of 1997. An updated food map was developed with use of a total of 306 core foods to map the USDA food consumption survey data for 1994 to 1996. The micronutrient contents of the 306 core foods were determined by FDA, USDA CFSII Code Book, Standard Reference 12, or literature published by individual laboratories. The intake data were not adjusted for day-to-day variation, and therefore do not represent usual intakes.

Appendix C provides the mean and the fifth through ninety-ninth percentiles of dietary intakes of vitamin A, vitamin K, boron, copper, iron, and zinc from NHANES III, adjusted by methods described by the National Research Council (NRC, 1986) and by Feinleib et al. (1993) and adjusted for day-to-day variation by the method of Nusser et al. (1996).

TABLE 2-2 Percentage of Persons Taking Vitamin and Mineral Supplements, by Sex and Age: National Health Interview Survey, United States, 1986

Vitamin/Mineral Supplement Taken	Women			
	All Adults 18+ y	18–44 y	45–64 y	65+ y
Vitamin A	25.9	26.3	26.3	24.4
Chromium	9.4	9.9	9.1	8.7
Copper	15.2	15.3	14.7	15.6
Iodine	15.3	15.7	14.3	15.5
Iron	23.1	24.5	22.0	20.7
Manganese	12.4	12.3	12.4	12.7
Zinc	17.2	17.0	17.2	17.9

NOTE: The high use of supplements by pregnant women is not reflected in this table.
SOURCE: Moss et al. (1989).

Appendix D provides comparable information from the 1994–1996 CSFII for boron, copper, iron, and zinc. Appendix E gives the mean and first through ninety-ninth percentiles of dietary intakes of vitamin K, arsenic, copper, iodine, iron, manganese, nickel, silicon, and zinc from the FDA Total Diet Study. Appendix F provides means and selected percentiles of dietary intakes of vitamin A, iron, and zinc for individuals in Québec and Nova Scotia.

Sources of Supplement Intake Data

Although subjects in the CSFII (1994–1996) were asked about the use of dietary supplements, quantitative information was not collected. Data on supplement intake obtained from NHANES III were reported as a part of total intake of vitamin K, copper, iron, and zinc (Appendix C). Intake, based on supplement intake alone for vitamin A, boron, chromium, iodine, manganese, molybdenum, nickel, silicon, and vanadium, is also reported in Appendix C. NHANES III data on overall prevalence of supplement use are also available (LSRO/FASEB, 1995). In 1986, the National Health Interview Survey queried 11,558 adults and 1,877 children on their intake of supplements during the previous 2 weeks (Moss et al., 1989). The composition of the supplement was obtained directly from the product label whenever possible. Table 2-2 shows the percentage of

Men			
All Adults 18+ y	18–44 y	45–64 y	65+ y
19.8	19.6	20.5	19.4
7.6	7.9	6.4	8.5
13.1	13.2	12.9	12.7
12.6	12.6	12.7	12.6
16.0	15.8	16.3	16.4
10.1	9.9	9.6	11.4
14.5	14.3	15.1	14.6

adults, by age, taking at least one of the micronutrients reviewed in this report.

Food Sources

For some nutrients, two types of information are provided about food sources: identification of the foods that are the major contributors of the nutrients to diets in the United States and the foods that contain the highest amounts of the nutrient. The determination of foods that are major contributors depends on both nutrient content of a food and the total consumption of the food (amount and frequency). Therefore, a food that has a relatively low concentration of the nutrient might still be a large contributor to total intake if that food is consumed in relatively large amounts.

SUMMARY

General methods for examining and interpreting the evidence on requirements for nutrients are presented in this chapter, with special attention given to infants, children, and pregnant and lactating women, methodological problems, and dietary intake data. Relevant detail is provided in the nutrient chapters.

REFERENCES

AAP (American Academy of Pediatrics). 1997. Breastfeeding and the use of human milk. *Pediatrics* 100:1035–1039.

Butte NF, Garza C, Smith EO, Nichols BL. 1984. Human milk intake and growth in exclusively breast-fed infants. *J Pediatr* 104:187–195.

Carmichael S, Abrams B, Selvin S. 1997. The pattern of maternal weight gain in women with good pregnancy outcomes. *Am J Public Health* 87:1984–1988.

Chandra RK. 1984. Physical growth of exclusively breast-fed infants. *Nutr Res* 2:275–276.

FAO/WHO/UNA (Food and Agriculture Organization of the United Nations/World Health Organization/United Nations). 1985. *Energy and Protein Requirements Report of a Joint FAO/WHO/UNA Expert Consultation*. Technical Report Series, No. 724. Geneva: WHO.

Feinleib M, Rifkind B, Sempos C, Johnson C, Bachorik P, Lippel K, Carroll M, Ingster-Moore L, Murphy R. 1993. Methodological issues in the measurement of cardiovascular risk factors: Within-person variability in selected serum lipid measures—Results from the Third National Health and Nutrition Survey (NHANES III). *Can J Cardiol* 9:87D–88D.

Health Canada. 1990. *Nutrition Recommendations. The Report of the Scientific Review Committee 1990*. Ottawa: Canadian Government Publishing Centre.

Heinig MJ, Nommsen LA, Peerson JM, Lonnerdal B, Dewey KG. 1993. Energy and protein intakes of breast-fed and formula-fed infants during the first year of life and their association with growth velocity: The DARLING Study. *Am J Clin Nutr* 58:152–161.

Heitmann BL, Lissner L. 1995. Dietary underreporting by obese individuals—Is it specific or non-specific? *Br Med J* 311:986–989.

Hill AB. 1971. *Principles of Medical Statistics*, 9th ed. New York: Oxford University Press.

Hofvander Y, Hagman U, Hillervik C, Sjolin S. 1982. The amount of milk consumed by 1–3 months old breast- or bottle-fed infants. *Acta Paediatr Scand* 71:953–958.

Hytten FE, Leitch I. 1971. *The Physiology of Human Pregnancy*, 2nd ed. Oxford: Blackwell Scientific.

IOM (Institute of Medicine). 1990. *Nutrition During Pregnancy*. Washington, DC: National Academy Press.

IOM. 1991. *Nutrition During Lactation*. Washington, DC: National Academy Press.

IOM 2000. *Dietary Reference Intakes: Applications in Dietary Assessment*. Washington, DC: National Academy Press.

Kleiber M. 1947. Body size and metabolic rate. *Physiol Rev* 27:511–541.

Lichtman SW, Pisarska K, Berman ER, Pestone M, Dowling H, Offenbacher E, Weisel H, Heshka S, Matthews DE, Heymsfield SB. 1992. Discrepancy between self-reported and actual caloric intake and exercise in obese subjects. *N Engl J Med* 327:1893–1898.

LSRO/FASEB (Life Sciences Research Office/Federation of American Societies for Experimental Biology). 1995. *Third Report on Nutrition Monitoring in the United States*. Washington, DC: US Government Printing Office.

Mertz W, Tsui JC, Judd JT, Reiser S, Hallfrisch J, Morris ER, Steele PD, Lashley E. 1991. What are people really eating? The relation between energy intake derived from estimated diet records and intake determined to maintain body weight. *Am J Clin Nutr* 54:291–295.

Moss AJ, Levy AS, Kim I, Park YK. 1989. *Use of Vitamin and Mineral Supplements in the United States: Current Users, Types of Products, and Nutrients*. Advance Data, Vital and Health Statistics of the National Center for Health Statistics, Number 174. Hyattsville, MD: National Center for Health Statistics.

Neville MC, Keller R, Seacat J, Lutes V, Neifert M, Casey C, Allen J, Archer P. 1988. Studies in human lactation: Milk volumes in lactating women during the onset of lactation and full lactation. *Am J Clin Nutr* 48:1375–1386.

NRC (National Research Council). 1986. *Nutrient Adequacy. Assessment Using Food Consumption Surveys*. Washington, DC: National Academy Press.

Nusser SM, Carriquiry AL, Dodd KW, Fuller WA. 1996. A semiparametric transformation approach to estimating usual daily intake distributions. *J Am Stat Assoc* 91:1440–1449.

Perloff BP, Rizek RL, Haytowitz DB, Reid PR. 1990. Dietary intake methodology. II. USDA's Nutrient Data Base for Nationwide Dietary Intake Surveys. *J Nutr* 120:1530–1534.

Rainey CJ, Nyquist LA, Christensen RA, Strong PL, Culver BD, Coughlin JR. 1999. Daily boron intake from the American diet. *J Am Diet Assoc* 99:335–340.

West GB, Brown JH, Enquist BJ. 1997. A general model for the origin of allometric scaling laws in biology. *Science* 276:122–126.

Willett WC, Sampson L, Stampfer MJ, Rosner B, Bain C, Witschi J, Hennekens CH, Speizer FE. 1985. Reproducibility and validity of a semiquantitative food frequency questionnaire. *Am J Epidemiol* 122:51–65.

3

A Model for
the Development of
Tolerable Upper Intake Levels

BACKGROUND

The *Tolerable Upper Intake Level* (UL) refers to the highest level of daily nutrient intake that is likely to pose no risk of adverse health effects for almost all individuals in the general population. As intake increases above the UL, the potential risk of adverse effects increases. The term *tolerable* is chosen because it connotes a level of intake that can, with high probability, be tolerated biologically by individuals; it does not imply acceptability of that level in any other sense. The setting of a UL does not indicate that nutrient intakes greater than the Recommended Dietary Allowance (RDA) or Adequate Intake (AI) are recommended as being beneficial to an individual. Many individuals are self-medicating with nutrients for curative or treatment purposes. It is beyond the scope of this report to address the possible therapeutic benefits of higher nutrient intakes that may offset the potential risk of adverse effects. The UL is not meant to apply to individuals who are treated with the nutrient under medical supervision or to individuals with predisposing conditions that modify their sensitivity to the nutrient. This chapter describes a model for developing ULs.

The term *adverse effect* is defined as any significant alteration in the structure or function of the human organism (Klaassen et al., 1986) or any impairment of a physiologically important function that could lead to a health effect that is adverse, in accordance with the definition set by the joint World Health Organization, Food and Agriculture Organization of the United Nations, and Interna-

60

tional Atomic Energy Agency Expert Consultation in *Trace Elements in Human Nutrition and Health* (WHO, 1996). In the case of nutrients, it is exceedingly important to consider the possibility that the intake of one nutrient may alter in detrimental ways the health benefits conferred by another nutrient. Any such alteration (referred to as an adverse nutrient-nutrient interaction) is considered an adverse health effect. When evidence for such adverse interactions is available, it is considered in establishing a nutrient's UL.

ULs are useful because of the increased interest in and availability of fortified foods, the increased use of dietary supplements, and the growing recognition of the health consequences of excesses, as well as inadequacies, of nutrient intakes. ULs are based on total intake of a nutrient from food, water, and supplements if adverse effects have been associated with total intake. However, if adverse effects have been associated with intake from supplements or food fortificants only, the UL is based on nutrient intake from those sources only, not on total intake. The UL applies to chronic daily use.

For many nutrients, there are insufficient data on which to develop a UL. This does not mean that there is no potential for adverse effects resulting from high intake. When data about adverse effects are extremely limited, extra caution may be warranted.

Like all chemical agents, nutrients can produce adverse health effects if their intake from a combination of food, water, nutrient supplements, and pharmacological agents is excessive. Some lower level of nutrient intake will ordinarily pose no likelihood (or risk) of adverse health effects in normal individuals even if the level is above that associated with any benefit. It is not possible to identify a single risk-free intake level for a nutrient that can be applied with certainty to all members of a population. However, it is possible to develop intake levels that are unlikely to pose risk of adverse health effects for most members of the general population, including sensitive individuals. For some nutrients, these intake levels pose a potential risk to subpopulations with extreme or distinct vulnerabilities.

Although members of the general population should not routinely exceed the UL, intake above the UL may be appropriate for investigation within well-controlled clinical trials. Clinical trials of doses above the UL should not be discouraged, as long as subjects participating in these trials have signed informed consent documents regarding possible toxicity and as long as these trials employ appropriate safety monitoring of trial subjects.

A MODEL FOR THE DERIVATION OF TOLERABLE UPPER INTAKE LEVELS

The possibility that the methodology used to derive Tolerable Upper Intake Levels (ULs) might be reduced to a mathematical model that could be generically applied to all nutrients was considered. Such a model might have several potential advantages, including ease of application and assurance of consistent treatment of all nutrients. It was concluded, however, that the current state of scientific understanding of toxic phenomena in general, and nutrient toxicity in particular, is insufficient to support the development of such a model. Scientific information about various adverse effects and their relationships to intake levels varies greatly among nutrients and depends on the nature, comprehensiveness, and quality of available data. The uncertainties associated with the unavoidable problem of extrapolating from the circumstances under which data are developed (e.g., in the laboratory or clinic) to other circumstances (e.g., to the healthy population) adds to the complexity.

Given the current state of knowledge, any attempt to capture in a mathematical model all of the information and scientific judgments that must be made to reach conclusions about ULs would not be consistent with contemporary risk assessment practices. Instead, the model for the derivation of ULs consists of a set of scientific factors that always should be considered explicitly. The framework by which these factors are organized is called *risk assessment*. Risk assessment (NRC, 1983, 1994) is a systematic means of evaluating the probability of occurrence of adverse health effects in humans from excess exposure to an environmental agent (in this case, a nutrient) (FAO/WHO, 1995; Health Canada, 1993). The hallmark of risk assessment is the requirement to be explicit in all of the evaluations and judgments that must be made to document conclusions.

RISK ASSESSMENT AND FOOD SAFETY

Basic Concepts

Risk assessment is a scientific undertaking having as its objective a characterization of the nature and likelihood of harm resulting from human exposure to agents in the environment. The characterization of risk typically contains both qualitative and quantitative information and includes a discussion of the scientific uncertainties in that information. In the present context, the agents of interest are nutrients, and the environmental media are food, water, and nonfood sources such as nutrient supplements and pharmacological preparations.

Performing a risk assessment results in a characterization of the relationships between exposure to an agent and the likelihood that adverse health effects will occur in members of exposed populations. Scientific uncertainties are an inherent part of the risk assessment process and are discussed below. Deciding whether the magnitude of exposure is *acceptable* or *tolerable* in specific circumstances is not a component of risk assessment; this activity falls within the domain of *risk management*. Risk management decisions depend on the results of risk assessments but may also involve the public health significance of the risk, the technical feasibility of achieving various degrees of risk control, and the economic and social costs of this control. Because there is no single, scientifically definable distinction between safe and unsafe exposures, risk management necessarily incorporates components of sound, practical decision making that are not addressed by the risk assessment process (NRC, 1983, 1994).

Risk assessment requires that information be organized in rather specific ways but does not require any specific scientific evaluation methods. Rather, risk assessors must evaluate scientific information using what they judge to be appropriate methods and must make explicit the basis for their judgments, the uncertainties in risk estimates, and, when appropriate, alternative scientifically plausible interpretations of the available data (NRC, 1994; OTA, 1993).

Risk assessment is subject to two types of scientific uncertainties: those related to data and those associated with inferences that are required when directly applicable data are not available (NRC, 1994). Data uncertainties arise during the evaluation of information obtained from the epidemiological and toxicological studies of nutrient intake levels that are the basis for risk assessments. Examples of inferences include the use of data from experimental animals to estimate responses in humans and the selection of uncertainty factors to estimate inter- and intraspecies variabilities in response to toxic substances. Uncertainties arise whenever estimates of adverse health effects in humans are based on extrapolations of data obtained under dissimilar conditions (e.g., from experimental animal studies). Options for dealing with uncertainties are discussed below and in detail in Appendix L.

Steps in the Risk Assessment Process

The organization of risk assessment is based on a model proposed by the National Research Council (NRC, 1983, 1994) that is widely

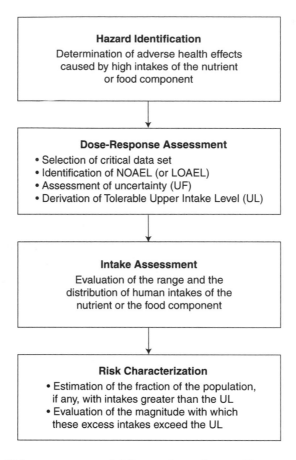

Hazard Identification

Determination of adverse health effects
caused by high intakes of the nutrient
or food component

Dose-Response Assessment

• Selection of critical data set
• Identification of NOAEL (or LOAEL)
• Assessment of uncertainty (UF)
• Derivation of Tolerable Upper Intake Level (UL)

Intake Assessment

Evaluation of the range and the
distribution of human intakes of the
nutrient or the food component

Risk Characterization

• Estimation of the fraction of the population,
if any, with intakes greater than the UL
• Evaluation of the magnitude with which
these excess intakes exceed the UL

FIGURE 3-1 Risk assessment model for nutrient adverse effects.

used in public health and regulatory decision making. The steps of risk assessment as applied to nutrients follow (see also Figure 3-1).

• Step 1. Hazard identification involves the collection, organization, and evaluation of all information pertaining to the adverse effects of a given nutrient. It concludes with a summary of the evidence concerning the capacity of the nutrient to cause one or more types of toxicity in humans.

• Step 2. Dose-response assessment determines the relationship between nutrient intake (dose) and adverse effect (in terms of incidence and severity). This step concludes with an estimate of the Tolerable Upper Intake Level (UL)—it identifies the highest level of daily nutrient intake that is likely to pose no risk of adverse health effects for almost all individuals in the general population. Different ULs may be developed for various life stage groups.

• Step 3. Intake assessment evaluates the distribution of usual total daily nutrient intakes for members of the general population. In cases where the UL pertains only to supplement use and does not pertain to usual food intakes of the nutrient, the assessment is directed at supplement intakes only. It does not depend on step 1 or 2.

• Step 4. Risk characterization summarizes the conclusions from steps 1 and 2 with step 3 to determine the risk. The risk is generally expressed as the fraction of the exposed population, if any, having nutrient intakes (step 3) in excess of the estimated UL (steps 1 and 2). If possible, characterization also covers the magnitude of any such excesses. Scientific uncertainties associated with both the UL and the intake estimates are described so that risk managers understand the degree of scientific confidence they can place in the risk assessment.

The risk assessment contains no discussion of recommendations for reducing risk; these are the focus of risk management.

Thresholds

A principal feature of the risk assessment process for noncarcinogens is the long-standing acceptance that no risk of adverse effects is expected unless a threshold dose (or intake) is exceeded. The adverse effects that may be caused by a nutrient almost certainly occur only when the threshold dose is exceeded (NRC, 1994; WHO, 1996). The critical issues concern the methods used to identify the approximate threshold of toxicity for a large and diverse human population. Because most nutrients are not considered to be carcinogenic in humans, approaches used for carcinogenic risk assessment are not discussed here.

Thresholds vary among members of the general population (NRC, 1994). For any given adverse effect, if the distribution of thresholds in the population could be quantitatively identified, it would be possible to establish ULs by defining some point in the lower tail of the distribution of thresholds that would protect some specified fraction of the population. The method for identifying thresholds for a general population described here is designed to ensure that almost all members of the population will be protected, but it is not based on an analysis of the theoretical (but practically unattainable) distribution of thresholds. By using the model to derive the threshold, however, there is considerable confidence that the threshold, which becomes the UL for nutrients or food components, lies very near the low end of the theoretical distribution and is the end representing the most sensitive members of the population. For some nutrients, there may be subpopulations that are not included in the general distribution because of extreme or distinct vulnerabilities to toxicity. Data relating to the effects observed in these groups are not used to derive ULs. Such distinct groups, whose conditions warrant medical supervision, may not be protected by the UL.

The Joint FAO/WHO Expert Committee on Food Additives and various national regulatory bodies have identified factors (called *uncertainty factors* [UFs]) that account for interspecies and intraspecies differences in response to the hazardous effects of substances and for other uncertainties (WHO, 1987). UFs are used to make inferences about the threshold dose of substances for members of a large and diverse human population from data on adverse effects obtained in epidemiological or experimental studies. These factors are applied consistently when data of specific types and quality are available. They are typically used to derive acceptable daily intakes for food additives and other substances for which data on adverse effects are considered sufficient to meet minimum standards of quality and completeness (FAO/WHO, 1982). These adopted or recognized UFs have sometimes been coupled with other factors to compensate for deficiencies in the available data and other uncertainties regarding data.

When possible, the UL is based on a no-observed-adverse-effect level (NOAEL), which is the highest intake (or experimental oral dose) of a nutrient at which no adverse effects have been observed in the individuals studied. This is identified for a specific circumstance in the hazard identification and dose-response assessment steps of the risk assessment. If there are no adequate data demonstrating a NOAEL, then a lowest-observed-adverse-effect level (LOAEL) may be used. A LOAEL is the lowest intake (or experimental oral dose) at which an adverse effect has been identified. The derivation of a UL from a NOAEL (or LOAEL) involves a series of choices about what factors should be used to deal with uncertainties. Uncertainty factors are applied in an attempt to deal both with gaps in data and with incomplete knowledge about the inferences required (e.g., the expected variability in response within the human population). The problems of both data and inference uncertainties arise in all steps of the risk assessment. A discussion of options available for dealing with these uncertainties is presented below and in greater detail in Appendix L.

A UL is not, in itself, a description or estimate of human risk. It is derived by application of the hazard identification and dose-response evaluation steps (steps 1 and 2) of the risk assessment model. To determine whether populations are at risk requires an intake or exposure assessment (step 3, evaluation of intakes of the nutrient by the population) and a determination of the fractions of these populations, if any, whose intakes exceed the UL. In the intake assessment and risk characterization steps (steps 3 and 4), the distribution of actual intakes for the population is used as a basis for determining whether and to what extent the population is at risk (Figure 3-1). A discussion of other aspects of the risk characterization that may be useful in judging the public health significance of the risk and in risk management decisions is provided in the final section of this chapter, "Risk Characterization."

APPLICATION OF THE RISK ASSESSMENT MODEL TO NUTRIENTS

This section provides guidance for applying the risk assessment framework (the model) to the derivation of Tolerable Upper Intake Levels (ULs) for nutrients.

Special Problems Associated with Substances Required for Human Nutrition

Although the risk assessment model outlined above can be applied to nutrients to derive ULs, it must be recognized that nutrients possess some properties that distinguish them from the types of agents for which the risk assessment model was originally developed (NRC, 1983). In the application of accepted standards for risk assessment of environmental chemicals to risk assessment of nutrients, a fundamental difference between the two categories must be recognized: within a certain range of intakes, nutrients are essential for human well-being and usually for life itself. Nonetheless, they may share with other chemicals the production of adverse effects at excessive exposures. Because the consumption of balanced diets is consistent with the development and survival of humankind over many millennia, there is less need for the large uncertainty factors that have been used for the risk assessment of nonessential chemicals. In addition, if data on the adverse effects of nutrients are available primarily from studies in human populations, there will be less uncertainty than is associated with the types of data available on nonessential chemicals.

There is no evidence to suggest that nutrients consumed at the recommended intake (the Recommended Dietary Allowance or Adequate Intake) present a potential risk of adverse effects to the general population.[1] It is clear, however, that the addition of nutrients to a diet through the ingestion of large amounts of highly fortified food, nonfood sources such as supplements, or both, (at some level) pose a potential risk of adverse health effects. The UL is the highest level of daily nutrient intake that is likely to pose no risk of adverse health effects for almost all individuals in the general population. As intake increases above the UL, the risk of adverse effects increases.

If adverse effects have been associated with total intake, ULs are based on total intake of a nutrient from food, water, and supplements. For cases in which adverse effects have been associated with intake only from supplements and food fortificants, the UL is based on intake from those sources only, rather than on total intake. The effects of nutrients from fortified foods or supplements may differ from those of naturally occurring constituents of foods because of the chemical form of the nutrient, the timing of the intake and amount consumed in a single bolus dose, the matrix supplied by the food, and the relation of the nutrient to the other constituents of the diet. Nutrient requirements and food intake are related to the metabolizing body mass, which is also at least an indirect measure of the space in which the nutrients are distributed. This relation between food intake and space of distribution supports homeostasis, which maintains nutrient concentrations in that space within a range compatible with health. However, excessive intake of a single nutrient from supplements or fortificants may compromise this homeostatic mechanism. Such elevations alone pose potential risk of adverse effects; imbalances among the nutrients may also be possible. These reasons and those discussed previously support the need to include the form and pattern of consumption in the assessment of risk from high nutrient or food component intake.

---

[1]It is recognized that possible exceptions to this generalization relate to specific geochemical areas with excessive environmental exposures to certain trace elements (e.g., selenium) and to rare case reports of adverse effects associated with highly eccentric consumption of specific foods. Data from such findings are generally not useful for setting ULs for the general North American population.

Consideration of Variability in Sensitivity

The risk assessment model outlined in this chapter is consistent with classical risk assessment approaches in that it must consider variability in the sensitivity of individuals to adverse effects of nutrients or food components. A discussion of how variability is dealt with in the context of nutritional risk assessment follows.

Physiological changes and common conditions associated with growth and maturation that occur during an individual's lifespan may influence sensitivity to nutrient toxicity. For example, sensitivity increases with declines in lean body mass and with declines in renal and liver function that occur with aging; sensitivity changes in direct relation to intestinal absorption or intestinal synthesis of nutrients; in the newborn infant sensitivity is also increased because of rapid brain growth and limited ability to secrete or biotransform toxicants; and sensitivity increases with decreases in the rate of metabolism of nutrients. During pregnancy, the increase in total body water and glomerular filtration results in lower blood levels of water-soluble vitamins dose for dose and therefore results in reduced susceptibility to potential adverse effects. However, in the unborn fetus this may be offset by active placental transfer, accumulation of certain nutrients in the amniotic fluid, and rapid development of the brain. Examples of life stage groups that may differ in terms of nutritional needs and toxicological sensitivity include infants and children, the elderly, and women during pregnancy and lactation.

Even within relatively homogeneous life stage groups, there is a range of sensitivities to toxic effects. The model described below accounts for normally expected variability in sensitivity but excludes subpopulations with extreme and distinct vulnerabilities. Such subpopulations consist of individuals needing medical supervision; they are better served through the use of public health screening, product labeling, or other individualized health care strategies. Such populations may not be at *negligible risk* when their intakes reach the UL developed for the healthy population. The decision to treat identifiable vulnerable subgroups as distinct (not protected by the UL) is a matter of judgment and is discussed in individual nutrient chapters, as applicable.

Bioavailability

In the context of toxicity, the bioavailability of an ingested nutrient can be defined as its accessibility to normal metabolic and physiological processes. Bioavailability influences a nutrient's beneficial effects at physiological levels of intake and also may affect the nature and severity of toxicity due to excessive intakes. The concentration and chemical form of the nutrient, the nutrition and health of the individual, and excretory losses all affect bioavailability. Bioavailability data for specific nutrients must be considered and incorporated by the risk assessment process.

Some nutrients may be less readily absorbed when part of a meal than when consumed separately. Supplemental forms of some nutrients may require special consideration if they have higher bioavailability and therefore may present a greater risk of producing adverse effects than equivalent amounts from the natural form found in food.

Nutrient-Nutrient Interactions

A diverse array of adverse health effects can occur as a result of the interaction of nutrients. The potential risks of adverse nutrient-nutrient interactions increase when there is an imbalance in the intake of two or more nutrients. Excessive intake of one nutrient may interfere with absorption, excretion, transport, storage, function, or metabolism of a second nutrient. Possible adverse nutrient-nutrient interactions are considered as a part of setting a UL. Nutrient-nutrient interactions may be considered either as a critical endpoint on which to base a UL or as supportive evidence for a UL based on another endpoint.

Other Relevant Factors Affecting the Bioavailability of Nutrients

In addition to nutrient interactions, other considerations have the potential to influence nutrient bioavailability, such as the nutritional status of an individual and the form of intake. These issues are considered in the risk assessment. With regard to the form of intake, fat soluble vitamins, such as vitamin A, are more readily absorbed when they are part of a meal that is high in fat. ULs must therefore be based on nutrients as part of the total diet, including the contribution from water. Nutrient supplements that are taken separately from food require special consideration, because they are likely to have different bioavailabilities and therefore may represent a greater risk of producing adverse effects in some cases.

STEPS IN THE DEVELOPMENT OF THE TOLERABLE UPPER INTAKE LEVEL

Hazard Identification

Based on a thorough review of the scientific literature, the hazard identification step outlines the adverse health effects that have been demonstrated to be caused by the nutrient. The primary types of data used as background for identifying nutrient hazards in humans are as follows:

- *Human studies.* Human data provide the most relevant kind of information for hazard identification and, when they are of sufficient quality and extent, are given greatest weight. However, the number of controlled human toxicity studies conducted in a clinical setting is very limited because of ethical reasons. Such studies are generally most useful for identifying very mild (and ordinarily reversible) adverse effects. Observational studies that focus on well-defined populations with clear exposures to a range of nutrient intake levels are useful for establishing a relationship between exposure and effect. Observational data in the form of case reports or anecdotal evidence are used for developing hypotheses that can lead to knowledge of causal associations. Sometimes a series of case reports, if it shows a clear and distinct pattern of effects, may be reasonably convincing on the question of causality.

- *Animal data.* Most of the available data used in regulatory risk assessments come from controlled laboratory experiments in animals, usually mammalian species other than humans (e.g., rodents). Such data are used in part because human data on nonessential chemicals are generally very limited. Moreover, there is a long-standing history of the use of animal studies to identify the toxic properties of chemical substances, and there is no inherent reason why animal data should not be relevant to the evaluation of nutrient toxicity. Animal studies offer several advantages over human studies. They can, for example, be readily controlled so that causal relationships can be recognized. It is possible to identify the full range of toxic effects produced by a chemical, over a wide range of exposures, and to establish dose-response relationships. The effects of chronic exposures can be identified in far less time than they can with the use of epidemiological methods. All these advantages of animal data, however, may not always overcome the fact that species differences in response to chemical substances can sometimes be profound, and any extrapolation of animal data to predict human response needs to take into account this possibility.

BOX 3-1 Development of Tolerable Upper Intake Levels (ULs)

COMPONENTS OF HAZARD IDENTIFICATION
- Evidence of adverse effects in humans
- Causality
- Relevance of experimental data
- Pharmacokinetic and metabolic data
- Mechanisms of toxic action
- Quality and completeness of the database
- Identification of distinct and highly sensitive subpopulations

COMPONENTS OF DOSE-RESPONSE ASSESSMENT
- Data selection and identification of critical endpoints
- Identification of no-observed-adverse-effect level (NOAEL) (or lowest-observed-adverse-effect level [LOAEL]) and critical endpoint
- Assessment of uncertainty and data on variability in response
- Derivation of a UL
- Characterization of the estimate and special considerations

Key issues that are addressed in the data evaluation of human and animal studies are described below (see Box 3-1).

Evidence of Adverse Effects in Humans

The hazard identification step involves the examination of human, animal, and in vitro published evidence addressing the likelihood of a nutrient's eliciting an adverse effect in humans. Decisions about which observed effects are adverse are based on scientific judgments. Although toxicologists generally regard any demonstrable structural or functional alteration as representing an adverse effect, some alterations may be considered to be of little or self-limiting biological importance. As noted earlier, adverse nutrient-nutrient interactions are considered in the definition of an adverse effect.

Causality

The identification of a hazard is strengthened by evidence of causality. As explained in Chapter 2, the criteria of Hill (1971) are considered in judging the causal significance of an exposure-effect association indicated by epidemiological studies.

Relevance of Experimental Data

Consideration of the following issues can be useful in assessing the relevance of experimental data.

Animal Data. Some animal data may be of limited utility in judging the toxicity of nutrients because of highly variable interspecies differences in nutrient requirements. Nevertheless, relevant animal data are considered in the hazard identification and dose-response assessment steps where applicable, and, in general, they are used for hazard identification unless there are data demonstrating they are not relevant to human beings, or it is clear that the available human data are sufficient.

Route of Exposure.[2] Data derived from studies involving oral exposure (rather than parenteral, inhalation, or dermal exposure) are most useful for the evaluation of nutrients. Data derived from studies involving parenteral, inhalation, or dermal routes of exposure may be considered relevant if the adverse effects are systemic and data are available to permit interroute extrapolation.

Duration of Exposure. Because the magnitude, duration, and frequency of exposure can vary considerably in different situations, consideration needs to be given to the relevance of the exposure scenario (e.g., chronic daily dietary exposure versus short-term bolus doses) to dietary intakes by human populations.

Pharmacokinetic and Metabolic Data

When available, data regarding the rates of nutrient absorption, distribution, metabolism, and excretion may be important in derivation of Tolerable Upper Intake Levels (ULs). Such data may provide significant information regarding the interspecies differences and similarities in nutrient behavior, and so may assist in identifying relevant animal data. They may also assist in identifying life stage differences in response to nutrient toxicity.

In some cases, there may be limited or even no significant data relating to nutrient toxicity. It is conceivable that in such cases,

---

[2]The terms *route of exposure* and *route of intake* refer to how a substance enters the body (e.g., by ingestion, injection, or dermal absorption). These terms should not be confused with *form of intake*, which refers to the medium or vehicle used (e.g., supplements, food, or drinking water).

pharmacokinetic and metabolic data may provide valuable insights into the magnitude of the UL. Thus, if there are significant pharmacokinetic and metabolic data over the range of intakes that meet nutrient requirements, and if it is shown that this pattern of pharmacokinetic and metabolic data does not change in the range of intakes greater than those required for nutrition, it may be possible to infer the absence of toxic risk in this range. In contrast, an alteration of pharmacokinetics or metabolism may suggest the potential for adverse effects. There has been no case encountered thus far in which sufficient pharmacokinetic and metabolic data are available for establishing ULs in this fashion, but it is possible such situations may arise in the future.

Mechanisms of Toxic Action

Knowledge of molecular and cellular events underlying the production of toxicity can assist in dealing with the problems of extrapolation between species and from high to low doses. It may also aid in understanding whether the mechanisms associated with toxicity are those associated with deficiency. In most cases, however, because knowledge of the biochemical sequence of events resulting from toxicity and deficiency is still incomplete, it is not yet possible to state with certainty whether these sequences share a common pathway.

Quality and Completeness of the Database

The scientific quality and quantity of the database are evaluated. Human or animal data are reviewed for suggestions that the substances have the potential to produce additional adverse health effects. If suggestions are found, additional studies may be recommended.

Identification of Distinct and Highly Sensitive Subpopulations

The ULs are based on protecting the most sensitive members of the general population from adverse effects of high nutrient intake. Some highly sensitive subpopulations have responses (in terms of incidence, severity, or both) to the agent of interest that are clearly distinct from the responses expected for the healthy population. The risk assessment process recognizes that there may be individuals within any life stage group who are more biologically sensitive than others, and thus their extreme sensitivities do not fall within the range of sensitivities expected for the general population. The UL for the general population may not be protective for these subgroups. As indicated earlier, the extent to which a distinct subpopulation will be included in the derivation of a UL for the general population is an area of judgment to be addressed on a case-by-case basis.

Dose-Response Assessment

The process for deriving the UL is described in this section and outlined in Box 3-1. It includes selection of the critical data set, identification of a critical endpoint with its no-observed-adverse-affect level (NOAEL) or lowest-observed-adverse-effect level (LOAEL), and assessment of uncertainty.

Data Selection and Identification of Critical Endpoints

The data evaluation process results in the selection of the most appropriate or critical data sets for deriving the UL. Selecting the critical data set includes the following considerations:

• Human data, when adequate to evaluate adverse effects, are preferable to animal data, although the latter may provide useful supportive information.
• In the absence of appropriate human data, information from an animal species with biological responses most like those of humans is most valuable. Pharmacokinetic, metabolic, and mechanistic data may be available to assist in the identification of relevant animal species.
• If it is not possible to identify such a species or to select such data, data from the most sensitive animal species, strain, and gender combination are given the greatest emphasis.
• The route of exposure that most resembles the route of expected human intake is preferable. This consideration includes the digestive state (e.g., fed or fasted) of the subjects or experimental animals. When this is not possible, the differences in route of exposure are noted as a source of uncertainty.
• The critical data set defines a dose-response relationship between intake and the extent of the toxic response known to be most relevant to humans. Data on bioavailability are considered and adjustments in expressions of dose-response are made to determine whether any apparent differences in response can be explained.
• The critical data set documents the route of exposure and the

magnitude and duration of the intake. Furthermore, the critical data set documents the NOAEL (or LOAEL).

Identification of a NOAEL (or LOAEL)

A nutrient can produce more than one toxic effect (or endpoint), even within the same species or in studies using the same or different exposure durations. The NOAELs and LOAELs for these effects will ordinarily differ. The critical endpoint used to establish a UL is the adverse biological effect exhibiting the lowest NOAEL (e.g., the most sensitive indicator of a nutrient's toxicity). Because the selection of uncertainty factors (UFs) depends in part upon the seriousness of the adverse effect, it is possible that lower ULs may result from the use of the most *serious* (rather than most *sensitive*) endpoint. Thus, it is often necessary to evaluate several endpoints independently to determine which leads to the lowest UL.

For some nutrients, such as vitamin K, arsenic, chromium, and silicon, there may be inadequate data on which to develop a UL. The lack of reports of adverse effects following excess intake of a nutrient does not mean that adverse effects do not occur. As the intake of any nutrient increases, a point (see Figure 3-2) is reached at which intake begins to pose a risk. Above this point, increased

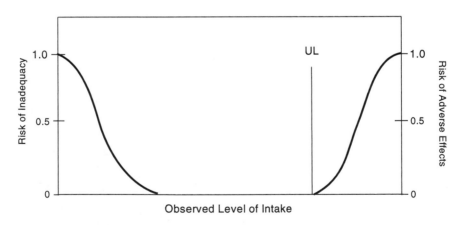

FIGURE 3-2 Theoretical description of health effects of a nutrient as a function of level of intake. The Tolerable Upper Intake Level (UL) is the highest level of daily nutrient intake that is likely to pose no risk of adverse health effects for almost all individuals in the general population. At intakes above the UL, the risk of adverse effects potentially increase.

intake increases the risk of adverse effects. For some nutrients and for various reasons, there are inadequate data to identify this point, or even to estimate its location.

Because adverse effects are almost certain to occur for any nutrient at some level of intake, it should be assumed that such effects may occur for nutrients for which a scientifically documentable UL cannot now be derived. Until a UL is set or an alternative approach to identifying protective limits is developed, intakes greater than the Recommended Dietary Allowance or Adequate Intake should be viewed with caution.

The absence of sufficient data to establish a UL points to the need for studies suitable for developing ULs.

Uncertainty Assessment

Several judgments must be made regarding the uncertainties and thus the UF associated with extrapolating from the observed data to the general population (see Appendix L). Applying a UF to a NOAEL (or LOAEL) results in a value for the derived UL that is less than the experimentally derived NOAEL, unless the UF is 1.0. The greater the uncertainty, the larger the UF and the smaller the resulting UL. This is consistent with the ultimate goal of the risk assessment: to provide an estimate of a level of intake that will protect the health of virtually all members of the healthy population (Mertz et al., 1994).

Although several reports describe the underlying basis for UFs (Dourson and Stara, 1983; Zielhuis and van der Kreek, 1979), the strength of the evidence supporting the use of a specific UF will vary. The imprecision of the UFs is a major limitation of risk assessment approaches and considerable leeway must be allowed for the application of scientific judgment in making the final determination. Because data are generally available regarding intakes of nutrients in human populations, the data on nutrient toxicity may not be subject to the same uncertainties as are data on nonessential chemical agents. The resulting UFs for nutrients and food components are typically less than the factors of 10 often applied to nonessential toxic substances. The UFs are lower with higher quality data and when the adverse effects are extremely mild and reversible.

In general, when determining a UF, the following potential sources of uncertainty are considered and combined in the final UF:

• *Interindividual variation in sensitivity.* Small UFs (close to 1) are used to represent this source of uncertainty if it is judged that little population variability is expected for the adverse effect, and larger factors (close to 10) are used if variability is expected to be great (NRC, 1994).

• *Extrapolation from experimental animals to humans.* A UF to account for the uncertainty in extrapolating animal data to humans is generally applied to the NOAEL when animal data are the primary data set available. While a default UF of 10 is often used to extrapolate animal data to humans for nonessential chemicals, a lower UF may be used because of data showing some similarities between the animal and human responses (NRC, 1994).

• *LOAEL instead of NOAEL.* If a NOAEL is not available, a UF may be applied to account for the uncertainty in deriving a UL from the LOAEL. The size of the UF involves scientific judgment based on the severity and incidence of the observed effect at the LOAEL and the steepness (slope) of the dose response.

• *Subchronic NOAEL to predict chronic NOAEL.* When data are lacking on chronic exposures, scientific judgment is necessary to determine whether chronic exposure is likely to lead to adverse effects at lower intakes than those producing effects after subchronic exposures (exposures of shorter duration).

Derivation of a UL

The UL is derived by dividing the NOAEL (or LOAEL) by a single UF that incorporates all relevant uncertainties. ULs, expressed as amount per day, are derived for various life stage groups using relevant databases, NOAELs, LOAELs, and UFs. In cases where no data exist with regard to NOAELs or LOAELs for the group under consideration, extrapolations from data in other age groups or animal data are made on the basis of known differences in body size, physiology, metabolism, absorption, and excretion of the nutrient. Generally, any age group adjustments are based solely on differences in body weight, unless there are data demonstrating age-related differences in nutrient pharmacokinetics, metabolism, or mechanism of action.

The derivation of the UL involves the use of scientific judgment to select the appropriate NOAEL (or LOAEL) and UF. The risk assessment requires explicit consideration and discussion of all choices made, regarding both the data used and the uncertainties accounted for. These considerations are discussed in the chapters on nutrients and food components. In this report, because of the lack of data to set a threshold, ULs could not be set for vitamin K, arsenic, chromium, and silicon.

Characterization of the Estimate and Special Considerations

If the data review reveals the existence of subpopulations having distinct and exceptional sensitivities to a nutrient's toxicity, these subpopulations are explicitly discussed and concerns related to adverse effects are noted; however, the use of the data is not included in the identification of the NOAEL or LOAEL, upon which the UL for the general population is based.

INTAKE ASSESSMENT

In order to assess the risk of adverse effects, information on the range of nutrient intakes in the general population is required. As noted earlier, in cases where the Tolerable Upper Intake Level pertains only to supplement use and does not pertain to usual food intakes of the nutrient, the assessment is directed at supplement intakes only.

RISK CHARACTERIZATION

As described earlier, the question of whether nutrient intakes create a risk of adverse effects requires a comparison of the range of nutrient intakes (food, supplements, and other sources or supplements alone, depending upon the basis for the Tolerable Upper Intake Level [UL]) with the UL.

Figure 3-3 illustrates a distribution of chronic nutrient intakes in a population; the fraction of the population experiencing chronic intakes above the UL represents the potential at-risk group. A policy decision is needed to determine whether efforts should be made to reduce risk. No precedents are available for such policy choices, although in the area of food additive or pesticide regulation, federal regulatory agencies have generally sought to ensure that the ninetieth or ninety-fifth percentile intakes fall below the UL (or its approximate equivalent measure of risk). If this goal is achieved, the fraction of the population remaining above the UL is likely to experience intakes only slightly greater than the UL and is likely to be at little or no risk.

For risk management decisions, it is useful to evaluate the public health significance of the risk, and information contained in the risk characterization is critical for that purpose.

Thus, the significance of the risk to a population consuming a nutrient in excess of the UL is determined by the following:

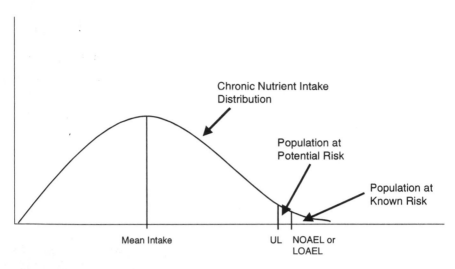

Chronic Nutrient Intake
Distribution

Population at
Potential Risk

Population at
Known Risk

Mean Intake   UL   NOAEL or
                                                LOAEL

FIGURE 3-3 Illustration of the population at risk from excessive nutrient intakes. The fraction of the population consistently consuming a nutrient at intake levels in excess of the Tolerable Upper Intake Level (UL) is potentially at risk of adverse health effects. See text for a discussion of additional factors necessary to judge the significance of the risk. LOAEL = lowest-observed-adverse-effect level, NOAEL = no-observed-adverse-effect level.

1. the fraction of the population consistently consuming the nutrient at intake levels in excess of the UL;

2. the seriousness of the adverse effects associated with the nutrient;

3. the extent to which the effect is reversible when intakes are reduced to levels less than the UL; and

4. the fraction of the population with consistent intakes above the NOAEL or even the LOAEL.

The significance of the risk of excessive nutrient intake cannot, therefore, be judged only by reference to Figure 3-3, but requires careful consideration of all of the above factors. Information on these factors is contained in this report's sections describing the bases for each of the ULs.

REFERENCES

Dourson ML, Stara JF. 1983. Regulatory history and experimental support of uncertainty (safety) factors. *Regul Toxicol Pharmacol* 3:224–238.

FAO/WHO (Food and Agriculture Organization of the United Nations/World Health Organization). 1982. *Evaluation of Certain Food Additives and Contaminants.* Twenty-sixth report of the Joint FAO/WHO Expert Committee on Food Additives. WHO Technical Report Series, No. 683. Geneva: WHO.

FAO/WHO. 1995. *The Application of Risk Analysis to Food Standard Issues.* Recommendations to the Codex Alimentarius Commission (ALINORM 95/9, Appendix 5). Geneva: WHO.

Health Canada. 1993. *Health Risk Determination—The Challenge of Health Protection.* Ottawa: Health Canada, Health Protection Branch.

Hill AB. 1971. *Principles of Medical Statistics,* 9th ed. New York: Oxford University Press.

Klaassen CD, Amdur MO, Doull J. 1986. *Casarett and Doull's Toxicology: The Basic Science of Poisons,* 3rd ed. New York: Macmillan.

Mertz W, Abernathy CO, Olin SS. 1994. *Risk Assessment of Essential Elements.* Washington, DC: ILSI Press.

NRC (National Research Council). 1983. *Risk Assessment in the Federal Government: Managing the Process.* Washington, DC: National Academy Press.

NRC. 1994. *Science and Judgment in Risk Assessment.* Washington, DC: National Academy Press.

OTA (Office of Technology Assessment). 1993. *Researching Health Risks.* Washington, DC: OTA.

WHO (World Health Organization). 1987. *Principles for the Safety Assessment of Food Additives and Contaminants in Food.* Environmental Health Criteria 70. Geneva: WHO.

WHO. 1996. *Trace Elements in Human Nutrition and Health.* Geneva: WHO.

Zielhuis RL, van der Kreek FW. 1979. The use of a safety factor in setting health-based permissible levels for occupational exposure. *Int Arch Occup Environ Health* 42:191–201.

4

Vitamin A

SUMMARY

Vitamin A is important for normal vision, gene expression, reproduction, embryonic development, growth, and immune function. There are a variety of foods rich in vitamin A and provitamin A carotenoids that are available to North Americans. Thus, current dietary patterns appear to provide sufficient vitamin A to prevent deficiency symptoms such as night blindness. The Estimated Average Requirement (EAR) is based on the assurance of adequate stores of vitamin A. The Recommended Dietary Allowance (RDA) for men and women is 900 and 700 µg retinol activity equivalents (RAE)/day, respectively. The Tolerable Upper Intake Level (UL) for adults is set at 3,000 µg/day of preformed vitamin A.

There are a number of sources of dietary vitamin A. Preformed vitamin A is abundant in some animal-derived foods, whereas provitamin A carotenoids are abundant in darkly colored fruits and vegetables, as well as oily fruits and red palm oil.

For dietary provitamin A carotenoids—β-carotene, α-carotene, and β-cryptoxanthin—RAEs have been set at 12, 24, and 24 µg, respectively. Using µg RAE, the vitamin A activity of provitamin A carotenoids is half the vitamin A activity assumed when using µg retinol equivalents (µg RE) (NRC, 1980, 1989). This change in equivalency values is based on data demonstrating that the vitamin A activity of purified β-carotene in oil is half the activity of vitamin A, and based on recent data demonstrating that the vitamin A activity of dietary β-carotene is one-sixth, rather than one-third, the vitamin activity of purified β-carotene in oil. This change in bioconversion means that a larger amount of provitamin A carotenoids, and therefore darkly colored, carotene-rich fruits and vegetables, is needed to meet the vitamin A requirement. It also means that in the past, vitamin A intake has been overestimated,

The median intake of vitamin A ranges from 744 to 811 µg RAE/day for men and 530 to 716 µg RAE/day for women. Using µg RAE, approximately 26 and 34 percent of vitamin A activity consumed by men and women, respectively, is provided from provitamin A carotenoids. Ripe, colored fruits and cooked, yellow tubers are more efficiently converted to vitamin A than equal amounts of dark green, leafy vegetables.

Although a large body of observational epidemiological evidence suggests that higher blood concentrations of β-carotenes and other carotenoids obtained from foods are associated with a lower risk of several chronic diseases, there is currently not sufficient evidence to support a recommendation that requires a certain percentage of dietary vitamin A to come from provitamin A carotenoids in meeting the vitamin A requirement. However, the existing recommendations for increased consumption of carotenoid-rich fruits and vegetables for their health-promoting benefits are strongly supported (see *Dietary Reference Intakes for Vitamin C, Vitamin E, Selenium, and Carotenoids* [IOM, 2000]).

BACKGROUND INFORMATION

Vitamin A is a fat-soluble vitamin that is essential for humans and other vertebrates. Vitamin A comprises a family of molecules containing a 20 carbon structure with a methyl substituted cyclohexenyl ring (beta-ionone ring) (Figure 4-1) and a tetraene side chain with a hydroxyl group (retinol), aldehyde group (retinal), carboxylic acid group (retinoic acid), or ester group (retinyl ester) at carbon-15. The term vitamin A includes provitamin A carotenoids that are dietary precursors of retinol. The term retinoids refers to retinol, its metabolites, and synthetic analogues that have a similar structure. Carotenoids are polyisoprenoids, of which more than 600 forms exist. Of the many carotenoids in nature, several have provitamin A nutritional activity, but food composition data are available for only three (α-carotene, β-carotene, and β-cryptoxanthin) (Figure 4-1). The all-*trans* isomer is the most common and stable form of each carotenoid; however, many *cis* isomers also exist. Carotenoids usually contain 40 carbon atoms, have an extensive system of conjugated double bonds, and contain one or two cyclic structures at the end

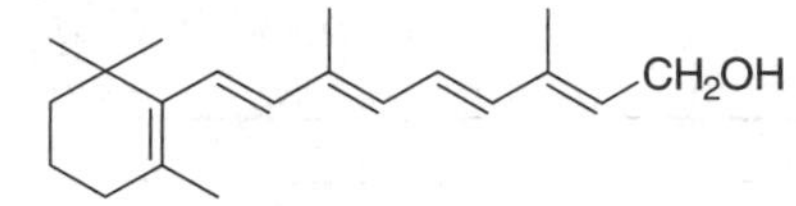

all trans-Retinol

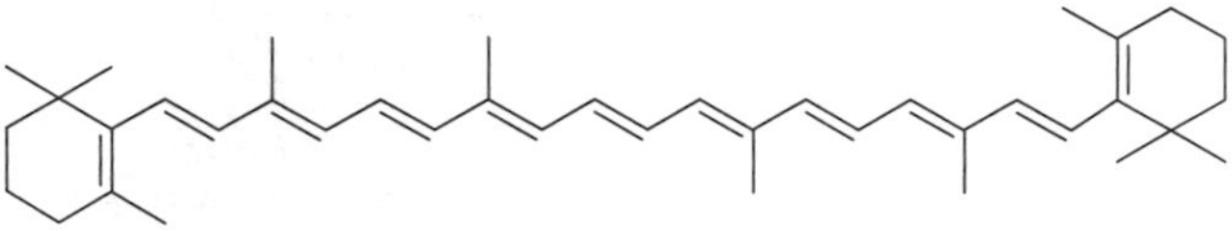

all trans-β-Carotene

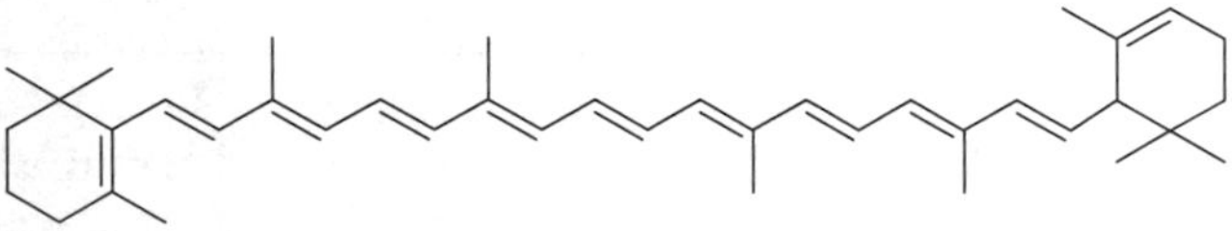

all trans-α-Carotene

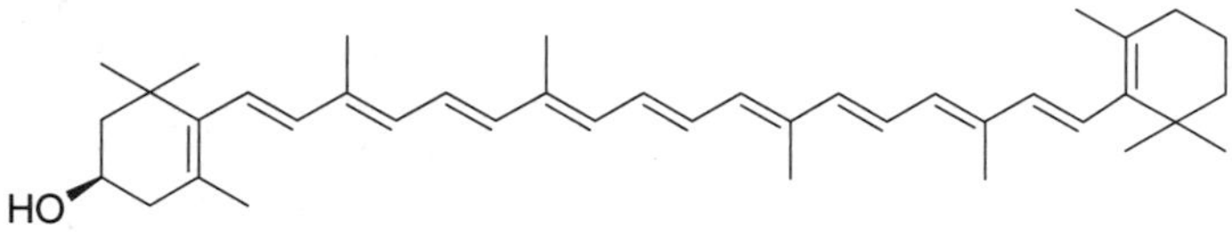

all trans-β-Cryptoxanthin

FIGURE 4-1 Structure of retinol and provitamin A carotenoids.

of their conjugated chain. An exception is lycopene, which has no ring structure and does not have vitamin A activity. Preformed vitamin A is found only in animal-derived food products, whereas dietary carotenoids are present primarily in oils, fruits, and vegetables.

Function

The 11-*cis*-retinaldehyde (retinal) form of vitamin A is required by the eye for the transduction of light into neural signals necessary for vision (Saari, 1994). The retinoic acid form is required to maintain normal differentiation of the cornea and conjunctival membranes, thus preventing xerophthalmia (Sommer and West, 1996), as well as for the photoreceptor rod and cone cells of the retina. Rods contain the visual pigment rhodopsin (opsin protein bound to 11-*cis*-retinal). The absorption of light catalyzes the photoisomerization of rhodopsin's 11-*cis*-retinal to all-*trans*-retinal in thousands of rods, which triggers the signaling to neuronal cells associated with the brain's visual cortex. After photoisomerization, all-*trans*-retinal is released, and for vision to continue, 11-*cis*-retinal must be regenerated. Regeneration of 11-*cis*-retinal requires the reduction of all-*trans* retinal to retinol, transport of retinol from the photoreceptor cells (rods) to the retinal pigment epithelium, and esterification of all-*trans*-retinol, thereby providing a local storage pool of retinyl esters. When needed, retinyl esters are hydrolyzed and isomerized to form 11-*cis*-retinol, which is oxidized to 11-*cis*-retinal and transported back to the photoreceptor cells for recombination with opsin to begin another photo cycle.

Vitamin A is required for the integrity of epithelial cells throughout the body (Gudas et al., 1994). Retinoic acid, through the activation of retinoic acid (RAR) and retinoid X (RXR) receptors in the nucleus, regulates the expression of various genes that encode for structural proteins (e.g., skin keratins), enzymes (e.g., alcohol dehydrogenase), extracellular matrix proteins (e.g., laminin), and retinol binding proteins and receptors.

Retinoic acid plays an important role in embryonic development. Retinoic acid, as well as RAR, RXR, cellular retinol-binding protein (CRBP), and cellular retinoic acid-binding proteins (CRABP-I and CRABP-II), is present in temporally specific patterns in the embryonic regions known to be involved in the development of structures posterior to the hindbrain (e.g., the vertebrae and spinal cord) (Morriss-Kay and Sokolova, 1996). Retinoic acid is also involved in the development of the limbs, heart, eyes, and ears (Dickman and Smith, 1996; Hofmann and Eichele, 1994; McCaffery and Drager, 1995).

Retinoids are necessary for the maintenance of immune function, which depends on cell differentiation and proliferation in response to immune stimuli. Retinoic acid is important in maintaining an adequate level of circulating natural killer cells that have antiviral and anti-tumor activity (Zhao and Ross, 1995). Retinoic acid has been shown to increase phagocytic activity in murine macrophages (Katz et al., 1987) and to increase the production of interleukin 1 and other cytokines, which serve as important mediators of inflammation and stimulators of T and B lymphocyte production (Trechsel et al., 1985). Furthermore, the growth, differentiation, and activation of B lymphocytes requires retinol (Blomhoff et al., 1992).

Proposed functions of provitamin A carotenoids are described in *Dietary Reference Intakes for Vitamin C, Vitamin E, Selenium, and Carotenoids* (IOM, 2000).

Physiology of Absorption, Metabolism, and Excretion

Absorption and Bioconversion

Absorption of Vitamin A. Intestinal absorption of preformed vitamin A occurs following the processing of retinyl esters in the lumen of the small intestine. Within the water-miscible micelles formed from bile salts, solubilized retinyl esters as well as triglycerides are hydrolyzed to retinol and products of lipolysis by various hydrolases (Harrison, 1993). A small percentage of dietary retinoids is converted to retinoic acid in the intestinal cell. In addition, the intestine actively synthesizes retinoyl β-glucuronide that is hydrolyzed to retinoic acid by β-glucuronidases (Barua and Olson, 1989). The efficiency of absorption of preformed vitamin A is generally high, in the range of 70 to 90 percent (Sivakumar and Reddy, 1972). A specific retinol transport protein within the brush border of the enterocyte facilitates retinol uptake by the mucosal cells (Dew and Ong, 1994). At physiological concentrations, retinol absorption is carrier mediated and saturable, whereas at high pharmacological doses, the absorption of retinol is nonsaturable (Hollander and Muralidhara, 1977). As the amount of ingested preformed vitamin A increases, its absorbability remains high (Olson, 1972). Vitamin A absorption and intestinal retinol esterification are not markedly different in the elderly compared to young adults, although hepatic uptake of newly absorbed vitamin A in the form of retinyl ester is slower in the elderly (Borel et al., 1998).

Absorption and Bioconversion of Provitamin A Carotenoids. Carotenoids are also solubilized into micelles in the intestinal lumen from which they are absorbed into duodenal mucosal cells by a passive diffusion mechanism. Percent absorption of a single dose of 45 μg to 39 mg β-carotene, measured by means of isotopic methods, has been reported to range from 9 to 22 percent (Blomstrand and Werner, 1967; Goodman et al., 1966; Novotny et al., 1995). However, the absorption efficiency decreases as the amount of dietary carotenoids increases (Brubacher and Weiser, 1985; Tang et al., 2000). The relative carotene concentration in micelles can vary in response to the physical state of the carotenoid (e.g., whether it is dissolved in oil or associated with plant matrix materials). A number of factors affect the bioavailability and bioconversion of carotenoids (Castenmiller and West, 1998). Carotene bioavailability can differ with different processing methods of the same foods and among different foods containing similar levels of carotenoids (Boileau et al., 1999; Hume and Krebs, 1949; Rock et al., 1998; Torronen et al., 1996; Van den Berg and van Vliet, 1998) (also see *Dietary Reference Intakes for Vitamin C, Vitamin E, Selenium, and Carotenoids* [IOM, 2000]).

Absorbed β-carotene is principally converted to vitamin A by the enzyme β-carotene-15, 15′-dioxygenase within intestinal absorptive cells. The central cleavage of β-carotene by this enzyme will, in theory, result in two molecules of retinal. β-Carotene can also be cleaved eccentrically to yield β-apocarotenals that can be further degraded to retinal or retinoic acid (Krinsky et al., 1993). The predominant form of vitamin A in human lymph, whether originating from ingested vitamin A or provitamin A carotenoids, is retinyl ester (retinol esterified with long-chain fatty acids, typically palmitate and stearate) (Blomstrand and Werner, 1967; Goodman et al., 1966). Along with exogenous lipids, the newly synthesized retinyl esters and nonhydrolyzed carotenoids are transported from the intestine to the liver in chylomicrons and chylomicron remnants. Derived from dietary retinoids, retinoic acid is absorbed via the portal system bound to albumin (Blaner and Olson, 1994; Olson, 1991).

Vitamin A Activity of Provitamin A Carotenoids: Rationale for Developing Retinol Activity Equivalents. The carotene:retinol equivalency ratio (μg:μg) of a low dose (less than 2 mg) of purified β-carotene in oil is approximately 2:1 (i.e., 2 μg of β-carotene in oil yields 1 μg of retinol) (Table 4-1). This ratio was derived from the relative amount of β-carotene required to *correct* abnormal dark adaptation in vitamin A-deficient individuals (Hume and Krebs, 1949; Sauberlich et al., 1974). The data by Sauberlich et al. (1974) were given greater consideration because (1) the actual amount (μg) of vitamin A and β-carotene consumed was cited, (2) varied amounts of vitamin A or β-carotene were consumed by each individual, and (3) a greater sample size was employed (six versus two subjects). In addition to these studies, an earlier study by Wagner (1940) estimated a carotene:retinol equivalency ratio of 4:1; however, the method employed for measuring dark adaptation was not standardized and used an imprecise outcome measure.

Studies have been performed to compare the efficiency of absorption of β-carotene after feeding physiological amounts of β-carotene

TABLE 4-1 Relative Absorption of Vitamin A and Supplemental β-Carotene

Reference	Study Group[a]	Study Design
Hume and Krebs, 1949	1 adult per treatment group, England	Depletion/repletion study; depletion phase ranged from 18 to 22 mo and the repletion phase ranged from 3 wk to 6 mo
Sauberlich et al., 1974	2 or 4 men per treatment group, United States	Depletion/repletion study; depletion phase ranged from 361 to 771 d and the repletion phase ranged from 2 to 455 d

[a] Treatment group received supplemental vitamin A or β-carotene.
[b] Based on the assumption that 1 IU is equivalent to 0.3 µg of vitamin A (WHO, 1950).
[c] One IU is equivalent to 0.6 µg of β-carotene (Hume and Krebs, 1949).

in oil, in individual foods, and as part of a mixed vegetable and fruit diet. Many of the earlier studies analyzed the fecal content of β-carotene after the consumption of a supplement, fruit, or vegetable. Data from these studies were not considered because the portion of unabsorbed β-carotene that is degraded by the intestinal microflora is not known. The efficiency of absorption of β-carotene in food is lower than the absorption of β-carotene in oil by a representative factor of a. Assuming that after absorption of β-carotene, whether from oil or food, the metabolism of the molecule is similar and that the retinol equivalency ratio of β-carotene in oil is 2:1, the vitamin A activity of β-carotene from food can be derived by multiplying a by 2:1.

Until recently it was thought that 3 µg of dietary β-carotene was equivalent to 1 µg of purified β-carotene in oil (NRC, 1989) due to a relative absorption efficiency of about 33 percent of β-carotene from food sources. Only one study has compared the relative absorption of β-carotene in oil versus its absorption in a principally mixed vegetable diet in healthy and nutritionally adequate individuals (Van het Hof et al., 1999). This study concluded that the relative absorption of β-carotene from the mixed vegetable diet compared to β-carotene in oil is only 14 percent, as assessed by the increase in plasma β-carotene concentration after dietary interven-

Diet/Dose	Results
Low (< 21 µg/d) vitamin A diet plus a single dose of supplemental vitamin A or β-carotene were provided to subjects after depletion period	Abnormal dark adaptation was reversed with 1,300 IU (390 µg)[b] of vitamin A and 2,500 IU (1,500 µg)[c] of β-carotene; thus the retinol equivalency ratio is assumed to be 3.8:1
Low vitamin A diet (< 23 µg) plus varying doses of supplemental vitamin A (37.5–25,000 µg/d) or β-carotene (150–2,400 µg/d) were provided after the depletion period	600 µg/d retinol corrected dark adaptation; 1,200 µg/d β-carotene corrected dark adaptation; therefore the retinol equivalency ratio was concluded to be 2:1

tion. Based on this finding, approximately 7 µg of dietary β-carotene is equivalent to 1 µg of β-carotene in oil. This absorption efficiency value of 14 percent is supported by the relative ranges in β-carotene absorption reported by others using similar methods for mixed green leafy vegetables (4 percent) (de Pee et al., 1995), carrots (18 to 26 percent) (Micozzi et al., 1992; Torronen et al., 1996), broccoli (11 to 12 percent) (Micozzi et al., 1992), and spinach (5 percent) (Castenmiller et al., 1999) (Table 4-2).

Only one study has been published to assess the relative bio-conversion of β-carotene from fruits versus vegetables by measuring the rise in serum retinol concentration after the provision of a diet high in vegetables, fruits, or retinol (de Pee et al., 1998). This study used methods similar to those employed by other researchers (Castenmiller et al. [1999], de Pee et al. [1995], Micozzi et al. [1992], Torronen et al. [1996], and Van het Hof et al. [1999]), and indicated that the vitamin A activity was approximately half the activity for dark, green leafy vegetables compared to equal amounts of β-carotene from orange fruits and some yellow tubers, such as pumpkin squash (de Pee et al., 1998) (Table 4-2). Because of the low content of fruits contained in the principally mixed vegetable diet of Van het Hof et al. (1999) and the low proportion of dietary β-carotene that is consumed from fruits compared to vegetables in

TABLE 4-2 Relative Absorption of Supplemental and Dietary β-Carotene

Reference	Subjects	Study Design
Micozzi et al., 1992	30 men, 20–45 y, United States	Diet/supplementation intervention, 6 wk
de Pee et al., 1995	173 children, 7–11 y, Indonesia	Diet intervention, 9 wk
Torronen et al., 1996	42 women, 20–53 y, Finland	Diet/supplementation intervention, 6 wk
de Pee et al., 1998	188 anemic school children, 7–11 y, Indonesia	Diet intervention, 9 wk
Castenmiller et al., 1999	72 men and women, 18–58 y, Netherlands	Diet/supplementation intervention, 3 wk
Van het Hof et al., 1999	55 men and women, 18–45 y, Netherlands	Diet/supplementation intervention, 1 mo

the United States (16 percent from the 14 major dietary contributors of β-carotene which provide a total of 70 percent of dietary β-carotene) (Chug-Ahuja et al., 1993), it is estimated that 6 μg, rather than 7 μg, of β-carotene from a mixed diet is nutritionally equivalent to 1 μg of β-carotene in oil. Therefore, the retinol activity equivalency (μg RAE) ratio for β-carotene from food is estimated to be 12:1 (6 × 2:1) (Figure 4-2). Unfortunately, studies using a positive control group (preformed vitamin A) at a level equivalent to β-carotene from a mixed vegetable and fruit diet using levels similar to the RAE have not been conducted in healthy and nutritionally adequate individuals. An RAE of 12 μg for dietary β-carotene is supported by Parker et al. (1999) who reported that 8 percent of ingested β-carotene from carrots was absorbed and converted to retinyl esters

Diet/Dose of β-Carotene	Results
Supplement, 30 mg/d Carrots, 30 mg/d Broccoli, 6 mg/d	Increase of plasma β-carotene from carrots compared to supplemental β-carotene in gelatin beadlets was 18% Increase of plasma β-carotene from broccoli compared to supplemental β-carotene in gelatin beadlets was 12%
Vegetable diet, 3.5 mg/d Fruit diet, 2.3 mg/d	Increase of serum β-carotene from fruit diet was 5–6 times higher than from vegetable diet
Low carotenoid diet + Raw carrots, 12 mg/d + Supplement, 12 mg/d	Increase of serum β-carotene from raw carrots was 26% compared to that from supplemental β-carotene in a gelatin beadlet
Fruit/squash diet, 509 µg/d Dark green leafy vegetables + carrots, 684 µg/d Low vitamin A/ß-carotene diet, 44 µg/d	Increase of serum β-carotene from fruit/squash diet was 3.5-fold greater than that for the dark green leafy vegetables + carrots diet
Control diet, 0.5 mg/d Supplement diet, 9.8 mg/d Spinach diet, 10.4 mg/d	Increase of serum β-carotene from spinach was 5% compared to that from supplemental β-carotene in oil
Supplement, 7.2 mg/day High vegetable diet, 5.1 mg/d	Increase of plasma β-carotene from high vegetable diet compared to supplemental β-carotene in oil was 14%

contained in chylomicrons, resulting in a carotene:retinol equivalency ratio of 13:1.

One RAE for dietary provitamin A carotenoids other than β-carotene is set at 24 µg on the basis of the observation that the vitamin A activity of β-cryptoxanthin and α-carotene is approximately half of that for β-carotene (Bauernfeind, 1972; Deuel et al., 1949). Therefore, the amount of vitamin A activity of provitamin A carotenoids in µg RAE is half the amount obtained if using µg RE (Table 4-3).

Example: A diet contains 500 µg retinol, 1,800 µg β-carotene and 2,400 µg α-carotene.

$$500 + (1,800 \div 12) + (2,400 \div 24) = 750 \text{ µg RAE.}$$

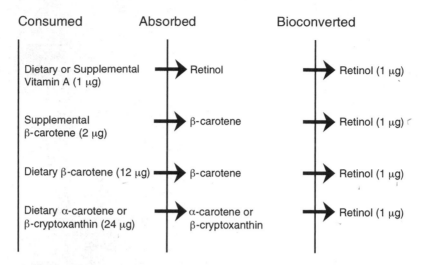

FIGURE 4-2 Absorption and bioconversion of ingested provitamin A carotenoids to retinol based on new equivalency factors (retinol activity equivalency ratio).

TABLE 4-3 Comparison of the 1989 National Research Council and 2001 Institute of Medicine Interconversion of Vitamin A and Carotenoid Units

NRC, 1989	IOM, 2001
1 retinol equivalent (µg RE) = 1 µg of all-*trans*-retinol = 2 µg of supplemental all-*trans*-β-carotene = 6 µg of dietary all-*trans*-β-carotene = 12 µg of other dietary provitamin A carotenoids	1 retinol activity equivalent (µg RAE) = 1 µg of all-*trans*-retinol = 2 µg of supplemental all-*trans*-β-carotene = 12 µg of dietary all-*trans*-β-carotene = 24 µg of other dietary provitamin A carotenoids

NOTE: 1 µg retinol = 3.33 IU vitamin A activity from retinol (WHO, 1966); 10 IU β-carotene = 3.33 IU retinol (WHO, 1966); 10 IU is based on 3.33 IU vitamin A activity × 3 (the relative vitamin activity of β-carotene in supplements versus in diets). Thus, when converting from IU β-carotene from fruits or vegetables to µg RAE, IU is divided by 20 (2 × 10).

Example: A diet contains 1,666 IU of retinol and 3,000 IU of β-carotene.

$$(1,666 \div 3.33) + (3,000 \div 20) = 650 \text{ μg RAE.}$$

Example: A supplement contains 5,000 IU of vitamin A (20 percent as β-carotene).

$$5,000 \div 3.33 = 1,500 \text{ μg RAE.}$$ ✎

The use of μg RAE rather than μg RE or international units (IU) is preferred when calculating and reporting the amount of the total vitamin A in mixed foods or assessing the amount of dietary and supplemental vitamin A consumed. Given the need to be able to calculate the intake of carotenoids, food composition data tables should report food content in amounts of each carotenoid whenever possible.

Metabolism, Transport, and Excretion

Retinyl esters and carotenoids are transported to the liver in chylomicron remnants. Apoprotein E is required for the uptake of chylomicron remnants by the liver. Some retinyl esters can also be taken up directly by peripheral tissues (Goodman et al., 1965). Several specific hepatic membrane receptors (low density lipoprotein [LDL] receptor, LDL receptor-related protein, lipolysis-stimulated receptor) have been proposed to also be involved with the uptake of chylomicron remnants (Cooper, 1997). The hydrolysis of retinyl ester to retinol is catalyzed by retinyl ester hydrolase following endocytosis. To meet tissue needs for retinoids, retinol binds to retinol-binding protein (RBP) for release into the circulation. In the blood, holo-RBP associates with transthyretin (a transport protein) to form a trimolecular complex with retinol in a 1:1:1 molar ratio. Retinol is transported in this trimolecular complex to various tissues, including the eye. The mechanism through which retinol is taken up from the circulation by peripheral cells has not been conclusively established. Retinol that is not immediately released into circulation by the liver is reesterified and stored in the lipid-containing stellate (Ito) cells of the liver until needed to maintain normal blood retinol concentrations.

Carotenoids are incorporated into very low density lipoproteins (VLDL) and exported from the liver into the blood. VLDL are converted to LDL by lipoprotein lipase on the surface of blood vessels.

Plasma membrane-associated receptors of peripheral tissue cells bind apolipoprotein B100 on the surface of LDL, initiating receptor-mediated uptake of LDL and their lipid contents. The liver, lung, adipose, and other tissues possess carotene 15, 15'-dioxygenase activity (Goodman and Blaner, 1984; Olson and Hayaishi, 1965), and thus it is presumed that carotenes may be converted to vitamin A as they are delivered to tissues. The major end products of the enzyme's activity are retinol and retinoic acid (Napoli and Race, 1988). It is unclear, however, whether carotenoids stored in tissues other than the intestinal mucosa cells are cleaved to yield retinol. Thatcher et al. (1998) demonstrated that β-carotene stored in liver is not utilized for vitamin A needs in gerbils.

Typically, the majority of vitamin A metabolites are excreted in the urine. Sauberlich et al. (1974) reported that the percentage of a radioactive dose of vitamin A recovered in breath, feces, and urine ranged from 18 to 30 percent, 18 to 37 percent, and 38 to 60 percent, respectively, after 400 days on a vitamin A-deficient diet. Almost all of the excreted metabolites are biologically inactive.

Retinol is metabolized in the liver to numerous products, some of which are conjugated with glucuronic acid or taurine for excretion in bile (Sporn et al., 1984). The portion of excreted vitamin A metabolites in bile increases as the liver vitamin A exceeds a critical concentration. This increased excretion has been suggested to serve as a protective mechanism for reducing the risk of excess storage of vitamin A (Hicks et al., 1984).

Body Stores

The hepatic vitamin A concentration can vary markedly depending on dietary intake. When vitamin A intake is adequate, over 90 percent of total body vitamin A is located in the liver (Raica et al., 1972) as retinyl ester (Schindler et al., 1988), where it is concentrated in the lipid droplets of perisinusoidal stellate cells (Hendriks et al., 1985). The average concentration of vitamin A in postmortem livers of American and Canadian adults is reported to range from 10 to as high as 1,400 µg/g liver (Furr et al., 1989; Hoppner et al., 1969; Mitchell et al., 1973; Raica et al., 1972; Schindler et al., 1988; Underwood et al., 1970). In developing countries where vitamin A deficiency is prevalent, the vitamin A concentration in liver biopsy samples is much lower (17 to 141 µg/g) (Abedin et al., 1976; Flores and de Araujo, 1984; Haskell et al., 1997; Olson, 1979; Suthutvoravoot and Olson, 1974). A concentration of at least 20 µg retinol/g of liver in adults is suggested to be the minimal acceptable reserve

(Loerch et al., 1979; Olson, 1982). The mean liver stores of vitamin A in children (1 to 10 years of age) have been reported to range from 171 to 723 µg/g (Flores and de Araujo, 1984; Mitchell et al., 1973; Money, 1978; Raica et al., 1972; Underwood et al., 1970), whereas the mean liver vitamin A stores in apparently healthy infants is lower, ranging from 0 to 320 µg/g of liver (Flores and de Araujo, 1984; Huque, 1982; Olson et al., 1979; Raica et al., 1972; Schindler et al., 1988).

With use of radio-isotopic methods, the efficiency of storage (retention) of vitamin A in liver has been estimated to be approximately 50 percent (Bausch and Rietz, 1977; Kusin et al., 1974; Sauberlich et al., 1974). More recently, stable-isotopic methods have shown an efficiency of storage of 42 percent for individuals with concentrations greater than or equal to 20 µg retinol/g of liver (Haskell et al., 1997). The efficiency of storage was lower in those with lower vitamin A status. The percentage of total body vitamin A stores lost per day was approximately 0.5 percent in adults consuming a vitamin A-free diet (Sauberlich et al., 1974).

Clinical Effects of Inadequate Intake

The most specific clinical effect of inadequate vitamin A intake is xerophthalmia. It is estimated that 3 to 10 million children, mostly in developing countries, become xerophthalmic, and 250,000 to 500,000 go blind annually (Sommer and West, 1996; WHO, 1995). The World Health Organization (WHO, 1982) classified various stages of xerophthalmia to include night blindness (impaired dark adaptation due to slowed regeneration of rhodopsin), conjunctival xerosis, Bitot's spots, corneal xerosis, corneal ulceration, and scarring, all related to vitamin A deficiency. Night blindness is the first ocular symptom to be observed with vitamin A deficiency (Dowling and Gibbons, 1961), and it responds rapidly to treatment with vitamin A (Sommer, 1982). High-dose (60 mg) vitamin A supplementation reduced the incidence of night blindness by 63 percent in Nepalese children (Katz et al., 1995). Similarly, night blindness was reduced by 50 percent in women after weekly supplementation with either 7,500 µg RE of vitamin A or β-carotene (Christian et al., 1998b).

An association of vitamin A deficiency and impaired embryonic development is well documented in animals (Morriss-Kay and Sokolova, 1996; Wilson et al., 1953). In laboratory animals, fetal resorption is common in severe vitamin A deficiency, while fetuses that survive have characteristic malformations of the eye, lungs, urogenital tract, and cardiovascular system. Similar abnormalities are observed in rat embryos lacking nuclear retinoid receptors (Wendling et al., 1999). Morphological abnormalities associated with vitamin A deficiency are not commonly found in humans; however, functional defects of the lungs have been observed (Chytil, 1996).

Because of the role of vitamin A in maintaining the structural integrity of epithelial cells, follicular hyperkeratosis has been observed with inadequate vitamin A intake (Chase et al., 1971; Sauberlich et al., 1974). Men who were made vitamin A deficient under controlled conditions were then supplemented with either retinol or β-carotene, which caused the hyperkeratosis to gradually clear (Sauberlich et al., 1974).

Vitamin A deficiency has been associated with a reduction in lymphocyte numbers, natural killer cells, and antigen-specific immunoglobulin responses (Cantorna et al., 1995; Nauss and Newberne, 1985). A decrease in leukocytes and lymphoid organ weights, impaired T cell function, and decreased resistance to immunogenic tumors have been observed with inadequate vitamin A intake (Dawson and Ross, 1999; Wiedermann et al., 1993). A generalized dysfunction of humoral and cell-mediated immunity is common in experimental animals and is likely to exist in humans.

In addition to xerophthalmia, vitamin A deficiency has been associated with increased risk of infectious morbidity and mortality in experimental animals and humans, especially in developing countries. A higher risk of respiratory infection and diarrhea has been reported among children with mild to moderate vitamin A deficiency (Sommer et al., 1984). Mortality rates were about four times greater among children with mild xerophthalmia than those without it (Sommer et al., 1983). The risk of severe morbidity and mortality decreases with vitamin A repletion. In children hospitalized with measles, case fatality (Barclay et al., 1987; Hussey and Klein, 1990) and the severity of complications on admission were reduced when they received high doses (60 to 120 mg) of vitamin A (Coutsoudis et al., 1991; Hussey and Klein, 1990). In some studies, vitamin A supplementation (30 to 60 mg) has been shown to reduce the severity of diarrhea (Barreto et al., 1994; Donnen et al., 1998) and *Plasmodium falciparum* malaria (Shankar et al., 1999) in young children, but vitamin A supplementation has had little effect on the risk or severity of respiratory infections, except when associated with measles (Humphrey et al., 1996).

In developing countries, vitamin A supplementation has been shown to reduce the risk of mortality among young children (Ghana VAST Study Team, 1993; Muhilal et al., 1988; Rahmathullah et al., 1990; Sommer et al., 1986; West et al., 1991), infants (Humphrey et al., 1996), and pregnant and postpartum women (West et al., 1999). Meta-analyses of the results from these and other community-based trials are consistent with a 23 to 30 percent reduction in mortality of young children beyond 6 months of age after vitamin A supplementation (Beaton et al., 1993; Fawzi et al., 1993, Glasziou and Mackerras, 1993). WHO recommends broad-based prophylaxis in vitamin A-deficient populations. It also recommends treating children who suffer from xerophthalmia, measles, prolonged diarrhea, wasting malnutrition, and other acute infections with vitamin A (WHO, 1997). Furthermore, the American Academy of Pediatrics (AAP, 1993) recommends vitamin A supplementation for children in the United States who are hospitalized with measles.

SELECTION OF INDICATORS FOR ESTIMATING THE REQUIREMENT FOR VITAMIN A

Dark Adaptation

The ability of the retina to adapt to dim light depends upon an adequate supply of vitamin A, because 11-*cis* retinal is an integral part of the rhodopsin molecule of the rods. Without adequate levels of vitamin A in the retina, the function of the rods in dim light situations becomes compromised, resulting in abnormal dark adaptation (night blindness). Before clinically apparent night blindness occurs, abnormal rod function may be detected by dark adaptation testing. In addition to vitamin A deficiency, zinc deficiency and severe protein deficiency also may affect dark adaptation responses (Bankson et al., 1989; Morrison et al., 1978).

Dark Adaptation Test

To perform a dark adaptation test, the eye is first dilated and the subject fixates on a point located approximately 15 degrees above the center of the test light. The test stimulus consists of light flashes of approximately 1-second duration separated by 1-second intervals of darkness. A tracking method is used with the luminance of the test light being increased or decreased depending upon the response of the subject. The ascending threshold is the intensity at which the subject first sees the test light as its luminance is increased. The descending threshold is the intensity at which the subject ceases to see the test light as its luminance is lowered. Each threshold intensity is plotted versus time and the values are read from the graph at the end of a test session. Testing is continued until the final threshold is stabilized. The final dark-adapted threshold is defined as the average of three ascending and three descending thresholds and is obtained after 35 to 40 minutes in darkness.

When the logarithm of the light perception is plotted as a function of time in darkness, the change in threshold follows a characteristic course. There is an initial rapid fall in threshold attributed to cones, followed by a plateau. A steeper descent, referred to as the rod-cone break, usually occurs at 3 to 9 minutes followed by a slower descent attributed to adaptation of the rods. The final threshold attained at about 35 to 40 minutes is the most constant indicator of dark adaptation. Among stable subjects, test results are reproducible over a 1- to 6-month interval with final threshold differences ranging from 0 to 0.1 log candela/meter^2. In one series, the dark adapted final threshold among 50 normal subjects (aged 20 to 60 years) was -5.0 ± 0.3 candela/ meter^2 (Carney and Russell, 1980).

Similar information on retinal function may be obtained by an electroretinogram or an electrooculorgram. However, these tests are more invasive than dark adaptation and there are not as many data relating these functional tests to dietary vitamin A levels.

There is literature relating dark adaptation test results to dietary levels of vitamin A under controlled experimental conditions (Table 4-4). Under controlled feeding conditions, dark adaptation, objectively measured by dark adaptometry, is one of the most sensitive indicators of a change in vitamin A deficiency status (Figure 4-3). Epidemiological evidence suggests that host resistance to infection is impaired at lesser stages of vitamin A deficiency, prior to clinical onset of night blindness (Arroyave et al., 1979; Arthur et al., 1992; Barreto et al., 1994; Bloem et al., 1990; Ghana VAST Study Team, 1993; Loyd-Puryear et al., 1991; Salazar-Lindo et al., 1993). Moreover, laboratory animals fed a vitamin A-deficient diet maintain ocular levels of vitamin A despite a significant reduction in hepatic vitamin A levels (Bankson et al., 1989; Wallingford and Underwood, 1987). Nevertheless, this approach can be used to estimate the average requirement for vitamin A but without assurance of adequate tissue levels to meet nonvisual needs for vitamin A.

Pupillary Response Test

Another test of ability to dark adapt, one that avoids reliance on psychophysical responses, is the pupillary response test that measures the threshold of light at which a pupillary reflex (contraction) first occurs under dark-adapted conditions (Stewart and Young, 1989). The retina of one eye is briefly exposed to incremental pulses of light while a trained observer monitors the consensual response of the other pupil under dark conditions. A high scotopic (vision in dim light) threshold indicates low retinal sensitivity, a pathophysiological response to vitamin A deficiency. An early report of pupillary nonresponse to candlelight among night blind Confederate soldiers in the Civil War (Hicks, 1867) led to the development and validation of instrumentation for this test as a reliable, functional measure of vitamin A deficiency in Indonesian (Congdon et al., 1995) and Indian (Sanchez et al., 1997) children. However, data do not currently exist relating pupillary threshold sensitivity as determined by this test to usual vitamin A intakes, and so measures of pupillary response cannot be used at the present to establish dietary vitamin A requirements.

Plasma Retinol Concentration

The concentration of plasma retinol is under tight homeostatic control in individuals and therefore is insensitive to liver vitamin A stores. The relationship is not linear and over a wide range of adequate hepatic vitamin A reserves there is little change in plasma retinol or retinol binding protein (RBP) concentrations (Underwood, 1984). When liver vitamin A reserves fall below a critical concentration, thought to be approximately 20 µg/g of liver (Olson, 1987), plasma retinol concentration declines. When dietary vitamin A is provided to vitamin A-deficient children, plasma retinol concentration increases rapidly, even before liver stores are restored (Devadas et al., 1978; Jayarajan et al., 1980). Thus, a low concentration of plasma retinol may indicate inadequacy of vitamin A status, although median or mean concentrations for plasma retinol may not be well correlated with valid indicators of vitamin A status.

In malnourished populations, often 25 percent or more individuals exhibit a plasma retinol concentration below 0.70 µmol/L (20 µg/dL), a level considered to reflect vitamin A inadequacy in a population (Flores, 1993; Underwood, 1994). However, a low plasma retinol concentration also may result from an inadequate supply of dietary protein, energy, or zinc, all of which are required for a normal rate of synthesis of RBP (Smith et al., 1974). Plasma retinol concentration may also be low during infection as a result of transient decreases in the concentrations of the negative acute phase proteins, RBP, and transthyretin, even when liver retinol is adequate (Christian et al., 1998a; Filteau et al., 1995; Golner et al., 1987; Rosales et al., 1996). The presence of one or more of these factors could lead to an overestimation of the prevalence of vitamin

TABLE 4-4 Correction of Abnormal Dark Adaptation with Vitamin A

Reference	Subject	Vitamin A Intake (µg/d)	Duration	Serum Retinol	Dark Adaptation[a]	ERG[b]
Blanchard and Harper, 1940	DA, man, 20 y	90–165 +450 +600	3 d 2 d		A C SI	
	JK, man, 23 y	90–165 +300 +1,081	4 d 2 d		A C C	
	TH, man, 20 y	90–165 +150 +721	3 d 4 d		A PC N	
Batchelder and Ebbs, 1943	GG, young adult woman	60 600 1,201			A A N	
	KY, young adult man	60 600 1,201			A A N	
	MW, young adult woman	60 600 1,200 1,200 3,000	6 d 17 d	440 and 620 IU/dL	A A TC A C	
Hume and Krebs, 1949	Golding, man, 32 y, vitamin A depleted	21 390	14 mo 1 mo 2 mo 6 mo	22 IU/dL 50 IU/dL 88 IU/dL 88 IU/dL	2.81, A 2.38, A 2.26, M 1.81, N	

continued

TABLE 4-4 Continued

Reference	Subject	Vitamin A Intake (µg/d)	Duration	Serum Retinol	Dark Adaptation[a]	ERG[b]
Sauberlich et al., 1974	Subject #1, man, 37 y, vitamin A depleted	< 24 37.5 75 150 300 600	771 d 14 d 14 d 15 d 14 d 11 d	 8 µg/dL 7 µg/dL 4 µg/dL 12 µg/dL 19 µg/dL	 A A C C C	 A A A PC
	Subject #5, man, 43 y, vitamin A depleted	< 24 150 300 600 1,200 2,400	359 d 82 d 372 d 14 d 14 d 14 d	 4 µg/dL 27 µg/dL 42 µg/dL 42 µg/dL 47 µg/dL	 C C C C C	 A PC C C
	Subject #7, man, 41 y, vitamin A depleted	< 24 150 300 600 1,200	505 d 82 d 42 d 16 d 9 d	 9 µg/dL 16 µg/dL 20 µg/dL 24 µg/dL	 C C C C	 A A
	Subject # 8, man, 32 y, vitamin A depleted	< 24 75 150 300	595 d 10 d 17 d 3 d	 8 µg/dL 9 µg/dL	 A C C	 A A
	KC, medical student, vitamin A depleted	60 570	40 d 10 d		A C	
	MS, medical student, vitamin A depleted	60 255	52 d 10 d		A C	

NOTE: Subjects from the four studies were included based on two rules: (1) only subjects with intake gaps less than 600 µg/day were used and (2) the lowest corrected/normal intake value was chosen as that level at which dark adaptation was corrected or normal and for which no abnormal ERG was recorded.

[a] Dark adaptation normal = 1.37 to 2.3 log µm lamberts. A = abnormal, C = corrected, SI = slight improvement, PC = partially corrected, N = normal, TC = temporarily corrected, M = marginal.

[b] ERG = electroretinogram.

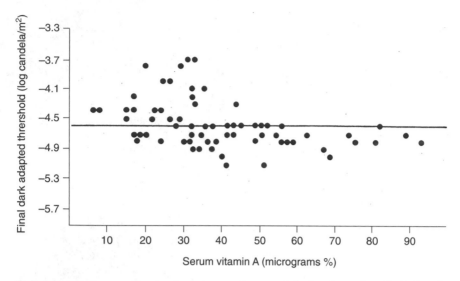

FIGURE 4-3 Serum vitamin A concentrations and dark adaptation final thresholds. Upper limit of normal final threshold = –4.6 log candela/m². Adapted from Carney and Russell (1980).

A deficiency when serum retinol concentration is used as an indicator. According to an analysis of the Third National Health and Nutrition Examination Survey, individuals in the highest quartile for vitamin A intake had only slightly higher serum retinol concentrations than those in the lowest quartile for vitamin A intake (Appendix Tables H-1 and H-2).

In the United States (Looker et al., 1988; Pilch, 1987) (Appendix Table G-4), serum retinol concentration is rarely low (< 0.7 µmol/ L) in more than 5 percent of preschool children, although 20 to 60 percent may exhibit concentrations between 0.70 and 1.05 µmol/L, a range that may be marginal for some individuals (Underwood, 1994). Excluding pregnant women, less than 5 percent of adults had a serum retinol concentration less than 1.05 µmol/L (Appendix Table G-4). The median concentration of serum retinol in adults was 1.7 to 2.2 µmol/L (48 to 63 µg/dL).

At the usual U.S. range of plasma retinol concentration, the concentration is neither related to observed levels of usual vitamin A intake, from either dietary preformed vitamin A or provitamin A carotenoid sources (Hallfrisch et al., 1994), nor responsive to supplement use (Krasinski et al., 1989; Nierenberg et al., 1997; Stauber et al., 1991). Because of the relatively insensitive relationship between plasma retinol concentration and liver vitamin A in the adequate range, and because of the potential for confounding factors to affect the level and interpretation of the concentration, it was not chosen as a primary status indicator for a population for estimating an average requirement for vitamin A.

Total Liver Reserves by Isotope Dilution

Body stores of vitamin A can be estimated directly by liver biopsy, but this is not an appropriate indicator of status, except at autopsy, for a population. Vitamin A stores can also be estimated by an indirect approach using an isotope dilution technique. This technique involves administering an oral dose of stable-isotopically labeled vitamin A and, after a period of equilibration, drawing blood for measurement of the isotopic ratio in plasma. The Bausch and Rietz (1977) equation used to calculate liver reserves is: TLR = F × dose × [(H:D) − 1] where *TLR* is the pretreatment total liver reserve of vitamin A in millimoles of retinol, *F* is a factor that expresses the efficacy of storage of an early administered dose, *dose* is the oral dose of labeled retinol in millimoles, *H:D* is the ratio of hydrogen to deuterated retinol in the plasma after an equilibration period, and −1 corrects TLR for the contribution of the administered dose to the total body pool. Furr et al. (1989) have suggested modification of this formula to: TLR = F × dose × (S × a × [H:D] −1]) where *S* is the ratio of the specific activities of retinol in serum to that in liver and *a* is the fraction of the absorbed dose of deuterated retinol remaining in the liver at the time of blood sampling. Liver reserves of vitamin A can be correlated with known dietary intake levels of vitamin A. An Estimated Average Requirement (EAR) could be derived by knowing the population median intake of vitamin A at which half the population has hepatic stores above a certain desired level (e.g., 20 µg/g) and half has stores below it. Although theoretically such an approach could be used to establish an EAR, no studies have been conducted in which detailed and long-term dietary data have been obtained in the tested subjects.

Relative Dose Response and Modified Relative Dose Response

In healthy individuals, approximately 90 percent of vitamin A in the body is stored in the liver and this percentage decreases to 50 percent or less in severely deficient individuals (Olson, 1987). Hepatic vitamin A stores can thus be interpreted to reflect nutrient adequacy to meet total body needs, barring factors that impede their release into circulation (e.g., liver disease and severe protein malnutrition). The relative dose response (RDR) is a method that permits indirect assessment of the relative adequacy of hepatic vitamin A stores. The RDR test was first demonstrated in rats where the release of RBP from liver was shown to depend on the availability of retinol (Loerch et al., 1979). In experimental vitamin A deficiency in rats, RBP accumulated in liver but was rapidly released after vitamin A (retinol) was administered (Carney et al., 1976; Keilson et al., 1979). This observation led Loerch et al. (1979) to propose that a positive plasma retinol response to a small test dose of vitamin A could be used as an indicator of inadequate liver vitamin A reserves.

The test was subsequently validated against measured liver retinol stores in humans (Amedee-Manesme et al., 1984, 1987; Mobarhan et al., 1981). For the test, a blood sample is drawn before retinol administration (zero time), and then a small dose of vitamin A is administered; a second blood sample is taken after an interval, generally 5 hours. The concentration of retinol in each sample is determined and the difference (response) in plasma retinol concentration (5 hours minus zero hours) is calculated and expressed as a percentage of the 5-hour concentration.

Although various cutoff levels have been used, a plasma retinol response greater than or equal to 20 percent is generally considered to indicate that liver vitamin A is inadequate (Tanumihardjo, 1993). The synthesis of RBP depends on the adequacy of other nutrients, and other deficiencies, such as zinc deficiency and protein energy malnutrition, can confound the results of the RDR test, particularly when a repeat test is conducted within a week or less after the first or baseline test. With proper controls the RDR test is considered a valid test to determine inadequate vitamin A status. However, just as plasma retinol concentration is insensitive across a wide range of "adequate" liver vitamin A reserves, the RDR test does not distinguish among different levels of adequate vitamin A reserves (Solomons et al., 1990).

The modified relative dose response (MRDR) test is a variation of the RDR test (Tanumihardjo and Olson, 1991). The MRDR requires a single blood sample and uses as the test dose vitamin A2 (dehydroretinol), which combines with RBP in the same manner as retinol but is not found endogenously in human plasma (with the possible exception of populations consuming high levels of fresh water fish). The test is subject to the same limitations as the RDR test. Neither the RDR nor the MRDR was chosen for estimating an EAR because little data exist relating usual dietary intakes of individuals or populations to RDR or MRDR test value distributions.

Conjunctival Impression Cytology

Before the clinical onset of xerophthalmia, mild vitamin A deficiency leads to early keratinizing metaplasia and losses of mucin-secreting goblet cells on the bulbar surface of the conjunctiva of the eye. These functional changes on the ocular surface can be detected by microscopic examination of PAS-hematoxylin stained epithelial cells obtained by briefly applying a cellulose acetate filter paper strip (Hatchell and Sommer, 1984; Natadisastra et al., 1987; Wittpenn et al., 1986) or disc (Keenum et al., 1990) against the temporal conjunctivum. An alternative approach involves transferring cell specimens from the filter paper to a glass slide before staining and examination (Carlier et al., 1991). Specimens are classified as normal or into degrees of abnormality, depending on the density and distribution of stained normal epithelial cells, goblet cells, and mucin "spots" (contents of goblet cells). Vitamin A status is defined by target tissue cellularity, integrity, and function, which, unlike biochemical measures, if compromised may take several weeks to normalize following vitamin A repletion (Keenum, 1993). In spite of that, there is an association between the prevalence of conjunctival impression cytology (CIC) abnormality and serum retinol and RDR test results (Sommer and West, 1996). Although CIC is used for assessment, there are few data that relate CIC status to dietary vitamin A intake in the United States, other well-nourished populations, or malnourished populations. As a result, CIC was not selected as the functional indicator for the EAR for vitamin A.

Immune Function

There is sound evidence for a role of vitamin A in the maintenance of both humoral antibody responses and cell-mediated immunity. In experimental animals, both nonspecific immunity (Butera and Krakowka, 1986; Cohen and Elin, 1974) and antigen-specific responses, including delayed-type hypersensitivity (Smith et al., 1987), blastogenesis (Butera and Krakowka, 1986; Friedman and Sklan, 1989), and antibody production (Carman et al., 1989, 1992; Pasatiempo et al., 1990; Ross, 1996; Stephensen et al., 1993), have been shown to be altered by a deficiency of vitamin A or enhanced by vitamin A supplementation. The number and cytotoxic activity of natural killer cells (Dawson et al., 1999; Zhao et al., 1994) is reduced in vitamin A deficiency, although responsiveness to activation is maintained.

Several human studies have linked impairment in immunity to

low plasma or serum vitamin A concentrations (Coutsoudis et al., 1992; Semba et al., 1992, 1996). However, there are no human studies using controlled diets that have evaluated immune function tests as a means to assess the adequacy of different levels of dietary vitamin A. In addition to a lack of relevant dietary studies, there are some inherent limitations to using immune functions as indicators to establish dietary recommendations. Most changes in immune functions that have been associated with a nutrient deficiency are not specific to the nutrient under study (e.g., low T cell-mediated immunity may be caused by a lack of vitamin A, but also by a deficiency of protein or energy, zinc, or other specific nutrient deficiencies or imbalances). Thus, human dietary studies would have to be highly controlled with respect to the contents of potentially confounding nutrients. Another limitation of many immune function tests is related to difficulties encountered in standardizing tests of immunity (e.g., proliferative responses to antigen or mitogen challenge which are often used within studies to assess T and B cell responses). These tests are affected by many factors, such as the type and quality of mitogen used, cell culture conditions, and how subjects' cells have been collected, that cannot be readily controlled among laboratories or over time. Thus, for these reasons, immune function tests could not be used as an indicator for establishing the EAR for vitamin A.

FACTORS AFFECTING THE VITAMIN A REQUIREMENT

Intestinal Absorption

Dietary Fat

Dietary vitamin A is digested in mixed micelles and absorbed with fat. In some studies, increasing the level of fat in a low fat diet has been shown to improve retinol and carotene absorption (Reddy and Srikantia, 1966) and vitamin A nutriture (Jalal et al., 1998; Roels et al., 1963). Other studies, however, have not demonstrated a beneficial effect of fat on vitamin A absorption (Borel et al., 1997; Figueira et al., 1969).

For optimal carotenoid absorption, a number of research groups have demonstrated that dietary fat must be consumed along with carotenoids. Roels and coworkers (1958) reported that the addition of 18 g/day of olive oil improved carotene absorption from 5 to 25 percent. Jayarajan and coworkers (1980) reported that the addition 5 g of fat to the diet significantly improved serum vitamin A concentrations among children after the consumption of a low fat vegetable diet. The addition of 10 g of fat did not improve serum vitamin A concentrations any more than did 5 g of fat.

Infections

Malabsorption of vitamin A can occur with diarrhea and intestinal infections and infestations. Sivakumar and Reddy (1972) demonstrated depressed absorption of labeled vitamin A in children with gastroenteritis and respiratory infections. Malabsorption of vitamin A is also associated with intestinal parasitism (Mahalanabis et al., 1979; Sivakumar and Reddy, 1975).

The malabsorption of vitamin A that is observed in children with *Ascaris lumbricoides* infection was associated with an altered mucosal morphology that was reversed with deworming (Jalal et al., 1998; Maxwell et al., 1968).

Food Matrix

The matrix of foods affects the ability of carotenoids to be released from food and therefore affects intestinal absorption. The rise in serum β-carotene concentration was significantly less when individuals consumed β-carotene from carrots than when they received a similar amount of β-carotene supplement (Micozzi et al., 1992; Tang et al., 2000; Torronen et al., 1996). This observation was similar for broccoli (Micozzi et al., 1992) and mixed green leafy vegetables (de Pee et al., 1995; Tang et al., 2000) as compared with a β-carotene supplement. The food matrix effect on β-carotene bioavailability has been reviewed (Boileau et al., 1999).

Food Processing

The processing of foods greatly affects the absorption of carotenoids (Van het Hof et al., 1998). The absorption of carotene was 24 percent from sliced carrots, whereas the absorption of carotene from homogenized carrots was 56 percent (Hume and Krebs, 1949). Rock et al. (1998) reported that the rise in serum β-carotene concentration was significantly greater in subjects consuming cooked carrots and spinach as compared with those consuming an equal amount of raw carrots and spinach. Similarly, the rise in serum β-carotene concentration was greater after the consumption of carrot juice than after the same amount of raw carrots (Torronen et al., 1996).

Nutrient-Nutrient Interactions

Iron

A direct correlation between hemoglobin and serum retinol concentrations has been observed (Suharno et al., 1993; Wolde-Gebriel et al., 1993). Anemic rats have been shown to have reduced plasma retinol concentrations when fed a vitamin A-rich diet (Amine et al., 1970), although normal hepatic stores of vitamin A were observed (Staab et al., 1984). Rosales and coworkers (1999) reported that iron deficiency in young rats alters the distribution of vitamin A concentration between plasma and liver. In a cross-sectional study of children in Thailand, serum retinol concentration was positively associated with serum iron and ferritin concentrations (Bloem et al., 1989). Intervention studies among Indonesian girls demonstrated that combining vitamin A with iron supplementation was more effective in increasing hemoglobin concentrations than was giving iron alone (Suharno et al., 1993). As discussed in further detail in Chapter 9, various studies suggest that vitamin A deficiency impairs iron mobilization from stores and therefore vitamin A supplementation improves hemoglobin concentrations (Lynch, 1997).

Zinc

Zinc is required for protein synthesis, including the hepatic synthesis and secretion of retinol binding protein (RBP) and transthyretin; therefore, zinc deficiency influences the mobilization of vitamin A from the liver and its transport into the circulation (Smith et al., 1974; Terhune and Sandstead, 1972). In animal models, circulating and hepatic concentrations of retinol decline and rise with experimental zinc deficiency and repletion, respectively (Baly et al., 1984; Duncan and Hurley, 1978). In humans, cross-sectional studies and supplementation trials have failed to establish a consistent relationship between zinc and vitamin A status (Christian and West, 1998). Because zinc is important in the biosynthesis of RBP, it has been suggested that zinc intake may positively affect vitamin A status only when individuals are moderately to severely protein-energy deficient (Shingwekar et al., 1979).

Although the alcohol dehydrogenase enzymes involved in the formation of retinal from retinol in the eye are not zinc dependent (Duester, 1996; Persson et al., 1995), zinc-deficient rats had a significant reduction in the synthesis of rhodopsin (Dorea and Olson,

1986), which was postulated to be due to impaired protein (opsin and alcohol dehydrogenase) synthesis. Morrison and coworkers (1978) reported that dark adaptation improved after the provision of 220 mg/day of zinc to zinc-deficient patients.

Carotenoids

Competitive interactions among different carotenoids have been observed. When subjects were given purified β-carotene and lutein in a combined dose, β-carotene significantly reduced lutein absorption, and therefore serum lutein concentration, compared to when lutein was given alone (Kostic et al., 1995). However, lutein given in combination with β-carotene significantly increased β-carotene serum concentrations compared to when β-carotene was given alone. Johnson et al. (1997) reported that lycopene does not affect the absorption of β-carotene, and β-carotene improved the absorption of lycopene.

Alcohol

Because both retinol and ethanol are alcohols, there is potential for overlap in the metabolic pathways of these two compounds. Competition with each other for similar enzymatic pathways has been reported (Leo and Lieber, 1999), while other retinol and alcohol dehydrogenases show greater substrate specificity (Napoli et al., 1995). Ethanol consumption results in a depletion of hepatic vitamin A concentrations in animals (Sato and Lieber, 1981) and in humans (Leo and Lieber, 1985). Although the effect on vitamin A is due, in part, to hepatic damage (Leo and Lieber, 1982) and malnutrition, the reduction in hepatic stores is also a direct effect of alcohol consumption. Patients with low vitamin A stores, in the study by Leo and Lieber (1982), were otherwise well nourished. Furthermore, the reduction in hepatic vitamin A stores was reduced before the onset of fibrosis or cirrhosis of the liver (Sato and Lieber, 1981). Results suggest that vitamin A is mobilized from the liver to other organs (Mobarhan et al., 1991) with ethanol consumption. Chronic ethanol intake resulted in increased destruction of retinoic acid through the induction of P450 enzymes, resulting in reduced hepatic retinoic acid concentrations (Wang, 1999).

FINDINGS BY LIFE STAGE AND GENDER GROUP

Infants Ages 0 through 12 Months

Method Used to Set the Adequate Intake

No functional criteria of vitamin A status have been demonstrated that reflect response to dietary intake in infants. Thus, recommended intakes of vitamin A are based on an Adequate Intake (AI) that reflects a calculated mean vitamin A intake of infants principally fed human milk.

Ages 0 through 6 Months. Using the method described in Chapter 2, the AI of vitamin A for infants ages 0 though 6 months is based on the average amount of vitamin A in human milk that is consumed. After rounding, an AI of 400 μg retinol activity equivalents (RAE)/day is set based on the average volume of milk intake of 0.78 L/day (see Chapter 2) and an average concentration of vitamin A in human milk of 1.70 μmol/L (485 μg/L) during the first 6 months of lactation (Canfield et al., 1997, 1998) (see Table 4-5). Because the bioconversion of carotenoids in milk and in infants is not known, the contribution of carotenoids in human milk to meeting the vitamin A requirement of infants was not considered.

TABLE 4-5 Vitamin A in Human Milk

Reference	Study Group	Average Maternal Intake
Butte and Calloway, 1981	23 Navajo women	Not reported
Chappell et al., 1985	12 women	Not reported
Canfield et al., 1997	6 women, 23–36 y	2,334 μg/d
Canfield et al., 1998	5 women, 23–36 y	2,544 μg/d

[a] Vitamin A intake based on reported data or concentration (μg/L) × 0.78 L/day.

Ages 7 through 12 Months. Using the method described in Chapter 2 to extrapolate from the AI for infants ages 0 through 6 months fed human milk, the intake from human milk for the older infants is 483 µg RAE/day of vitamin A.

The vitamin A intake for older infants can also be determined by estimating the intake from human milk (concentration × 0.6 L/day) and complementary foods (Chapter 2). Vitamin A intake data ($n = 45$) from complementary foods was estimated to be 244 µg/day based on data from the Third National Health and Nutrition Examination Survey. The average intake from human milk is approximately 291 µg/day (485 µg/L × 0.6 L/day). Thus, the total vitamin A intake is estimated to be 535 µg RAE/day (244 µg/day + 291 µg/day).

On the basis of these two approaches and rounding, the AI was set at 500 µg RAE/day. The AI for infants is greater than the Recommended Dietary Allowance (RDA) for young children because the RDA is based on extrapolation of adult data (see "Children and Adolescents Ages 1 through 18 Years").

Vitamin A AI Summary, Ages 0 through 12 Months

AI for Infants
0–6 months	**400 µg RAE/day of vitamin A**
7–12 months	**500 µg RAE/day of vitamin A**

Stage of Lactation	Milk Concentration (µg/L)	Estimated Vitamin A Intake of Infants (µg/d)[a]
1 mo	329	256
3–4 d	2,000	1,560
37 d	≈600	468
< 6 mo	314	245
	485	380
> 1 mo	640	500

Special Considerations

Concentrations of 520 to 590 µg/L of vitamin A in milk from Holstein cows have been reported (Tomlinson et al., 1976), which is significantly less than the levels observed in human milk (Table 4-5). The majority of vitamin A and carotenes are located in the fat globule and fat globule membrane in cow milk (Patton et al., 1980; Zahar et al., 1995). The concentrations of retinol and β-carotene in cow milk averaged 18 to 27 µg/g of milk fat in one study (Jensen and Nielsen, 1996). Retinol in cow milk is bound to β-lactoglobulin, which has a structure very similar to retinol binding protein (Papiz et al., 1986). There is minimal isomerization of *trans*-retinol to *cis*-retinol in unheated cow milk (Panfili et al., 1998), the latter being less well absorbed. Cow milk submitted to pasteurization resulted in 3 to 6 percent isomerization to *cis*-retinol. Greater isomerization was observed with severe heat treatments (16 percent in ultra high temperature milk and 34 percent in sterilized milk).

Children and Adolescents Ages 1 through 18 Years

Method Used to Estimate the Average Requirement

No data are available to estimate an average requirement for children and adolescents. A computational method is used that includes an allowance for adequate liver vitamin A stores to set the Estimated Average Requirement (EAR) (see "Adults Ages 19 Years and Older"). The EAR for children and adolescents is extrapolated from adults by using metabolic body weight and the method described in Chapter 2. If total body weight is used, the RDA for children 1 through 3 years would be 200 µg RAE/day. If metabolic weight ($kg^{0.75}$) is used, the RDA would be 300 µg RAE/day. Studies conducted in developing countries indicate that xerophthalmia and serum retinol concentrations of less than 20 µg/dL exist among preschool children with daily intakes of up to 200 µg of vitamin A, whereas 300 µg/day of vitamin A is associated with serum retinol concentrations greater than 30 µg/dL (Reddy, 1985). Although similar data are lacking in developed countries, to ensure that the RDA will meet the requirement of almost all North American preschool children, metabolic weight was used to extrapolate from adults.

Vitamin A EAR and RDA Summary, Ages 1 through 18 Years

EAR for Children
    1–3 years   210 µg RAE/day of vitamin A
    4–8 years   275 µg RAE/day of vitamin A

EAR for Boys
    9–13 years   445 µg RAE/day of vitamin A
    14–18 years   630 µg RAE/day of vitamin A

EAR for Girls
    9–13 years   420 µg RAE/day of vitamin A
    14–18 years   485 µg RAE/day of vitamin A

The RDA for vitamin A is set by using a coefficient of variation (CV) of 20 percent based on the calculated half-life values for liver vitamin A (see "Adults Ages 19 Years and Older"). The RDA is defined as equal to the EAR plus twice the CV to cover the needs of 97 to 98 percent of individuals in the group (therefore, for vitamin A the RDA is 140 percent of the EAR). The calculated values for the RDAs have been rounded to the nearest 100 µg.

RDA for Children
    1–3 years   300 µg RAE/day of vitamin A
    4–8 years   400 µg RAE/day of vitamin A

RDA for Boys
    9–13 years   600 µg RAE/day of vitamin A
    14–18 years   900 µg RAE/day of vitamin A

RDA for Girls
    9–13 years   600 µg RAE/day of vitamin A
    14–18 years   700 µg RAE/day of vitamin A

Adults Ages 19 Years and Older

Evidence Considered in Estimating the Average Requirement

The calculation described below can be used for estimating the vitamin A requirement and is calculated on the basis of the amount of dietary vitamin A required to maintain a given body-pool size in well-nourished subjects. Olson (1987) determined the average requirement of vitamin A by this approach using the calculation:

$$A \times B \times C \times D \times E \times F$$

A = Percent of body vitamin A stores lost per day when ingesting a vitamin A-free diet
B = Minimum acceptable liver vitamin A reserve
C = The liver weight:body weight ratio
D = Reference weight for a specific age group and gender
E = Ratio of total body:liver vitamin A reserves
F = Efficiency of storage of ingested vitamin A.

By using this approach, a daily vitamin A intake can be determined that will assure vitamin A reserves to cover increased needs during periods of stress and low vitamin A intake. That value can be used for estimating the average requirement for vitamin A.

The portion of body vitamin A stores lost per day has been estimated to be 0.5 percent based on the rate of excretion of radioactivity from radiolabeled vitamin A and by the calculation of the half-life of vitamin A. The minimal acceptable liver reserve is estimated to be 20 µg/g and is based on the concentration at which (1) no clinical signs of a deficiency are observed, (2) adequate plasma retinol concentrations are maintained (Loerch et al., 1979), (3) induced biliary excretion of vitamin A is observed (Hicks et al., 1984), and (4) there is a protection against a vitamin A deficiency for approximately 4 months while the person consumes a vitamin A-deficient diet. The liver weight:body weight ratio is 1:33 (0.03) and is an average of ratios for infants and adults. The reference weights for adult women and men are 61 and 76 kg, respectively (see Chapter 1). The ratio of total body:liver vitamin A reserves is 10:9 (1.1) and is based on individuals with adequate vitamin A status. Finally, the efficiency of storage can be determined by isotope dilution methods following the administration of either radioactive or stable-isotopically labeled vitamin A to subjects adequate in vitamin A (Bausch and Reitz, 1977; Haskell et al., 1997). Recent studies by Haskell and coworkers (1997) suggest that the efficiency of storage is approximately 40 percent, rather than the 50 percent that was previously reported (Olson, 1987). Based on these current estimations, the EAR of preformed vitamin A required to assure an adequate body reserve in an adult man is 0.005×20 µg/g $\times 0.03 \times 76$ kg $\times 1.1 \times 2.5$, or 627 µg RAE/day. With a reference weight of 61 kg for women, the EAR would be 503 µg RAE/day.

Based on the study of Sauberlich and coworkers (1974), Olson (1987) estimated that the liver vitamin A concentration was less than 10 µg/g at the time the first clinical signs of vitamin A deficiency appeared. From this assumption, it was estimated that the half-life of vitamin A is approximately 128 days, and the CV is 21 percent. Because the portion of this variability that is due to experimental error is not known, a CV of 20 percent is used for setting the RDA.

Vitamin A EAR and RDA Summary, Ages 19 Years and Older

EAR for Men
19–30 years	625 µg RAE/day of vitamin A
31–50 years	625 µg RAE/day of vitamin A
51–70 years	625 µg RAE/day of vitamin A
> 70 years	625 µg RAE/day of vitamin A

EAR for Women
19–30 years	500 µg RAE/day of vitamin A
31–50 years	500 µg RAE/day of vitamin A
51–70 years	500 µg RAE/day of vitamin A
> 70 years	500 µg RAE/day of vitamin A

The RDA for vitamin A is set by using a CV of 20 percent (see Chapter 1) using the EAR for adequate body stores of vitamin A. The RDA is defined as equal to the EAR plus twice the CV to cover the needs of 97 to 98 percent of the individuals in the group (therefore, for vitamin A the RDA is 140 percent of the EAR). The calculated values for the RDAs have been rounded to the nearest 100 µg.

RDA for Men
19–30 years	900 µg RAE/day of vitamin A
31–50 years	900 µg RAE/day of vitamin A
51–70 years	900 µg RAE/day of vitamin A
> 70 years	900 µg RAE/day of vitamin A

RDA for Women
19–30 years	700 µg RAE/day of vitamin A
31–50 years	700 µg RAE/day of vitamin A
51–70 years	700 µg RAE/day of vitamin A
> 70 years	700 µg RAE/day of vitamin A

Pregnancy

Evidence Considered in Estimating the Average Requirement

Direct studies of the requirement for vitamin A during pregnancy are lacking. The model used to establish the EAR is based on the accumulation of vitamin A in the liver of the fetus during gestation and an assumption that liver contains approximately half of the body's vitamin A when liver stores are low, as in the case of newborns. Liver vitamin A concentrations for full-term stillborn infants (Dorea et al., 1984; Hoppner et al., 1968; Montreewasuwat and Olson, 1979; Olson, 1979) have ranged from less than 10 to greater than 100 μg/g liver, with values tending to be skewed towards the lower range (Olson, 1979). A vitamin A concentration of 1,800 μg per liver for 37 to 40 week gestation age (Montreewasuwat and Olson, 1979) was used to calculate a concentration of 3,600 μg per fetus. Assuming the efficiency of maternal vitamin A absorption to average 70 percent and vitamin A to be accumulated mostly in the last 90 days of pregnancy, the mother's requirement would be increased by approximately 50 μg/day during the last trimester. Because vitamin A in the mother's diet may be stored and mobilized later as needed and some vitamin A may be retained in the placenta, the EAR is estimated to be ~50 μg/day in addition to the EAR for nonpregnant adolescent girls and women for the entire pregnancy period.

Vitamin A EAR and RDA Summary, Pregnancy

EAR for Pregnancy
14–18 years	530 μg RAE/day of vitamin A
19–30 years	550 μg RAE/day of vitamin A
31–50 years	550 μg RAE/day of vitamin A

The RDA for vitamin A is set by using a CV of 20 percent based on the calculated half-life values for liver vitamin A (see "Adults Ages 19 Years and Older"). The RDA is defined as equal to the EAR plus twice the CV to cover the needs of 97 to 98 percent of individuals in the group (therefore, for vitamin A the RDA is 140 percent of the EAR). The calculated values for the RDAs have been rounded up to the nearest 10 μg.

RDA for Pregnancy

14–18 years	750 μg RAE/day of vitamin A
19–30 years	770 μg RAE/day of vitamin A
31–50 years	770 μg RAE/day of vitamin A

Lactation

Evidence Considered in Estimating the Average Requirement

As indicated earlier in the section on infants, human milk-fed infants consume on average 400 μg/day of vitamin A in the first 6 months of life. The carotenoid content of human milk has been summarized in *Dietary Reference Intakes for Vitamin C, Vitamin E, Selenium, and Carotenoids* (IOM, 2000). Because the bioconversion of carotenoids in milk and in infants is not known, the contribution of carotenoids in human milk to meeting the vitamin A requirement of infants was not considered. To set an EAR during pregnancy, 400 μg RAE/day is added to the EAR for nonpregnant adolescent girls and women to assure adequate body stores of vitamin A.

Vitamin A EAR and RDA Summary, Lactation

EAR for Lactation

14–18 years	885 μg RAE/day of vitamin A
19–30 years	900 μg RAE/day of vitamin A
31–50 years	900 μg RAE/day of vitamin A

The RDA for vitamin A is set by using a CV of 20 percent based on the calculated half-life values for liver vitamin A (see "Adults Ages 19 Years and Older"). The RDA is defined as equal to the EAR plus twice the CV to cover the needs of 97 to 98 percent of individuals in the group (therefore, for vitamin A the RDA is 140 percent of the EAR). The calculated values for the RDAs have been rounded to the nearest 100 μg.

RDA for Lactation

14–18 years	1,200 μg RAE/day of vitamin A
19–30 years	1,300 μg RAE/day of vitamin A
31–50 years	1,300 μg RAE/day of vitamin A

Requirement for Provitamin A Carotenoids

Although a large body of observational epidemiological evidence suggests that higher blood concentrations of β-carotene and other carotenoids obtained from foods are associated with a lower risk of several chronic diseases (see *Dietary Reference Intakes for Vitamin C, Vitamin E, Selenium, and Carotenoids* [IOM, 2000]), no evidence pointed to the need for a certain percentage of dietary vitamin A to come from provitamin A carotenoids to meet the vitamin A requirement. In view of the health benefits associated with consumption of fruits and vegetables, existing recommendations for increased consumption of carotenoid-rich fruits and vegetables are strongly supported (see IOM, 2000). Consumption of five servings of fruits and vegetables per day could provide 5.2 to 6 mg/day of provitamin A carotenoids (Lachance, 1997), which would contribute approximately 50 to 65 percent of the men's RDA for vitamin A.

Special Considerations

Alcohol Consumption

Excessive alcohol consumption results in a depletion of liver vitamin A stores (Leo and Lieber, 1985). Depletion is partly due to the reduced consumption of foods. Furthermore, mobilization of vitamin A out of the liver may be increased with excessive alcohol consumption (Lieber and Leo, 1986). Because alcohol intake has been shown to enhance the toxicity of vitamin A (Leo and Lieber, 1999) (see "Tolerable Upper Intake Levels"), individuals who consume alcohol may be distinctly susceptible to the adverse effects of vitamin A and any increased intake to meet one's needs should be in the context of maintaining health.

Developing Countries and Vegetarian Diets

A number of factors can influence the requirement for vitamin A, including iron status, the presence and severity of infection and parasites, the level of dietary fat, protein energy malnutrition, and the available sources for preformed vitamin A and provitamin A carotenoids.

Parasites and Infection. Malabsorption of vitamin A can occur with diarrhea and intestinal infestations (Jalal et al., 1998; Sivakumar and Reddy, 1972). Furthermore, the urinary excretion of vitamin A is increased with infection, and especially with fever (Alvarez et al., 1995; Stephensen et al., 1994). For these reasons, with parasitic infestation and during infection, the requirement for vitamin A may be greater than the requirements set in this report, which are based on generally healthy individuals.

Protein Energy Malnutrition. Protein synthesis generally, and specifically retinol binding protein synthesis, is reduced with severe protein energy malnutrition (PEM) (marasmus and kwashiorkor), and therefore release of retinol from the liver (assuming stores are present) is also reduced (Large et al., 1980). With successful dietary treatment of PEM, growth and tissue weight gain will be stimulated, and the relative requirement of vitamin A will increase during the recovery period.

Vegetarianism. Preformed vitamin A is found only in animal-derived food products. A clinical sign of vitamin A deficiency, night blindness, is prevalent in developing countries where animal and vitamin A-fortified products are not commonly available. Although carotenoids such as β-carotene are abundant in green leafy vegetables and certain fruits, because it takes 12 µg of dietary β-carotene to provide 1 retinol activity equivalent (RAE) (as compared to previous recommendations where 1 µg of retinol was thought to be provided by 6 µg of β-carotene [NRC, 1989 and Table 4-3]), a greater amount of fruits and vegetables than previously recommended are required to meet the daily vitamin A requirement for vegetarians and those whose primary source of vitamin A is green leafy vegetables.

Analyzing intakes of vitamin A and β-carotene and using an RAE of 12 µg for dietary β-carotene indicate that the RDA for vitamin A can be met by those consuming a strict vegetarian diet containing the deeply colored fruits and vegetables (1,262 µg RAE) that are major sources of β-carotene in the United States (Chug-Ahuja et al., 1993) (Table 4-6). The United States has several vitamin A-fortified foods, including milk, cereals, and infant formula. Furthermore, certain food products, such as sugar, are being fortified with vitamin A in some developing countries. If menus are restricted in the amounts of provitamin A carotenoids consumed and such fortified products are not part of routine diets, then vitamin A supplements may be required.

Populations Where Consumption of Vitamin A-Rich Foods is Limited. Three major intervention trials have been conducted in developing countries to evaluate the efficacy of provitamin A carotenoids in

TABLE 4-6 Vitamin A Intake from a Vegan Diet High in
Carotene-Rich Fruits and Vegetables

Meal	Foods Eaten	β-Carotene Equivalents Intake[a] (µg)	Retinol Intake (µg)	Vitamin A Intake (µg RAE[b])
Breakfast	Bagel (1 medium)	0	0	0
	Peanut butter (2 T)	1	0	0
	Canned pineapple, juice pack (1/2 cup)	40	0	3
	Orange juice (3/4 cup)	103	0	9
	Total for meal	143	0	12
Snack	Banana (1 medium)	28	0	2
	Total for snack	28	0	2
Lunch	Vegetable soup, prepared from ready-to-serve can (1 cup)	1,195	0	166
	Hummus (2 T)	2	0	0
	White pita (1 large)	0	0	0
	Soy milk (1 cup)	0	0	0
	Apple, with skin (1 medium)	70	0	6
	Total for meal	2,067	0	172
Dinner	Lettuce salad: romaine lettuce (1 cup) with tomato (2 wedges) and oil and vinegar dressing (2 T)	850	0	71
	Baked sweet potato (1 medium)	10,195	0	850
	Bean burrito (1 medium) with avocado (3 slices) and salsa (2 T)	165	0	13
	Soy milk (1 cup)	0	0	0
	Total for meal	11,210	0	934
Snack	Vegetable juice (3/4 cup)	1,697	0	141
	Nuts, seeds and dried fruit mixture (1/4 cup)	2	0	0
	Total for snack	1,699	0	141
Daily Totals		15,148	0	1,262

NOTE: Source of food composition data: NDS-R Food and Nutrient Data Base, Version 30, 1999, Nutrition Coordinating Center, University of Minnesota. Nutrient totals may not equal the sum of the parts.
[a] β-Carotene equivalents (µg) = µg β-carotene + 1/2(µg α-carotene + µg β-cryptoxanthin).
[b] RAE = retinol activity equivalents; 1 RAE = 1 µg retinol + 1/12(µg β-carotene equivalents).

maintaining or improving vitamin A status in lactating women (de Pee et al., 1995), preschool children (Jalal et al., 1998), and young children (Takyi, 1999). Vitamin A status, as determined by serum retinol concentration, was not improved in Indonesian lactating women after the consumption of dark green leafy vegetables (de Pee et al., 1995). These women had hemoglobin concentrations less than 13 mg/dL. There is evidence that iron deficiency impairs the metabolism of vitamin A in laboratory animals (Jang et al., 2000; Rosales et al., 1999). In some, but not all, studies (Suharno et al., 1993), iron supplementation improved vitamin A status in humans (Munoz et al., 2000). Therefore the presence of iron deficiency, which is prevalent in developing countries, may impair the efficacy of dark green leafy vegetables. Jalal and coworkers (1998) reported that the addition of β-carotene-rich foods to the diets of preschool children improved vitamin A status, however, vitamin A status improved almost as well when fat was added to the diet and an anthelmintic drug to destroy parasitic worms was provided. This finding demonstrates the importance of dietary fat, which is often low in the diets of developing countries and the importance of intestinal parasites on vitamin A status. Takyi (1999) reported that the vitamin A status of young children improved similarly when fed either a pureed β-carotene-rich diet or provided a similar amount of β-carotene as a supplement. Here, in contrast to the findings of Jalal et al. (1998), dietary fat and anthelmentic drugs did not appear to have a beneficial effect on vitamin A status, possibly because the carotenoid was already provided in a highly absorbable, pureed form.

The EARs that have been set for the North American population are achievable through diet because of the abundance of vitamin A-rich foods. Populations of less developed countries may have difficulty in meeting the EAR that ensures adequate vitamin A stores. Therefore, an EAR that does not assure adequate vitamin A stores has been determined on the basis of the level of vitamin A for correction of abnormal dark adaptation in adults. This approach does not assure adequate stores of vitamin A because animal studies indicate that vitamin A depletion of the eye occurs after the depletion of hepatic vitamin A reserves (Bankson et al., 1989; Lewis et al., 1942). Furthermore, epidemiological studies in children suggest impaired host resistance to infection, presumably reflecting compromised immunity and represented by increased risk of morbidity and mortality at lesser stages of depletion (Arroyave et al., 1979; Arthur et al., 1992; Barreto et al., 1994; Bloem et al., 1990; Ghana

VAST Study Team, 1993; Loyd-Puryear et al., 1991; Rahmathullah et al., 1990; Salazar-Lindo et al., 1993; West et al., 1991).

An EAR of 300 µg RAE/day can be calculated based on the dark adaptation data obtained from 13 individuals from four studies on adults (Table 4-4). The duration of depletion and repletion varied among these four studies and the majority of the studies were conducted on men. Interpolation of the level of vitamin A at which dark adaptation of each individual was corrected in these four studies results in a median intake of 300 µg RAE/day, which can be used to set an EAR based on dark adaptation for adults. Using this method, there was insufficient evidence to support setting a different EAR for men and for women, as there were too few women studied. EARs using dark adaptation as the indicator for children (1–3 years, 112 µg RAE/day; 4–8 years, 150 µg RAE/day; 9–13 years, 230 µg RAE/day) and adolescents (14–18 years, 300 µg RAE/day) are based on extrapolation from the adult EAR as described in Chapter 2.

INTAKE OF VITAMIN A

Food Sources

Common dietary sources of preformed vitamin A in the United States and Canada include liver, dairy products, and fish. Chug-Ahuja et al. (1993) reported that carrots were the major contributor of β-carotene (25 percent). Other major contributors to β-carotene intakes included cantaloupe, broccoli, squash, peas, and spinach. Carrots were also the major contributor (51 percent) of α-carotene. Fruits were the sole contributors of β-cryptoxanthin. According to data collected from the 1994–1996 Continuing Survey of Food Intakes by Individuals (CFSII), the major contributors of vitamin A from foods were grains and vegetables (approximately 55 percent), followed by dairy and meat products (approximately 30 percent).

Dietary Intake

The Third National Health and Nutrition Examination Survey (NHANES III) (Appendix Table C-8) estimated that the median dietary intake of vitamin A is 744 to 811 µg/day for men and 530 to 716 µg/day for women using the new provitamin A carotenoid conversion factors for calculating retinol activity equivalents (RAE) (see Table 4-3). When one examines Appendix Table C-8 to determine the proportion of individuals with intakes that were less than the EAR (500 µg RAE/day for women and 625 µg RAE/day for men), it is apparent that for most age groups between 25 and 50 percent of adults fell in this category. The EAR for vitamin A is based on a criterion of adequate liver stores; thus, these data suggest that considerable proportions of adults have liver vitamin A stores that are less than desirable. It should be recognized that this does not represent a clinical deficiency state, such as abnormal dark adaptation.

Because the level of vitamin A intake varies greatly (Beaton et al., 1983), it is very important that the daily intake distribution be adjusted for day-to-day variability in intakes when assessing intake distributions of groups to determine the proportion with intakes below the EAR. This adjustment can be carried out using the methods of Nusser et al. (1986) and the National Research Council (NRC, 1986).

When reporting as RAE, the vitamin A activity of provitamin A carotenoids is half the activity given as retinol equivalents (RE) (Table 4-3). Therefore, vitamin A intakes calculated using RAE are less than intakes determined using RE (compare Appendix Tables C-7 and C-8) resulting in a higher percentage of certain groups who consume levels of vitamin A less than the EAR. Thus, a greater amount of provitamin A carotenoids, and therefore darkly colored, carotene-rich fruits and vegetables, is needed to meet the vitamin A requirement.

Data from NHANES III indicate that for men 31 to 50 years of age, the median intakes of the provitamin A carotenoids α-carotene, β-carotene, and β-cryptoxanthin, were 51 (2 µg RAE), 1,942 (162 µg RAE), and 39 (1.6 µg RAE) µg/day, respectively (Appendix Tables C-1, C-2 and C-3). Using RAE, dietary β-carotene contributes approximately 21 percent of the total vitamin A intake. All provitamin A carotenoids contributed 26 and 34 percent of vitamin A consumed by men and women, respectively.

The median intake of other carotenoids, lutein and zeaxanthin, ranged from 1,353 µg/day to 1,966 µg/day for men and women (Appendix Table C-4). For men and women, the median intake of lycopene ranged from 842 to 5,079 µg/day (Appendix Table C-5).

The menus in Table 4-7 show that the total day's vitamin A intake (1,168 µg RAE/day) exceeds the Recommended Dietary Allowance (RDA) when consuming an omnivorous diet and choosing five fruits and vegetables that are major contributors of β-carotene in the United States. The RDA can also be achieved for individuals consuming vegetarian diets high in carotene-rich fruits and vegetables (Table 4-6).

TABLE 4-7 Vitamin A Intake from an Omnivorous Diet High in Carotene-Rich Fruits and Vegetables

Meal	Foods Eaten	β-Carotene Equivalents Intake[a] (μg)	Retinol Intake (μg)	Vitamin A Intake (μg RAE[b])
Breakfast	Ready-to-eat oat cereal (1 cup)	1	150	150
	Skim milk (1/2 cup)	0	75	75
	Toasted wheat bread (2 medium slices) with margarine (2 pats)	53	95	99
	Orange juice (3/4 cup)	103	0	9
	Total for meal	157	319	332
Lunch	Roast beef sandwich (1 medium)	49	0	4
	Vegetable soup, prepared from ready-to-serve can (1 cup)	1,195	0	166
	Nectarine (1 medium)	177	0	15
	Cola (12 fl oz)	0	0	0
	Total for meal	2,221	0	185
Dinner	Lettuce salad: iceberg lettuce (1 cup) with tomato (2 wedges) and creamy dressing (2 T)	247	6	27
	Chicken pot pie (8 oz)	2,333	3	197
	Cooked broccoli (1/2 cup)	943	0	79
	White dinner roll (1 medium) with margarine (1 pat)	23	47	49
	Skim milk (1 cup)	0	149	149
	Total for meal	3,547	205	501
Snack	Skim milk (1 cup)	0	149	149
	Oatmeal cookie (1 medium)	0	0	0
	Total for snack	0	149	149
Daily Totals		5,925	647	1,168

NOTE: Source of food composition data: NDS-R Food and Nutrient Data Base, Version 30, 1999, Nutrition Coordinating Center, University of Minnesota. Nutrient totals may not equal the sum of the parts.
[a] β-Carotene equivalents (μg) = μg β-carotene + 1/2(μg α-carotene + μg β-cryptoxanthin).
[b] RAE = retinol activity equivalents; 1 RAE = μg retinol + 1/12(μg β-carotene equivalents).

Intake from Supplements

Information from NHANES III on Americans' use of supplements containing vitamin A is given in Appendix Table C-9. The median intake of vitamin A from supplements was approximately 1,430 µg RAE/day for men and women. In 1986, approximately 26 percent of adults in the United States took supplements that contained vitamin A (Moss et al., 1989; see Table 2-2).

TOLERABLE UPPER INTAKE LEVELS

The Tolerable Upper Intake Level (UL) is the highest level of daily vitamin A intake that is likely to pose no risk of adverse health effects in almost all individuals. Although members of the general population should be advised not to routinely exceed the UL, intake above the UL may be appropriate for investigation within well-controlled clinical trials. Clinical trials of doses above the UL should not be discouraged as long as subjects participating in these trials have signed informed consent documents regarding possible toxicity and as long as these trials employ appropriate safety monitoring of trial subjects. In addition, the UL is not meant to apply to individuals who are receiving vitamin A under medical supervision. The UL for provitamin A carotenoids has been addressed in the report *Dietary Reference Intakes for Vitamin C, Vitamin E, Selenium, and Carotenoids* (IOM, 2000).

Hazard Identification

There are substantial data on the adverse effects of high vitamin A intakes. Acute toxicity is characterized by nausea, vomiting, headache, increased cerebrospinal fluid pressure, vertigo, blurred vision, muscular incoordination (Olson, 1983), and bulging fontanel in infants (Persson et al., 1965). These are usually transient effects involving single or short-term large doses of greater than or equal to 150,000 µg in adults and proportionately less in children (Bendich and Langseth, 1989). The clinical picture for chronic hypervitaminosis A is varied and nonspecific and may include central nervous system effects, liver abnormalities, bone and skin changes, and other adverse effects. Chronic toxicity is usually associated with ingestion of large doses greater than or equal to 30,000 µg/day for months or years. Both acute and chronic vitamin A toxicity are associated with increased plasma retinyl ester concentrations (Krasinski et al., 1989; Ross, 1999).

For the purpose of deriving a UL, three primary adverse effects of chronic vitamin A intake are discussed below: (1) reduced bone mineral density, (2) teratogenicity, and (3) liver abnormalities. High β-carotene intake has not been shown to cause hypervitaminosis A. Therefore, this review is limited to the adverse effects of preformed vitamin A or retinol. The terms *vitamin A* and *retinol* will be used interchangeably in the following sections. Because provitamin A carotenoids were not included in vitamin A supplements until the late 1980s, it is assumed that studies and case reports published before 1990 used preformed vitamin A in supplements. The UL derived here applies to chronic intake of preformed vitamin A from food, fortified food, and/or supplements.

Adverse Effects in Adults

Bone Mineral Density. Chronic, excessive vitamin A intake has been shown to lead to bone mineral loss in animals (Rohde et al., 1999), making such a consequence in humans biologically plausible. Most human case reports are not well described and epidemiological studies are inadequate in design. However, four studies provide interpretable evidence relating changes in bone mineral density (BMD) and risk of hip fracture with variation in dietary intake of preformed vitamin A (Freudenheim et al., 1986; Houtkooper et al., 1995; Melhus et al., 1998). The studies are distinguished by their well-described study designs and populations, adequate dietary intake estimates, and accurate methods for measuring BMD at multiple sites.

One two-part study (Melhus et al., 1998) suggests that a chronic intake of 1.5 mg/day of preformed vitamin A is associated with osteoporosis and increased risk of hip fracture. The first part, a cross-sectional multivariate regression analysis in 175 Swedish women 28 to 74 years of age, showed a consistent loss in BMD at four sites and in total BMD with increased preformed vitamin A intake. Numerous nutritional and non-nutritional exposures were concurrently assessed, allowing substantial control of potential confounders. With the use of stratified estimates of retinol intake in a univariate regression analysis, BMD was shown to increase with each 0.5 mg/day increment in intake above a reference intake of less than 0.5 mg/day, until intakes exceeded 1.5 mg/day. Above this level, mean BMD decreased markedly at each site. In a multivariate model, adjusting for effects of 14 other covariates, similar results were found. It is not clear whether the findings are equally applicable to pre- and postmenopausal women.

The second part was a nested case-control study on the risk factors for hip fracture. Cases were mostly postmenopausal women with first hip fracture within 2 to 64 months after entry into the large cohort study, or 5 to 67 months after the mid-point of the recalled dietary assessment. Four matched control subjects were selected for each case. A total of 247 cases and 873 control subjects completed the study. Univariate and multivariate conditional logistic regression analysis showed a dose-dependent increase in the risk of hip fracture with each 0.5 mg/day increment in reported retinol intake above 0.5 mg/day (baseline). The odds ratio was 2.05 (95 percent confidence interval, 1.05–3.98) at intakes above 1.5 mg/day.

In contrast to the results of Melhus and coworkers (1998), which suggest that risk of bone mineral loss and hip fracture occurs at estimated intakes above 1.5 mg/day, two U.S. studies provide no evidence of increased bone mineral loss in women with intakes of preformed vitamin A up to 1.5 to 2.0 mg/day (Freudenheim et al., 1986; Houtkooper et al., 1995). Freudenheim and coworkers (1986) evaluated the correlation between mean 3-year vitamin A intakes ranging from approximately 2 to 3 mg/day and rates of change in BMD in 84 women, 35 to 65 years of age (17 pre- and 67 post-menopausal). No consistent relationship was reported between vitamin A intake and the rate of bone mineral content loss in pre- and postmenopausal women. The single subject who showed rapid bone mineral loss with very high vitamin A intake also appeared to have consumed large amounts of other micronutrients as well, obscuring the significance of this relationship. Further, this study suffers from a small sample size in each of the four key groups (i.e., pre- and postmenopausal women by calcium supplement status), making correlations of potential nutritional or pathological importance indeterminate.

Houtkooper and coworkers (1995), in a longitudinal study of 66 women 28 to 39 years of age, showed that vitamin A intake was significantly associated with the increased annual rate of change in total body BMD. The mean rate of change in total body BMD over the 18-month study was negative, although several sites (lumbar spine, trochanter, and Ward's triangle) showed small positive slopes. The estimated mean intake of preformed vitamin A from the diet was 1,220 ± 472 (standard deviation [SD]) µg/day. The estimated vitamin A intake from provitamin A carotenoids was 595 ± 352 (SD) µg/day. In multivariable regression models that included covariables for body composition and treatment (exercise versus sedentary) status, the slopes for vitamin A and carotene (two separate models) were both positive [b = 0.007 and 0.008 mg/(cm^2-year)] with r^2 values of ~0.30 for each model. While the positive association between vitamin A and carotene intake and change in BMD may not be causal, the data provide evidence that vitamin A does not adversely affect premenopausal bone health within this range of intake.

The findings from these studies are provocative but conflicting, and therefore, they are not useful for setting a UL for vitamin A. More research is needed to clarify whether chronic vitamin A intake, at levels that characterize upper-usual intake ranges for many American and European populations, may lead to loss in BMD and consequent increased risk of hip fracture in certain population groups, particularly among pre- and postmenopausal women.

Teratogenicity. Concern for the possible teratogenicity of high vitamin A intake in humans is based on the unequivocal demonstration of human teratogenicity of 13-*cis*-retinoic acid (Lammer et al., 1985) after supplementation with high doses of vitamin A (Eckhoff and Nau, 1990; Eckhoff et al., 1991). Numerous studies in experimental animals clearly establish the teratogenic potential of excessive intakes of vitamin A (Cohlan, 1953, 1954; Geelen, 1979; Hutchings and Gaston, 1974; Hutchings et al., 1973; Kalter and Warkany, 1961; Pinnock and Alderman, 1992).

Epidemiological data show the possibility of teratogenic effects with high intakes of preformed vitamin A (Table 4-8). The critical period for susceptibility appears to be the first trimester of pregnancy and the primary birth defects associated with excess vitamin A intake are those derived from cranial neural crest (CNC) cells such as craniofacial malformations and abnormalities of the central nervous system (except neural tube defects), thymus, and heart. Examination of the data suggests a likely dose-dependent association between vitamin A intake at excessive levels and the risk of birth defects. One case-control report showed a statistically nonsignificant association between a reported maternal intake of greater than 12,000 µg/day and malformations, but not below that level (Martinez-Frias and Salvador, 1990). Two other large case-control studies showed no relationship between risk of malformation and likely supplemental daily doses of 2,400 to 3,000 µg by mothers (Khoury et al., 1996; Shaw et al., 1996). An observational study by Rothman and co-workers (1995) involving 22,748 pregnant women found that those who ingested greater than 4,500 µg/day of preformed vitamin A from food and supplements were at greater risk of delivering infants with malformations of CNC cell origin (e.g., cleft lip or palate) than were women consuming less than 1,500 µg/day. But questions have been raised about the accuracy of intake estimates and birth defects diagnosed. It has been argued further that the limited number of excess cases used to identify a toxicity threshold of 4,500 μg/day of preformed vitamin A (or 3,000 μg from supplements) permits the study's findings to be consistent with a larger threshold than other studies would suggest (Brent et al., 1996; Mastroiacovo et al., 1999; Watkins et al., 1996; Werler et al., 1996). Thus, while few dispute a causal association between excessive periconceptual vitamin A intake and risk of malformation, the threshold at which risk increases remains a matter of debate. However, in the context of the totality of data on vitamin A and birth defects, the data of Rothman and coworkers (1995) provide supportive evidence of a causal association. Case reports of malformations exist to support an increased risk of birth defects above a maternal intake of 7,800 μg/day of vitamin A (Bauernfcind, 1980; Bernhardt and Dorsey, 1974). Human case reports support a temporal association between maternal exposure to elevated vitamin A intakes and birth defects (Bernhardt and Dorsey, 1974; Von Lennep et al., 1985).

Liver Abnormalities. There is a strong causal association shown by human and animal data between excess vitamin A intake and liver abnormalities because the liver is the main storage site and target organ for vitamin A toxicity. The wide spectrum of vitamin A-induced liver abnormalities ranges from reversibly elevated liver enzymes to widespread fibrosis, cirrhosis, and sometimes death. Table 4-9 shows consistency and specificity of the following effects in liver pathology: spontaneous green fluorescence of sinusoidal cells, perisinusoidal fibrosis, hyperplasia, and hypertrophy of Ito cells. Human data are potentially confounded by other factors related to liver damage such as alcohol intake, hepatitis A, B, and C, hepatotoxic medications, or preexisting liver disease. A thorough evaluation of the liver data is provided in the later section, "Dose-Response Assessment".

Adverse Interactions. Alcohol intake has been shown to enhance the toxicity of vitamin A (Leo and Lieber, 1999). In particular, the hepatotoxicity of vitamin A may be potentiated by alcohol use. Therefore, alcohol drinkers may be distinctly susceptible to the adverse effects of vitamin A.

Adverse Effects in Infants and Children

There are numerous case reports of infants (Table 4-10), toddlers, and children who have demonstrated toxic effects due to ex-

TABLE 4-8 The Relationship Between Reproductive Risk and Excess Preformed Vitamin A in Humans

Study	Design	Subjects	Daily Dose (µg/day)
Martinez-Frias and Salvador, 1990	Case control study	11,293 cases of birth defects 11,193 controls	< 12,000 ≥ 12,000 (supplemental forms)
Dudas and Czeizel, 1992	Letter	1,203 exposed 1,510 nonexposed	1,800
Rothman et al., 1995	Cohort study	22,748 pregnant women	≤ 1,500 control > 3,000 supplement > 4,500 supplement + food
Khoury et al., 1996	Case control study	1,623 cases[b] 3,029 controls[b]	< 2,400[c]
Shaw et al., 1996	Case control study	925 cases of birth defects 871 controls	≥ 3,000 (presumed)
Mills et al., 1997	Case control study	89 cases 573 controls	< 1,500 (supplement + fortification) > 2,400 (supplement + fortification) > 3,000 (supplement + fortification)
Czeizel and Rockenbauer, 1998	Case control pair analysis	20,830 cases 35,727 controls	Estimated range: 150–30,000 Most < 3,000

Time of Exposure	Results	Conclusions
NA	Risk ratio for birth defects 0.5 ($p = 0.15$) 2.7 ($p = 0.06$)	This suggests women of reproductive age may be at increased risk of teratogenicity at vitamin A exposures $\geq$ 12,000 µg/day
-1 to 3 mo gestation	Cranial neural crest defects not observed in exposed group	The comparison of the rate and pattern of congenital abnormalities in exposed and nonexposed groups did not indicate any teratogenic effect of vitamin A
First trimester	Risk ratio for neural crest defects 1.0 4.8 3.5[a]	Vitamin A intakes > 3,000 µg/d, significant increased risk of cranial neural crest defects
-1 to 3 mo gestation	Risk ratio for cranial neural crest defects 1.36 vitamin A supplement 0.69 vitamin A + multivitamin supplement	No increased risks of defects from cranial neural crest among vitamin A and multivitamin users
-1 to 3 mo gestation	Risk ratio 0.55	No increased risk of orofacial clefts at vitamin A intakes $\geq$ 3,000 µg/d compared to controls
-15 d to 1 mo gestation	Risk ratio 1.0 0.76 1.09	No association between periconceptional vitamin A at doses > 2,400 or > 10,000 µg/d and malformations in general and cranial neural crest defects
1 to 9 mo gestation	Fewer cases were treated with vitamin A (1,642 or 7.9%) than controls (3,399 or 9.5%) ($p < 0.001$)	Vitamin A doses < 3,000 µg/d during the first trimester of pregnancy is not teratogenic

continued

TABLE 4-8 Continued

Study	Design	Subjects	Daily Dose (µg/day)
Mastroiacovo et al., 1999	Cohort study	311 infants evaluated	Median: 15,000 Range: 3,000–100,000

[a] 3.5 = the ratio of the prevalence among babies born to women who consumed more than 4,500 µg/d of preformed vitamin A/d from food and supplements to the prevalence among the babies whose mothers consumed 1,500 µg or less/d. For vitamin A from supplements alone, the ratio of the prevalence among the babies born to women who consumed more than 3,000 µg/day to that among the babies whose mothers consumed 1,500 µg/d or less was 4.8.

cess vitamin A intakes for months to years. Of particular concern are intracranial (bulging fontanel) and skeletal abnormalities that can result in infants given vitamin A doses of 5,500 to 6,750 µg/day (Persson et al., 1965). The clinical presentation of vitamin A toxicity in infants and young children varies widely. The more commonly recognized signs and symptoms include skeletal abnormalities, bone tenderness and pain, increased intracranial pressure, desquamation, brittle nails, mouth fissures, alopecia, fever, headache, lethargy, irritability, weight loss, vomiting, and hepatomegaly (Bush and Dahms, 1984). Furthermore, tolerance to excess vitamin A intake also appears to vary (Carpenter et al., 1987). Carpenter and coworkers (1987) described two boys who developed hypervitaminosis A by age 2 years for one and by age 6 years for the other. Both were given chicken liver that supplied about 690 µg/day of vitamin A and various supplements that supplied another 135 to 750 µg/day. An older sister who had been treated similarly remained completely healthy.

Summary

Based on considerations of causality, quality, and completeness of the database, teratogenicity was selected as the critical adverse effect on which to base a UL for women of childbearing age. For all other adults, liver abnormalities were the critical adverse effect. Abnormal

Time of Exposure	Results	Conclusions
0 to 9 wk gestation	Risk ratio of prevalence of major malformations in treated group vs. controls was 0.5	Daily intake of preformed vitamin A supplement ≥ 3,000 µg/d does not seem to increase risk of serious anomalies of structures with a cranial neural crest cell contribution

[b] Cases refer to mothers of infants with cranial neural crest-derived defects ascertained within the first year of life. Controls represent mothers of infants without birth defects, frequency-matched to cases by period of birth, race, and hospital of birth.

[c] There was no information to quantify the actual vitamin A content of the supplements or multivitamins. During the period of the study, most were expected to contain under 2,400 µg and contained preformed vitamin A.

liver pathology, characteristic of vitamin A intoxication (or grossly elevated hepatic vitamin A levels), was selected rather than elevated liver enzymes because of the uncertainties regarding other possible causes such as concurrent use of hepatotoxic drugs, alcohol intake, and hepatitis B and C. Bone changes were not used because of the conflicting findings and the lack of other data confirming the findings of Melhus et al. (1998).

Dose-Response Assessment

Women of Reproductive Age

Data Selection. Epidemiological studies evaluating the teratogenicity of vitamin A intake shortly before or during pregnancy (Table 4-8) were used to derive a UL for women of reproductive age. Because adequate human data were available, animal data were not used to derive a UL.

Identification of a No-Observed-Adverse-Effect Level (NOAEL). A NOAEL of approximately 4,500 µg/day of preformed vitamin A from food and supplements was based on a critical evaluation of the data in Table 4-8. There are numerous reports showing no adverse effects at doses below 3,000 µg/day of vitamin A from supplements (Czeizel and Rockenbauer, 1998; Dudas and Czeizel, 1992; Khoury et al.,

TABLE 4-9 Evidence of Liver Abnormalities After Excess Preformed Vitamin A Intakes (< 30,000 µg/day), Based on Increasing Dose

Case Reports	Subject	Dose (µg/d)	Duration (y)	Outcome[a]
Oren and Ilan, 1992	Woman, 56 y	1,515	10	Severe fibrosis to portal areas; ALP (870 U/L)
Weber et al., 1982	Man, 62 y	6,000 (supplement) 10,000 (food[b]) 4,500 (food[c]) 7,500 (supplement)	6 1	Increase of vitamin A in liver (5,700 µg/g); decrease in serum vitamin A & RBP; liver biopsy: lipid vacuoles within hepatocyte cytoplasm; sinusoidal fibrosis; lipid-filled Ito cells
Hatoff et al., 1982	Vegetarian man, 42 y	7,600[d] (supplement) 7,600 (food[e])	10	Acute hypervitaminosis A precipitated by viral hepatitis B infection; liver biopsy showed many lipid-filled Ito cells; enlarged Kupffer cells; perisinusoidal fibrosis; increase in liver and serum vitamin A; headache, skin desquamation, hypercalcemia, and confusion
Kowalski et al., 1994	Woman, 45 y	7,600	6	Severe hepatotoxicity
Eaton, 1978	Woman, 51 y	8,300–10,600 (diet + supplements)	30	Cirrhosis; portal hypertension; marked fibrosis
	Woman, 63 y	14,000 from supplements (information on diet not provided)	10	AST (73 U/L), ALT (96 U/L), ALP (258 U/L); vacuolated, lipid-filled Ito cells

Hepatitis	Increased Alcohol Use	Other Factors
No history of hepatitis or blood transfusions; negative immunological profiles	No	None
Hepatitis B	No	It is possible that effects were due to protein deficiency
Hepatitis B	Limited (3 beers/ wk)	
Hepatitis A, B, and C	No	Patient's health status; meds
Unknown	No	
Two blood transfusions 30 y previously Hepatitis A HbsAg anti-HBc	Extremely rare	

continued

TABLE 4-9 Continued

Case Reports	Subject	Dose (μg/d)	Duration (y)	Outcome[a]
Minuk et al., 1988	Man, 62 y	14,000 from supplement (diet contained no raw meat or seafood)	10	AST (124 U/L), ALT (256 U/L), ALP (76 U/L), albumin (46 g/L), increase in total bilirubin; tests for IgM antibody to hepatitis A virus, HbsAg and anti-HBc were negative
Zafrani et al., 1984	Man, 36 y	15,000 from supplement	12	Increase in liver vitamin A concentration; spontaneous green fluorescence of sinusoidal cells; perisinusoidal fibrosis and hyperplasia; hypertrophy of Ito cells; portal and periportal fibrosis; lesions of hepatic sinusoids randomly distributed areas of sinusoidal dilation; RBCs present in Disse's spaces; sinusoidal barrier abnormalities mimicking peliosis hepatitis
Zafrani et al., 1984	Woman, 25 y	26,000	8	Hepatic lesions; spontaneous green fluorescence of sinusoidal cells; perisinusoidal fibrosis, hyperplasia, and hypertrophy of Ito cells; randomly distributed areas of sinusoidal dilation; RBCs present in Disse's spaces; sinusoidal barrier abnormalities mimicking peliosis hepatitis

Hepatitis	Increased Alcohol Use	Other Factors
Hepatitis A virus infection 5 y earlier	Not excessive	No meds
Negative hepatitis B surface antigen; positive serum hepatitis B surface and core antibodies	No	No meds
Negative hepatitis B surface antigen; negative serum hepatitis B surface and core antibodies	No	None

continued

TABLE 4-9 Continued

Case Reports	Subject	Dose (μg/d)	Duration (y)	Outcome[a]
Geubel et al., 1991	41 cases, 9–76 y	Mean, 29,000	Mean, 4.6	Cirrhosis ($n = 9$); mild, chronic hepatitis ($n = 10$); noncirrhotic portal hypertension ($n = 5$); fat storing cell hyperplasia and hypertrophy ($n = 9$); death ($n = 6$)
Farrell et al., 1977	Woman, 57 y	30,000 (supplement) 1,600 (food)	4	Serum ALP (108 U/L); serum AST (72 U/L); increased size and number of fat storing cells

[a] ALP = alkaline phosphatase (normal range = 0–36 U/L), AST = aspartate aminotransferase (normal range = 45–110 U/L), ALT = alanine aminotransferase (normal range = 0–41 U/L).
[b] Ingestion of sweet potatoes, carrots, peaches, tomatoes, and desiccated beef liver accounted for this high vitamin A intake.
[c] Diet included sweet potatoes, carrots, peaches, tomatoes, and desiccated beef liver.

1996; Rothman et al., 1995) or 4,500 μg/day of preformed vitamin A from food and supplements (Rothman et al., 1995). Rothman and coworkers (1995) showed a significantly increased risk of birth defects at the cranial neural crest sites among women who consumed greater than 4,500 μg of preformed vitamin A/day from food and supplements during the first trimester compared to those who took 1,500 μg/day or less. Most of the human data on teratogenicity of vitamin A involve doses equal to or greater than 7,800 μg/day. There are limited epidemiological data to clearly define a dose-response relationship in the dose range of 3,000 to 7,800 μg/day. Nevertheless, 4,500 μg/day represents a conservative value for a NOAEL in light of the evidence of no adverse effects at or below that level.

Hepatitis	Increased Alcohol Use	Other Factors
No hepatitis B virus	No	Meds
Not reported		Unknown

d Subject took an additional vitamin A capsule (7,500 µg/d) "when under stress" or not feeling well.
e Diet included carrot and raisin salad daily, large amounts of leafy, green vegetables. Subject also took 1,000 IU vitamin D/d and unknown quantities of vitamin E, B-complex, and bone meal.

Uncertainty Assessment. An uncertainty factor (UF) of 1.5 was selected on the basis of inter-individual variability in susceptibility. Because there are substantial data (Table 4-8) showing no adverse effects at doses up to 3,000 µg/day of vitamin A supplements, a higher UF was not justified.

Derivation of a UL. The NOAEL of 4,500 µg/day was divided by the UF of 1.5 to obtain a UL value of 3,000 µg/day for women of reproductive age.

$$UL = \frac{NOAEL}{UF} = \frac{4,500 \text{ µg/day}}{1.5} = 3,000 \text{ µg/day}$$

TABLE 4-10 Cases of Subchronic and Chronic, Low-Dose Vitamin A Toxicity in Infants, Based on Increasing Dose

Report	Age, Gender	Dose (μg/kg/day)	Dose (μg/day)	Form
Persson et al., 1965	4.5 mo, F	840	5,500[a]	Drops[b]
	4.5 mo, M	1,100	6,750	Drops
	4 mo, M	1,200	6,750	Drops
	5.5 mo, M	820	6,750	Drops
Mahoney et al., 1980	7 mo, F	1,700[c]	12,100 (total)	Chicken liver (11,000 μg)[d]; milk (600 μg); supplement (600 μg)
Arena et al., 1951	6.5 mo, F	1,650–4,400[e]	9,100–24,200	Drops in oil solution
Persson et al., 1965	2.5 mo, F	4,250[f]	18,200	Drops
Woodard et al., 1961	2 mo, M	5,250[g]	21,200	Aqueous drops
Bush and Dahms, 1984	11 d, M	14,000	27,300	Drops-Aqualsol A
Naz and Edwards, 1952	9 mo, F	28,570[h]	60,000	Drops in oil

[a] 50 capsules (38,000 μg vitamin A) were consumed over a period of several weeks. The daily dose was not specified.

[b] AD-vimin®. Astra, aqueous suspension. Ten drops correspond to 2,300 μg of vitamin A and 1,500 IU of vitamin D.

[c] Calculation of 1,700 μg/kg/d is based on a reference body weight of 7 kg (for infants 2–6 mo). Because these infants weighed slightly more than 7 kg at 7 mo, using the reference weight of 9 kg would have been inappropriate. Therefore, 12,000 μg/day (total preformed vitamin A intake) ÷ 7 kg = 1,700 μg/kg/d.

[d] The source of 11,000 μg/d of vitamin A was homogenized chicken livers. The actual total vitamin A intake was higher as the children were also consuming a vitamin supple-

Duration (mo)	Adverse Effect
3	Bulging fontanels
2	Bulging fontanels, anorexia, hyperirritability, edema of occipital area, bone changes, skin lesions, desquamation
1	Bulging fontanels, hyperirritability, anorexia, occipital edema, increased head circumference
2.5	Anorexia, hyperirritability, edema of the occipital area, pronounced craniotabes, increased intracranial pressure, skin lesions, skin desquamation, x-ray findings: epiphyseal line changes
4	Bulging anterior fontanels, irritability, vomiting
4	Anorexia, hyperirritability, pronounced craniotabes, x-ray findings: cortical hyperostosis
1.5	Anorexia, hyperirritability, edema of the occipital area, pronounced craniotabes, increased intracranial pressure, skin lesions, skin desquamation, x-ray findings: epiphyseal line changes
2	Anorexia, hyperirritability, edema of the occipital area, pronounced craniotabes, increased intracranial pressure, skin lesions, skin desquamation, falling out of hair, x-ray findings: cortical hyperostosis
0.4	Hypercalcemia, metastatic calcification of the lungs, kidneys, stomach, soft tissue, and skin; peeling skin; erythematous rash; hyperphosphatemia, bleeding disorder; pulmonary insufficiency; and death after 2-week hospital stay
5.5	Anorexia, hyperirritability, edema of the occipital area, increased intracranial pressure, skin lesions, skin desquamation, x-ray findings: cortical hyperostosis

ment containing 600 µg vitamin A, along with a mixed diet high in fruits and vegetables. When the use of the chicken livers was discontinued, the children recovered with no lingering effects.
e Dose in µg/kg/d was calculated assuming the average body weight equaled the arithmetic mean of 3.5 (weight at birth) and 7.5 kg (weight on admission to hospital) = 5.5 kg.
f Dose in µg/kg/d was calculated using the arithmetic mean of the body weight at birth (2,850 g) and the body weight on admission to the hospital (5,590 g) or about 4.2 kg.
g Dose in µg/kg/d was calculated assuming a body weight of 4 kg (body weight at birth).
h Dose in µg/kg/d was calculated using the standard reference weight of 7 kg for infants 0 to 6 mo.

The UL for adolescent girls was adjusted on the basis of relative body weight as described in Chapter 3 with the use of reference weights from Chapter 1 (Table 1-1).

Vitamin A UL Summary, Adolescent Girls and Women Ages 14 through 50 Years, Pregnancy, Lactation

UL for Women
    14–18 years   **2,800 µg/day of preformed vitamin A**
    19–50 years   **3,000 µg/day of preformed vitamin A**

UL for Pregnancy
    14–18 years   **2,800 µg/day of preformed vitamin A**
    19–50 years   **3,000 µg/day of preformed vitamin A**

UL for Lactation
    14–18 years   **2,800 µg/day of preformed vitamin A**
    19–50 years   **3,000 µg/day of preformed vitamin A**

All Other Adults Ages 19 Years and Older, Excluding Women of Childbearing Age

Data Selection. Data on liver abnormalities in humans were used to derive a UL. Because clear toxicity has been demonstrated in numerous studies at doses above 15,000 µg/day, only data involving doses less than 30,000 µg/day of vitamin A were included in Table 4-9. Data were thoroughly evaluated for other potential causes of liver abnormalities. The following criteria for selecting the data sets were used: (1) data must show grossly elevated liver vitamin A levels or hypertrophy of Ito cells, (2) no alcoholism, (3) no concomitant liver hepatitis, and (4) no hepatotoxic drug use. While hepatitis A and B status are known in most cases, testing for hepatitis C did not begin until the early 1990s and is unknown in most cases. Therefore, hepatitis C was not used as a criterion for exclusion.

Two case studies reported hypertrophy of Ito cells in a 63-year-old woman after vitamin A intake of 14,000 µg/day for 10 years (Minuk et al., 1988) and in a 36-year-old man who took about 15,000 µg/day for 12 years (Zafrani et al., 1984). Neither of these reports appear to be confounded by hepatitis A or B viral infections or concomitant exposure to other hepatotoxic agents including alcohol. Reports of vitamin A-induced hepatotoxicity at doses less than 14,000 µg/day were found (Eaton, 1978; Hatoff et al., 1982; Kowalski et al., 1994; Oren and Ilan, 1992). However, as Table 4-9 shows, these studies fail to provide information on other predisposing or confounding factors such as alcohol intake, drugs and medications used, and history of viral hepatitis infection.

Uncertainty Assessment. A UF of 5.0 was selected to account for the severe, irreversible nature of the adverse effect, extrapolation from a lowest-observed-adverse-effect level (LOAEL) to a NOAEL, and interindividual variation in sensitivity.

Derivation of a UL. Hepatotoxicity was reported at vitamin A supplement doses of 14,000 µg/day. A LOAEL of 14,000 µg/day was divided by a UF of 5 to obtain a UL after rounding of 3,000 µg/day for adults other than women of reproductive age. This UL is the same as that set for women of reproductive age, given that the UL is defined as the highest level of daily nutrient intake likely to pose no risk of adverse health effects to almost all of the general population.

$$UL = \frac{LOAEL}{UF} = \frac{14{,}000 \text{ µg/day}}{5} \cong 3{,}000 \text{ µg/day}$$

Vitamin A UL Summary, Ages 19 Years and Older, Excluding Women of Childbearing Age

UL for Men
  ≥ 19 years   **3,000 µg/day of preformed vitamin A**

UL for Women
  ≥ 51 years   **3,000 µg/day of preformed vitamin A**

Infants, Children, and Adolescent Boys

Data Selection. Case reports of hypervitaminosis A in infants were used to identify a LOAEL and derive a UL. Data were not available to identify a NOAEL.

Identification of a LOAEL. A LOAEL of 6,460 µg/day of vitamin A (which was rounded to 6,000 µg/day) was identified by averaging the lowest doses of four case reports (Persson et al., 1965). Four cases of hypervitaminosis A occurred after doses of 5,500 to 6,750 µg/day of vitamin A for 1 to 3 months (Table 4-10). The age of onset of symptoms ranged from 2.5 to 5.5 months and included anorexia, hyperirritability, occipital edema, pronounced craniotabes, bulging fontanels, increased intracranial pressure, and skin lesions and desquamation. The lowest dose associated with a bulging fontanel involved a 4-month-old girl given a daily dose of 24 drops of AD-vimin (about 5,500 µg of vitamin A) for 3 months. Her fontanels bulged 0.5 centimeters above the plane of the skull. The other three cases involved a dose of 6,750 µg/day of vitamin A for 1 to 2.5 months. Increased intracranial pressure and bulging fontanels were observed in these cases as well. Other effects observed at the higher dose included anorexia, hyperirritability, occipital edema, pronounced craniotabes, skin lesions, skin desquamation, epiphyseal line changes, and cortical hyperostosis on x-rays.

Uncertainty Assessment. A UF of 10 was selected to account for the uncertainty of extrapolating a LOAEL to a NOAEL for a nonsevere and reversible effect (i.e., bulging fontanel) and the interindividual variability in sensitivity.

Derivation of a UL. The LOAEL of 6,000 µg/day was divided by a UF of 10 to calculate a UL of 600 µg/day of preformed vitamin A for infants.

Children and Adolescent Boys. There are limited case report data of hypervitaminosis A (e.g., bulging anterior fontanels, increased intracranial pressure, hair loss, increased suture markings on the skull, and periosteal new bone formation) in children and adolescents after doses ranging from 7,000 µg/day in young children to 15,000 µg/day in older children and adolescents (Farris and Erdman, 1982; Siegel and Spackman, 1972; Smith and Goodman, 1976). Given the dearth of information and the need for conservativism, the UL values for children and adolescents are extrapolated from those established for adults. Thus, the adult UL of 3,000 µg/day of preformed vitamin A was adjusted for children and adolescents on the basis of relative body weight as described in Chapter 2 with use of reference weights from Chapter 1 (Table 1-1). Values have been rounded.

Vitamin A UL Summary, Infants, Children, and Adolescent Boys

UL for Infants
  0–12 months   **600 µg/day of preformed vitamin A**

UL for Children
  1–3 years   **600 µg/day of preformed vitamin A**
  4–8 years   **900 µg/day of preformed vitamin A**
  9–13 years   **1,700 µg/day of preformed vitamin A**

UL for Boys
   14–18 years   2,800 µg/day of preformed vitamin A

Special Considerations

A review of the literature revealed that individuals with high alcohol intake, pre-existing liver disease, hyperlipidemia, or severe protein malnutrition may be distinctly susceptible to the adverse effects of excess preformed vitamin A intake (Ellis et al., 1986; Hathcock et al., 1990; Leo and Lieber, 1999). These individuals may not be protected by the UL for vitamin A for the general population.

Intake Assessment

Based on data from the Third National Health and Nutrition Survey (NHANES III), the highest median intake of preformed vitamin A for any gender and life stage group was 895 µg/day (Appendix Table C-6). This intake was being consumed by lactating women. The highest reported intake at the ninety-fifth percentile was 1,503 µg/day in lactating women. For adult Americans who take supplements containing vitamin A, intakes at the ninety-fifth percentile ranged from approximately 1,500 to 3,000 µg/day (Appendix Table C-9). Less than 5 percent of pregnant women had dietary and supplemental intake levels exceeding the UL.

Risk Characterization

The risk of exceeding the UL for vitamin A appears to be small based on the intakes cited above. There is not a large difference between the UL for infants (600 µg/day) and the Adequate Intake for older infants (500 µg/day). There is a body of evidence supporting the reversibility of bulging fontanels following the elimination of intermittent supplementation (de Francisco et al., 1993) or chronic ingestion (Naz and Edwards, 1952; Persson et al., 1965; Woodard et al., 1961) of high doses of vitamin A.

The UL is based on healthy populations in developed countries. Supplemental doses exceeding the UL for vitamin A (60 to 120 mg) are currently used in fortification and supplementation programs for the prevention and treatment of vitamin A deficiency, especially in developing countries. The UL is not meant to apply to communities of malnourished individuals receiving vitamin A prophylactically, either periodically or through fortification, as a means to prevent vitamin A deficiency or for individuals being treated for diseases, such as retinitis pigmentosa, with vitamin A.

RESEARCH RECOMMENDATIONS FOR VITAMIN A

• Effects of food matrices (e.g., carotenoids in milk and supplements) on the bioavailability of provitamin A carotenoids.

• Age-related differences in the bioavailability of vitamin A.

• Defined critical endpoints for population assessment for vitamin A and evaluation of their association with liver vitamin A stores.

• Effect of dietary vitamin A and vitamin A status on turnover and utilization of vitamin A. Is there significant adaptation to low vitamin A intakes? Is vitamin A absorption increased in response to low vitamin A intake? Is catabolism upregulated as body stores increase?

• Relationship of bioactive vitamin A indicators (e.g., retinoic acid) to dietary vitamin A intake.

• Effects of pregnancy and lactation on maternal vitamin A turnover.

• Effect of the interaction of vitamin A with other nutrients and food processing on the bioavailability of vitamin A.

REFERENCES

AAP (American Academy of Pediatrics Committee on Infectious Diseases). 1993. Vitamin A treatment of measles. *Pediatrics* 91:1014–1015.

Abedin Z, Hussain MA, Ahmad K. 1976. Liver reserve of vitamin A from medicolegal cases in Bangladesh. *Bangladesh Med Res Counc Bull* 2:43–51.

Alvarez JO, Salazar-Lindo E, Kohatsu J, Miranda P, Stephensen CB. 1995. Urinary excretion of retinol in children with acute diarrhea. *Am J Clin Nutr* 61:1273–1276.

Amedee-Manesme O, Anderson D, Olson JA. 1984. Relation of the relative dose response to liver concentrations of vitamin A in generally well-nourished surgical patients. *Am J Clin Nutr* 39:898–902.

Amedee-Manesme O, Mourey MS, Hanck A, Therasse J. 1987. Vitamin A relative dose response test: Validation by intravenous injection in children with liver disease. *Am J Clin Nutr* 46:286–289.

Amine EK, Corey J, Hegsted DM, Hayes KC. 1970. Comparative hematology during deficiencies of iron and vitamin A in the rat. *J Nutr* 100:1033–1040.

Arena JM, Sarazen P, Baylin GJ. 1951. Hypervitaminosis A: Report of an unusual case with marked craniotabes. *Pediatrics* 8:788–794.

Arroyave G, Aguilar JR, Flores M, Guzman MA. 1979. *Evaluation of Sugar Fortification with Vitamin A at the National Level*. Scientific Publication No. 384. Washington, DC: Pan American Health Organization.

Arthur P, Kirkwood B, Ross D, Morris S, Gyapong J, Tomkins A, Addy H. 1992. Impact of vitamin A supplementation on childhood morbidity in northern Ghana. *Lancet* 339:361–362.

Baly DL, Golub MS, Gershwin ME, Hurley LS. 1984. Studies of marginal zinc deprivation in rhesus monkeys. III. Effects on vitamin A metabolism. *Am J Clin Nutr* 40:199–207.

Bankson DD, Ellis JK, Russell RM. 1989. Effects of a vitamin-A-free diet on tissue vitamin A concentration and dark adaptation of aging rats. *Exp Gerontol* 24:127–136.

Barclay AJ, Foster A, Sommer A. 1987. Vitamin A supplements and mortality related to measles: A randomised clinical trial. *Br Med J* 294:294–296.

Barreto ML, Santos LM, Assis AM, Araujo MP, Farenzena GG, Santos PA, Fiaccone RL. 1994. Effect of vitamin A supplementation on diarrhoea and acute lower-respiratory-tract infections in young children in Brazil. *Lancet* 344:228–231.

Barua AB, Olson JA. 1989. Chemical synthesis of all-trans [11-^{3}H]-retinoyl β-glucuronide in its metabolism in rats in vivo. *Biochem J* 263:403–409.

Batchelder EL, Ebbs JC. 1943. Some observations of dark adaptation in man and their bearing on the problem of human requirement for vitamin A. *Rhode Island Agricultural Experiment Station Bulletin,* No. 645.

Bauernfeind JC. 1972. Carotenoid vitamin A precursors and analogs in foods and feeds. *J Agric Food Chem* 20:456–473.

Bauernfeind JC. 1980. *The Safe Use of Vitamin A.* A report of the International Vitamin A Consultative Group. Washington, DC: The Nutrition Foundation.

Bausch J, Rietz P. 1977. Method for the assessment of vitamin A liver stores. *Acta Vitaminol Enzymol* 31:99–112.

Beaton GH, Martorell R, Aronson KJ, Edmonston B, McCabe G, Ross AC, Harvey B. 1993. *Effectiveness of Vitamin A Supplementation in the Control of Young Child Morbidity and Mortality in Developing Countries.* Geneva: Subcommittee on Nutrition, Administrative Committee on Coordination, World Health Organization.

Beaton GH, Milner J, McGuire V, Feather TE, Little JA. 1983. Source of variance in 24-hour dietary recall data: Implications for nutrition study design and interpretation. Carbohydrate source, vitamins and minerals. *Am J Clin Nutr* 37:986–995.

Bendich A, Langseth L. 1989. Safety of vitamin A. *Am J Clin Nutr* 49:358–371.

Bernhardt IB, Dorsey DJ. 1974. Hypervitaminosis A and congenital renal anomalies in a human infant. *Obstet Gynecol* 43:750–755.

Blanchard EL, Harper HA. 1940. Measurement of vitamin A status of young adults by the dark adaptation technic. *Arch Int Med* 66:661–669.

Blaner WS, Olson JA. 1994. Retinol and retinoic acid metabolism. In: Sporn MB, Roberts AB, Goodman DS, eds. *The Retinoids: Biology, Chemistry, and Medicine,* 2nd ed. New York: Raven Press. Pp. 229–255.

Bloem MW, Wedel M, Egger RJ, Speek AJ, Schrijver J, Saowakontha S, Schreurs WH. 1989. Iron metabolism and vitamin A deficiency in children in northeast Thailand. *Am J Clin Nutr* 50:332–338.

Bloem MW, Wedel M, Egger RJ, Speek AJ, Schrijver J, Saowakontha S, Schreurs WH. 1990. Mild vitamin A deficiency and risk of respiratory tract diseases and diarrhea in preschool and school children in northeastern Thailand. *Am J Epidemiol* 131:332–339.

Blomhoff HK, Smeland EB, Erikstein B, Rasmussen AM, Skrede B, Skjonsberg C, Blomhoff R. 1992. Vitamin A is a key regulator for cell growth, cytokine production, and differentiation in normal B cells. *J Biol Chem* 267:23988–23992.

Blomstrand RM, Werner B. 1967. Studies on the intestinal absorption of radioactive β-carotene and vitamin A in man. *Scand J Clin Lab Invest* 19:339–345.

Boileau TW, Moore AC, Erdman JW Jr. 1999. Carotenoids and vitamin A. In: Papas AM, ed. *Antioxidant Status, Diet, Nutrition and Health*. Boca Raton, FL: CRC Press. Pp. 133–158.

Borel P, Dubois C, Mekki N, Grolier P, Partier A, Alexandre-Gouabau MC, Lairon D, Azais-Braesco V. 1997. Dietary triglycerides, up to 40 g/meal, do not affect preformed vitamin A bioavailability in humans. *Eur J Clin Nutr* 51:717–722.

Borel P, Mekki N, Boirie Y, Partier A, Alexandre-Gouabau MC, Grolier P, Beaufrere B, Portugal H, Lairon D, Azais-Braesco V. 1998. Comparison of the postprandial plasma vitamin A response in young and older adults. *J Gerontol A Biol Sci Med Sci* 53:B133–B140.

Brent RL, Hendrickx AG, Holmes LB, Miller RK. 1996. Teratogenicity of high vitamin A intake. *N Engl J Med* 334:1196–1197.

Brubacher G, Weiser H. 1985. The vitamin A activity of beta-carotene. *Int J Vitam Nutr Res* 55:5–15.

Bush ME, Dahms BB. 1984. Fatal hypervitaminosis A in a neonate. *Arch Pathol Lab Med* 108:838–842.

Butera ST, Krakowka S. 1986. Assessment of lymphocyte function during vitamin A deficiency. *Am J Vet Res* 47:850–855.

Butte NF, Calloway DH. 1981. Evaluation of lactational performance of Navajo women. *Am J Clin Nutr* 34:2210–2215.

Canfield LM, Giuliano AR, Neilson EM, Yap HH, Graver EJ, Cui HA, Blashill BM. 1997. Beta-carotene in breast milk and serum is increased after a single beta-carotene dose. *Am J Clin Nutr* 66:52–61.

Canfield LM, Giuliano AR, Neilson EM, Blashil BM, Graver EJ, Yap HH. 1998. Kinetics of the response of milk and serum beta-carotene to daily beta-carotene supplementation in healthy, lactating women. *Am J Clin Nutr* 67:276–283.

Cantorna MT, Nashold FE, Hayes CE. 1995. Vitamin A deficiency results in a priming environment conducive for TH1 cell development. *Eur J Immunol* 25:1673–1679.

Carlier C, Moulia-Pelat J-P, Ceccon J-F, Mourey MS, Fall M, N'Diaye M, Amedee-Manesme. 1991. Prevalence of malnutrition and vitamin A deficiency in the Diourbel, Fatick and Kaolack regions of Senegal: Feasibility of the method of impression cytology with transfer. *Am J Clin Nutr* 53:66–69.

Carman JA, Smith SM, Hayes CE. 1989. Characterization of a helper T-lymphocyte defect in vitamin A deficient mice. *J Immunol* 142:388–393.

Carman JA, Pond L, Nashold F, Wassom DL, Hayes CE. 1992. Immunity to Trichinella spiralis infection in vitamin A-deficient mice. *J Exp Med* 175:111–120.

Carney EA, Russell RM. 1980. Correlation of dark adaptation test results with serum vitamin A levels in diseased adults. *J Nutr* 110:552–557.

Carney SM, Underwood BA, Loerch JD. 1976. Effects of zinc and vitamin A deficient diets on the hepatic mobilization and urinary excretion of vitamin A in rats. *J Nutr* 106:1773–1781.

Carpenter TO, Pettifor JM, Russell RM, Pitha J, Mobarhan S, Ossip MS, Wainer S, Anast CS. 1987. Severe hypervitaminosis A in siblings: Evidence of variable tolerance to retinol intake. *J Pediatr* 111:507–512.

Castenmiller JJ, West CE. 1998. Bioavailability and bioconversion of carotenoids. *Ann Rev Nutr* 18:19–38.

Castenmiller JJ, West CE, Linssen JP, Van het Hof KH, Voragen AG. 1999. The food matrix of spinach is a limiting factor in determining the bioavailability of beta-carotene and to a lesser extent of lutein in humans. *J Nutr* 129:349–355.

Chappell JE, Francis T, Clandinin MT. 1985. Vitamin A and E content of human milk at early stages of lactation. *Early Hum Dev* 11:157–167.

Chase HP, Kumar V, Dodds JM, Sauberlich HE, Hunter RM, Burton RS, Spalding V. 1971. Nutritional status of preschool Mexican-American migrant farm children. *Am J Dis Child* 122:316–324.

Christian P, West KP Jr. 1998. Interactions between zinc and vitamin A: An update. *Am J Clin Nutr* 68:435S–441S.

Christian P, Schulze K, Stoltzfus RJ, West KP Jr. 1998a. Hyporetinolemia, illness symptoms, and acute phase protein response in pregnant women with and without night blindness. *Am J Clin Nutr* 67:1237–1243.

Christian P, West KP Jr, Khatry SK, Katz J, LeClerq S, Pradhan EK, Shrestha SR. 1998b. Vitamin A or beta-carotene supplementation reduces but does not eliminate maternal night blindness in Nepal. *J Nutr* 128:1458–1463.

Chug-Ahuja JK, Holden JM, Forman MR, Mangels AR, Beecher GR, Lanza E. 1993. The development and application of a carotenoid database for fruits, vegetables, and selected multicomponent foods. *J Am Diet Assoc* 93:318–323.

Chytil F. 1996. Retinoids in lung development. *FASEB J* 10:986–992.

Cohen BE, Elin RJ. 1974. Vitamin A-induced nonspecific resistance to infection. *J Infect Dis* 129:597–600.

Cohlan SQ. 1953. Excessive intake of vitamin A as a cause of congenital anomalies in the rat. *Science* 117:535–536.

Cohlan SQ. 1954. Congenital anomalies in the rat produced by excessive intake of vitamin A during pregnancy. *Pediatrics* 13:556–567.

Congdon N, Sommer A, Severns M, Humphrey J, Friedman D, Clement L, Wu LS, Natadisastra G. 1995. Pupillary and visual thresholds in young children as an index of population vitamin A status. *Am J Clin Nutr* 61:1076–1082.

Cooper AD. 1997. Hepatic uptake of chylomicron remnants. *J Lipid Res* 38:2173–2192.

Coutsoudis A, Broughton M, Coovadia HM. 1991. Vitamin A supplementation reduces measles morbidity in young African children: A randomized, placebo-controlled, double-blind trial. *Am J Clin Nutr* 54:890–895.

Coutsoudis A, Kiepiela P, Coovadia HM, Broughton M. 1992. Vitamin A supplementation enhances specific IgG antibody levels and total lymphocyte numbers while improving morbidity in measles. *Pediatr Infect Dis J* 11:203–209.

Czeizel AE, Rockenbauer M. 1998. Prevention of congenital abnormalities by vitamin A. *Int J Vitam Nutr Res* 68:219–231.

Dawson HD, Ross AC. 1999. Chronic marginal vitamin A status effects the distribution and function of T cells and natural T cells in aging Lewis rats. *J Nutr* 129:1782–1790.

Dawson HD, Li NQ, DeCicco KL, Nibert JA, Ross AC. 1999. Chronic marginal vitamin A status reduces natural killer cell number and function in aging Lewis rats. *J Nutr* 129:1510–1517.

de Francisco A, Chakraborty J, Chowdhury HR, Yunus M, Baqui AH, Siddique AK, Sack RB. 1993. Acute toxicty of vitamin A given with vaccines in infancy. *Lancet* 342:526–527.

de Pee S, West CE, Muhilal, Karyadi D, Hautvast JG. 1995. Lack of improvement in vitamin A status with increased consumption of dark-green leafy vegetables. *Lancet* 346:75–81.

de Pee S, West CE, Permaesih D, Martuti S, Muhilal, Hautvast JG. 1998. Orange fruit is more effective than dark-green, leafy vegetables in increasing serum concentrations of retinol and beta-carotene in schoolchildren in Indonesia. *Am J Clin Nutr* 68:1058–1067.

Deuel HJ, Greenberg SM, Straub E, Fukui T, Chatterjee A, Zechmeister L. 1949. Stereochemical configuration and provitamin A activity. VII. Neocryptoxanthin U. *Arch Biochem* 23:239–240.

Devadas R, Premakumari S, Subramanian G. 1978. Biological availability of β-carotene from fresh and dried green leafy vegetables on preschool children. *Ind J Nutr Dietet* 15:335–340.

Dew SE, Ong DE. 1994. Specificity of the retinol transporter of the rat small intestine brush border. *Biochemistry* 33:12340–12345.

Dickman ED, Smith SM. 1996. Selective regulation of cardiomyocyte gene expression and cardiac morphogenesis by retinoic acid. *Dev Dyn* 206:39–48.

Donnen P, Dramaix M, Brasseur D, Bitwe R, Vertongen F, Hennart P. 1998. Randomized placebo-controlled clinical trial of the effect of a single high dose or daily low doses of vitamin A on the morbidity of hospitalized, malnourished children. *Am J Clin Nutr* 68:1254–1260.

Dorea JG, Olson JA. 1986. The rate of rhodopsin regeneration in the bleached eyes of zinc-deficient rats in the dark. *J Nutr* 116:121–127.

Dorea JG, Souza JA, Galvao MO, Iunes MA. 1984. Concentration of vitamin A in the liver of foetuses and infants dying of various causes in Brasilia, Brazil. *Int J Vitam Nutr Res* 54:119–123.

Dowling JE, Gibbons IR. 1961. In: Smelser GK, ed. *The Structure of the Eye*. New York: Academic Press.

Dudas I, Czeizel AE. 1992. Use of 6,000 IU vitamin A during early pregnancy without teratogenic effect. *Teratology* 45:335–336.

Duester G. 1996. Involvement of alcohol dehydrogenase, short-chain dehydrogenase/reductase, aldehyde dehydrogenase, and cytochrome P450 in the control of retinoid signaling by activation of retinoic acid synthesis. *Biochemistry* 35:12221–12227.

Duncan JR, Hurley LS. 1978. An interaction between zinc and vitamin A in pregnant and fetal rats. *J Nutr* 108:1431–1438.

Eaton ML. 1978. Chronic hypervitaminosis A. *Am J Hosp Pharm* 35:1099–1102.

Eckhoff C, Nau H. 1990. Vitamin A supplementation increases levels of retinoic acid compounds in human plasma: Possible implications for teratogenesis. *Arch Toxicol* 64:502–503.

Eckhoff C, Bailey JR, Collins MD, Slikker W Jr, Nau H. 1991. Influence of dose and pharmaceutical formulation of vitamin A on plasma levels of retinyl esters and retinol and metabolic generation of retinoic acid compounds and beta-glucuronides in the cynomolgus monkey. *Toxicol Appl Pharmacol* 111:116–127.

Ellis JK, Russell RM, Makrauer FL, Schaefer EJ. 1986. Increased risk for vitamin A toxicity in severe hypertriglyceridemia. *Ann Intern Med* 105:877–879.

Farrell GC, Bhathal PS, Powell LW. 1977. Abnormal liver function in chronic hypervitaminosis A. *Am J Dig Dis* 22:724–728.

Farris WA, Erdman JW Jr. 1982. Protracted hypervitaminosis A following long-term, low-level intake. *J Am Med Assoc* 247:1317.

Fawzi WW, Chalmers TC, Herrera MG, Mosteller F. 1993. Vitamin A supplementation and child mortality. A meta-analysis. *J Am Med Assoc* 269:898–903.

Figueira F, Mendonca S, Rocha J, Azevedo M, Bunce GE, Reynolds JW. 1969. Absorption of vitamin A by infants receiving fat-free or fat-containing dried skim milk formulas. *Am J Clin Nutr* 22:588–593.

Filteau SM, Morris SS, Raynes JG, Arthur P, Ross DA, Kirkwood BR, Tomkins AM, Gyapong JO. 1995. Vitamin A supplementation, morbidity, and serum acute-phase proteins in young Ghanaian children. *Am J Clin Nutr* 62:434–438.

Flores H. 1993. Frequency distributions of serum vitamin A levels in cross-sectional surveys and in surveys before and after vitamin A supplementation. In: *A Brief Guide to Current Methods of Assessing Vitamin A Status*. A report of the International Vitamin A Consultative Group (IVACG). Washington, DC: The Nutrition Foundation. Pp. 9–11.

Flores H, de Araujo RC. 1984. Liver levels of retinol in unselected necropsy specimens: A prevalence survey of vitamin A deficiency in Recife, Brazil. *Am J Clin Nutr* 40:146–152.

Freudenheim JL, Johnson NE, Smith EL. 1986. Relationships between usual nutrient intake and bone-mineral content of women 35–65 years of age: Longitudinal and cross-sectional analysis. *Am J Clin Nutr* 44:863–876.

Friedman A, Sklan D. 1989. Impaired T lymphocyte immune response in vitamin A depleted rats and chicks. *Br J Nutr* 62:439–449.

Furr HC, Amedee-Manesme O, Clifford AJ, Bergen HR, Jones AD, Anderson LD, Olson JA. 1989. Vitamin A concentrations in liver determined by isotope dilution assay with tetradeuterated vitamin A and by biopsy in generally healthy adult humans. *Am J Clin Nutr* 49:713–716.

Geelen JA. 1979. Hypervitaminosis A induced teratogenesis. *CRC Crit Rev Toxicol* 6:351–375.

Geubel AP, De Galocsy C, Alves N, Rahier J, Dive C. 1991. Liver damage caused by therapeutic vitamin A administration: Estimate of dose-related toxicity in 41 cases. *Gastroenterology* 100:1701–1709.

Ghana VAST Study Team. 1993. Vitamin A supplementation in northern Ghana: Effects on clinic attendances, hospital admissions, and child mortality. *Lancet* 342:7–12.

Glasziou PP, Mackerras DE. 1993. Vitamin A supplementation and infectious disease: A meta-analysis. *Br Med J* 306:366–370.

Golner BB, Reinhold RB, Jacob RA, Sadowski JA, Russell RM. 1987. The short and long term effect of gastric partitioning surgery on serum protein levels. *J Am Coll Nutr* 6:279–285.

Goodman DS, Blaner WS. 1984. Biosynthesis, absorption, and hepatic metabolism of retinol. In: Sporn MB, Roberts AB, Goodman DS, eds. *The Retinoids*, Vol. 2. Orlando: Academic Press. Pp 1–39.

Goodman DS, Huang HS, Shiratori T. 1965. Tissue distribution and metabolism of newly absorbed vitamin A in the rat. *J Lipid Res* 6:390–396.

Goodman DS, Blomstrand R, Werner B, Huang HS, Shiratori T. 1966. The intestinal absorption and metabolism of vitamin A and β-carotene in man. *J Clin Invest* 45:1615–1623.

Gudas LJ, Sporn MB, Roberts AB. 1994. Cellular biology and biochemistry of the retinoids. In: Sporn MB, Roberts AB, Goodman DS, eds. *The Retinoids: Biology, Chemistry, and Medicine,* 2nd ed. New York: Raven Press. Pp. 443–520.

Hallfrisch J, Muller DC, Singh VN. 1994. Vitamin A and E intakes and plasma concentrations of retinol, beta-carotene, and alpha-tocopherol in men and women of the Baltimore Longitudinal Study of Aging. *Am J Clin Nutr* 60:176–182.

Harrison EH. 1993. Enzymes catalyzing the hydrolysis of retinyl esters. *Biochim Biophys Acta* 1170:99–108.

Haskell MJ, Handelman GJ, Peerson JM, Jones AD, Rabbi MA, Awal MA, Wahed MA, Mahalanabis D, Brown KH. 1997. Assessment of vitamin A status by the deuterated-retinol-dilution technique and comparison with hepatic vitamin A concentration in Bangladeshi surgical patients. *Am J Clin Nutr* 66:67–74.

Hatchell DL, Sommer A. 1984. Detection of ocular surface abnormalities in experimental vitamin A deficiency. *Arch Ophthalmol* 102:1389–1393.

Hathcock JN, Hattan DG, Jenkins MY, McDonald JT, Sundaresan PR, Wilkening VL. 1990. Evaluation of vitamin A toxicity. *Am J Clin Nutr* 52:183–202.

Hatoff DE, Gertler SL, Miyai K, Parker BA, Weiss JB. 1982. Hypervitaminosis A unmasked by acute viral hepatitis. *Gastroenterology* 82:124–128.

Hendriks HF, Verhoofstad WA, Brouwer A, de Leeuw AM, Knook DL. 1985. Perisinusoidal fat-storing cells are the main vitamin A storage sites in rat liver. *Exp Cell Res* 160:138–149.

Hicks RJ. 1867. Night-blindness in the Confederate Army. *Richmond Med J* 3:34–38.

Hicks VA, Gunning DB, Olson JA. 1984. Metabolism, plasma transport, and biliary excretion of radioactive vitamin A and its metabolites as a function of liver reserves of vitamin A in the rat. *J Nutr* 114:1327–1333.

Hofmann C, Eichele G. 1994. Retionoids in development. In: Sporn MB, Roberts AB, Goodman DS, eds. *The Retinoids: Biology, Chemistry, and Medicine*, 2nd ed. New York: Raven Press. Pp. 387–441.

Hollander D, Muralidhara KS. 1977. Vitamin A1 intestinal absorption in vivo: Influence of luminal factors on transport. *Am J Physiol* 232:E471–E477.

Hoppner K, Phillips WE, Murray TK, Campbell JS. 1968. Survey of liver vitamin A stores of Canadians. *Can Med Assoc J* 99:983–986.

Hoppner K, Phillips WE, Erdody P, Murray TK, Perrin DE. 1969. Vitamin A reserves of Canadians. *Can Med Assoc J* 101:84–86.

Houtkooper LB, Ritenbaugh C, Aickin M, Lohman TG, Going SB, Weber JL, Greaves KA, Boyden TW, Pamenter RW, Hall MC. 1995. Nutrients, body composition and exercise are related to change in bone mineral density in premenopausal women. *J Nutr* 125:1229–1237.

Hume EM, Krebs HA. 1949. *Vitamin A Requirement of Human Adults. An Experimental Study of Vitamin A Deprivation in Man.* Medical Research Council Special Report Series No. 264. London: His Majesty's Stationery Office.

Humphrey JH, Agoestina T, Wu L, Usman A, Nurachim M, Subardja D, Hidayat S, Tielsch J, West KP Jr, Sommer A. 1996. Impact of neonatal vitamin A supplementation on infant morbidity and mortality. *J Pediatr* 128:489–496.

Huque T. 1982. A survey of human liver reserves of retinol in London. *Br J Nutr* 47:165–172.

Hussey GD, Klein M. 1990. A randomized, controlled trial of vitamin A in children with severe measles. *N Engl J Med* 323:160–164.

Hutchings DE, Gaston J. 1974. The effects of vitamin A excess administered during the mid-fetal period on learning and development in rat offspring. *Dev Psychobiol* 7:225–233.

Hutchings DE, Gibbon J, Kaufman MA. 1973. Maternal vitamin A excess during the early fetal period: Effects on learning and development in the offspring. *Dev Psychobiol* 6:445–457.

IOM (Institute of Medicine). 2000. *Dietary Reference Intakes for Vitamin C, Vitamin E, Selenium, and Carotenoids.* Washington, DC: National Academy Press.

Jalal F, Nesheim MC, Agus Z, Sanjur D, Habicht JP. 1998. Serum retinol concentrations in children are affected by food sources of beta-carotene, fat intake, and anthelmintic drug treatment. *Am J Clin Nutr* 68:623–629.

Jang JT, Green JB, Beard JL, Green MH. 2000. Kinetic analysis shows that iron deficiency decreases liver vitamin A mobilization in rats. *J Nutr* 130:1291–1296.

Jayarajan P, Reddy V, Mohanram M. 1980. Effect of dietary fat on absorption of β-carotene from green leafy vegetables in children. *Indian J Med Res* 71:53–56.

Jensen SK, Nielsen KN. 1996. Tocopherols, retinol, beta-carotene and fatty acids in fat globule membrane and fat globule core in cows' milk. *J Dairy Sci* 63:565–574.

Johnson EJ, Qin J, Krinsky NI, Russell RM. 1997. Ingestion by men of a combined dose of β-carotene and lycopene does not affect the absorption of β-carotene but improves that of lycopene. *J Nutr* 127:1833–1837.

Kalter H, Warkany J. 1961. Experimental production of congenital malformations in strains of inbred mice by maternal treatment with hypervitaminosis A. *Am J Pathol* 38:1–14.

Katz DR, Dizymala M, Turton JA, Hicks RM, Hunt R, Palmer L, Malkovsky M. 1987. Regulation of accessory cell function by retinoids in murine immune responses. *Br J Exp Pathol* 68:343–350.

Katz J, West KP Jr, Khatry SK, Thapa MD, LeClerq SC, Pradhan EK, Pokhrel RP, Sommer A. 1995. Impact of vitamin A supplementation on prevalence and incidence of xerophthalmia in Nepal. *Invest Ophthalmol Vis Sci* 36:2577–2583.

Keenum D. 1993. Conjunctival impression cytology. In: *A Brief Guide to Current Methods of Assessing Vitamin A Status. A report* of the International Vitamin A Consultative Group (IVACG). Washington, DC: The Nutrition Foundation. Pp. 19–21.

Keenum D, Semba RD, Wirasasmita S, Natadisastra G, Muhilal, West KP Jr, Sommer A. 1990. Assessment of vitamin A status by a disk applicator for conjunctival impression cytology. *Arch Ophthalmol* 108:1436–1441.

Keilson B, Underwood BA, Loerch JD. 1979. Effects of retinoic acid on the mobilization of vitamin A from the liver in rats. *J Nutr* 109:787–795.

Khoury MJ, Moore CA, Mulinare J. 1996. Vitamin A and birth defects. *Lancet* 347:322.

Kostic D, White WS, Olson JA. 1995. Intestinal absorption, serum clearance, and interactions between lutein and beta-carotene when administered to human adults in separate or combined oral doses. *Am J Clin Nutr* 62:604–610.

Kowalski TE, Falestiny M, Furth E, Malet PF. 1994. Vitamin A hepatotoxicity: A cautionary note regarding 25,000 IU supplements. *Am J Med* 97:523–528.

Krasinski SD, Russell RM, Otradovec CL, Sadowski JA, Hartz SC, Jacob RA, McGandy RB. 1989. Relationship of vitamin A and vitamin E intake to fasting plasma retinol, retinol-binding protein, retinyl ester, carotene, alpha-tocopherol, and cholesterol among elderly people and young adults: Increased plasma retinyl esters among vitamin A-supplement users. *Am J Clin Nutr* 49:112–120.

Krinsky NI, Wang X-D, Tang G, Russell RM. 1993. Mechanism of carotenoid cleavage to retinoids. *Ann NY Acad Sci* 691:167–176.

Kusin JA, Reddy V, Sivakumar B. 1974. Vitamin E supplements and the absorption of a massive dose of vitamin A. *Am J Clin Nutr* 27:774–776.

Lachance PA. 1997. Nutrient addition to foods: The public health impact in countries with rapidly westernizing diets. In: Bendich A, Deckelbaum RJ, eds. *Preventive Nutrition: The Comprehensive Guide for Health Professionals.* Totowa, NJ: Humana Press. Pp. 441–454.

Lammer EJ, Chen DT, Hoar RM, Agnish ND, Benke PJ, Braun JT, Curry CJ, Fernhoff PM, Grix AW Jr, Lott IT, Richard JM, Sun SC. 1985. Retinoic acid embryopathy. *N Engl J Med* 313:837–841.

Large S, Neal G, Glover J, Thanangkul O, Olson RE. 1980. The early changes in retinol-binding protein and prealbumin concentrations in plasma of protein-energy malnourished children after treatment with retinol and an improved diet. *Br J Nutr* 43:393–402.

Leo MA, Lieber CS. 1982. Hepatic vitamin A depletion in alcoholic liver injury. *N Engl J Med* 307:597–601.

Leo MA, Lieber CS. 1985. New pathway for retinol metabolism in liver microsomes. *J Biol Chem* 260:5228–5231.

Leo MA, Lieber CS. 1999. Alcohol, vitamin A, and beta-carotene: Adverse interactions, including hepatotoxicity and carcinogenicity. *Am J Clin Nutr* 69:1071–1085.

Lewis JM, Bodansky O, Falk KG, McGuire G. 1942. Vitamin A requirements in the rat. The relation of vitamin A intake to growth and to concentration of vitamin A in the blood plasma, liver and retina. *J Nutr* 23:351–363.

Lieber CS, Leo MA. 1986. Interaction of alcohol and nutritional factors with hepatic fibrosis. *Prog Liver Dis* 8:253–272.

Loerch JD, Underwood BA, Lewis KC. 1979. Response of plasma levels of vitamin A to a dose of vitamin A as an indicator of hepatic vitamin A reserves in rat. *J Nutr* 109:778–786.

Looker AC, Johnson CL, Woteki CE, Yetley EA, Underwood BA. 1988. Ethnic and racial differences in serum vitamin A levels of children aged 4–11 years. *Am J Clin Nutr* 47:247–252.

Loyd-Puryear MA, Mahoney J, Humphrey JH, Mahoney F, Siren N, Moorman C, West KP Jr. 1991. Vitamin A deficiency in Micronesia: A statewide survey in Chuuk. *Nutr Res* 11:1101–1110.

Lynch SR. 1997. Interaction of iron with other nutrients. *Nutr Rev* 55:102–110.

Mahalanabis D, Simpson TW, Chakraborty ML, Ganguli C, Bhattacharjee AK, Mukherjee KL. 1979. Malabsorption of water miscible vitamin A in children with giardiasis and ascariasis. *Am J Clin Nutr* 32:313–318.

Mahoney CP, Margolis MT, Knauss TA, Labbe RF. 1980. Chronic vitamin A intoxication in infants fed chicken liver. *Pediatrics* 65:893–897.

Martinez-Frias ML, Salvador J. 1990. Epidemiological aspects of prenatal exposure to high doses of vitamin A in Spain. *Eur J Epidemiol* 6:118–123.

Mastroiacovo P, Mazzone T, Addis A, Elephant E, Carlier P, Vial T, Garbis H, Robert E, Bonati M, Ornoy A, Finardi A, Schaffer C, Caramelli L, Rodriguez-Pinilla E, Clementi M. 1999. High vitamin A intake in early pregnancy and major malformations: A multicenter prospective controlled study. *Teratology* 59:7–11.

Maxwell JD, Murray D, Ferguson A, Calder E. 1968. Ascaris lumbricoides infestation associated with jejunal mucosal abnormalities. *Scott Med J* 13:280–281.

McCaffery P, Drager UC. 1995. Retinoic acid synthesizing enzymes in the embryonic and adult vertebrate. In: Weiner H, Holmes RS, Wermuth B, eds. *Enzymology and Molecular Biology of Carbonyl Metabolism 5*. New York: Plenum Press. Pp. 173–183.

Melhus H, Michaelsson K, Kindmark A, Bergstrom R, Holmberg L, Mallmin H, Wolk A, Ljunghall S. 1998. Excessive dietary intake of vitamin A is associated with reduced bone mineral density and increased risk for hip fracture. *Ann Intern Med* 129:770–778.

Micozzi MS, Brown ED, Edwards BK, Bieri JG, Taylor PR, Khachik F, Beecher GR, Smith JC. 1992. Plasma carotenoid response to chronic intake of selected foods and β-carotene supplements in men. *Am J Clin Nutr* 55:1120–1125.

Mills JL, Simpson JL, Cunningham GC, Conley MR, Rhoads GG. 1997. Vitamin A and birth defects. *Am J Obstet Gynecol* 177:31–36.

Minuk GY, Kelly JK, Hwang WS. 1988. Vitamin A hepatotoxicity in multiple family members. *Hepatology* 8:272–275.

Mitchell GV, Young M, Seward CR. 1973. Vitamin A and carotene levels of a selected population in metropolitan Washington, D.C. *Am J Clin Nutr* 26:992–997.

Mobarhan S, Russell RM, Underwood BA, Wallingford J, Mathieson RD, Al-Midani H. 1981. Evaluation of the relative dose response test for vitamin A nutriture in cirrhotics. *Am J Clin Nutr* 34:2264–2270.

Mobarhan S, Seitz HK, Russell RM, Mehta R, Hupert J, Friedman H, Layden TJ, Meydani M, Langenberg P. 1991. Age-related effects of chronic ethanol intake on vitamin A status in Fisher 344 rats. *J Nutr* 121:510–517.

Money DF. 1978. Vitamin E, selenium, iron, and vitamin A content of livers from Sudden Infant Death Syndrome cases and control children: Interrelationships and possible significance. *NZ J Sci* 21:41–45.

Montreewasuwat N, Olson JA. 1979. Serum and liver concentrations of vitamin A in Thai fetuses as a function of gestational age. *Am J Clin Nutr* 32:601–606.

Morrison SA, Russell RM, Carney EA, Oaks EV. 1978. Zinc deficiency: A cause of abnormal dark adaptation in cirrhotics. *Am J Clin Nutr* 31:276–281.

Morriss-Kay GM, Sokolova N. 1996. Embryonic development and pattern formation. *FASEB J* 10:961–969.

Moss AJ, Levy AS, Kim I, Park YK. 1989. *Use of Vitamin and Mineral Supplements in the United States: Current Users, Types of Products, and Nutrients.* Advance Data, Vital and Health Statistics of the National Center for Health Statistics, Number 174. Hyattsville, MD: National Center for Health Statistics.

Muhilal, Permeisih D, Idjradinata YR, Muherdiyantiningsih, Karyadi D. 1988. Vitamin A-fortified monosodium glutamate and health, growth, and survival of children: A controlled field trial. *Am J Clin Nutr* 48:1271–1276.

Munoz EC, Rosado JL, Lopez P, Furr HC, Allen LH. 2000. Iron and zinc supplementation improves indicators of vitamin A status of Mexican preschoolers. *Am J Clin Nutr* 71:789–794.

Napoli JL, Race KR. 1988. Biogenesis of retinoic acid from β-carotene: Differences between the metabolism of β-carotene and retinal. *J Biol Chem* 263:17372–17377.

Napoli JL, Boerman MH, Chai X, Zhai Y, Fiorella PD. 1995. Enzymes and binding proteins affecting retinoic acid concentrations. *J Steroid Biochem Mol Biol* 53:497–502.

Natadisastra G, Wittpenn JR, West KP Jr, Muhilal, Sommer A. 1987. Impression cytology for detection of vitamin A deficiency. *Arch Ophthalmol* 105:1224–1228.

Nauss KM, Newberne PM. 1985. Local and regional immune function of vitamin A-deficient rats with ocular herpes simplex virus (HSV) infections. *J Nutr* 115:1316–1324.

Naz JF, Edwards WM. 1952. Hypervitaminosis A: A case report. *N Engl J Med* 246:87–89.

Nierenberg DW, Dain BJ, Mott LA, Baron JA, Greenberg ER. 1997. Effects of 4 y of oral supplementation with beta-carotene on serum concentrations of retinol, tocopherol, and five carotenoids. *Am J Clin Nutr* 66:315–319.

Novotny JA, Dueker SR, Zech LA, Clifford AJ. 1995. Compartmental analysis of the dynamics of β-carotene metabolism in an adult volunteer. *J Lipid Res* 36:1825–1838.

NRC (National Research Council). 1980. *Recommended Dietary Allowances*, 9th ed. Washington, DC: National Academy Press.

NRC. 1986. *Nutrient Adequacy: Assessment Using Food Consumption Surveys*. Washington, DC: National Academy Press.

NRC. 1989. *Recommended Dietary Allowances*, 10th ed. Washington, DC: National Academy Press.

Nusser SM, Carriquiry AL, Dodd KW, Fuller WA. 1986. A semiparametric transformation approach to estimating usual daily intake distributions. *J Am Stat Assoc* 91:1440–1449.

Olson JA. 1972. The prevention of childhood blindness by the administration of massive doses of vitamin A. *Isr J Med Sci* 8:1199–1206.

Olson JA. 1979. Liver vitamin A reserves of neonates, preschool children and adults dying of various causes in Salvador, Brazil. *Arch Latinoam Nutr* 29:521–545.

Olson JA. 1982. New approaches to methods for the assessment of nutritional status of the individual. *Am J Clin Nutr* 35:1166–1168.

Olson JA. 1983. Adverse effects of large doses of vitamin A and retinoids. *Semin Oncol* 10:290–293.

Olson JA. 1987. Recommended dietary intakes (RDI) of vitamin A in humans. *Am J Clin Nutr* 45:704–716.

Olson JA. 1991. Vitamin A. In: Machlin LJ, ed. *Handbook of Vitamins*, 2nd ed. New York: Marcel Dekker. Pp. 1–57.

Olson JA, Hayaishi O. 1965. The enzymatic cleavage of β-carotene into vitamin A by soluble enzymes of rat liver and intestine. *Proc Nat Acad Sci USA* 54:1364–1370.

Olson JA, Gunning D, Tilton R. 1979. The distribution of vitamin A in human liver. *Am J Clin Nutr* 32:2500–2507.

Oren R, Ilan Y. 1992. Reversible hepatic injury induced by long-term vitamin A ingestion. *Am J Med* 93:703–704.

Panfili G, Manzi P, Pizzoferrato L. 1998. Influence of thermal and other manufacturing stresses on retinol isomerization in milk and dairy products. *J Dairy Res* 65:253–260.

Papiz MZ, Sawyer L, Eliopoulos EE, North AC, Findlay JB, Sivaprasadarao R, Jones TA, Newcomer ME, Kraulis PJ. 1986. The structure of beta-lactoglobulin and its similarity to plasma retinol-binding protein. *Nature* 324:383–385.

Parker RS, Swanson JE, You CS, Edwards AJ, Huang T. 1999. Bioavailability of carotenoids in human subjects. *Proc Nutr Soc* 58:155–162.

Pasatiempo AM, Kinoshita M, Taylor CE, Ross AC. 1990. Antibody production in vitamin A-depleted rats is impaired after immunization with bacterial polysaccharide or protein antigens. *FASEB J* 4:2518–2527.

Patton S, Kelly JJ, Keenan TW. 1980. Carotene in bovine milk fat globules: Observations on origin and high content in tissue mitochondria. *Lipids* 15:33–38.

Persson B, Tunell R, Ekengren K. 1965. Chronic vitamin A intoxication during the first half year of life. *Acta Paediatr Scand* 54:49–60.

Persson B, Krook M, Jornvall H. 1995. Short-chain dehydrogenases/reductases. In: Weiner H, Holmes RS, Wermuth B, eds. *Enzymology and Molecular Biology of Carbonyl Metabolism 5*. New York: Plenum Press. Pp. 383–395.

Pilch SM. 1987. Analysis of vitamin A data from the health and nutrition examination surveys. *J Nutr* 117:636–640.

Pinnock CB, Alderman CP. 1992. The potential for teratogenicity of vitamin A and its congeners. *Med J Aust* 157:804–809.

Rahmathullah L, Underwood BA, Thulasiraj RD, Milton RC, Ramaswamy K, Rahmathullah R, Babu G. 1990. Reduced mortality among children in southern India receiving a small weekly dose of vitamin A. *N Engl J Med* 323:929–935.

Raica N Jr, Scott J, Lowry L, Sauberlich HE. 1972. Vitamin A concentration in human tissues collected from five areas in the United States. *Am J Clin Nutr* 25:291–296.

Reddy V. 1985. *Vitamin A Requirements of Preschool Children.* Joint FAO/WHO Expert Group on Requirement for Vitamin A, Iron, Folate and Vitamin B12, Doc. No. 6. Geneva: World Health Organization.

Reddy V, Srikantia SG. 1966. Serum vitamin A in kwashiorkor. *Am J Clin Nutr* 18:105–109.

Rock CL, Lovalvo JL, Emenhiser C, Ruffin MT, Flatt SW, Schwartz SJ. 1998. Bioavailability of β-carotene is lower in raw than in processed carrots and spinach in women. *J Nutr* 128:913–916.

Roels OA, Trout M, Dujacquier R. 1958. Carotene balances on boys in Ruanda where vitamin A deficiency is prevalent. *J Nutr* 65:115–127.

Roels OA, Djaeni S, Trout ME, Lauw TG, Heath A, Poey SH, Tarwotjo MS, Suhadi B. 1963. The effect of protein and fat supplements on vitamin A deficient children. *Am J Clin Nutr* 12:380–387.

Rohde CM, Manatt M, Clagett-Dame M, DeLuca HF. 1999. Vitamin A antagonizes the action of vitamin D in rats. *J Nutr* 129:2246–2250.

Rosales FJ, Ritter SJ, Zolfaghari R, Smith JE, Ross AC. 1996. Effects of acute inflammation on plasma retinol, retinol-binding protein, and its mRNA in the liver and kidneys of vitamin A-sufficient rats. *J Lipid Res* 37:962–971.

Rosales FJ, Jang JT, Pinero DJ, Erikson KM, Beard JL, Ross AC. 1999. Iron deficiency in young rats alters the distribution of vitamin A between plasma and liver and between hepatic retinol and retinyl esters. *J Nutr* 129:1223–1228.

Ross AC. 1996. Vitamin A deficiency and retinoid repletion regulate the antibody response to bacterial antigens and the maintenance of natural killer cells. *Clin Immunol Immunopathol* 80:S63–S72.

Ross AC. 1999. Vitamin A and retinoids. In: Shils ME, Olson JA, Shike M, Ross AC, eds. *Modern Nutrition in Health and Disease,* 9th ed. Baltimore, MD: Williams & Wilkins. Pp. 305–328.

Rothman KJ, Moore LL, Singer MR, Nguygen UDT, Mannino S, Milunsky B. 1995. Teratogenicity of high vitamin A intake. *N Engl J Med* 333:1369–1373.

Saari JC. 1994. Retinoids in photosensitive systems. In: Sporn MB, Roberts AB, Goodman DS, eds. *The Retinoids: Biology, Chemistry, and Medicine,* 2nd ed. New York: Raven Press. Pp. 351–385.

Salazar-Lindo E, Salazar M, Alvarez JO. 1993. Association of diarrhea and low serum retinol in Peruvian children. *Am J Clin Nutr* 58:110–113.

Sanchez AM, Congdon NG, Sommer A, Rahmathullah L, Venkataswamy PG, Chandravathi PS, Clement L. 1997. Pupillary threshold as an index of population vitamin A status among children in India. *Am J Clin Nutr* 65:61–66.

Sato M, Lieber CS. 1981. Hepatic vitamin A depletion after chronic ethanol consumption in baboons and rats. *J Nutr* 111:2015–2023.

Sauberlich HE, Hodges HE, Wallace DL, Kolder H, Canham JE, Hood J, Raica N, Lowry LK. 1974. Vitamin A metabolism and requirements in the human studied with the use of labeled retinol. *Vitam Horm* 32:251–275.

Schindler R, Friedrich DH, Kramer M, Wacker HH, Feldheim W. 1988. Size and composition of liver vitamin A reserves of human beings who died of various causes. *Int J Vitam Nutr Res* 58:146–154.

Semba RD, Muhilal, Scott AL, Natadisastra G, Wirasasmita S, Mele L, Ridwan E, West KP Jr, Sommer A. 1992. Depressed immune response to tetanus in children with vitamin A deficiency. *J Nutr* 122:101–107.

Semba RD, Bulterys M, Munyeshuli V, Gatsinzi T, Saah A, Chao A, Dushimimana A. 1996. Vitamin A deficiency and T-cell subpopulations in children with meningococcal disease. *J Trop Pediatr* 42:287–290.

Shankar AH, Genton B, Semba RD, Baisor M, Paino J, Tamja S, Adiguma T, Wu L, Rare L, Tielsch JM, Alpers MP, West KP Jr. 1999. Effect of vitamin A supplementation on morbidity due to *Plasmodium falciparum* in young children in Papua, New Guinea: A randomised trial. *Lancet* 354:203–209.

Shaw GM, Wasserman CR, Block G, Lammer EJ. 1996. High maternal vitamin A intake and risk of anomalies of structures with a cranial neural crest cell contribution. *Lancet* 347:899–900.

Shingwekar AG, Mohanram M, Reddy V. 1979. Effect of zinc supplementation on plasma levels of vitamin A and retinol-binding protein in malnourished children. *Clin Chim Acta* 93:97–100.

Siegel NJ, Spackman TJ. 1972. Chronic hypervitaminosis A with intracranial hypertension and low cerebrospinal fluid concentration of protein. Two illustrative cases. *Clin Pediatr* 11:580–584.

Sivakumar B, Reddy V. 1972. Absorption of labelled vitamin A in children during infection. *Br J Nutr* 27:299–304.

Sivakumar B, Reddy V. 1975. Absorption of vitamin A in children with ascariasis. *J Trop Med Hyg* 78:114–115.

Smith FR, Goodman DS. 1976. Vitamin A transport in human vitamin A toxicity. *N Engl J Med* 294:805–808.

Smith JE, Brown ED, Smith JC Jr. 1974. The effect of zinc deficiency on the metabolism of retinol-binding protein in the rat. *J Lab Clin Med* 84:692–697.

Smith SM, Levy NL, Hayes CE. 1987. Impaired immunity in vitamin A-deficient mice. *J Nutr* 117:857–865.

Solomons NW, Morrow FD, Vasquez A, Bulux J, Guerrero AM, Russell RM. 1990. Test-retest reproducibility of the relative dose response for vitamin A status in Guatemalan adults: Issues of diagnostic sensitivity. *J Nutr* 120:738–744.

Sommer A. 1982. *Nutritional Blindness. Xerophthalmia and Keratomalacia.* New York: Oxford University Press.

Sommer A, West KP Jr. 1996. *Vitamin A Deficiency: Health, Survival, and Vision.* New York: Oxford University Press.

Sommer A, Tarwotjo I, Hussaini G, Susanto D. 1983. Increased mortality in children with mild vitamin A deficiency. *Lancet* 2:585–588.

Sommer A, Katz J, Tarwotjo I. 1984. Increased risk of respiratory disease and diarrhea in children with pre-existing mild vitamin A deficiency. *Am J Clin Nutr* 40:1090–1095.

Sommer A, Tarwotjo I, Djunaedi E, West KP Jr, Loeden AA, Tilden R, Mele L. 1986. Impact of vitamin A supplementation on childhood mortality: A randomized controlled community trial. *Lancet* 1:1169–1173.

Sporn MB, Roberts AB, Goodman DS. 1984. *The Retinoids.* Orlando: Academic Press.

Staab DB, Hodges RE, Metcalf WK, Smith JL. 1984. Relationship between vitamin A and iron in the liver. *J Nutr* 114:840–844.

Stauber PM, Sherry B, VanderJagt DJ, Bhagavan HN, Garry PJ. 1991. A longitudinal study of the relationship between vitamin A supplementation and plasma retinol, retinyl esters, and liver enzyme activities in a healthy elderly population. *Am J Clin Nutr* 54:878–883.

Stephensen CB, Blount SR, Schoeb TR, Park JY. 1993. Vitamin A deficiency impairs some aspects of the host response to influenza A virus infection in BALB/c mice. *J Nutr* 123:823–833.

Stephensen CB, Alvarez JO, Kohatsu J, Hardmeier R, Kennedy JI, Gammon RB. 1994. Vitamin A is excreted in the urine during acute infection. *Am J Clin Nutr* 60:388–392.

Stewart BE, Young RS. 1989. Pupillary response: An index of visual threshold. *Appl Optics* 28:1122–1127.

Suharno D, West CE, Muhilal, Karyadi D, Hautvast JG. 1993. Supplementation with vitamin A and iron for nutritional anaemia in pregnant women in West Java, Indonesia. *Lancet* 342:1325–1328.

Suthutvoravoot S, Olson JA. 1974. Plasma and liver concentration of vitamin A in a normal population of urban Thai. *Am J Clin Nutr* 27:883–891.

Takyi EE. 1999. Children's consumption of dark green, leafy vegetables with added fat enhances serum retinol. *J Nutr* 129:1549–1554.

Tang G, Qin J, Dolnikowski GG, Russell RM. 2000. Vitamin A equivalence of β-carotene in a woman as determined by a stable isotope reference method. *Eur J Nutr* 39:7–11.

Tanumihardjo SA. 1993. The modified relative dose-response assay. In: *A Brief Guide to Current Methods of Assessing Vitamin A Status.* A report of the International Vitamin A Consultative Group (IVACG). Washington, DC: The Nutrition Foundation. Pp. 14–15.

Tanumihardjo SA, Olson JA. 1991. The reproducibility of the modified relative dose response (MRDR) assay in healthy individuals over time and its comparison with conjunctival impression cytology (CIC). *Eur J Clin Nutr* 45:407–411.

Terhune MW, Sandstead HH. 1972. Decreased RNA polymerase activity in mammalian zinc deficiency. *Science* 177:68–69.

Thatcher AJ, Lee CM, Erdman JW Jr. 1998. Tissue stores of β-carotene are not conserved for later use as a source of vitamin A during compromised vitamin A status in Mongolian gerbils (Meriones unguiculatus). *J Nutr* 128:1179–1185.

Tomlinson JE, Hemken RW, Mitchell GE, Tucker RE. 1976. Mammary transfer of vitamin A alcohol and ester in lactating dairy cows. *J Dairy Sci* 59:607–613.

Torronen R, Lehmusaho M, Hakkinen S, Hanninen O, Mykkanen H. 1996. Serum β-carotene response to supplementation with raw carrots, carrot juice or purified β-carotene in healthy non-smoking women. *Nutr Res* 16:565–575.

Trechsel U, Evequoz V, Fleisch H. 1985. Stimulation of interleukin 1 and 3 production by retinoic acid in vitro. *Biochem J* 230:339–344.

Underwood BA. 1984. Vitamin A in animal and human nutrition. In: Sporn MB, Roberts AB, Goodman DS, eds. *The Retinoids,* Vol. 1. New York: Academic Press. Pp. 281–392.

Underwood BA. 1994. Hypovitaminosis A: International programmatic issues. *J Nutr* 124:1467S–1472S.

Underwood BA, Siegel H, Weisell RC, Dolinski M. 1970. Liver stores of vitamin A in a normal population dying suddenly or rapidly from unnatural causes in New York City. *Am J Clin Nutr* 23:1037–1042.

Van den Berg H, van Vliet T. 1998. Effect of simultaneous, single oral doses of β-carotene with lutein or lycopene on the β-carotene and retinyl ester responses in the triacylglycerol-rich lipoprotein fraction of men. *Am J Clin Nutr* 68:82–89.

Van het Hof KH, Gartner C, West CE, Tijburg LB. 1998. Potential of vegetable processing to increase the delivery of carotenoids to man. *Int J Vitam Nutr Res* 68:366–370.

Van het Hof KH, Brouwer IA, West CE, Haddeman E, Steegers-Theunissen RP, van Dusseldorp M, Weststrate JA, Ekes TK, Hautvast JG. 1999. Bioavailability of lutein from vegetables is five times higher than that of β-carotene. *Am J Clin Nutr* 70:261–268.

Von Lennep E, El Khazen N, De Pierreux G, Amy JJ, Rodesch F, Van Regemorter N. 1985. A case of partial sirenomelia and possible vitamin A teratogenesis. *Prenat Diagn* 5:35–40.

Wagner KH. 1940. Die experimentelle avitaminose a bein menschen. *Ztschf Physiol Chem* 264:153–188.

Wallingford JC, Underwood BA. 1987. Vitamin A status needed to maintain vitamin A concentrations in nonhepatic tissues of the pregnant rat. *J Nutr* 117:1410–1415.

Wang XD. 1999. Chronic alcohol intake interfers with retinoid metabolism and signaling. *Nutr Rev* 57:51–59.

Watkins M, Moore C, Mulinare J. 1996. Teratogenicity of high vitamin A intake. *N Engl J Med* 334:1196–1197.

Weber FL Jr, Mitchell GE Jr, Powell DE, Reiser BJ, Banwell JG. 1982. Reversible hepatotoxicity associated with hepatic vitamin A accumulation in a protein-deficient patient. *Gastroenterology* 82:118–123.

Wendling O, Chambon P, Mark M. 1999. Retinoid X receptors are essential for early mouse development and placentogenesis. *Proc Natl Acad Sci USA* 96:547–551.

Werler MM, Lammer EJ, Mitchell AA. 1996. Teratogenicity of high vitamin A intake. *N Engl J Med* 334:1195–1196.

West KP Jr, Pokhrel RP, Katz J, LeClerq SC, Khatry SK, Shrestha SR, Pradhan EK, Tielsch JM, Pandey MR, Sommer A. 1991. Efficacy of vitamin A in reducing preschool child mortality in Nepal. *Lancet* 338:67–71.

West KP Jr, Katz J, Khatry SK, LeClerq SC, Pradhan EK, Shrestha SR, Conner PB, Dali SM, Christian P, Pokhrel RP, Sommer A. 1999. Double blind, cluster randomized trial of low dose supplementation with vitamin A or beta carotene on mortality related to pregnancy in Nepal. *Br Med J* 318:570–575.

WHO (World Health Organization). 1950. *Expert Committee on Biological Standardisation.* Technical Report Series, No. 3. Geneva:WHO.

WHO. 1966. *WHO Expert Committee on Biological Standardization Eighteenth Report.* Technical Report Series, No. 329. Geneva: WHO.

WHO. 1982. *Control of Vitamin A Deficiency and Xerophthalmia.* Technical Report Series No. 672. Geneva: WHO.

WHO. 1995. *Global Prevalence of Vitamin A Deficiency.* Micronutrient Deficiency Information System Working Paper, No. 2. Geneva: WHO.

WHO. 1997. *Vitamin A Supplements: A Guide to Their Use in the Treatment of Vitamin A Deficiency and Xerophthalmia.* Geneva: WHO.

Wiedermann U, Hanson LA, Kahu H, Dahlgren UI. 1993. Aberrant T-cell function in vitro and impaired T-cell dependent antibody response in vivo in vitamin A-deficient rats. *Immunology* 80:581–586.

Wilson JG, Roth CB, Warkany J. 1953. An analysis of the syndrome of malformations induced by maternal vitamin A deficiency. Effects of restoration of vitamin A at various times during gestation. *Am J Anat* 92:189–217.

Wittpenn JR, Tseng SC, Sommer A. 1986. Detection of early xerophthalmia by impression cytology. *Arch Ophthalmol* 104:237–239.

Wolde-Gebriel Z, West CE, Gebru H, Tadesse AS, Fisseha T, Gabre P, Aboye C, Ayana G, Hautvast JG. 1993. Interrelationship between vitamin A, iodine and iron status in schoolchildren in Shoa Region, central Ethiopia. *Br J Nutr* 70:593–607.

Woodard WK, Miller LJ, Legant O. 1961. Acute and chronic hypervitaminosis in a 4-month-old infant. *J Pediatr* 59:260–264.

Zafrani ES, Bernuau D, Feldmann G. 1984. Peliosis-like ultrastructural changes of the hepatic sinusoids in human chronic hypervitaminosis A: Report of three cases. *Hum Pathol* 15:1166–1170.

Zahar M, Smith DE, Martin F. 1995. Vitamin A distribution among fat globule core, fat globule membrane, and serum fraction in milk. *J Dairy Sci* 78:498–505.

Zhao Z, Ross AC. 1995. Retinoic acid repletion restores the number of leukocytes and their subsets and stimulates natural cytotoxicity in vitamin A-deficient rats. *J Nutr* 125:2064–2073.

Zhao Z, Murasko DM, Ross AC. 1994. The role of vitamin A in natural killer cell cytotoxicity, number and activation in the rat. *Nat Immun* 13:29–41.

5
Vitamin K

SUMMARY

Vitamin K functions as a coenzyme during the synthesis of the biologically active form of a number of proteins involved in blood coagulation and bone metabolism. Because of the lack of data to estimate an average requirement, an Adequate Intake (AI) is set based on representative dietary intake data from healthy individuals. The AI for men and women is 120 and 90 µg/day, respectively. No adverse effect has been reported for individuals consuming higher amounts of vitamin K, so a Tolerable Upper Intake Level (UL) was not established.

BACKGROUND INFORMATION

Compounds with vitamin K activity are 3-substituted 2-methyl-1,4-naphthoquinones. Phylloquinone, the plant form of the vitamin, contains a phytyl group; "long chain" menaquinones (MK-n), produced by bacteria in the lower bowel, contain a polyisoprenyl side chain with 6 to 13 isoprenyl units at the 3-position (Suttie, 1992). A specific menaquinone, MK-4, is not a major bacterial product, but can be formed by the cellular alkylation of menadione (2-methyl-1,4-naphthoquinone). Recently, MK-4 has been shown to be produced from phylloquinone in germ-free animals and in tissue culture (Davidson et al., 1998).

162

Function

Vitamin K plays an essential role in the posttranslational conversion of specific glutamyl residues in a limited number of proteins to γ-carboxyglutamyl (Gla) residues (Suttie, 1993). These proteins include plasma prothrombin (coagulation factor II) and the plasma procoagulants, factors VII, IX, and X. Because under-γ-carboxylated forms of these proteins lack biological activity, the classical sign of a vitamin K deficiency has been a vitamin K-responsive increase in prothrombin time and, in severe cases, a hemorrhagic event. Two structurally related vitamin K-dependent proteins (Price, 1988), osteocalcin found in bone and matrix Gla protein originally found in bone but now known to be more widely distributed, have received recent attention as proteins with possible roles in the prevention of chronic disease (Ferland, 1998). No relationship between a decreased biological activity of any of the other vitamin K-dependent proteins and a disease-related physiological response has been postulated.

Physiology of Absorption, Metabolism, and Excretion

Phylloquinone, the major form of vitamin K in the diet, is absorbed in the jejunum and ileum in a process that is dependent on the normal flow of bile and pancreatic juice and is enhanced by dietary fat (Shearer et al., 1974). Absorption of free phylloquinone is nearly quantitative (Shearer et al., 1970), but recent studies (Garber et al., 1999; Gijsbers et al., 1996) suggest that the vitamin in food sources is less well absorbed. Absorbed phylloquinone is secreted into lymph as a component of chylomicrons and enters the circulation in this form. Circulating phylloquinone is present in the very low density triglyceride-rich lipoprotein fractions and chylomicrons (Kohlmeier et al., 1996; Lamon-Fava et al., 1998). A dependence of plasma phylloquinone concentrations (Kohlmeier et al., 1995) on the distribution of lipoprotein apoE isoforms suggests that the vitamin enters the liver through the endocytosis of chylomicron remnants. The liver rapidly accumulates ingested phylloquinone and contains the highest concentration. Skeletal muscle contains little phylloquinone, but significant concentrations are found in the heart and some other tissues (Davidson et al., 1998; Thijssen and Drittij-Reijnders, 1994). It is not known how or if hepatic phylloquinone is secreted and transported from the liver to peripheral tissues.

The vitamin is rapidly catabolized and excreted from the liver, mainly in bile. A smaller amount appears in urine (Shearer et al.,

1974). The excretion products have not been extensively character-ized but are known to proceed through the oxidative degradation of the phytyl side chain of phylloquinone, followed by glucuronide conjugation. Turnover in the liver is rapid and hepatic reserves are rapidly depleted when dietary intake of vitamin K is restricted (Usui et al., 1990).

The human gut contains a large amount of bacterially produced menaquinones, but their contribution to the maintenance of vita-min K status has been difficult to assess (Suttie, 1995). Although the content is extremely variable, human liver contains about 10 times as much vitamin K as a mixture of menaquinones than as phyllo-quinone (Shearer, 1992; Thijssen and Drittij-Reijnders, 1996; Usui et al., 1990). Absorption of these very lipophilic membrane-associated compounds from the distal bowel has been difficult to demonstrate (Ichihashi et al., 1992). Evidence of vitamin K inadequacy in normal human subjects following dietary restriction of vitamin K also suggests that this source of the vitamin is not utilized in sufficient amounts to maintain maximal γ-carboxylation of vitamin K-dependent pro-teins. One specific menaquinone, MK-4, appears to have a unique yet unidentified role. MK-4 can be formed from menadione (2-methyl-1,4-naphthoquinone) but is also formed in animal tissues from phylloquinone (Davidson et al., 1998; Thijssen and Drittij-Reijnders, 1994). It is present in much higher concentrations than phylloquinone in tissues such as pancreas, salivary gland, brain, and sternum, and its concentration in these tissues is to some degree dependent on phylloquinone intake.

Clinical Effects of Inadequate Intake

A clinically significant vitamin K deficiency has usually been defined as a vitamin K-responsive hypoprothrombinemia and is asso-ciated with an increase in prothrombin time (PT) and, in severe cases, bleeding. Spontaneous cases have been rare and have usually been associated with various lipid malabsorption syndromes (Savage and Lindenbaum, 1983). There are numerous case reports of bleed-ing episodes in antibiotic-treated patients, and these have often been ascribed to an acquired vitamin K deficiency resulting from a suppression of menaquinone-synthesizing organisms. However, these reports are complicated by the possibility of general malnutri-tion in this patient population and by the antiplatelet action of many of the same drugs (Suttie, 1995).

Reports of experimentally induced, clinically significant vitamin K deficiencies are scant. Udall (1965) fed 10 healthy subjects a diet that probably contained less than 10 µg /day of phylloquinone. After 3 weeks, a statistically significant increase in the PT was observed, but it was still within the normal range. In another study, Frick and coworkers (1967) administered a parenteral nutrient solution to a small number of neomycin-treated adults for 4 weeks and observed prolonged PT that responded to the parenteral administration of phylloquinone. They concluded that the minimal daily requirement was between 0.3 and 1.05 µg per kg body weight of phylloquinone. In more recent studies (Allison et al., 1987; Ferland et al., 1993), feeding healthy individuals diets containing 5 to 10 µg/day of phylloquinone for 14- to 16-day periods failed to induce any change in PT measurements.

These limited studies, conducted over a number of years, indicate that the simple restriction of vitamin K intake to levels almost impossible to achieve in any nutritionally adequate, self-selected diet do not impair normal hemostatic control in healthy subjects. Although there is some interference in the hepatic synthesis of the vitamin K-dependent clotting factors that can be measured by sensitive assays, standard clinical measures of procoagulant potential are not changed.

SELECTION OF INDICATORS FOR ESTIMATING THE REQUIREMENT FOR VITAMIN K

Various indicators have been used to assess vitamin K status in humans (Booth and Suttie, 1998). Of these, only one, prothrombin time (PT), has been associated with adverse clinical effects. All other indicators have been shown to respond to alterations in dietary vitamin K, but the physiological significance of these diet-induced changes is lacking. Therefore, these indicators have been used to assess relative changes in vitamin K status but do not provide, by themselves or collectively, an adequate basis on which to estimate an average requirement for vitamin K.

Prothrombin Time

The classical PT used to measure the procoagulant potential of plasma is not a sensitive indicator of vitamin K status because plasma prothrombin concentration must be decreased by approximately 50 percent before a value is outside of the "normal" range (Suttie, 1992). Furthermore, studies conducted thus far clearly indicate that PT does not respond to a change in dietary vitamin K in healthy subjects (Allison et al., 1987; Bach et al., 1996; Binkley et al., 1999; Booth et al., 1999a; Suttie et al., 1988).

Factor VII

On the basis of its relatively short half-life (approximately 6 hours), factor VII activity has been used to assess vitamin K status. Allison and colleagues (1987) maintained 33 healthy subjects, some given antibiotics, for 2 weeks on a low vitamin K diet (less than 5 µg/day of phylloquinone) and observed a decrease from the normal range of plasma factor VII in seven of the subjects. However, in the absence of antibiotic treatment, factor VII activity is not a sensitive indicator of vitamin K status as it does not usually respond to changes in vitamin K intake in healthy individuals (Bach et al., 1996; Ferland et al., 1993).

Plasma and Serum Phylloquinone Concentration

Both phylloquinone and the menaquinones have been used to assess status, with phylloquinone as the vitamer usually studied because it is the primary source of dietary vitamin K in western countries (Booth and Suttie, 1998). Serum or plasma phylloquinone concentration reflects recent intakes and has been shown to respond to changes in dietary intake within 24 hours (Sokoll et al., 1997). However, given the distribution of vitamin K in the food supply, a single day plasma (serum) phylloquinone concentration may not reflect normal dietary intake. Positive correlations between circulating phylloquinone concentration and dietary intake have been reported, but the strength of this association has varied according to studies, possibly due to differences in intake assessment methodology (i.e., number of diet record days) (Booth et al., 1995, 1997b). In healthy individuals, phylloquinone concentrations are higher in older subjects than in younger subjects, irrespective of dietary intake (Booth et al., 1997b; Ferland et al., 1993; Sokoll and Sadowski, 1996). Strong positive correlations between plasma (serum) phylloquinone and triglyceride concentrations have been reported (Kohlmeier et al., 1995; Sadowski et al., 1989; Saupe et al., 1993), a finding that likely explains the higher vitamin K concentrations observed in older individuals (Sadowski et al., 1989). Normal ranges for plasma phylloquinone concentration in healthy adults aged 20 to 49 years ($n = 131$) was 0.25 to 2.55 nmol/L; for those aged 65 to 92 years ($n = 195$), 0.32 to 2.67 nmol/L (Sadowski et al., 1989).

Urinary γ-Carboxyglutamyl Residues

After protein catabolism, γ-carboxyglutamyl (Gla) residues contained in the vitamin K-dependent proteins are not further metabolized and are excreted via urine (Shah et al., 1978). As a result, urinary Gla excretion has been used as an indicator of vitamin K status. Urinary Gla responds to alterations in dietary intake, but periods of several days are needed before any change can be observed (Ferland et al., 1993; Suttie et al., 1988). In a study by Suttie and coworkers (1988), 10 college-age men were asked to eliminate the major sources of vitamin K from their diet, thereby reducing their intake to less than 40 μg/day of phylloquinone. Urinary Gla excretion decreased 22 percent after 3 weeks and returned to baseline values 12 days after supplementation with 50 or 500 μg of phylloquinone. In a recent study, increasing phylloquinone intakes from 100 μg/day to a range of 377 to 417 μg/day for 5 days did not induce significant changes in urinary Gla (Booth et al., 1999a).

Response of urinary Gla to vitamin K intake alterations appears to be age-specific. In a study by Ferland and coworkers (1993), 32 subjects were divided into four groups of eight (men or women, 20 to 40 or 60 to 80 years old) and housed in a metabolic research unit. They were fed 80 μg of phylloquinone for 4 days followed by a low vitamin K diet (approximately 10 μg phylloquinone/day) for 16 days. At the end of the depletion period, urinary Gla excretion had decreased significantly in the younger, but not the older subjects. Short-term supplementation with 45 μg/day of phylloquinone reversed the decline to near baseline values. In another study involving 263 healthy individuals (127 men, 136 women) aged 18 to 55 years, urinary Gla/creatinine excretion ratios increased significantly with age in both men and women with values 20 percent higher in women over the age span (Sokoll and Sadowski, 1996). To date, there are insufficient data for using urinary Gla excretion for estimating an average requirement.

Undercarboxylated Prothrombin

In humans, an insufficiency of vitamin K leads to the secretion into plasma of biologically inactive, under-γ-carboxylated forms of the vitamin K-dependent clotting factors. These proteins are referred to as protein induced by vitamin K absence or antagonism (PIVKA). In reference to prothrombin (factor II), the term used is PIVKA-II. This protein has been measured by specific immunoassay (Blanchard et al., 1981), by thrombin generation after the removal of normal prothrombin by adsorption to barium or calcium salts (Francis, 1988), or by an indirect assay that compares biologically active prothrombin to the amount of thrombin that can be generated by a nonphysiological activator (Allison et al., 1987). A number of immunochemical assays, which are very sensitive and are capable of measuring very small increases of this indicator of vitamin K insufficiency, are now commercially available. Typically, these kits will detect changes of a few ng/mL whereas plasma prothrombin concentration averages 100 µg/mL.

Concentrations of PIVKA-II vary little with aging in healthy subjects (Sokoll and Sadowski, 1996) but respond to dietary alterations. In two independent studies using immunological assays (Booth et al., 1999b; Ferland et al., 1993), intakes of 10 µg/day of phylloquinone were associated with abnormal PIVKA-II concentrations (greater than 2 ng/mL) in the great majority of subjects, whereas an intake of 100 µg/day was associated with normal (less than 2 ng/mL) PIVKA-II concentrations in 15 of 16 subjects (Booth et al., 1999b). In older studies that used indirect colorimetric assays, abnormal PIVKA-II concentrations were observed with diets containing 40 to 60 µg/day of phylloquinone but were normal when intakes were approximately 80 µg/day (Jones et al., 1991; Suttie et al., 1988).

Although it is clear from these data that PIVKA-II concentrations can be influenced by vitamin K intake, results from these studies cannot be used to set dietary vitamin K recommendations. This is because there have been no studies to compare the immunoassay and colorimetric studies for determining whether the data given above can be used collectively. Therefore, at the present there are inadequate dose-response data from a single procedure. Intervention studies using graded intakes of vitamin K and protocols of longer duration need to be conducted before this indicator can be used to establish dietary recommendations for vitamin K.

Under-γ-carboxylated Osteocalcin

Small amounts of the bone protein, osteocalcin, circulate in plasma, and like PIVKA-II, under-γ-carboxylated osteocalcin (ucOC) has been considered an indicator of suboptimal vitamin K status. Assays for measuring the degree of carboxylation of osteocalcin have been indirect and have relied on the lower affinity of ucOC for hydroxyapatite (Knapen et al., 1989) or barium sulfate (Sokoll et al., 1995). Only recently has direct assessment of ucOC been possible with the development of a monoclonal antibody specific for the undercarboxylated form of osteocalcin (Vergnaud et al., 1997).

As discussed below, a number of reports have correlated decreased bone mineral density (BMD) or increased fracture rate with a five- to eight-fold increase in ucOC. Concurrently, it has been observed that vitamin K intakes similar to those reported for the general population did not ensure complete carboxylation of osteocalcin (Bach et al., 1996; Sokoll and Sadowski, 1996) and that ucOC could be decreased by increasing vitamin K intake (Binkley et al., 1999; Booth et al., 1999b; Douglas et al., 1995; Knapen et al., 1989, 1993). These reports have led to the suggestion that vitamin K requirements for bone function are probably much higher than those needed to maintain normal hemostasis and that the recommendation for vitamin K should be much higher than current recommendations (Weber, 1997).

However, a number of issues must be considered before a minimal ucOC concentration can be used as an indicator to estimate an average requirement for vitamin K. Because osteocalcin is used clinically as a marker of bone turnover, there are a number of commercial kits currently marketed. Although they may all be internally reproducible, they react with different epitopes and have different reactivity with osteocalcin degradation fragments. Therefore, they do not give the same "normal" values (Delmas et al., 1990a, 1990b; Gundberg et al., 1998). Because of this, most investigators interested in the influence of vitamin K status on bone have expressed measurements of ucOC as percent ucOC. In apparently healthy subjects, ucOC has ranged from 3 to 45 percent, depending on the assay. The basis for these higher values has not been established but in many cases may reflect the fact that the assay is recognizing some osteocalcin fragments that do not contain potential Gla sites as ucOC. This interpretation of the data is supported by the high ucOC values that have been seen in some studies after vitamin K supplementation (Booth et al., 1999a; Douglas et al., 1995; Knapen et al., 1993). Other investigators have reported nearly complete elimination of ucOC by vitamin K supplementation. Bach and coworkers (1996) reduced ucOC from 8 to 3 percent and from 2 to 1 percent in small groups ($n = 9$) of younger and older subjects, respectively, with 1 mg phylloquinone for 5 days. Binkley and coworkers (1999) supplemented a larger ($n = 107$) group of both younger and older subjects by supplementation with 1 mg phylloquinone for 2 weeks and reduced ucOC from 8 to 3 percent and from 7 to 3 percent, respectively.

The wide variations in percent ucOC reported for vitamin K-sufficient subjects have made it essentially impossible to compare studies. The emphasis that investigators have placed on ucOC, an indicator of a nonfunctional protein, has also influenced thinking in this field. If percent ucOC in the apparently healthy population is as low as indicated in the more recent studies, about 90 to 95 percent of osteocalcin is in its biologically active form. Whether it is reasonable to assume that an increase in this value to 100 percent would be expected to have any physiological significance is a question that must be considered.

Although there is little doubt that vitamin K intake affects the degree of osteocalcin λ-carboxylation, the technical problems associated with the current assays and the uncertainty surrounding the physiological significance of diet-induced changes prevent the use of ucOC for estimating an average requirement for vitamin K.

Relationship of Vitamin K Intake to Chronic Disease

Vitamin K and Osteoporosis

The possibility that vitamin K may have a role in osteoporosis was first suggested with reports of lower circulating phylloquinone concentrations in osteoporotic patients having suffered a spinal crush fracture or fracture of the femur (Hart et al., 1985; Hodges et al., 1991, 1993). More recently, lower circulating phylloquinone and menaquinone concentrations have been observed in subjects with reduced BMD (Kanai et al., 1997; Tamatani et al., 1998) though other studies have not confirmed this finding (Rosen et al., 1993). As the circulating vitamin K concentration can be altered through diet within a few days, the clinical significance of these relationships remains to be established.

The role of vitamin K in bone metabolism has also been investigated by studying the vitamin K bone protein osteocalcin and its undercarboxylated form, ucOC. The extent to which osteocalcin is undercarboxylated has been assessed with respect to age, bone status, and risk of hip fracture (Binkley and Suttie, 1995; Vermeer et al., 1996). Although ucOC was reported to increase with age in some studies (Knapen et al., 1998; Liu and Peacock, 1998; Plantalech et al., 1991), other reports have not confirmed this finding (Sokoll and Sadowski, 1996). Negative correlations have also been reported between ucOC and BMD, but the strength of the associations has varied depending on the population studied (Knapen et al., 1998; Liu and Peacock, 1998; Vergnaud et al., 1997). Although the observed relationship between ucOC and BMD is of interest, it requires further investigation as significant inverse relationships have also been observed between BMD and total osteocalcin (Liu and Peacock, 1998; Ravn et al., 1996) and between BMD and the active (carboxylated) form of osteocalcin (Knapen et al., 1998).

Undercarboxylated osteocalcin has also been associated with increased risk of hip fracture. In a series of reports involving institutionalized elderly women studied for periods of up to 3 years, women with elevated ucOC at the start of the study had a three- to six-fold higher risk of suffering a hip fracture during the follow-up period (Szulc et al., 1993, 1996). It is of interest that in these studies the concentration of carboxylated osteocalcin, presumably the biologically active form, also was highest in the hip fracture group. Similar results subsequently were observed in a 22-month follow-up study involving a group of 359 independently living women (104 women having suffered a hip fracture and 255 controls) (Vergnaud et al., 1997). When the risk of hip fracture was related to levels of ucOC, increased baseline ucOC levels were associated with increased hip fracture risk with an odds ratio of 2. Although it is not possible to calculate carboxylated osteocalcin by quartiles from the data presented, this biologically active form of osteocalcin was not reduced in the hip fracture group. These studies are of interest with respect to a potential role of vitamin K in bone health, but they should be interpreted with caution given that in most cases they did not control for confounding factors such as overall quality of the diet or for nutrients known to influence bone metabolism (i.e., vitamin D and calcium). The increased concentration of circulating carboxylated osteocalcin in the fracture-prone population would also suggest that if vitamin K status has a role in bone health, it is not mediated through the action of osteocalcin.

Vitamin K intake has been associated with bone health in an epidemiological study. Utilizing the Nurse's Health Study cohort, researchers found that vitamin K intakes were inversely related to the risk of hip fractures in a 10-year follow-up period (Feskanich et al., 1999). Vitamin K intakes of 71,327 women aged 38 to 63 years were assessed through the use of a food frequency questionnaire. Women in quintiles two through five of vitamin K intake had a lower age-adjusted relative risk of hip fracture (relative risk, 0.70; 95 percent confidence interval, 0.53–0.93) than women in the lowest quintile (vitamin K intake less than 109 µg/day). Risk did not decrease between quintiles two and five, a finding that should be explored further.

Intervention studies using different K vitamers in physiological and pharmacological dosages have also been performed. In a study involving a group of secluded nuns, 2-week supplementation with 1 mg of phylloquinone was associated with significant decreases in urinary hydroxyproline and calcium excretion in subjects characterized as being "fast losers" of calcium (calcium/creatinine greater than 0.6) (Knapen et al., 1989). These results were subsequently confirmed in a larger group of free-living women, but the effect was again limited to postmenopausal, "fast loser" subjects (Knapen et al., 1993). The fact that in these two studies the positive effect of phylloquinone supplementation was restricted to subgroups of the populations limits the generalizability of the results.

More recently, administration of pharmacological doses (45 mg/day) of menoquinone (MK-4) to osteoporotic patients for 6 months was associated with an increase in metacarpal bone density, increased total osteocalcin, and reduced urinary calcium excretion. Interestingly, MK-4 treatment was associated with increased parathyroid hormone and had no effect on BMD of the lumbar spine (Orimo et al., 1992). Although this study is probably the most rigorous one conducted thus far with respect to study design and clinical outcomes, it has little relevance to vitamin K nutrition as the action of MK-4 in bone may be quite different from that of phylloquinone. Studies have indeed shown that the action of MK-4 may be independent of its usual role in the γ-carboxylation of the Gla proteins (Hara et al., 1995).

Although many of the studies discussed so far point to a role for vitamin K in bone, results from studies involving patients undergoing anticoagulant therapy with warfarin, a vitamin K antagonist, tend not to support this possibility. Because patients treated with warfarin are in a constant state of relative vitamin K deficiency by virtue of the drug's action, these patients would likely be at risk of bone disorders. In a recent meta-analysis (nine studies), long-term exposure to oral anticoagulants, including warfarin, was assessed in relation to bone density (Caraballo et al., 1999). Oral anticoagulant exposure was found to be associated with lower bone density in the ultradistal radius; however, there was no significant effect on the distal radius, lumbar spine, femoral neck, or femoral trochanter.

Finally, it should be mentioned that mice lacking the gene that codes for osteocalcin were recently studied (Ducy et al., 1996). The phenotype was not that of decreased mineralization; but rather these animals were found to present greater bone mass and stronger bones than the wild-type animals.

Whether vitamin K intake is a significant etiological component of osteoporosis is difficult to establish on the basis of the studies performed thus far. However, clinical intervention studies presently being conducted in North America and in Europe will help elucidate this question within the next few years.

Vitamin K and Atherosclerosis

A role for vitamin K in atherosclerosis was hypothesized when proteins containing Gla residues were isolated from hardened atherosclerotic plaque (Gijsbers et al., 1990; Levy et al., 1979). These were later identified as osteocalcin and matrix Gla proteins (Ferland, 1998). In a more recent study involving 113 postmenopausal women, lower vitamin K intakes and higher ucOC levels were associated with the presence of atherosclerotic calcification in the abdominal aorta (Jie et al., 1995). Although these results are interesting, they should be considered with caution as the assessment of vitamin K status was performed 5 years after the diagnosis of atherosclerosis was made. To what extent this time lag affected the findings is unknown. Furthermore, the vitamin K intake reported for this population is quite high, in fact much higher than what is usually reported for subjects of similar age (Booth and Suttie, 1998).

A role of vitamin K in vascular health is supported by the finding of extensive arterial calcification in the matrix Gla protein knockout mouse (Luo et al., 1997). Whether vitamin K status within the range of normal intake plays a significant role in the development of atherosclerosis requires further investigation and should be verified in studies using rigorous experimental designs.

FACTORS AFFECTING THE VITAMIN K REQUIREMENT

Bioavailability

The predominant form of vitamin K in the North American diet is phylloquinone from green leafy vegetables, and the available data on the vitamin K content of foods have been reviewed (Booth and Suttie, 1998). These data are comprehensive, but little information on the relative bioavailability of phylloquinone from various foods in human subjects is available. Gijsbers and colleagues (1996) have compared the relative bioavailability, measured as area under an absorption curve, of 1,000 µg of phylloquinone from a synthetic preparation and from a food matrix. Phylloquinone in the form of cooked spinach was reported to be 4 percent as bioavailable as that from a phylloquinone supplement. Three times as much phylloquinone was absorbed when butter was consumed with the spinach. Garber and coworkers (1999) observed that when 500 µg of phylloquinone was consumed with a 400 kcal (27 percent energy from fat) meal, the relative absorption was between five and six times lower from spinach than from a phylloquinone tablet. In this study, phylloquinone absorption from fresh spinach, broccoli, or romaine lettuce did not differ and was highly variable between subjects. It is apparent from these limited studies that until more data are available, the bioavailability of phylloquinone from vegetable sources should not be considered to be more than 20 percent as available as phylloquinone consumed as a supplement.

Approximately 34 percent of phylloquinone in the American diet is consumed from fats and oils (Booth et al., 1995). It might be expected that phylloquinone dissolved in oil would be more available than from a food matrix, but this may not be true. Vitamin K is not well absorbed by patients exhibiting lipid malabsorption syndromes (Savage and Lindenbaum, 1983), and efficient absorption of this fat-soluble vitamin from the digestive tract does require dietary fat. Although direct measures of bioavailabilty have not been reported, a recent study reported no difference in fasting plasma phylloquinone concentrations when 400 µg of phylloquinone as broccoli or as phylloquinone-fortified oil was added to a diet containing 100 µg of phylloquinone (Booth et al., 1999a). Hydrogenated fats contain significant amounts of 2',3'-dihydrophylloquinone formed from phylloquinone during processing. Dietary intake of this form of the vitamin in the United States is estimated to be about 20 percent of phylloquinone (Booth et al., 1999c). Neither the biological activity nor the bioavailability of this form of vitamin K is known. The amount of dietary fat needed for optimal absorption has not been determined.

Drug-Nutrient Interactions

Oral 4-hydroxycoumarin derivatives such as warfarin are widely prescribed anticoagulants for the prevention of thrombotic disorders. These drugs function through the inhibition of a hepatic vitamin K-epoxide reductase. This enzyme reduces the coproduct of the λ-glutamyl carboxylase reaction, the vitamin K 2,3-epoxide, to the hydronaphthoquinone form of the vitamin, which is the substrate for the enzyme. The result is an acquired cellular vitamin K deficiency and a decrease in the synthesis of the vitamin K-dependent plasma clotting factors. Alterations in vitamin K intake can, therefore, influence warfarin efficacy, and numerous case reports of these occurrences have been reviewed (Booth et al., 1997a). Short-term, day-to-day variations in vitamin K intake do not appear to alter anticoagulant status, and there are few data on the extent to which long-term differences in dietary vitamin K intake modulate the response to warfarin. Lubetsky and coworkers (1999) studied a population of 46 patients with an estimated (by food frequency recall) median intake of 179 μg/day of phylloquinone. Patients with intakes greater than 250 μg/day were maintained at the targeted international normalized ratio with 5.8 mg/day warfarin, while patients with an intake of less than 250 μg/day of phylloquinone were maintained on a lower warfarin intake of 4.4 mg/day. These data suggest that alterations in vitamin K intake might influence warfarin dosage. As an effective warfarin dose varies widely within individuals, patients are closely monitored. Once a dose has been established, patients can avoid any complications resulting from variations in vitamin K intake by continuing to follow their normal dietary patterns.

Nutrient-Nutrient Interactions

The ability of elevated intakes of vitamin E to antagonize vitamin K action has been clearly established. Woolley (1945) first demonstrated that increased dietary or parenteral α-tocopherol or α-tocopherol quinone could induce a hemorrhagic syndrome in the rat, and vitamin K administration was demonstrated to reverse this response (Rao and Mason, 1975). Studies of the microsomal vitamin K-dependent carboxylase have demonstrated that the enzyme can be inhibited by α-tocopherol and that it is even more sensitive to α-tocopherol quinone (Bettger and Olson, 1982; Dowd and Zheng, 1995).

Increased intakes of vitamin E have not been reported to antagonize vitamin K status in healthy humans. However, in one study, oral supplementation of anticoagulated patients (50 percent plasma prothrombin concentrations) with approximately 360 mg/day (400 IU/day) of α-tocopherol resulted in nonstatistically significant decreases in prothrombin concentrations over a 4-week period, and a statistically significant decrease in the ratio of biologically active prothrombin to prothrombin antigen (Corrigan and Ulfers, 1981). More sensitive measures of vitamin K status are now available and should be used to assess the potential impact of vitamin E supplementation in anticoagulated patients or subjects with low vitamin K intakes.

The metabolic basis for vitamin E antagonism of vitamin K function has not been completely elucidated. Recent data from a study using a rat model have demonstrated an adverse effect of dietary α-tocopherol on phylloquinone absorption (Alexander and Suttie, 1999), and it is likely that both this response and cellular interactions are responsible for the antagonism that has been observed in both animals and human subjects.

Antagonism of vitamin K action in animal models by retinoids (retinyl acetate, 13-*cis* retinoic acid, and N-(7-hydroxyphenyl) retinamide) has been reported by a group of investigators (McCarthy et al., 1989). High doses of these compounds have been used in animal studies, and adverse responses in humans have not been reported. The metabolic basis for this interaction has not been determined.

FINDINGS BY LIFE STAGE AND GENDER GROUP

Infants Ages 0 through 12 Months

Vitamin K is poorly transported across the placenta, which puts newborn infants at risk for vitamin K deficiency (Greer, 1995). Concentrations of vitamin K in cord blood are usually less than 0.1 nmol/L or undetectable (Mandelbrot et al., 1988; Widdershoven et al., 1988), and elevated concentrations of undercarboxylated prothrombin (PIVKA-II) have been reported (Greer, 1995). Poor vitamin K status added to the fact that the concentrations of most plasma clotting factors are low at the time of birth increases the risk of bleeding during the first weeks of life, a condition known as hemorrhagic disease of the newborn (HDNB). Because HDNB can be effectively prevented by administration of vitamin K, infants born in the United States and in Canada routinely receive 0.5 to 1 mg of phylloquinone intramuscularly or 2.0 mg orally within 6 hours of birth. Compared to oral prophylaxis, intramuscular (IM) treatment has been shown to be more efficacious in the prevention of HDNB (Greer, 1995). In light of this and because an oral dosage form of vitamin K has not been readily available in North America, newborns have typically been administered vitamin K via the IM route. Studies published in the early nineties reporting an association between IM prophylaxis and childhood cancer created some concern and questioned the safety of this practice. In two studies, Golding and coworkers (1990, 1992) reported an increased risk (odds ratio, 1.97–2.6) of leukemia and other forms of cancer in children who had received vitamin K intramuscularly at birth. Subsequent studies conducted in the United States and European countries (Ansell et al., 1996; Ekelund et al., 1993; Klebanoff et al., 1993; Olsen et al., 1994; von Kries et al., 1996) have failed to confirm Golding's findings and quieted the debate. Recently, both the American and the

Canadian pediatric societies reaffirmed their confidence in the IM prophylaxis, encouraging its general use (AAP, 1993; CPS, 1998).

Method Used to Set the Adequate Intake

No functional criteria of vitamin K status have been demonstrated that reflect response to dietary intake in infants. Thus, recommended intakes of vitamin K are based on an Adequate Intake (AI) that reflects a calculated mean vitamin K intake of infants principally fed human milk and provided vitamin K prophylaxis.

Although vitamin K prophylaxis at birth offers good protection with respect to HDNB during the first few weeks of life, infants become increasingly dependent on vitamin K intake in subsequent weeks. Though not a major concern in the United States or Canada, late HDNB occurs between 3 and 8 weeks of life and is usually associated with breast-feeding (Lane and Hathaway, 1985; von Kries et al., 1993). Milk intake appears to be an important factor in the etiology of late HDNB as inverse correlations have been reported between human milk intake and undercarboxylated prothrombin (Motohara et al., 1989; von Kries et al., 1987a).

Vitamin K concentrations in mature human milk have ranged from 0.85 to 9.2 µg/L with a mean concentration of 2.5 µg/L (Table 5-1) (Canfield et al., 1990, 1991; Greer et al., 1991, 1997; Haroon et al., 1982; Hogenbirk et al.,1993; von Kries et al., 1987b). Vitamin K content of colostrum is slightly higher than that of mature milk, but concentrations do not vary significantly through the first 6 months of lactation (Canfield et al., 1991; Greer et al., 1991; von Kries et al., 1987b). Vitamin K content of human milk can be increased by maternal intakes of pharmacological doses of vitamin K (Greer et al., 1991; Haroon et al., 1982). In a study by Greer and coworkers (1997), supplementing mothers with a dose of 5 mg/day of phylloquinone for 12 weeks increased the vitamin K concentration of milk by 70-fold (82.1 versus 1.17 µg/mL in unsupplemented mothers). In another study, supplementing one mother with 0.1 mg/day of phylloquinone, an amount that can be obtained in the diet, raised milk concentrations from 2.5 to 4.9 ng/L (von Kries et al., 1987b).

Ages 0 through 6 Months. The AI for infants 0 through 6 months of age is based on a reported average intake of milk of 0.78 L/day (Chapter 2) and on an average phylloquinone concentration of 2.5 mg/L in human milk. This gives an AI of 2.0 µg/day after rounding. The AI assumes that infants also receive prophylactic vitamin K at birth in amounts suggested by the American and Canadian pedi-

TABLE 5-1 Vitamin K in Human Milk

Reference	Study Group	Maternal Intake (µg/d)
Haroon et al., 1982	60 women	Not reported
von Kries et al., 1987b	9 women, 17–34 y	Not reported
Canfield et al., 1990	15 women, 20–35 y	Not reported
Canfield et al., 1991	15 women, 20–35 y	Not reported
Greer et al., 1991	23 women, 31 ± 3.6 y	Not reported
		302 ± 361 (SD)[b]
		296 ± 169 (SD)
		436 ± 667 (SD)
Hogenbirk et al., 1993	26 women	Not reported
Greer et al., 1997	22 women	No vitamin K supplements taken

[a] Vitamin K intake based on reported data or concentration (µg/L) × 0.78 L/day for 0–6 months postpartum.
[b] SD = standard deviation.

atric societies. The AI agrees with intakes of 0.6 to 2.3 µg/day reported for infants exclusively fed human milk (Canfield et al., 1991; Greer et al., 1991; Pietschnig et al., 1993).

The AI is significantly lower than recently reported intakes based on the Food and Drug Administration Total Diet Study of 77 µg/day (Booth et al., 1996b) and 111 µg/day (Appendix Table E-1). However, these values exclude intakes from human milk and include only intakes from other food sources. Booth and coworkers (1996b) reported that 87 percent of the estimated intake of 77 µg/day was attributed to infant formulas, which on average contain 50 to 100 mg/L of phylloquinone (Greer, 1995; Haroon et al., 1982).

Ages 7 through 12 Months. Using the method described in Chapter 2 to extrapolate from the AI for infants ages 0 through 6 months, the AI for older infants is 2.5 µg/day after rounding. Because complementary foods become a more important part of the infant diet in the second 6 months of life, vitamin K intake for this age category is expected to be higher than the AI based solely on human milk consumption. However, data concerning the vitamin K content of

Stage of Lactation	Milk Concentration	Estimated Vitamin K Intake of Infants (µg/d)[a]
Mature	2.5 µg/L	1.95
8–36 d	1.2 µg/L	0.94
1 mo	3.15 µg/L	2.45
Colostrum 30–81 h	3.39 µg/L	2.64
1 mo	3.14 µg/L	2.45
3 mo	2.31 µg/L	1.81
6 mo	2.59 µg/L	2.03
1 wk	0.64 µg/L	0.50
6 wk	0.86 µg/L	0.67
12 wk	1.14 µg/L	0.88
26 wk	0.87 µg/L	0.52
1 wk	1.21 µg/L	0.94
6 wk	0.9 µg/L	0.7
3 d	1.10 µg/L	0.86
2 wk	1.17 µg/L	0.92
6 wk	1.14 µg/L	0.89
12 wk	1.17 µg/L	0.92

weaning foods and their contribution to daily vitamin K intake are not presently available. Alternatively, if the adult AI of 80 µg/day is extrapolated down by means of the method described in Chapter 2, the AI would be 23 µg/day. Because older infant vitamin K intakes of 2.5 µg/day have not been associated with adverse clinical outcomes (Greer et al., 1991), the AI is set at the level obtained by extrapolating up from young infants.

Vitamin K AI Summary, Ages 0 through 12 Months

AI for Infants
0–6 months	**2.0 µg/day of vitamin K**
7–12 months	**2.5 µg/day of vitamin K**

Special Considerations

Human milk does not contain as much vitamin K as cow milk (5 µg/mL) or infant formulas (50–100 µg/L) (Greer, 1995; Haroon et al., 1982). Significant amounts of menaquinone-4 have been detected in cow milk, yet its physiological function in infant nutrition is unknown (Indyk and Woollard, 1997). Vitamin K has been shown to specifically and reversibly bind to a protein complex in cow milk (Fournier et al., 1987). There is no information on the bioavailability of vitamin K in infant formula.

Children and Adolescents Ages 1 through 18 Years

Method Used to Set the Adequate Intake

No data were found on which to base an Estimated Average Requirement (EAR) for vitamin K for children or adolescents. Therefore AIs are set on the basis of the highest median intake for each age group reported by the Third National Health and Nutrition Examination Survey (NHANES III) (Appendix Table C-10) and rounding. The significant increase in the AI from infancy to early childhood is most likely due to the method used to set the AI for older infants and the increased portion of the diet containing vitamin K-rich fruits and vegetables as the diet becomes more diversified.

Vitamin K AI Summary, Ages 1 through 18 Years

AI for Children
1–3 years   30 µg/day of vitamin K
4–8 years   55 µg/day of vitamin K

AI for Boys
9–13 years   60 µg/day of vitamin K
14–18 years   75 µg/day of vitamin K

AI for Girls
9–13 years   60 µg/day of vitamin K
14–18 years   75 µg/day of vitamin K

Adults Ages 19 Years and Older

Method Used to Set the Adequate Intake

Clinically significant vitamin K deficiency is extremely rare in the general population, with cases being limited to individuals with malabsorption syndromes or those treated with drugs known to interfere with vitamin K metabolism. The recent development of indicators sensitive to vitamin K intake, though useful to describe relative diet-induced changes in vitamin K status, were not used for establishing an EAR because of the uncertainty surrounding their true physiological significance and the lack of sufficient dose-response data.

Therefore, the AI for adults is based on reported vitamin K dietary intakes in apparently healthy population groups. In a recent paper, Booth and Suttie (1998) reviewed 11 studies in which phylloquinone intakes ranged from 61 to 210 µg/day with average intakes of approximately 80 µg/day for adults younger than 45 years and approximately 150 µg/day for adults older than 55 years (Table 5-2). NHANES III data (Appendix Table C-10) indicate that median vitamin K intakes of adults varied between 82 and 117 µg/day.

Studies have demonstrated that abnormal PIVKA-II concentrations were observed in individuals consuming 40 to 60 µg/day of vitamin K but were normal when intakes were approximately 80 µg/

TABLE 5-2 Dietary Phylloquinone Intake in Healthy Men and Women

Reference	Sex	Age (y)	Subjects	Method	Mean Intake (µg/day)
Suttie et al., 1988	Men	20–35	10	Duplicate portion	77
Jones et al., 1991	Men and women	18–55	221	Diet record	61
Booth et al., 1995	Women	41–71	362	Diet record	156
Vermeer et al., 1995	Women	60–79	80	Food frequency questionnaire	210
Bach et al., 1996	Men	20–28	9	Diet record	83
Bach et al., 1996	Men	55–75	9	Diet record	164
Booth et al., 1996b	Men and women	25–30, 40–45	1,490	Diet recall and record	71
Booth et al., 1996b	Men and women	60–65, > 70	1,216	Diet recall and record	80
Price et al., 1996	Men and women	22–54	65	Diet record	68
Booth et al., 1997b	Men and women	20–40	17	Diet record	111
Booth et al., 1997b	Men and women	60–80	17	Diet record	143

SOURCE: Booth and Suttie (1998).

day (Jones et al., 1991; Suttie et al., 1988). Healthy individuals with phylloquinone intakes approaching 80 µg/day have been investigated and have shown no signs of a deficiency, a finding that suggests this level of intake is probably adequate for the majority of the adult population (Bach et al., 1996; Ferland et al., 1993; Suttie et al., 1988). Reported vitamin K intakes are slightly lower for women than men (Booth et al., 1996b; Appendix Table C-10).

Reported phylloquinone intakes of older adults have generally been higher than those of younger individuals, a finding explained by their higher intakes of vegetables (Booth et al., 1996b). Older subjects have been found to be more resistant to vitamin K deficiency than younger adults (Ferland et al., 1993).

The AI is based on median intake data from NHANES III (Appendix Table C-10). Because dietary intake assessment methods tend to underestimate the actual daily intake of foods, the highest intake value reported for the four adult age groups was used to set the AI for each gender; numbers are rounded up to the nearest 5 µg.

Vitamin K AI Summary, Ages 19 Years and Older

AI for Men
19–30 years	**120 µg/day of vitamin K**
31–50 years	**120 µg/day of vitamin K**
51–70 years	**120 µg/day of vitamin K**
> 70 years	**120 µg/day of vitamin K**

AI for Women
19–30 years	**90 µg/day of vitamin K**
31–50 years	**90 µg/day of vitamin K**
51–70 years	**90 µg/day of vitamin K**
> 70 years	**90 µg/day of vitamin K**

Pregnancy

Method Used to Set the Adequate Intake

Data pertaining to vitamin K status of pregnant women are limited but suggest that status is not different from that of nonpregnant women, that is, lack of signs of clinical deficiency and comparable circulating vitamin K concentrations (Mandelbrot et al., 1988; von Kries et al., 1992). Furthermore, there are no data on the vitamin K content of fetal tissue for estimating additional needs during pregnancy. Therefore, median vitamin K intake was used for setting the

AI. In the Total Diet Study, phylloquinone intakes of pregnant women were lower than those of nonpregnant women (Appendix Table E-1). Similarly, the median vitamin K intake for pregnant women was approximately 80 µg/day, whereas the vitamin K intake of premenopausal women was approximately 85 to 90 µg/day from NHANES III (Appendix Table C-10). In a recent report by Booth and coworkers (1999c), phylloquinone intakes were estimated from 14-day food diaries for a small group of pregnant women ($n = 17$) and were found to be similar (72 ± 56 µg/day [SD]) to those of nonpregnant women (73 ± 46 µg/day [SD]).

Although supplementation with pharmacological doses of vitamin K during the later stages of pregnancy has been shown to increase plasma concentrations of vitamin K and improve coagulation function of pregnant women in some studies (Anai et al., 1993; Morales et al., 1988), the impact of antenatal supplementation on status of the newborn has been mixed (Dickson et al., 1994; Kazzi et al., 1990; Morales et al., 1988). Until more data are available, there is no evidence to suggest that the AI for pregnant women should be different from that for nonpregnant women. Therefore, the AI is based on median NHANES III intake estimates of nonpregnant women.

Vitamin K AI Summary, Pregnancy

AI for Pregnancy
14–18 years	**75 µg/day of vitamin K**
19–30 years	**90 µg/day of vitamin K**
31–50 years	**90 µg/day of vitamin K**

Lactation

Method Used to Set the Adequate Intake

Available studies suggest the vitamin K status of lactating women is comparable to that of nonlactating women. Reported vitamin K intake of pregnant women does not differ significantly from those of nonlactating women. In a study by Greer and coworkers (1991) involving 23 lactating mothers, phylloquinone intakes at 6, 12, and 26 weeks were 302 ± 361 (standard deviation [SD]), 296 ± 169 (SD), and 436 ± 667 (SD) µg/day, respectively. There was no significant correlation between phylloquinone intake and breast milk concentration. Based on NHANES III intake estimates, median phylloquinone intakes of 99 lactating women was 74 µg/day, which is lower than the median intake of premenopausal women (approximately 85 to 90 µg/day) (Appendix Table C-10).

Although the phylloquinone content in maternal milk can be increased after treatment of mothers with pharmacological doses of vitamin K (Greer et al., 1997; Haroon et al., 1982; von Kries et al., 1987b), results from Greer and coworkers (1991) suggest that vitamin K content of milk is little affected by intake of lactating women who consume typical diets. Because vitamin K is not significantly secreted in milk, there is no evidence to suggest that the AI for lactating women should be different from that for nonlactating women. Therefore, the AI is the same as for nonpregnant women.

Vitamin K AI Summary, Lactation

AI for Lactation

14–18 years	**75 µg/day of vitamin K**
19–30 years	**90 µg/day of vitamin K**
31–50 years	**90 µg/day of vitamin K**

INTAKE OF VITAMIN K

Food Sources

Early data obtained by chick bioassay on the vitamin K content of foods were unreliable and a limited number of foods were assayed. Over the last decade, rapid and reliable chromatographic procedures for vitamin K have been developed, and data for the phylloquinone content of most commonly consumed foods are available (Booth et al., 1995). Only a relatively small number of food items (Table 5-3) contribute substantially to the dietary phylloquinone intake of most people. A few green vegetables (collards, spinach, and salad greens) contain in excess of 300 µg of phylloquinone/100 g, while broccoli, brussels sprouts, cabbage, and bib lettuce contain between 100 and 200 µg of phylloquinone/100 g. Other green vegetables contain smaller amounts. Plant oils and margarine are the second major source of phylloquinone in the diet. The phylloquinone content of plant oils is variable, with soybean and canola oils containing greater than 100 µg of phylloquinone/100 g. Cottonseed oil and olive oil contain about 50 µg/100 g, and corn oil contains less than 5 µg/100 g. Prepared foods contain variable amounts of vitamin K depending on their content of green vegetables and the source and amount of oil used in their preparation. Information relative to the important food sources of vitamin K for infants

TABLE 5-3 Phylloquinone Concentration of Common Foods[a]

Food Item	μg/100 g	Food Item	μg/100 g
Vegetables		*Protein sources*	
Collards	440	Dry soybeans	47
Spinach	380	Dry lentils	22
Salad greens	315	Liver	5
Broccoli	180	Eggs	2
Brussels sprouts	177	Fresh meats	< 1
Cabbage	145	Fresh fish	< 1
Bib lettuce	122	Whole milk	< 1
Asparagus	60	Tuna in oil	24
Okra	40		
Iceberg lettuce	35	*Prepared foods[b]*	
Green beans	33	Salad dressings	100
Green peas	24	Coleslaw	80
Cucumbers	20	Mayonnaise	41
Cauliflower	20	Beef chow mein	31
Carrots	10	Muffins	25
Tomatoes	6	Doughnuts	10
Potatoes	1	Apple pie	11
		Potato chips	15
Fats and oils		French fries	5
Soybean oil	193	Macaroni/cheese	5
Canola oil	127	Lasagna	5
Cottonseed oil	60	Pizza	4
Olive oil	55	Hamburger/bun	4
Corn oil	3	Hot dog/bun	3
Margarine	42	Baked beans	3
Butter	7	Bread	3

[a] Median value obtained from Booth et al. (1993, 1995), Koivu et al. (1997), Piironen et al. (1997), and Shearer et al. (1996). Both cooked and raw food values were used.
[b] Phylloquinone content may vary widely depending on the source of oil used in preparation.

and children of various age groups and for adults by gender and age group are available from data obtained from the U.S. Food and Drug Administration Total Diet Study (Booth et al., 1996b). Spinach, collards, broccoli, and iceberg lettuce are the major contributors of vitamin K in the diet of U.S. adults and children.

Hydrogenation of plant oils to form solid shortenings results in some conversion of phylloquinone to 2′,3′-dihydrophylloquinone (Davidson et al., 1996). This form of the vitamin is most prevalent in margarines, infant formulas, and prepared foods (Booth et al., 1996a) and can represent a substantial portion of the total vitamin

K in some diets. The bioavailability and the relative biological activity of dihydrophylloquinone have not been determined with any certainty. The long-chain menaquinones, which are produced in substantial amounts by intestinal microorganisms, can also serve as active forms of vitamin K, but they are not widely distributed in commonly consumed foods. Green vegetables and plant oils, the major dietary sources of vitamin K, do not contain menaquinones, and only small amounts are found in animal products. Relatively large amounts (40–80 µg/100 g) can, however, be obtained from some cheeses (Schurgers et al., 1999).

Dietary Intake

The availability of reliable data on the vitamin K content of foods has now made it possible to obtain reasonable estimates of the dietary phylloquinone intake of the North American population. The results of a number of studies on phylloquinone intake that used dietary records, with or without recall or a food frequency questionnaire, have been summarized by Booth and Suttie (1998) and are presented in Table 5-2. These data are somewhat variable but indicate a mean phylloquinone intake of about 150 µg/day for older (above 55 years) and 80 µg/day for younger men and women. Gender differences were not apparent in these studies.

Data from nationally representative U.S. surveys are available to estimate vitamin K intakes (Appendix Tables C-10, C-11, E-1). Data from the Third National Health and Nutrition Examination Survey (NHANES III) shows that median intakes of dietary vitamin K ranged from 79 to 88 µg/day for women and 89 to 117 µg/day for men (Appendix Table C-10). Because of the relatively small number of foods that provide significant amounts of phylloquinone in the diet, the daily variation in intake is high, and Booth and co-workers (1995) have estimated that a 5-day record of intake is needed to get a true measure of dietary intake. Data on phylloquinone intake have recently been calculated (Booth et al., 1999c) from 14-day food diaries collected by the Market Research Corporation of America. These data reflect the intake of nearly 4,000 men and women aged 13 years or older with a demographic profile similar to that of the U.S. census. These data clearly demonstrate the large daily variation in phylloquinone intake and indicate an average intake of 70 to 80 µg/day for the U.S. adult population. The same data provide an estimate of the dihydrophylloquinone intake of this population (19 µg/day for men and 15 µg/day for women) that is about 20 to 25 percent as much as the intake of phylloquinone.

The adult phylloquinone intake in The Netherlands has been reported to be two to three times higher than that of the U.S. population (Schurgers et al., 1999). Whether this represents a real difference in the consumption of phylloquinone-rich foods or differences in methods used to estimate foods consumed is not known at the present time. This study has also provided an estimate of the average intake of long-chain menaquinones of 21 µg/day. Comprehensive data on menaquinone intake are not available for the U.S. population.

Intake from Supplements

The median intakes of vitamin K from food and supplements for the four adult age groups was 93 to 119 µg/day for American men who took supplements (Appendix Table C-11). The median vitamin K intake from food and supplements for women who reported consuming supplements was 82 to 90 µg/day.

TOLERABLE UPPER INTAKE LEVELS

The Tolerable Upper Intake Level (UL) is the highest level of daily nutrient intake that is likely to pose no risk of adverse health effects for almost all individuals. Although members of the general population should be advised not to routinely exceed the UL, intake above the UL may be appropriate for investigation within well-controlled clinical trials. Clinical trials of doses above the UL should not be discouraged, as long as subjects participating in these trials have signed informed consent documents regarding possible toxicity and as long as these trials employ appropriate safety monitoring of trial subjects.

Hazard Identification

No adverse effects associated with vitamin K consumption from food or supplements have been reported in humans or animals. Therefore, a quantitative risk assessment cannot be performed and a UL cannot be derived for vitamin K.

A search of the literature revealed no evidence of toxicity associated with the intake of either the phylloquinone or menaquinone forms of vitamin K. A synthetic form of vitamin K, menadione, has been associated with liver damage (Badr et al., 1987; Chiou et al., 1998) and therefore is no longer used therapeutically.

One study showed a significant association between intramuscularly (IM) administered vitamin K and childhood cancer, particularly leukemia (Golding et al., 1992). This study compared 195 children diagnosed with cancer between 1971 and 1991 and born in one of two major hospitals (between 1965 and 1987) with 558 controls. Golding and coworkers (1992) reported a significant association between IM vitamin K and cancer incidence ($p = 0.002$; observed risk, 1.97; 95 percent confidence interval, 1.3–3.0). No significantly increased risk was reported for children who had been given oral vitamin K. These findings on IM vitamin K doses have limited relevance to ULs based on oral intake.

Furthermore, evidence from other population studies fails to confirm an association between vitamin K and cancer (Ansell et al., 1996; Klebanoff et al., 1993; McKinney et al., 1998; Parker et al., 1998; Passmore et al., 1998). In a nested case-control study that used data from a large, multicenter prospective study (54,795 children), Klebanoff and coworkers (1993) found no association between vitamin K exposure and an increased risk of any childhood cancer or of all childhood cancers combined. Ansell and coworkers (1996) assessed associations between leukemia and prenatal and neonatal exposures and failed to show an increased risk of childhood leukemia in neonates receiving IM-administered vitamin K. The findings of Ansell and coworkers (1996) were confirmed by three similar case-control studies (McKinney et al., 1998; Parker et al., 1998; Passmore et al., 1998).

Data from animal models have shown no toxicity of vitamin K (NRC, 1987). No adverse effects were reported with administration of up to 25 g/kg of phylloquinone either parenterally or orally to laboratory animals (Molitor and Robinson, 1940).

Dose-Response Assessment

The data on adverse effects from high vitamin K intakes are not sufficient for a quantitative risk assessment, and a UL cannot be derived.

Intake Assessment

The highest intake of dietary vitamin K reported for the U.S. population was 340 µg/day in women aged 19 through 30 years (Appendix Table C-10). The highest intake of vitamin K from food and supplements was 367 µg/day, also in women aged 19 through 30 years (Appendix Table C-11).

Risk Characterization

No adverse effects have been reported with high intakes of vitamin K.

RESEARCH RECOMMENDATIONS FOR VITAMIN K

• Clinical studies of vitamin K supplementation aimed at elucidating the physiological significance of undercarboxylated osteocalcin; these studies should be designed so as to relate this indicator to overall bone health and integrity.

• Knowledge of the function of all of the vitamin K-dependent proteins and their role in human physiology.

• Knowledge of a possible role of vitamin K in promoting human health other than that mediated by the known Gla-containing vitamin K-dependent proteins.

• Further knowledge of the bioavailability of dietary vitamin K.

REFERENCES

AAP (American Academy of Pediatrics). 1993. Controversies concerning vitamin K and the newborn. *Pediatrics* 91:1001–1003.

Alexander GD, Suttie JW. 1999. The effects of vitamin E on vitamin K activity. *FASEB J* 13:A535.

Allison PM, Mummah-Schendel LL, Kindberg CG, Harms CS, Bang NU, Suttie JW. 1987. Effects of a vitamin K-deficient diet and antibiotics in normal human volunteers. *J Lab Clin Med* 110:180–188.

Anai T, Hirota Y, Yoshimatsu J, Oga M, Miyakawa I. 1993. Can prenatal vitamin K1 (phylloquinone) supplementation replace prophylaxis at birth? *Obstet Gynecol* 81:251–254.

Ansell P, Bull D, Roman E. 1996. Childhood leukaemia and intramuscular vitamin K: Findings from a case-control study. *Br Med J* 313:204–205.

Bach AU, Anderson SA, Foley AL, Williams EC, Suttie JW. 1996. Assessment of vitamin K status in human subjects administered "minidose" warfarin. *Am J Clin Nutr* 64:894–902.

Badr M, Yoshihara H, Kauffman F, Thurman R. 1987. Menadione causes selective toxicity to periportal regions of the liver lobule. *Toxicol Lett* 35:241–246.

Bettger WJ, Olson RE. 1982. Effect of alpha-tocopherol and alpha-tocopherolquinone on vitamin K-dependent carboxylation in the rat. *Fed Proc* 41:344.

Binkley NC, Suttie JW. 1995. Vitamin K nutrition and osteoporosis. *J Nutr* 125:1812–1821.

Binkley NC, Krueger D, Todd H, Foley A, Engelke J, Suttie J. 1999. Serum undercarboxylated osteocalcin concentration is reduced by vitamin K supplementation. *FASEB J* 13:A238.

Blanchard RA, Furie BC, Jorgensen M, Kruger SF, Furie B. 1981. Acquired vitamin K-dependent carboxylation deficiency in liver disease. *N Engl J Med* 305:242–248.

Booth SL, Suttie JW. 1998. Dietary intake and adequacy of vitamin K. *J Nutr* 128:785–788.

Booth SL, Sadowski JA, Weihrauch JL, Ferland G. 1993. Vitamin K1 (phylloquinone) content of foods: A provisional table. *J Food Comp Anal* 6:109–120.

Booth SL, Sokoll LJ, O'Brien ME, Tucker K, Dawson-Hughes B, Sadowski JA. 1995. Assessment of dietary phylloquinone intake and vitamin K status in post-menopausal women. *Eur J Clin Nutr* 49:832–841.

Booth SL, Pennington JA, Sadowski JA. 1996a. Dihydro-vitamin K1: Primary food sources and estimated dietary intakes in the American diet. *Lipids* 31:715–720.

Booth SL, Pennington JA, Sadowski JA. 1996b. Food sources and dietary intakes of vitamin K-1 (phylloquinone) in the American diet: Data from the FDA Total Diet Study. *J Am Diet Assoc* 96:149–154.

Booth SL, Charnley JM, Sadowski JA, Saltzman E, Bovill EG, Cushman M. 1997a. Dietary vitamin K1 and stability of oral anticoagulation: Proposal of a diet with constant vitamin K1 content. *Thromb Haemost* 77:504–509.

Booth SL, Tucker KL, McKeown NM, Davidson KW, Dallal GE, Sadowski JA. 1997b. Relationships between dietary intakes and fasting plasma concentrations of fat-soluble vitamins in humans. *J Nutr* 127:587–592.

Booth SL, O'Brien-Morse ME, Dallal GE, Davidson KW, Gundberg CM. 1999a. Response of vitamin K status to different intakes and sources of phylloquinone-rich foods: Comparison of younger and older adults. *Am J Clin Nutr* 70:368–377.

Booth SL, O'Brien-Morse ME, Saltzman E, Lichtenstein AH, McKeown NM, Wood RJ, Gundberg CM. 1999b. Influence of dietary vitamin K1 (phylloquinone) on bone resorption. *FASEB J* 13:A580.

Booth SL, Webb DR, Peters JC. 1999c. Assessment of phylloquinone and dihydro-phylloquinone dietary intakes among a nationally representative sample of US consumers using 14-day food diaries. *J Am Diet Assoc* 99:1072–1076.

Canfield LM, Hopkinson JM, Lima AF, Martin GS, Sugimoto K, Burr J, Clark L, McGee DL. 1990. Quantitation of vitamin K in human milk. *Lipids* 25:406–411.

Canfield LM, Hopkinson JM, Lima AF, Silva B, Garza C. 1991. Vitamin K in colostrum and mature human milk over the lactation period—A cross-sectional study. *Am J Clin Nutr* 53:730–735.

Caraballo PJ, Gabriel SE, Castro MR, Atkinson EJ, Melton LJ III. 1999. Changes in bone density after exposure to oral anticoagulants: A meta-analysis. *Osteoporos Int* 9:441–448.

Chiou TJ, Chou YT, Tzeng WF. 1998. Menadione-induced cell degeneration is related to lipid peroxidation in human cancer cells. *Proc Natl Sci Counc Repub China B* 22:13–21.

Corrigan JJ Jr, Ulfers LL. 1981. Effect of vitamin E on prothrombin levels in warfarin-induced vitamin K deficiency. *Am J Clin Nutr* 34:1701–1705.

CPS (Canadian Paediatric Society). 1998. Routine administration of vitamin K to newborns. Joint position paper of the Canadian Paediatric Society and the Committee on Child and Adolescent Health of the College of Family Physicians of Canada. *Can Fam Physician* 44:1083–1090.

Davidson KW, Booth SL, Dolnikowski GG, Sadowski JA. 1996. The conversion of phylloquinone to 2',3'-dihydrophylloquinone during hydrogenation of vegetable oils. *J Agric Food Chem* 44:980–983.

Davidson RT, Foley AL, Engelke JA, Suttie JW. 1998. Conversion of dietary phylloquinone to tissue menaquinone-4 in rats is not dependent on gut bacteria. *J Nutr* 128:220–223.

Delmas PD, Christiansen C, Mann KG, Price PA. 1990a. Bone Gla protein (osteocalcin) assay standardization report. *J Bone Miner Res* 5:5–11.

Delmas PD, Price PA, Mann KG. 1990b. Validation of the bone Gla protein (osteocalcin) assay. *J Bone Miner Res* 5:3–4.

Dickson RC, Stubbs TM, Lazarchick J. 1994. Antenatal vitamin K therapy of the low-birth-weight infant. *Am J Obstet Gynecol* 170:85–89.

Douglas AS, Robins SP, Hutchison JD, Porter RW, Stewart A, Reid DM. 1995. Carboxylation of osteocalcin in post-menopausal osteoporotic women following vitamin K and D supplementation. *Bone* 17:15–20.

Dowd P, Zheng ZB. 1995. On the mechanism of the anticlotting action of vitamin E quinone. *Proc Natl Acad Sci* 92:8171–8175.

Ducy P, Desbois C, Boyce B, Pinero G, Story B, Dunstan C, Smith E, Bonadio J, Goldstein S, Gundberg C, Bradley A, Karsenty G. 1996. Increased bone formation in osteocalcin-deficient mice. *Nature* 382:448–452.

Ekelund H, Finnstrom O, Gunnarskog J, Kallen B, Larsson Y. 1993. Administration of vitamin K to newborn infants and childhood cancer. *Br Med J* 307:89–91.

Ferland G. 1998. The vitamin K-dependent proteins: An update. *Nutr Rev* 56:223–230.

Ferland G, Sadowski JA, O'Brien ME. 1993. Dietary induced subclinical vitamin K deficiency in normal human subjects. *J Clin Invest* 91:1761–1768.

Feskanich D, Weber P, Willett WC, Rockett H, Booth SL, Colditz GA. 1999. Vitamin K intake and hip fractures in women: A prospective study. *Am J Clin Nutr* 69:74–79.

Fournier B, Leclercq M, Audigier-Petit C, Letoublon R, Got R, Frot-Coutaz J. 1987. Vitamin K1 binding protein in milk. *Int J Vitamin Nutr Res* 57:145–150.

Francis JL. 1988. A rapid and simple micromethod for the specific determination of descarboxylated prothrombin (PIVKA II). *Med Lab Sci* 45:69–73.

Frick PG, Riedler G, Brogli H. 1967. Dose response and minimal daily requirement for vitamin K in man. *J Appl Physiol* 23:387–389.

Garber AK, Binkley NC, Krueger DC, Suttie JW. 1999. Comparison of phylloquinone bioavailability from food sources or a supplement in human subjects. *J Nutr* 129:1201–1203.

Gijsbers BL, van Haarlem LJ, Soute BA, Ebberink RH, Vermeer C. 1990. Characterization of a Gla-containing protein from calcified human atherosclerotic plaques. *Arteriosclerosis* 10:991–995.

Gijsbers BL, Jie KS, Vermeer C. 1996. Effect of food composition on vitamin K absorption in human volunteers. *Br J Nutr* 76:223–229.

Golding J, Paterson M, Kinlen LJ. 1990. Factors associated with childhood cancer in a national cohort study. *Br J Cancer* 62:304–308.

Golding J, Greenwood R, Birmingham K, Mott M. 1992. Childhood cancer, intramuscular vitamin K, and pethidine given during labour. *Br Med J* 305:341–346.

Greer FR. 1995. The importance of vitamin K as a nutrient during the first year of life. *Nutr Res* 15:289–310.

Greer FR, Marshall S, Cherry J, Suttie JW. 1991. Vitamin K status of lactating mothers, human milk, and breast-feeding infants. *Pediatrics* 88:751–756.

Greer FR, Marshall SP, Foley AL, Suttie JW. 1997. Improving the vitamin K status of breastfeeding infants with maternal vitamin K supplements. *Pediatrics* 99:88–92.

Gundberg CM, Nieman SD, Abrams S, Rosen H. 1998. Vitamin K status and bone health: An analysis of methods for determination of undercarboxylated osteocalcin. *J Clin Endocrinol Metab* 83:3258–3266.

Hara K, Akiyama Y, Nakamura T, Murota S, Morita I. 1995. The inhibitory effect of vitamin K2 (menatetrenone) on bone resorption may be related to its side chain. *Bone* 16:179–184.

Haroon Y, Shearer MJ, Rahim S, Gunn WG, McEnery G, Barkhan P. 1982. The content of phylloquinone (vitamin K1) in human milk, cows' milk and infant formula foods determined by high-performance liquid chromatography. *J Nutr* 112:1105–1117.

Hart JP, Shearer MJ, Klenerman L, Catterall A, Reeve J, Sambrook PN, Dodds RA, Bitensky L, Chayen J. 1985. Electrochemical detection of depressed circulating levels of vitamin K1 in osteoporosis. *J Clin Endocrinol Metab* 60:1268–1269.

Hodges SJ, Pilkington MJ, Stamp TC, Catterall A, Shearer MJ, Bitensky L, Chayen J. 1991. Depressed levels of circulating menaquinones in patients with osteoporotic fractures of the spine and femoral neck. *Bone* 12:387–389.

Hodges SJ, Akesson K, Vergnaud P, Obrant K, Delmas PD. 1993. Circulating levels of vitamins K1 and K2 decreased in elderly women with hip fracture. *J Bone Miner Res* 8:1241–1245.

Hogenbirk K, Peters M, Bouman P, Sturk A, Buller HA. 1993. The effect of formula versus breast feeding and exogenous vitamin K1 supplementation on circulating levels of vitamin K1 and vitamin K-dependent clotting factors in newborns. *Eur J Pediatr* 152:72–74.

Ichihashi T, Takagishi Y, Uchida K, Yamada H. 1992. Colonic absorption of menaquinone-4 and menaquinone-9 in rats. *J Nutr* 122:506–512.

Indyk HE, Woollard DC. 1997. Vitamin K and infant formulas: Determination and distribution of phylloquinone and menaquinone-4. *Analyst* 122:465–469.

Jie KS, Bots ML, Vermeer C, Witteman JC, Grobbee DE. 1995. Vitamin K intake and osteocalcin levels in women with and without aortic atherosclerosis: A population-based study. *Atherosclerosis* 116:117–123.

Jones DY, Koonsvitsky BP, Ebert ML, Jones MB, Lin PY, Will BH, Suttie JW. 1991. Vitamin K status of free-living subjects consuming olestra. *Am J Clin Nutr* 53:943–946.

Kanai T, Takagi T, Masuhiro K, Nakamura M, Iwata M, Saji F. 1997. Serum vitamin K level and bone mineral density in post-menopausal women. *Int J Gynaecol Obstet* 56:25–30.

Kazzi NJ, Ilagan NB, Liang KC, Kazzi GM, Grietsell LA, Brans YW. 1990. Placental transfer of vitamin K1 in preterm pregnancy. *Obstet Gynecol* 75:334–337.

Klebanoff MA, Read JS, Mills JL, Shiono PH. 1993. The risk of childhood cancer after neonatal exposure to vitamin K. *N Engl J Med* 329:905–908.

Knapen MH, Hamulyak K, Vermeer C. 1989. The effect of vitamin K supplementation on circulating osteocalcin (bone Gla protein) and urinary calcium excretion. *Ann Intern Med* 111:1001–1005.

Knapen MH, Jie KS, Hamulyak K, Vermeer C. 1993. Vitamin K-induced changes in markers for osteoblast activity and urinary calcium loss. *Calcif Tissue Int* 53:81–85.

Knapen MH, Nieuwenhuijzen Kruseman AC, Wouters RS, Vermeer C. 1998. Correlation of serum osteocalcin fractions with bone mineral density in women during the first 10 years after menopause. *Calcif Tissue Int* 63:375–379.

Kohlmeier M, Saupe J, Drossel HJ, Shearer MJ. 1995. Variation of phylloquinone (vitamin K1) concentrations in hemodialysis patients. *Thromb Haemost* 74:1252–1254.

Kohlmeier M, Salomon A, Saupe J, Shearer MJ. 1996. Transport of vitamin K to bone in humans. *J Nutr* 126:1192S–1196S.

Koivu TJ, Piironen VI, Henttonen SK, Mattila PH. 1997. Determination of phylloquinone in vegetables, fruits, and berries by high-performance liquid chromatography with electrochemical detection. *J Agric Food Chem* 45:4644–4649.

Lamon-Fava S, Sadowski JA, Davidson KW, O'Brien ME, McNamara JR, Schaefer EJ. 1998. Plasma lipoproteins as carriers of phylloquinone (vitamin K1) in humans. *Am J Clin Nutr* 67:1226–1231.

Lane PA, Hathaway WE. 1985. Vitamin K in infancy. *J Pediatr* 106:351–359.

Levy RJ, Lian JB, Gallop P. 1979. Atherocalcin, a gamma-carboxyglutamic acid containing protein from atherosclerotic plaque. *Biochem Biophys Res Commun* 91:41–49.

Liu G, Peacock M. 1998. Age-related changes in serum undercarboxylated osteocalcin and its relationships with bone density, bone quality, and hip fracture. *Calcif Tissue Int* 62:286–289.

Lubetsky A, Dekel-Stern E, Chetrit A, Lubin F, Halkin H. 1999. Vitamin K intake and sensitivity to warfarin in patients consuming regular diets. *Thromb Haemost* 81:396–399.

Luo G, Ducy P, McKee MD, Pinero GJ, Loyer E, Behringer RR, Karsenty G. 1997. Spontaneous calcification of arteries and cartilage in mice lacking matrix GLA protein. *Nature* 386:78–81.

Mandelbrot L, Guillaumont M, Leclercq M, Lefrere JJ, Gozin D, Daffos F, Forestier F. 1988. Placental transfer of vitamin K1 and its implications in fetal hemostasis. *Thromb Haemost* 60:39–43.

McCarthy DJ, Lindamood C 3d, Gundberg CM, Hill DL. 1989. Retinoid-induced hemorrhaging and bone toxicity in rats fed diets deficient in vitamin K. *Toxicol Appl Pharmacol* 97:300–310.

McKinney PA, Juszczak E, Findlay E, Smith K. 1998. Case-control study of childhood leukaemia and cancer in Scotland: Findings for neonatal intramuscular vitamin K. *Br Med J* 316:173–177.

Molitor H, Robinson J. 1940. Oral and parenteral toxicity of vitamin K1, phthiocol, and 2 methyl 1,4 naphthoquinone. *Proc Soc Exp Biol Med* 43:125–128.

Morales WJ, Angel JL, O'Brien WF, Knuppel RA, Marsalisi F. 1988. The use of antenatal vitamin K in the prevention of early neonatal intraventricular hemorrhage. *Am J Obstet Gynecol* 159:774–779.

Motohara K, Matsukane I, Endo F, Kiyota Y, Matsuda I. 1989. Relationship of milk intake and vitamin K supplementation to vitamin K status in newborns. *Pediatrics* 84:90–93.

NRC (National Research Council). 1987. *Vitamin Tolerance of Animals.* Washington, DC: National Academy Press.

Olsen JH, Hertz H, Blinkenberg K, Verder H. 1994. Vitamin K regimens and incidence of childhood cancer in Denmark. *Br Med J* 308:895–896.

Orimo H, Shiraki M, Fujita T, Onomura T, Inoue T, Kushida K. 1992. Clinical evaluation of menatetrenone in the treatment of involutional osteoporosis—A double-blind multicenter comparative study with 1-α-hydroxyvitamin D$_3$. *J Bone Miner Res* 7:S122.

Parker L, Cole M, Craft AW, Hey EN. 1998. Neonatal vitamin K administration and childhood cancer in the north of England: Retrospective case-control study. *Br Med J* 316:189–193.

Passmore SJ, Draper G, Brownbill P, Kroll M. 1998. Case-control studies of relation between childhood cancer and neonatal vitamin K administration. *Br Med J* 316:178–184.

Pietschnig B, Haschke F, Vanura H, Shearer M, Veitl V, Kellner S, Schuster E. 1993. Vitamin K in breast milk: No influence of maternal dietary intake. *Eur J Clin Nutr* 47:209–215.

Piironen V, Koivu T, Tammisalo O, Mattila P. 1997. Determination of phylloquinone in oils, margarines and butter by high-performance liquid chromatography with electrochemical detection. *Food Chem* 59:473–480.

Plantalech L, Guillaumont M, Vergnaud P, Leclercq M, Delmas PD. 1991. Impairment of gamma carboxylation of circulating osteocalcin (bone gla protein) in elderly women. *J Bone Miner Res* 6:1211–1216.

Price PA. 1988. Role of vitamin K-dependent proteins in bone metabolism. *Annu Rev Nutr* 8:565–583.

Price R, Fenton S, Shearer MJ, Bolton-Smith C. 1996. Daily and seasonal variation in phylloquinone (vitamin K1) intake in Scotland. *Proc Nutr Soc* 55:244A.

Rao GH, Mason KE. 1975. Antisterility and antivitamin K activity of d-alpha-tocopheryl hydroquinone in the vitamin E-deficient female rat. *J Nutr* 105:495–498.

Ravn P, Fledelius C, Rosenquist C, Overgaard K, Christiansen C. 1996. High bone turnover is associated with low bone mass in both pre- and postmenopausal women. *Bone* 19:291–298.

Rosen HN, Maitland LA, Suttie JW, Manning WJ, Glynn RJ, Greenspan SL. 1993. Vitamin K and maintenance of skeletal integrity in adults. *Am J Med* 94:62–68.

Sadowski JA, Hood SJ, Dallal GE, Garry PJ. 1989. Phylloquinone in plasma from elderly and young adults: Factors influencing its concentration. *Am J Clin Nutr* 50:100–108.

Saupe J, Shearer MJ, Kohlmeier M. 1993. Phylloquinone transport and its influence on gamma-carboxyglutamate residues of osteocalcin in patients on maintenance hemodialysis. *Am J Clin Nutr* 58:204–208.

Savage D, Lindenbaum J. 1983. Clinical and experimental human vitamin K deficiency. In: Lindenbaum J, ed. *Nutrition in Hematology.* New York: Churchill Livingstone. Pp. 271–320.

Schurgers LJ, Geleijnse JM, Grobbee DE, Pols HAP, Hofman A, Witteman JCM, Vermeer C. 1999. Nutritional intake of vitamins K1 (phylloquinone) and K2 (menaquinone) in The Netherlands. *J Nutr Environ Med* 9:115–122.

Shah DV, Tews JK, Harper AE, Suttie JW. 1978. Metabolism and transport of gamma-carboxyglutamic acid. *Biochim Biophys Acta* 539:209–217.

Shearer MJ. 1992. Vitamin K metabolism and nutriture. *Blood Rev* 6:92–104.

Shearer MJ, Barkhan P, Webster GR. 1970. Absorption and excretion of an oral dose of tritiated vitamin K1 in man. *Br J Haematol* 18:297–308.

Shearer MJ, McBurney A, Barkhan P. 1974. Studies on the absorption and metabolism of phylloquinone (vitamin K1) in man. *Vitam Horm* 32:513–542.

Shearer MJ, Bach A, Kohlmeier M. 1996. Chemistry, nutritional sources, tissue distribution and metabolism of vitamin K with special reference to bone health. *J Nutr* 126:1181S–1186S.

Sokoll LJ, Sadowski JA. 1996. Comparison of biochemical indexes for assessing vitamin K nutritional status in a healthy adult population. *Am J Clin Nutr* 63:566–573.

Sokoll LJ, O'Brien ME, Camilo ME, Sadowski JA. 1995. Undercarboxylated osteocalcin and development of a method to determine vitamin K status. *Clin Chem* 41:1121–1128.

Sokoll LJ, Booth SL, O'Brien ME, Davidson KW, Tsaioun KI, Sadowski JA. 1997. Changes in serum osteocalcin, plasma phylloquinone, and urinary gamma-carboxyglutamic acid in response to altered intakes of dietary phylloquinone in human subjects. *Am J Clin Nutr* 65:779–784.

Suttie JW. 1992. Vitamin K and human nutrition. *J Am Diet Assoc* 92:585–590.

Suttie JW. 1993. Synthesis of vitamin K-dependent proteins. *FASEB J* 7:445–452.

Suttie JW. 1995. The importance of menaquinones in human nutrition. *Annu Rev Nutr* 15:399–417.

Suttie JW, Mummah-Schendel LL, Shah DV, Lyle BJ, Greger JL. 1988. Vitamin K deficiency from dietary vitamin K restriction in humans. *Am J Clin Nutr* 47:475–480.

Szulc P, Chapuy MC, Meunier PJ, Delmas PD. 1993. Serum undercarboxylated osteocalcin is a marker of the risk of hip fracture in elderly women. *J Clin Invest* 91:1769–1774.

Szulc P, Chapuy MC, Meunier PJ, Delmas PD. 1996. Serum undercarboxylated osteocalcin is a marker of the risk of hip fracture: A three year follow-up study. *Bone* 18:487–488.

Tamatani M, Morimoto S, Nakajima M, Fukuo K, Onishi T, Kitano S, Niinobu T, Ogihara T. 1998. Decreased circulating levels of vitamin K and 25-hydroxyvitamin D in osteopenic elderly men. *Metabolism* 47:195–199.

Thijssen HHI, Drittij-Reijnders MJ. 1994. Vitamin K distribution in rat tissues: Dietary phylloquinone is a source of tissue menaquinone-4. *Br J Nutr* 72:415–425.

Thijssen HH, Drittij-Reijnders MJ. 1996. Vitamin K status in human tissues: Tissue-specific accumulation of phylloquinone and menaquinone-4. *Br J Nutr* 75:121–127.

Udall JA. 1965. Human sources and absorption of vitamin K in relation to anticoagulation stability. *J Am Med Assoc* 194:107–109.

Usui Y, Tanimura H, Nishimura N, Kobayashi N, Okanoue T, Ozawa K. 1990. Vitamin K concentrations in the plasma and liver of surgical patients. *Am J Clin Nutr* 51:846–852.

Vergnaud P, Garnero P, Meunier PJ, Breart G, Kamihagi K, Delmas PD. 1997. Undercarboxylated osteocalcin measured with a specific immunoassay predicts hip fracture in elderly women: The EPIDOS Study. *J Clin Endocrinol Metab* 82:719–724.

Vermeer C, Jie KS, Knapen MH. 1995. Role of vitamin K in bone metabolism. *Annu Rev Nutr* 15:1–22.

Vermeer C, Gijsbers BL, Craciun AM, Groenen-van Dooren MM, Knapen MH. 1996. Effects of vitamin K on bone mass and bone metabolism. *J Nutr* 126:1187S–1191S.

von Kries R, Kreppel S, Becker A, Tangermann R, Gobel U. 1987a. Acarboxyprothrombin concentration after oral prophylactic vitamin K. *Arch Dis Child* 62:938–940.

von Kries R, Shearer M, McCarthy PT, Haug M, Harzer G, Gobel U. 1987b. Vitamin K1 content of maternal milk: Influence of the stage of lactation, lipid composition, and vitamin K1 supplements given to the mother. *Pediatr Res* 22:513–517.

von Kries R, Shearer MJ, Widdershoven J, Motohara K, Umbach G, Gobel U. 1992. Des-gamma-carboxyprothrombin (PIVKA II) and plasma vitamin K1 in newborns and their mothers. *Thromb Haemost* 68:383–387.

von Kries R, Kordass U, Shearer M, Gobel U. 1993. Idiopathic late hemorrhagic disease of newborn and conjugated hyperbilirubinemia. *J Pediatr Gastroenterol Nutr* 16:328–330.

von Kries R, Gobel U, Hachmeister A, Kaletsch U, Michaelis J. 1996. Vitamin K and childhood cancer: A population based case-control study in Lower Saxony, Germany. *Br Med J* 313:199–203.

Weber P. 1997. Management of osteoporosis: Is there a role for vitamin K? *Int J Vitam Nutr Res* 67:350–356.

Widdershoven J, Lambert W, Motohara K, Monnens L, de Leenheer A, Matsuda I, Endo F. 1988. Plasma concentrations of vitamin K1 and PIVKA-II in bottle-fed and breast-fed infants with and without vitamin K prophylaxis at birth. *Eur J Pediatr* 148:139–142.

Woolley DW. 1945. Some biological effects produced by α-tocopheral quinone. *J Biol Chem* 159:59–66.

6

Chromium

SUMMARY

Chromium potentiates the action of insulin in vivo and in vitro. There was not sufficient evidence to set an Estimated Average Requirement (EAR) for chromium. Therefore, an Adequate Intake (AI) was set based on estimated mean intakes. The AI is 35 µg/day and 25 µg/day for young men and women, respectively. Few serious adverse effects have been associated with excess intake of chromium from food. Therefore, a Tolerable Upper Intake Level (UL) was not established.

BACKGROUND INFORMATION

Chromium occurs most commonly in valance states of +3 (III) and +6 (VI). Chromium III is the most stable oxidation state (Greenwood and Earnshaw, 1997) and presumably is the form in the food supply due to the presence of reducing substances in foods. Even a bolus dose of 5 mg chromium VI was reduced to chromium III in 0.5 L of orange juice (Kuykendall et al., 1996), and endogenous reducing agents within the upper gastrointestinal tract and the blood also serve to prevent systemic uptake of chromium VI (Kerger et al., 1997). However, chromium VI, which is a by-product of manufacturing stainless steel, pigments, chromate chemicals, and numerous other products, is strongly oxidizing, produces local irritation or corrosion, and is recognized as a carcinogen when inhaled (Greenwood and Earnshaw, 1997; O'Flaherty, 1994).

197

Function

Chromium potentiates the action of insulin in vivo and in vitro (Mertz, 1969, 1993; Mertz et al., 1961). Schwarz and Mertz (1959) identified chromium as the element that restored glucose tolerance in rats. Impaired glucose tolerance of malnourished infants responded to an oral dose of chromium chloride (Hopkins and Majaj, 1967; Hopkins et al., 1968); subsequently, benefits of chromium chloride were reported in a patient receiving total parenteral nutrition (TPN) (Jeejeebhoy et al., 1977).

A number of studies have demonstrated beneficial effects of chromium on circulating glucose, insulin, and lipids in a variety of human subjects and animal species; however, not all reports of supplementation are positive (Anderson, 1997; Anderson et al., 1991) (for reviews see Anderson, 1997; Mertz, 1993; Offenbacher et al., 1997; Stoecker, 1996). Progress in the field has been limited by lack of a simple, widely accepted method for identification of subjects who are chromium depleted, and thus who would be expected to respond to chromium supplementation, and by the difficulty in producing chromium deficiency in animals.

Recent work by Davis and Vincent (1997a, 1997b) and Vincent (1999) suggests that a low molecular weight chromium-binding substance (LMWCr) may amplify insulin receptor tyrosine kinase activity in response to insulin. It is proposed that the inactive form of the insulin receptor (IR) is converted to the active form by binding insulin, which stimulates the movement of chromium from the blood into the insulin-dependent cells and results in the binding of apoLMWCr to chromium (Figure 6-1). The holoLMWCr then binds to the insulin receptor activating the tyrosine kinase. The ability of LMWCr to activate insulin receptor tyrosine kinase depends on its chromium content. When insulin concentration drops, the holoLMWCr is possibly released from the cell to terminate its effects.

Physiology of Absorption, Metabolism, and Excretion

Absorption estimates for chromium III, based on metabolic balance studies or on urinary excretion from physiological intakes, range from 0.4 to 2.5 percent (Anderson and Kozlovsky, 1985; Anderson et al., 1983, 1991, 1993a; Bunker et al., 1984; Doisy et al., 1971; Offenbacher et al., 1986).

Most chromium compounds are soluble at the pH of the stomach, but less soluble hydroxides may form as pH is increased (Mertz,

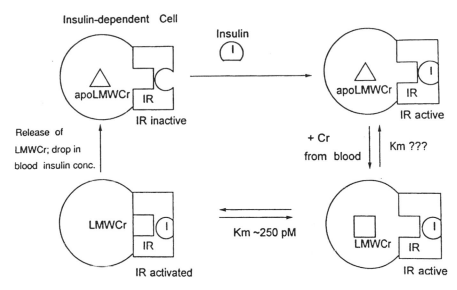

FIGURE 6-1 Proposed mechanism for the activation of insulin receptor by LMWCr in response to insulin. LMWCr = low molecular weight chromium-binding substance, I – insulin, IR = insulin receptor. Adapted from Vincent (1999).

1969). The environment of the gastrointestinal tract and ligands provided by foods and supplements are important for mineral absorption (Clydesdale, 1988). Several dietary factors that affect chromium absorption will be discussed in the bioavailability section of this chapter.

In humans consuming approximately 10 µg/day of chromium, about 2 percent was excreted in urine, but only 0.5 percent was excreted when intakes approached 40 µg/day (Anderson and Kozlovsky, 1985). These data suggest regulation of chromium absorption in these intake ranges.

A number of studies have reported increased urinary excretion of chromium with aerobic exercise (Anderson et al., 1982, 1984, 1988b). A recent study using ^{53}Cr demonstrated that acute and chronic resistive exercise may increase chromium absorption as determined by the increased urinary excretion of the ^{53}Cr isotope (Rubin et al., 1998). Further studies will be needed to clarify how much of the observed beneficial effects of exercise on glucose and insulin metabolism may be due to improved chromium absorption.

Chromium competes for one of the binding sites on transferrin (Harris, 1977). In rats fed physiological levels of ^{51}CrCl$_3$, more than

80 percent of the ^{51}Cr in blood precipitated with the transferrin. Several studies have investigated possible interactions between iron and chromium. Human apo-transferrin in Earle's medium bound chromium in the presence of citric acid, and iron uptake by apo-transferrin was reduced by either aluminum or chromium (Moshtaghie et al., 1992). The excessive iron in hemochromatosis has been hypothesized to interfere with the transport of chromium, thereby contributing to the diabetes associated with this condition (Lim et al., 1983; Sargent et al., 1979). Supplementation of 925 µg/ day of chromium for 12 weeks did not significantly affect indexes of iron status in older adult men (Campbell et al., 1997), but one study in young men that provided a daily 200 µg supplement for 8 weeks found a tendency for a decrease in transferrin saturation (Lukaski et al., 1996). No long-term studies have addressed this question.

In humans, chromium concentrates in liver, spleen, soft tissue, and bone (Lim et al., 1983). Similar patterns are seen in rats with accumulation in kidney, spleen, and bone as well as liver and testes (Hopkins, 1965; Kamath et al., 1997; Onkelinx, 1977). A three-compartment model with half-lives of 0.5, 5.9, and 83 days was originally proposed based on the distribution of ^{51}Cr from $^{51}CrCl_3$ in rats (Mertz et al., 1965). Onkelinx (1977) also proposed a three-compartment model in rats, but suggested different characteristics for the third compartment. Additional modeling work with patients having adult onset diabetes and normal control subjects utilized a compartment within the blood and slow and fast tissue compartments (Do Canto et al., 1995). A half-life for urinary excretion of chromium of 0.97 days for the diabetic group and 1.51 days for control subjects was calculated. The compartment that represented long-term tissue deposition had an extremely slow return rate of 231 days for patients with diabetes and 346 days for control subjects.

Most ingested chromium is excreted unabsorbed in the feces (Mertz, 1969; Offenbacher et al., 1986). Excretion via bile is not a major contributor to fecal chromium (Davis-Whitenack et al., 1996; Hopkins, 1965). Most absorbed chromium is excreted rapidly in the urine (Anderson et al., 1983). A recent report from England indicated significant age-related decreases in the chromium concentrations in hair, sweat, and urine (Davies et al., 1997).

Clinical Effects of Inadequate Intake

Chromium deficiency has been reported in three patients who did not receive supplemental chromium in their TPN solutions

(Brown et al., 1986; Freund et al., 1979; Jeejeebhoy et al., 1977). The first, a female who had received TPN for more than 3 years, developed unexplained weight loss and peripheral neuropathy. Her plasma glucose removal was impaired, plasma free fatty acids were elevated, and her low respiratory quotient indicated poor utilization of carbohydrates. The addition of 250 µg of chromium to the daily TPN solution for 2 weeks restored the glucose removal rate, increased her respiratory quotient, and allowed an insulin infusion to be discontinued. The other two patients responded similarly to chromium supplementation (Brown et al., 1986; Freund et al., 1979)

Because chromium potentiates the action of insulin and chromium deficiency in TPN patients, impairs glucose utilization, and raises insulin requirements, it has been hypothesized that poor chromium status is a factor contributing to the incidence of impaired glucose tolerance and Type II diabetes. Prevalence of impaired glucose tolerance was 15.8 percent in adults from 40 to 74 years of age in the Third National Health and Nutrition Examination Survey (1988–1994) (Harris et al., 1998). Addressing this question is difficult because of the current lack of information about variability in dietary chromium intakes and because there is not an easily usable clinical indicator to identify potential study subjects with poor chromium status.

There is considerable interest in chromium supplementation in Type II diabetes, but no large-scale controlled trials have been reported in the United States. In China, 180 subjects with Type II diabetes took either a placebo, 200 µg, or 1,000 µg of chromium as chromium picolinate daily for 4 months. Mean body weight of the subjects was 69 kg. Data collected at baseline and after 2 and 4 months of supplementation included standard health histories, fasting glucose and insulin, glycosylated hemoglobin, and glucose and insulin concentrations 2 hours after a 75-g glucose load. After 2 months, fasting and 2-hour insulin concentrations were decreased significantly at both supplement levels. Glycosylated hemoglobin and fasting and 2-hour glucose concentration decreased significantly in the higher (1,000 µg/day) dose group. The reductions in glucose and insulin concentrations were maintained for 4 months; additionally, glycosylated hemoglobin became significantly lower in both dose groups at 4 months (Anderson et al., 1997b). There are no data available on the basal dietary intake of chromium in these diabetic subjects. Also, no doses between 200 and 1,000 µg were tested in this study, nor were other forms of chromium supplemented.

SELECTION OF INDICATORS FOR ESTIMATING THE REQUIREMENT FOR CHROMIUM

Balance Studies

Two men were monitored for 12 days in a metabolic ward and were in apparent balance when fed 37 µg/day of chromium (Offenbacher et al., 1986). Bunker and coworkers (1984) conducted metabolic balance studies with 22 apparently healthy elderly people between 69 and 86 years of age. These subjects had mean chromium intakes of 24.5 µg/day (12.8 µg/1,000 kcal) with a range of 13.6 to 47.7 µg/day for men and 14.5 to 30.3 µg/day for women. Of the 22 subjects, 16 were in equilibrium, three were in positive balance, and three were in negative balance.

Urinary Chromium Excretion

For healthy, free-living adults, the average urinary chromium excretion is typically 0.22 µg/L (Paschal et al., 1998) or 0.2 µg/day (Anderson et al., 1982, 1983) for both men and women. In another study, urinary chromium excretion was found to be approximately 0.5 percent of the amount in the diet when diets contained 40 µg of chromium. For persons whose diets contained only 10 µg of chromium, urinary excretion was approximately 2 percent. There was a negative linear relationship between dietary chromium in this range and percent urinary chromium excretion (Anderson and Kozlovsky, 1985). However, urinary chromium excretion appears to be related to recent chromium intake but has not been useful as a predictor of chromium status (Anderson et al., 1983). Further investigation of urinary chromium in response to very low levels of intake is warranted (Anderson et al., 1991).

Plasma Chromium Concentration

Reported plasma chromium concentrations have declined from greater than 3,000 nmol/L in the 1950s to 2 to 3 nmol/L in well-controlled studies conducted since 1978 (Anderson, 1987). This change can be attributed to improved analytic methods and better control of contamination. Because plasma chromium is very close to the detection limits for graphite furnace atomic absorption and easily contaminated, it is unlikely to be a viable clinical indicator (Veillon, 1989).

Blood Glucose and Insulin Concentration

There is only one study in which subjects were given controlled low chromium diets (Anderson et al., 1991). Seventeen adults were provided diets that contained 5 µg of chromium per 1,000 kcal for 14 weeks. Glucose and insulin concentrations in response to a glucose load were monitored at baseline, 4, 9, and 14 weeks. After adapting to the diet for 4 weeks, subjects were assigned to placebo or chromium supplementation groups for 5 weeks followed by a crossover without washout for another 5 weeks (Anderson et al., 1991).

As one approach to the analysis of these data (Anderson et al., 1991), the subjects who received the placebo for the first 9 weeks were analyzed separately. After 4 weeks on the diet containing 5 µg/1,000 kcal, there were no significant changes in variables measured. However, after subjects consumed 5 µg of chromium per 1,000 kcal for 9 weeks, a significant increase from baseline was observed in sums of glucose and in glucose at 90 minutes after the glucose load (Table 6-1). Supplementation with 200 µg of chromium as $CrCl_3$ for 5 weeks tended ($p < 0.10$) to reduce sums of glucose and insulin concentrations in these subjects. Although this study suggests a role of chromium in regulating blood glucose concentrations, further studies using graded levels of intake between less than

TABLE 6-1 Glucose and Insulin Concentrations of Eight Subjects Fed Low Chromium (5 µg/1,000 kcal) Diets for 14 Weeks and Supplemented with Placebo for 9 Weeks Followed by 200 µg $CrCl_3$ for 5 Weeks

	Week			
	0	4	9	14
Glucose (mmol/L)				
Fasting	4.9 ± 0.2	4.8 ± 0.1	4.9 ± 0.1	5.1 ± 0.1
90 minute	4.2 ± 0.4	4.5 ± 0.4	5.0 ± 0.6[a]	4.4 ± 0.4
Sums (0–240 min)	33.6 ± 1.6	35.1 ± 1.4	37.0 ± 2.2	34.6 ± 1.6[b]
Insulin (pmol/L)				
Fasting	38 ± 5	33 ± 5	48 ± 6	49 ± 7
Sums (0–240 min)	1,146 ± 130	1,214 ± 167	1,577 ± 354	1,319 ± 281[b]

[a] Different from baseline by paired t-test, $p < 0.05$.
[b] Week 9 (end of placebo) vs. supplement by paired t-test, $p < 0.10$.
SOURCE: Reanalysis of Anderson et al. (1991), by personal communication.

5 µg/1,000 kcal and the usual dietary chromium levels (13 to 20 µg/1,000 kcal) and with different age groups are needed to estimate the average requirement for chromium.

FACTORS AFFECTING THE CHROMIUM REQUIREMENT

A number of dietary factors affect chromium absorption. Offenbacher (1994) noted plasma chromium concentrations in three women were consistently higher when they were given 1 mg chromium as $CrCl_3$ with 100 mg ascorbic acid than when given 1 mg chromium without ascorbic acid. In rats, concurrent dosing with $^{51}CrCl_3$ and ascorbic acid, as compared to dosing in water, produced significantly higher ^{51}Cr in urine without decreasing ^{51}Cr in tissues, a finding that suggests ascorbic acid enhanced ^{51}Cr absorption (Davis et al., 1995; Seaborn and Stoecker, 1990).

Consumption of diets high in simple sugars (35 percent of total kcal) increased urinary chromium excretion in adults (Kozlovsky et al., 1986). Urinary chromium excretion was found to be related to the insulinogenic properties of carbohydrates (Anderson et al., 1990). Carbohydrate source also had a significant effect on tissue chromium concentration in mice, with values generally being higher in those fed a starch diet (Seaborn and Stoecker, 1989). When amino acids were added to a test meal perfused through the intestinal lumen of rats, the absorption of chromium was increased twofold (Dowling et al., 1990).

In rats, phytate at high levels had adverse effects on ^{51}Cr absorption (Chen et al., 1973), but lower levels of phytate did not have detrimental effects on chromium status (Keim et al., 1987). Oxalate (present in some vegetables and grains) enhanced ^{51}Cr uptake (Chen et al., 1973). Bunker and coworkers (1984) commented that one subject in severe negative chromium balance ate a diet very high in fiber, but effects of high fiber diets on chromium absorption have not been investigated systematically.

Habitual consumption of certain medications that alter stomach acidity or gastrointestinal prostaglandins may affect chromium absorption and retention in rats. When rats were dosed with physiological doses (less than 100 ng) of $^{51}CrCl_3$ and prostaglandin inhibitors such as aspirin, ^{51}Cr in blood, tissues, and urine was markedly increased (Davis et al., 1995). Medications, such as antacids or dimethylprostaglandin E_2, reduced ^{51}Cr absorption and retention in rats (Kamath et al., 1997).

FINDINGS BY LIFE STAGE AND GENDER GROUP

Infants Ages 0 through 12 Months

Method Used to Set the Adequate Intake

No functional criteria of chromium status have been demonstrated that indicate response to dietary intake in infants. Thus, the recommended intakes of chromium are based on an Adequate Intake (AI) that reflects the observed mean chromium intake of infants principally fed human milk.

Ages 0 through 6 Months. According to the method described in Chapter 2, the AI for chromium is based on the milk content from healthy, well-nourished mothers who are not taking supplements. The average concentration of chromium in human milk was estimated to be 0.25 µg/L (Anderson et al., 1993a; Casey and Hambidge, 1984; Casey et al., 1985; Engelhardt et al., 1990; Mohamedshah et al., 1998) (Table 6-2). Based on the consumption of 0.78 L/day of human milk (Chapter 2), the AI for chromium for infants ages 0 through 6 months is 0.2 µg/day after rounding.

Ages 7 through 12 Months. Schroeder and coworkers (1962) reported a rapid decline in tissue chromium concentrations after birth. These tissue concentrations were generated before chromium measurement techniques were reliable (Anderson, 1987); nonetheless, the possibility that infants deplete their stores during the early months of life suggests that the AI possibly should not be based solely on human milk consumption.

There are no specific data on the chromium concentration of weaning foods; this indicates an area of needed research. An average daily caloric intake for this age group is 845 kcal and human milk provides 750 kcal/L (Fomon, 1974). During the second 6 months of lactation, the average volume of human milk consumed by the infant is 0.6 L/day (Chapter 2). Therefore, calories provided by human milk would be 450 kcal (0.6 L of human milk × 750 kcal/L) and the caloric content of the usual intake of complementary weaning foods would be 395 kcal (845 − 450).

Based on an average concentration of 0.25 µg/L, the chromium intake from human milk would be 0.15 µg/day (0.6 × 0.25). With an additional 400 kcal from complementary foods and the chromium content of well balanced meals containing approximately 13.4 µg/ 1,000 kcal (Anderson et al., 1992), the amount of chromium

TABLE 6-2 Chromium Concentration in Human Milk

Reference[a]	Study Group	Stage of Lactation	Milk Concentration (µg/L)	Estimated Chromium Intake of Infants (µg/d)[b]
Casey and Hambidge, 1984	45 women	0–14 d	0.29	0.22
		15–28 d	0.27	0.21
		1–3 mo	0.28	0.22
		4–6 mo	0.26	0.16
		7+ mo	0.46	0.27
Casey et al., 1985	11 women, 26–39 y	8 d	0.27	0.21
		14 d	0.22	0.17
		21 d	0.28	0.22
		28 d	0.26	0.20
Engelhardt et al., 1990			0.28	0.22
Anderson et al., 1993a	17 women	2 mo	0.18	0.14
Aquilio et al., 1996	14 women	21 d	1.2	0.93
Mohamedshah et al., 1998	6 women, 25–38 y	1–2 mo	0.09–0.46	0.07–0.36

[a] Maternal intakes were not reported in these studies.
[b] Chromium intake based on reported data or concentration (µg/L) × 0.78 L/day for 0–6 months postpartum and concentration (µg/L) × 0.6 L/day for 7–12 months postpartum.

consumed from weaning foods is estimated to be 5.36 µg/day. Therefore the amount of chromium consumed from human milk and complementary foods would be 5.5 µg/day (0.15 + 5.36). Downward extrapolation from an adult, according to the method in Chapter 2, would yield an average intake of 10 µg/day.

An AI of 5.5 µg/day is set for infants ages 7 through 12 months based on consumption of chromium from human milk and complementary foods.

Chromium AI Summary, Ages 0 through 12 Months

AI for Infants
    0–6 months   0.2 µg/day of chromium   29 ng/kg/day
    7–12 months   5.5 µg/day of chromium   611 ng/kg/day

Special Considerations

The mean concentration of chromium in cow milk and infant formula was reported to be 0.83 and 4.84 µg/L, respectively (Cocho et al., 1992). There is no information on the bioavailability of chromium in infant formula.

Children and Adolescents Ages 1 through 18 Years

Method Used to Set the Adequate Intake

No data were found on which to base an Estimated Average Requirement for children and adolescents; therefore AIs have been set. In the absence of information on the chromium content of children's diets, AIs for these age groups have been extrapolated from adults, ages 19 through 30 years, with use of the method described in Chapter 2 and rounding to the nearest 1 µg. Because urinary excretion of chromium is increased with exercise (Anderson et al., 1982, 1984, 1988b), metabolic weight ($kg^{0.75}$) was used to extrapolate from the adult AI.

Chromium AI Summary, Ages 1 through 18 Years

AI for Children
    1–3 years   11 µg/day of chromium
    4–8 years   15 µg/day of chromium

AI for Boys
    9–13 years   25 µg/day of chromium
    14–18 years   35 µg/day of chromium

AI for Girls
    9–13 years   21 µg/day of chromium
    14–18 years   24 µg/day of chromium

Adults Ages 19 through 50 Years

Method Used to Set the Adequate Intake

Data, as described earlier, are lacking for estimating an average requirement for adults. Furthermore, no national survey data are available on chromium intakes.

The mean chromium content of 22 well-balanced adult diets, designed by nutritionists, was 13.4 ± 1.1 µg/1,000 kcal (standard error of the mean [SEM]) (range 8.4 to 23.7 µg/1,000 kcal) (Anderson et al., 1992). The mean chromium intake of 13.4 µg/1,000 kcal and an energy intake estimate of 1,850 kcal/day for women and 2,800 kcal for men aged 19 through 30 years (Briefel et al., 1995) has been used as a basis for deriving AI estimates for chromium. For women and men aged 31 through 50 years, median energy intakes of 1,750 and 2,550 kcal/day, respectively, have been used (Briefel et al., 1995). Although there is no method available to adjust for the underreporting of intake, it is recognized that as much as 20 percent of energy intake may be underreported (Mertz et al., 1991). For this reason, the highest intake value for adults 19 through 30 years and 31 through 50 years was used to set the AI for each gender. Therefore, the AI for men is 35 µg/day ($2,800 \times 13.4$) and 25 µg/day ($1,850 \times 13.4$), after rounding.

Chromium AI Summary, Ages 19 through 50 Years

AI for Men
19–30 years	**35 µg/day of chromium**
31–50 years	**35 µg/day of chromium**

AI for Women
19–30 years	**25 µg/day of chromium**
31–50 years	**25 µg/day of chromium**

Adults Ages 51 Years and Older

Method Used to Set the Adequate Intake

As discussed for adults 19 through 50 years, the mean chromium content of 22 well-balanced daily diets, designed by nutritionists, was 13.4 ± 1.1 µg/1,000 kcal (SEM) (range 8.4 to 23.7 µg/1,000 kcal) (Anderson et al., 1992). The median energy intakes for men and women, 50 through 70 years of age, were 2,100 and 1,500 kcal/

day, respectively (Briefel et al., 1995). The energy needs for men and women older than 70 years of age are 1,700 and 1,300 kcal/day, respectively (Briefel et al., 1995). Although there is no method available to adjust for the underreporting of intake, it is recognized that as much as 20 percent of energy intake is underreported (Mertz et al., 1991). For this reason, the highest intake value for adults 51 through 70 years and greater than 70 years was used to set the AI for each gender. Therefore, the AI for men is 30 µg/day (2,100 × 13.4) and 20 µg/day (1,500 × 13.4) after rounding.

Research is imperative on chromium needs for this age group because of the paucity of data. Increased nutrient density is generally recommended for the elderly, and several factors suggest that the elderly might be more vulnerable to chromium depletion than younger adults. These factors include the severely negative chromium balance produced by a high fiber diet (Bunker et al., 1984), the possible impacts of medications on chromium absorption (Kamath et al., 1997; Martinez et al., 1985), the decrease with age of chromium concentrations in hair and sweat (Davies et al., 1997), and the increased prevalence of impaired glucose tolerance with aging (Harris et al., 1998).

Chromium AI Summary, Ages 51 Years and Older

AI for Men
  51–70 years   **30 µg/day of chromium**
  > 70 years   **30 µg/day of chromium**

AI for Women
  51–70 years   **20 µg/day of chromium**
  > 70 years   **20 µg/day of chromium**

Pregnancy

Method Used to Set the Adequate Intake

There are several reports that chromium is depleted throughout pregnancy and with multiple pregnancies (Hambidge, 1971; Mahalko and Bennion, 1976; Saner, 1981). Tissue analyses conducted before current instruments were available indicated that chromium is higher in tissues at birth (Schroeder et al., 1962) and declines rapidly with age. This suggests the need for deposition in the fetus from the mother. The low concentration of chromium in human milk also indicates that the infant may use stored chromium during the early months of life. These earlier estimates of the chromium concentrations, however, cannot be used to accurately predict the additional needs of chromium during pregnancy.

Because of the lack of data to estimate the additional chromium requirement during pregnancy, the AI is determined by extrapolating up from adolescent girls and adult women, as described in Chapter 2. Carmichael and coworkers (1997) reported that the median weight gain of 7,002 women who had good pregnancy outcomes was 16 kg. In six studies of U.S. women, no consistent relationship between maternal age and weight gain was observed (IOM, 1990). Therefore, 16 kg is added to the reference weight for adolescent girls and adult women for extrapolation.

Chromium AI Summary, Pregnancy

AI for Pregnancy
14–18 years	29 µg/day of chromium
19–30 years	30 µg/day of chromium
31–50 years	30 µg/day of chromium

Lactation

Method Used to Set the Adequate Intake

The AI for lactation is estimated on the basis of the chromium intake necessary to replace chromium secreted in human milk plus the AI for women. The amount that must be absorbed to replace the chromium secreted in milk is 0.252 µg/L × 0.78 L/day, or 200 ng/day. If absorption is estimated at 1 percent, 20 µg/day of chromium must be consumed beyond the usual intake to compensate for the milk losses. If absorption is only 0.5 percent, an additional 40 µg/day would be required. In the one study available on dietary intakes of lactating women, chromium intake was 41 µg/day (Anderson et al., 1993a).

Women do not appear to reduce urinary chromium excretion during lactation to compensate for increased needs (Mohamedshah et al., 1998). To calculate an AI for chromium during lactation, it is assumed that 1 percent of chromium is absorbed and 0.2 µg/day is secreted in human milk. Therefore 20 µg is added to the AI for adolescent girls and adult women, and the AI is rounded.

Chromium AI Summary, Lactation

AI for Lactation
14–18 years	**44 µg/day of chromium**
19–30 years	**45 µg/day of chromium**
31–50 years	**45 µg/day of chromium**

INTAKE OF CHROMIUM

Food Sources

Chromium is widely distributed throughout the food supply, but many foods contribute less than 1 to 2 µg per serving (Anderson et al., 1992). Determining the chromium content in foods requires rigorous contamination control because standard methods of sample preparation contribute substantial amounts of chromium to the foods being analyzed. In addition, chromium is quite variable among different lots of foods (Anderson et al., 1992) and may be influenced by geochemical factors (Welch and Cary, 1975). Consequently dietary chromium intakes cannot be determined from any currently existing databases.

The chromium content in foods may increase or decrease with processing. Early reports indicated chromium losses when grains and sugars were refined (Anderson, 1987). However, acidic foods accumulate chromium during preparation and processing, particularly when heated in stainless steel containers (Offenbacher and Pi-Sunyer, 1983). Cereals contribute variable, but potentially important, amounts of chromium to the total diet. The chromium content of a 50 g serving (dry weight) of 43 brands of cereal varied from 0.15 to 35 µg. High-bran cereals are generally, but not always, high in chromium. The bioavailability of chromium in these cereals was not evaluated (Anderson et al., 1988a). Most dairy products are low in chromium and provide less than 0.6 µg/serving. Meats, poultry, and fish generally contribute 1 to 2 µg per serving, but processed meats are higher in chromium and may acquire it from exogenous sources. Chromium concentrations of fruits and vegetables are highly variable (Anderson et al., 1992). Some brands of beer contain significant amounts of chromium, some of which presumably is exogenous (Anderson and Bryden, 1983). Cabrera-Vique and coworkers (1997) estimated that wine provides 4.1 µg chromium daily per resident in France, with red wines having the highest concentrations. Wines have not been analyzed for chromium in the United States.

Dietary Intake

Because chromium in foods cannot be analyzed from existing databases, paired food or duplicate meal analyses are required, and data are available from only a few laboratories and locations. In one study, self-selected diets were composited for 7 days and analyzed for chromium content. The mean chromium intake of 10 adult men was 33 µg/day (range 22 to 48 µg/day), and the chromium intake for 22 women was 25 µg/day (range 13 to 36 µg/day) (Anderson and Kozlovsky, 1985). Mean chromium intake was approximately 15.6 µg/1,000 kcal. The chromium content of 22 daily diets, designed by nutritionists to be well balanced, ranged from 8.4 to 23.7 µg/1,000 kcal with a mean of 13.4 µg/1,000 kcal (Anderson et al., 1992). In another study, a group of adults self-selected a mean chromium intake of 14.4 µg/1,000 kcal (Anderson et al., 1991), and lactating mothers consumed foods containing 18.8 µg/1,000 kcal (Anderson et al., 1993a). Chromium intake studies in Canadian women suggest median chromium intakes two or more times higher than the values reported from the eastern United States (Gibson and Scythes, 1984; Gibson et al., 1985). Further research is needed to define the contributions of differences in dietary patterns, regional variation in food chromium concentrations, and possible sample contamination in these disparate values.

Derivation of dietary intake based on duplicate meal analyses assumes that subjects do not change their intakes because of the collection; however, this assumption may underestimate actual food intake (Kim et al., 1984). In a controlled study in which actual energy requirements of subjects were estimated, Anderson and co-workers (1993b) found that the ratio of energy requirement to energy intake measured from the duplicate meal analysis was 1.29 for women and 1.46 for men. Applying these correction factors to chromium intakes would increase the estimated chromium intake of women in this study from 23.1 to 28.7 µg/day and of men from 38.8 to 54.1 µg/day. This correction raises the question of whether some of the current estimates of dietary chromium intake are too low.

Intake from Supplements

In 1986, 8 percent of adults consumed supplements that contained chromium (Moss et al., 1989; see Table 2-2). Based on the Third National Health and Nutrition Examination Survey data, the median supplemental intake of chromium was 23 µg/day for those who took supplements, which is similar to the average dietary chromium intake (Appendix Table C-14).

TOLERABLE UPPER INTAKE LEVELS

The Tolerable Upper Intake Level (UL) is the highest level of daily nutrient intake that is likely to pose no risk of adverse health effects for almost all individuals. Although members of the general population should be advised not to routinely exceed the UL, intake above the UL may be appropriate for investigation within well-controlled clinical trials. Clinical trials of doses above the UL should not be discouraged, as long as subjects participating in these trials have signed informed consent documents regarding possible toxicity and as long as these trials employ appropriate safety monitoring of trial subjects. In addition, the UL is not meant to apply to individuals who are receiving chromium under medical supervision.

Hazard Identification

The toxicity of chromium differs widely depending on the valence state. This review is limited to evaluating trivalent chromium (III) because this is the principal form of chromium found in food and supplements. Hexavalent chromium (VI), which has a much higher level of toxicity than trivalent chromium, is not found in food. Ingested chromium III has a low level of toxicity which is due, partially, to its very poor absorption (Stoecker, 1999). Chromium supplement use (particularly chromium picolinate) has increased in popularity as a result of reports that chromium potentiates the action of insulin and reduces hyperglycemia and hyperlipidemia (Flodin, 1990). Several studies have demonstrated the safety of large doses of chromium III (Anderson et al., 1997a; Hathcock, 1997). The data on the potential adverse effects of excess intake of chromium III compounds are reviewed below.

Chronic Renal Failure

Chronic interstitial nephritis in humans has been attributed to ingestion of chromium picolinate in two case reports (Cerulli et al., 1998; Wasser et al., 1997). However, there is no evidence of kidney damage in experimental animals exposed for up to 2 years to oral chromium as chromium chloride, chromium trichloride, chromium picolinate, or chromium acetate (Anderson et al., 1997a; Schroeder et al., 1962).

Genotoxicity

Chromium VI is a well established human carcinogen, mutagen, and clastogen, but chromium III compounds are not. In vivo genotoxicity assays for chromium III have been negative (Cupo and Wetterhahn, 1985; Hamamy et al., 1987; Itoh and Shimada, 1996). Most studies of genotoxicity in cellular systems have yielded negative results as well (ATSDR, 1998), which in some cases may be due to poor uptake by cells. In eukaryotic cells, negative results were obtained for DNA fragmentation, unscheduled DNA synthesis, and forward mutation (Raffetto et al., 1977; Whiting et al., 1979). Mostly negative results were obtained in sister chromatid exchange assays (Levis and Majone, 1979; Stella et al., 1982; Venier et al., 1982), but both positive and negative results have been found for chromosomal aberrations (Fornace et al., 1981; Levis and Majone, 1979; Nakamuro et al., 1978; Newbold et al., 1979; Raffetto et al., 1977; Stella et al., 1982; Tsuda and Kato, 1977; Umeda and Nishimura, 1979). In prokaryotic cells, the genotoxicity results were mostly negative. Positive results of chromium III were found in intact cells; however, these results could be due to contamination of the test compounds with traces of chromium VI, which is readily taken up by cells (ATSDR, 1998). Several studies suggest that chromium III picolinate and tri-picolinate may cause DNA damage through the generation of hydroxyl radicals (Bagchi et al., 1997; Speetjens et al., 1999; Stearns et al., 1995).

Carcinogenicity

There is little evidence of carcinogenicity in humans or animals after oral intake of chromium III. Kusiak and coworkers (1993) reported increased mortality due to stomach cancer in gold miners in Canada. Although the authors suggest that chromium dust may be the causative agent, the study did not adjust for possible important confounding factors (e.g., role of dietary habits) and failed to show a clear pattern of disease incidence with increasing exposure. A 2-year feeding study in rats by Ivankovic and Preussmann (1975) showed no carcinogenicity after intake (5 days/week for 2 years) of 1, 2, or 5 percent chromium oxide (Cr_2O_3) baked in bread.

Hepatic Dysfunction

There are reports of hepatic adverse effects in humans (Fristedt et al., 1965; Kaufman et al., 1970; Loubieres et al., 1999). Several rat studies show no morphological changes in livers following long-term ingestion of chromium compounds (Ivankovic and Preussmann, 1975; Mackenzie et al., 1958; Schroeder et al., 1965).

Reproductive Effects

There are no studies in humans to suggest that chromium III is a reproductive or developmental toxicant. However, various chromium III compounds have been studied in mice and rats with respect to their reproductive system toxicity. Chromium chloride (in drinking water) administered over 12 weeks reduced fertility in male mice, reduced the number of implantation sites and the number of viable fetuses, and delayed sexual maturity (Al-Hamood et al., 1998; Elbetieha and Al-Hamood, 1997). Intraperitoneal injections of chromium chloride (1, 2, or 4 mg/kg) for 5 days to male rats had no effect on testicular histology or sperm counts (Ernst, 1990). The ingestion of 1,000 µg/mL of chromium as chromium chloride in drinking water for 12 weeks led to significant reductions in the weight of the rat's testes and seminal vesicles (Bataineh et al., 1997).

Other Adverse Effects

Other adverse effects observed after high chromium intakes include rhabdomyolysis (Martin and Fuller, 1998). Rhabdomyolysis is characterized by skeletal muscle injury and release of muscle cell contents into the plasma. Reports of chromium-induced rhabdomyolysis failed to account for other potential etiologic factors including strenuous exercise, weight lifting, trauma, seizure, sepsis, and alcohol and drug abuse.

Identification of Distinct and Highly Sensitive Subpopulations

Data suggest that individuals with preexisting renal and liver disease may be particularly susceptible to adverse effects from excess chromium intake (ATSDR, 1998). These individuals should be particularly careful to limit chromium intake.

Dose-Response Assessment

The limited studies on renal, hepatic, reproductive, and DNA damaging effects of chromium III do not provide dose-response information or clear indications of a lowest-observed-adverse-effect level (LOAEL) or no-observed-adverse-effect level (NOAEL). Thus, there are insufficient data to establish a UL for soluble chromium III salts. Because of the current widespread use of chromium supplements, more research is needed to assess the safety of high-dose chromium intake from supplements. Data from randomized, double-blind, controlled clinical trials and surveillance studies would be most useful for assessing the safety of chromium intake in humans.

Intake Assessment

National survey data are not available on the intake of chromium at various percentiles. According to data from the Third National Health and Nutrition Examination Survey, the average supplemental intake of chromium at the ninety-fifth percentile was 100 µg/day for men and 127 µg/day for women (Appendix Table C-14).

Risk Characterization

No adverse effects have been convincingly associated with excess intake of chromium from food or supplements, but this does not mean that there is no potential for adverse effects resulting from high intakes. Since data on the adverse effects of chromium intake are limited, caution may be warranted.

RESEARCH RECOMMENDATIONS FOR CHROMIUM

• Controlled studies with low dietary intakes (less than 5 to 15 µg/1,000 kcal) to determine an Estimated Average Requirement.

• Chromium absorption, metabolism, and requirements during pregnancy and lactation.

• Information on variability in chromium concentration in the food and water supply.

• Development and validation of a useful clinical indicator to identify persons with marginal chromium status and investigation of effects of physiological levels of chromium supplementation in these patients.

• Investigation of possible relationships between chromium status and insulin resistance, impaired glucose tolerance, and Type II diabetes.

• Monitoring of any adverse effects of self-supplementation and of the design of controlled studies to assess potential beneficial, as well as adverse, effects of large-dose supplementation of chromium.

REFERENCES

Al-Hamood MH, Elbetieha A, Bataineh H. 1998. Sexual maturation and fertility of male and female mice exposed prenatally and postnatally to trivalent and hexavalent chromium compounds. *Reprod Fertil Dev* 10:179–183.

Anderson RA. 1987. Chromium. In: Mertz W, ed. *Trace Elements in Human and Animal Nutrition,* Vol. I. San Diego: Academic Press. Pp. 225–244.

Anderson RA. 1997. Chromium as an essential nutrient for humans. *Regul Toxicol Pharmacol* 26:S35–S41.

Anderson R, Bryden NA. 1983. Concentration, insulin potentiation, and absorption of chromium in beer. *J Agric Food Chem* 31:308–311.

Anderson RA, Kozlovsky AS. 1985. Chromium intake, absorption and excretion of subjects consuming self-selected diets. *Am J Clin Nutr* 41:1177–1183.

Anderson RA, Polansky MM, Bryden NA, Roginski EE, Patterson KY, Reamer DC. 1982. Effect of exercise (running) on serum glucose, insulin, glucagon, and chromium excretion. *Diabetes* 31:212–216.

Anderson RA, Polansky MM, Bryden NA, Patterson KY, Veillon C, Glinsmann WH. 1983. Effects of chromium supplementation on urinary Cr excretion of human subjects and correlation of Cr excretion with selected clinical parameters. *J Nutr* 113:276–281.

Anderson RA, Polansky MM, Bryden NA. 1984. Strenuous running: Acute effects on chromium, copper, zinc, and selected clinical variables in urine and serum of male runners. *Biol Trace Elem Res* 6:327–336.

Anderson RA, Bryden NA, Polansky MM. 1988a. Chromium content of selected breakfast cereals. *J Food Comp Anal* 1:303–308

Anderson RA, Bryden NA, Polansky MM, Deuster PA. 1988b. Exercise effects on chromium excretion of trained and untrained men consuming a constant diet. *J Appl Physiol* 64:249–252.

Anderson RA, Bryden NA, Polansky MM, Reiser S. 1990. Urinary chromium excretion and insulinogenic properties of carbohydrates. *Am J Clin Nutr* 51:864–868.

Anderson RA, Polansky MM, Bryden NA, Canary JJ. 1991. Supplemental-chromium effects on glucose, insulin, glucagon, and urinary chromium losses in subjects consuming controlled low-chromium diets. *Am J Clin Nutr* 54:909–916.

Anderson RA, Bryden NA, Polansky MM. 1992. Dietary chromium intake. Freely chosen diets, institutional diets, and individual foods. *Biol Trace Elem Res* 32:117–121.

Anderson RA, Bryden NA, Patterson KY, Veillon C, Andon MB, Moser-Veillon PB. 1993a. Breast milk chromium and its association with chromium intake, chromium excretion, and serum chromium. *Am J Clin Nutr* 57:519–523.

Anderson RA, Bryden NA, Polansky MM. 1993b. Dietary intake of calcium, chromium, copper, iron, magnesium, manganese, and zinc: Duplicate plate values corrected using derived nutrient intake. *J Am Diet Assoc* 93:462–464.

Anderson RA, Bryden NA, Polansky MM. 1997a. Lack of toxicity of chromium chloride and chromium picolinate in rats. *J Am Coll Nutr* 16:273–279.

Anderson RA, Cheng N, Bryden NA, Polansky MM, Cheng N, Chi J, Feng J. 1997b. Elevated intakes of supplemental chromium improve glucose and insulin variables in individuals with type 2 diabetes. *Diabetes* 46:1786–1791.

Aquilio E, Spagnoli R, Seri S, Bottone G, Spennati G. 1996. Trace element content in human milk during lactation of preterm newborns. *Biol Trace Elem Res* 51:63–70.

ATSDR (Agency for Toxic Substances and Disease Registry). 1998. *Toxicolgical Profile for Chromium (Update)*. Atlanta: Centers for Disease Control and Prevention.

Bagchi D, Bagchi M, Balmoori J, Ye X, Stohs SJ. 1997. Comparative induction of oxidative stress in cultured J774A.1 macrophage cells by chromium picolinate and chromium nicotinate. *Res Comm Mol Pathol Pharmacol* 97:335–346.

Bataineh H, Al-Hamood MH, Elbetieha A, Bani Hani I. 1997. Effect of long-term ingestion of chromium compounds on aggression, sex behavior and fertility in adult male rat. *Drug Chem Toxicol* 20:133–149.

Briefel RR, McDowell MA, Alaimo K, Caughman CR, Bischof AL, Carroll MD, Johnson CL. 1995. Total energy intake of the US population: The Third National Health and Nutrition Examination Survey, 1988–1991. *Am J Clin Nutr* 62:1072S–1080S.

Brown RO, Forloines-Lynn S, Cross RE, Heizer WD. 1986. Chromium deficiency after long-term parenteral nutrition. *Dig Dis Sci* 31:661–664.

Bunker VW, Lawson MS, Delves HT, Clayton BE. 1984. The uptake and excretion of chromium by the elderly. *Am J Clin Nutr* 39:797–802.

Cabrera-Vique C, Teissedre PL, Cabanis MT, Cabanis JC. 1997. Determination and levels of chromium in French wine and grapes by graphite furnace atomic absorption spectrometry. *J Agric Food Chem* 45:1808–1811.

Campbell WW, Beard JL, Joseph LJ, Davey SL, Evans WJ. 1997. Chromium picolinate supplementation and resistive training by older men: Effects on ironstatus and hematologic indexes. *Am J Clin Nutr* 66:944–949.

Carmichael S, Abrams B, Selvin S. 1997. The pattern of maternal weight gain in women with good pregnancy outcomes. *Am J Pub Health* 87:1984–1988.

Casey CE, Hambidge KM. 1984. Chromium in human milk from American mothers. *Br J Nutr* 52:73–77.

Casey CE, Hambidge KM, Neville MC. 1985. Studies in human lactation: Zinc, copper, manganese and chromium in human milk in the first month of lactation. *Am J Clin Nutr* 41:1193–1200.

Cerulli J, Grabe DW, Gauthier I, Malone M, McGoldrick MD. 1998. Chromium picolinate toxicity. *Ann Pharmacotherapy* 32:428–431.

Chen NSC, Tsai A, Dyer IA. 1973. Effect of chelating agents on chromium absorption in rats. *J Nutr* 103:1182–1186.

Clydesdale FM. 1988. Mineral interactions in foods. In: Bodwell CE, Erdman JW, eds. *Nutrient Interactions*. New York: Marcel Dekker. Pp. 73–113.

Cocho JA, Cervilla JR, Rey-Goldar ML, Fdez-Lorenzo JR, Fraga JM. 1992. Chromium content in human milk, cow's milk, and infant formulas. *Biol Trace Elem Res* 32:105–107.

Cupo DY, Wetterhahn KE. 1985. Binding of chromium to chromatin and DNA from liver and kidney of rats treated with sodium dichromate and chromium(III) chloride in vivo. *Cancer Res* 45:1146–1151.

Davies S, McLaren Howard J, Hunnisett A, Howard M. 1997. Age-related decreases in chromium levels in 51,665 hair, sweat, and serum samples from 40,872 patients—Implications for the prevention of cardiovascular disease and type II diabetes mellitus. *Metabolism* 46:469–473.

Davis CM, Vincent JB. 1997a. Chromium oligopeptide activates insulin receptor tyrosine kinase activity. *Biochemistry* 36:4382–4385.

Davis CM, Vincent JB. 1997b. Isolation and characterization of a biologically active chromium oligopeptide from bovine liver. *Arch Biochem Biophys* 339:335–343.

Davis ML, Seaborn CD, Stoecker BJ. 1995. Effects of over-the-counter drugs on [51]chromium retention and urinary excretion in rats. *Nutr Res* 15:201–210.

Davis-Whitenack ML, Adeleye BO, Rolf LL, Stoecker BJ. 1996. Biliary excretion of [51]chromium in bile-duct cannulated rats. *Nutr Res* 16:1009–1015.

Do Canto OM, Sargent T III, Liehn JC. 1995. Chromium (III) metabolism in diabetic patients. In: Sive Subrananian KN, Wastney ME, eds. *Kinetic Models of Trace Element and Mineral Metabolism during Development.* Boca Raton, FL: CRC Press. Pp. 205–219.

Doisy RJ, Streeten DHP, Souma ML, Kalafer ME, Rekant SI, Dalakos TG. 1971. Metabolism of chromium-51 in human subjects—Normal, elderly, and diabetic subjects. In: Mertz W, Cornatzer WE, eds. *Newer Trace Elements in Nutrition.* New York: Marcel Dekker. Pp 155–168.

Dowling HJ, Offenbacher EG, Pi-Sunyer FX. 1990. Effects of amino acids on the absorption of trivalent chromium and its retention by regions of the rat small intestine. *Nutr Res* 10:1261–1271.

Elbetieha A, Al-Hamood MH. 1997. Long-term exposure of male and female mice to trivalent and hexavalent chromium compounds: Effect on fertility. *Toxicology* 116:39–47.

Engelhardt S, Moser-Veillon PB, Mangels AR, Patterson KY, Veillon C. 1990. Appearance of an oral dose of chromium ([53]Cr) in breast milk? In: Atkinson SA, Hanson LA, Chandra RK, eds. *Human Lactation 4. Breastfeeding, Nutrition, Infection and Infant Growth in Developed and Emerging Countries.* St. Johns, Newfoundland: ARTS Biomedical. Pp. 485–487.

Ernst E. 1990. Testicular toxicity following short-term exposure to tri- and hexavalent chromium: An experimental study in the rat. *Toxicol Lett* 51:269–275.

Flodin NW. 1990. Micronutrient supplements: Toxicity and drug interactions. *Prog Food Nutr Sci* 14:277–331.

Fomon SJ. 1974. *Infant Nutrition,* 2nd ed. Philadelphia: WB Saunders. Pp. 24–25.

Fornace AJ Jr, Seres DS, Lechner JF, Harris CC. 1981. DNA-protein cross-linking by chromium salts. *Chem Biol Interact* 36:345–354.

Freund H, Atamian S, Fischer JE. 1979. Chromium deficiency during total parenteral nutrition. *J Am Med Assoc* 241:496–498.

Fristedt B, Lindqvist B, Schutz A, Ovrum P. 1965. Survival in a case of acute oral chromic acid poisoning with acute renal failure treated by haemodialysis. *Acta Med Scand* 177:153–159.

Gibson RS, Scythes CA. 1984. Chromium, selenium, and other trace element intakes of a selected sample of Canadian premenopausal women. *Biol Trace Elem Res* 6:105–116.

Gibson RS, MacDonald AC, Martinez OB. 1985. Dietary chromium and manganese intakes of a selected sample of Canadian elderly women. *Hum Nutr Appl Nutr* 39:43–52.

Greenwood NN, Earnshaw A. 1997. *Chemistry of the Elements,* 2nd ed. Oxford: Butterworth-Heinemann. Pp. 1002–1039.

Hamamy HA, Al-Hakkak ZS, Hussain AF. 1987. Chromosome aberrations in workers at a tannery in Iraq. *Mutat Res* 189:395–398.

Hambidge KM. 1971. Chromium nutrition in the mother and the growing child. In: Mertz W, Cornatzer WE, eds. *Newer Trace Elements in Nutrition.* New York: Marcel Dekker. Pp. 169–194.

Harris DC. 1977. Different metal-binding properties of the two sites of human transferrin. *Biochemistry* 16:560–564.

Harris MI, Flegal KM, Cowie CC, Eberhardt MS, Goldstein DE, Little RR, Wiedmeyer HM, Byrd-Holt DD. 1998. Prevalence of diabetes, impaired fasting glucose, and impaired glucose tolerance in U.S. adults. *Diabetes Care* 21:518–524.

Hathcock JN. 1997. Vitamins and minerals: Efficacy and safety. *Am J Clin Nutr* 66:427–437.

Hopkins LL Jr. 1965. Distribution in the rat of physiological amounts of injected Cr^{51}(III) with time. *Am J Physiol* 209:731–735.

Hopkins LL Jr, Majaj AS. 1967. Improvements of impaired glucose tolerance by chromium(III) in malnourished infants. In: Kuhnau J, ed. *Proceedings of the Seventh International Congress of Nutrition. Vol. 5: Physiology and Biochemistry of Food Components.* London: Pergamon Press. Pp. 721–723.

Hopkins LL Jr, Ransome-Kuti O, Majaj AS. 1968. Improvement of impaired carbohydrate metabolism by chromium (III) in malnourished infants. *Am J Clin Nutr* 21:203–211.

IOM (Institute of Medicine). 1990. *Nutrition During Pregnancy.* Washington, DC: National Academy Press. Pp. 96–120.

Itoh S, Shimada H. 1996. Micronucleus induction by chromium and selenium, and suppression by metallothionein inducer. *Mutat Res* 367:233–236.

Ivankovic S, Preussmann R. 1975. Absence of toxic and carcinogenic effects after administration of high doses of chromic oxide pigment in subacute and long-term feeding experiments in rats. *Food Cosmet Toxicol* 13:347–351.

Jeejeebhoy KN, Chu RC, Marliss EB, Greenberg GR, Bruce-Robertson A. 1977. Chromium deficiency, glucose intolerance, and neuropathy reversed by chromium supplementation, in a patient receiving long-term total parenteral nutrition. *Am J Clin Nutr* 30:531–538.

Kamath SM, Stoecker BJ, Davis-Whitenack ML, Smith MM, Adeleye BO, Sangiah S. 1997. Absorption, retention and urinary excretion of chromium-51 in rats pretreated with indomethacin and dosed with dimethylprostaglandin E$_2$, misoprostol or prostacyclin. *J Nutr* 127:478–482.

Kaufman DB, DiNicola W, McIntosh R. 1970. Acute potassium dichromate poisoning. Treated by peritoneal dialysis. *Am J Dis Child* 119:374–376.

Keim KS, Stoecker BJ, Henley S. 1987. Chromium status of the rat as affected by phytate. *Nutr Res* 7:253–263.

Kerger BD, Finley BL, Corbett GE, Dodge DG, Paustenbach DJ. 1997. Ingestion of chromium(VI) in drinking water by human volunteers: Absorption, distribution, and excretion of single and repeated doses. *J Toxicol Environ Health* 50:67–95.

Kim WW, Mertz W, Judd JT, Marshall MW, Kelsay JL, Prather ES. 1984. Effect of making duplicate food collections on nutrient intakes calculated from diet records. *Am J Clin Nutr* 40:1333–1337.

Kozlovsky AS, Moser PB, Reiser S, Anderson RA. 1986. Effects of diets high in simple sugars on urinary chromium losses. *Metabolism* 35:515–518.

Kusiak RA, Ritchie AC, Springer J, Muller J. 1993. Mortality from stomach cancer in Ontario miners. *Br J Ind Med* 50:117–126.

Kuykendall JR, Kerger BD, Jarvi EJ, Corbett GE, Paustenbach DJ. 1996. Measurement of DNA-protein cross-links in human leukocytes following acute ingestion of chromium in drinking water. *Carcinogenesis* 17:1971–1977.

Levis AG, Majone F. 1979. Cytotoxic and clastogenic effects of soluble chromium compounds on mammalian cell cultures. *Br J Cancer* 40:523–533.

Lim TH, Sargent T III, Kusubov N. 1983. Kinetics of trace element chromium(III) in the human body. *Am J Physiol* 244:R445–R454.

Loubieres Y, de Lassence A, Bernier M, Vieillard-Baron A, Schmitt JM, Page B, Jardin F. 1999. Acute, fatal, oral chromic acid poisoning. *J Toxicol Clin Toxicol* 37:333–336.

Lukaski HC, Bolonchuk WW, Siders WA, Milne DB. 1996. Chromium supplementation and resistance training: Effects on body composition, strength, and trace element status of men. *Am J Clin Nutr* 63:954–965.

Mackenzie RD, Byerrum RU, Decker CF, Hoppert CA, Langham RF. 1958. Chronic toxicity studies. II. Hexavalent and trivalent chromium administered in drinking water to rats. *AMA Arch Industr Health* 18:232–234.

Mahalko JR, Bennion M. 1976. The effect of parity and time between pregnancies on maternal hair chromium concentration. *Am J Clin Nutr* 29:1069–1072.

Martin WR, Fuller RE. 1998. Suspected chromium picolinate-induced rhabdomyolysis. *Pharmacotherapy* 18:860–862.

Martinez OB, MacDonald AC, Gibson RS, Bourn D. 1985. Dietary chromium and effect of chromium supplementation on glucose tolerance of elderly Canadian women. *Nutr Res* 5:609–620.

Mertz W. 1969. Chromium occurrence and function in biological systems. *Physiol Rev* 49:163–239.

Mertz W. 1993. Chromium in human nutrition: A review. *J Nutr* 123:626–633.

Mertz W, Roginski EE, Schwarz K. 1961. Effect of trivalent chromium complexes on glucose uptake by epididymal fat tissue of rats. *J Biol Chem* 236:318–322.

Mertz W, Roginski EE, Reba RC. 1965. Biological activity and fate of trace quantities of intravenous chromium(III) in the rat. *Am J Physiol* 209:489–494.

Mertz W, Tsui JC, Judd JT, Reiser S, Hallfrisch J, Morris ER, Steele PD, Lashley E. 1991. What are people really eating? The relation between energy intake derived from estimated diet records and intake determined to maintain body weight. *Am J Clin Nutr* 54:291–295.

Mohamedshah FY, Moser-Veillon PB, Yamini S, Douglass LW, Anderson RA, Veillon C. 1998. Distribution of a stable isotope of chromium (^{53}Cr) in serum, urine, and breast milk in lactating women. *Am J Clin Nutr* 67:1250–1255.

Moshtaghie AA, Ani M, Bazrafshan MR. 1992. Comparative binding study of aluminum and chromium to human transferrin: Effect of iron. *Biol Trace Elem Res* 32:39–46.

Moss AJ, Levy AS, Kim I, Park YK. 1989. *Use of Vitamin and Mineral Supplements in the United States: Current Users, Types of Products, and Nutrients.* Advance Data, Vital and Health Statistics of the National Center for Health Statistics, No. 174. Hyattsville, MD: National Center for Health Statistics.

Nakamuro K, Yoshikawa K, Sayato Y, Kurata H. 1978. Comparative studies of chromosomal aberration and mutagenicity of the trivalent and hexavalent chromium. *Mutat Res* 58:175–181.

Newbold RF, Amos J, Connell JR. 1979. The cytotoxic, mutagenic and clastogenic effects of chromium-containing compounds on mammalian cells in culture. *Mutat Res* 67:55–63.

Offenbacher EG. 1994. Promotion of chromium absorption by ascorbic acid. *Trace Elem Elect* 11:178–181.

Offenbacher EG, Pi-Sunyer FX. 1983. Temperature and pH effects on the release of chromium from stainless steel into water and fruit juices. *J Agric Food Chem* 31:89–92.

Offenbacher EG, Spencer H, Dowling HJ, Pi-Sunyer FX. 1986. Metabolic chromium balances in men. *Am J Clin Nutr* 44:77–82.

Offenbacher EG, Pi-Sunyer FX, Stoecker BJ. 1997. Chromium. In: O'Dell BL, Sunde RA, eds. *Handbook of Nutritionally Essential Mineral Elements.* New York: Marcel Dekker. Pp. 389–411.

O'Flaherty EJ. 1994. Comparison of reference dose with estimated safe and adequate daily dietary intake for chromium. In: Mertz W, Abernathy CO, Olin SS, eds. *Risk Assessment of Essential Elements*. Washington, DC: ILSI Press. Pp. 213–218.

Onkelinx C. 1977. Compartment analysis of metabolism of chromium(III) in rats of various ages. *Am J Physiol* 232:E478–E484.

Paschal DC, Ting BG, Morrow JC, Pirkle JL, Jackson RJ, Sampson EJ, Miller DT, Caldwell KL. 1998. Trace metals in the urine of United States residents: reference range concentrations. *Environ Res* 76:53-59.

Raffetto G, Parodi S, Parodi C, De Ferrari M, Troiano R, Brambilla G. 1977. Direct interaction with cellular targets as the mechanism for chromium carcinogenesis. *Tumori* 63:503–512.

Rubin MA, Miller JP, Ryan AS, Treuth MS, Patterson KY, Pratley RE, Hurley BF, Veillon C, Moser-Veillon PB, Anderson RA. 1998. Acute and chronic resistive exercise increase urinary chromium excretion in men as measured with an enriched chromium stable isotope. *J Nutr* 128:73–78.

Saner G. 1981. The effect of parity on maternal hair chromium concentration and the changes during pregnancy. *Am J Clin Nutr* 34:853–855.

Sargent T III, Lim TH, Jenson RL. 1979. Reduced chromium retention in patients with hemochromatosis, a possible basis of hemochromatotic diabetes. *Metabolism* 28:70–79.

Schroeder HA, Balassa JJ, Tipton IH. 1962. Abnormal trace metals in man—Chromium. *J Chron Dis* 15:941–964.

Schroeder HA, Balassa JJ, Vinton WH Jr. 1965. Chromium, cadmium and lead in rats: Effects on life span, tumors and tissue levels. *J Nutr* 86:51–66.

Schwarz K, Mertz W. 1959. Chromium(III) and the glucose tolerance factor. *Arch Biochem Biophys* 85:292–295.

Seaborn CD, Stoecker BJ. 1989. Effects of starch, sucrose, fructose, and glucose on chromium absorption and tissue concentrations in obese and lean mice. *J Nutr* 119:1444–1451.

Seaborn CD, Stoecker BJ. 1990. Effects of antacid or ascorbic acid on tissue accumulation and urinary excretion of [51]chromium. *Nutr Res* 10:1401–1407.

Speetjens JK, Collins RA, Vincent JB, Woski SA. 1999. The nutritional supplement chromium (III) tris(picolinate) cleaves DNA. *Chem Res Toxicol* 12:483–487.

Stearns DM, Wise JP, Patierno SR, Wetterhahn KE. 1995. Chromium(III) picolinate produces chromosome damage in Chinese hamster ovary cells. *FASEB J* 9:1643–1648.

Stella M, Montaldi A, Rossi R, Rossi G, Levis AG. 1982. Clastogenic effects of chromium on human lymphocytes in vitro and in vivo. *Mutat Res* 101:151–164.

Stoecker BJ. 1996. Chromium. In: Ziegler EE, Filer LJ Jr, eds. *Present Knowledge in Nutrition*, 7th ed. Washington, DC: ILSI Press. Pp. 344–352.

Stoecker BJ. 1999. Chromium. In: Shils ME, Olson JA, Shike M, Ross AC, eds. *Modern Nutrition in Health and Disease*, 9th ed. Baltimore, MD: Williams & Wilkins. Pp. 281.

Tsuda H, Kato K. 1977. Chromosomal aberrations and morphological transformation in hamster embryonic cells treated with potassium dichromate in vitro. *Mutat Res* 46:87–94.

Umeda M, Nishimura M. 1979. Inducibility of chromosomal aberrations by metal compounds in cultured mammalian cells. *Mutat Res* 67:221–229.

Veillon C. 1989. Analytical chemistry of chromium. *Sci Total Environ* 86:65–68.

Venier P, Montaldi A, Majone F, Bianchi V, Levis AG. 1982. Cytotoxic, mutagenic and clastogenic effects of industrial chromium compounds. *Carcinogenesis* 3:1331–1338.

Vincent JB. 1999. Mechanisms of chromium action: Low-molecular-weight chromium-binding substance. *J Am Coll Nutr* 18:6–12.

Wasser WG, Feldman NS, D'Agati VD. 1997. Chronic renal failure after ingestion of over-the-counter chromium picolinate. *Ann Intern Med* 126:410.

Welch RM, Cary EE. 1975. Concentration of chromium, nickel, and vanadium in plant materials. *J Agric Food Chem* 23:479–482.

Whiting RF, Stich HF, Koropatnick DJ. 1979. DNA damage and DNA repair in cultured human cells exposed to chromate. *Chem Biol Interact* 26:267–280.

7

Copper

SUMMARY

Copper functions as a component of a number of metalloenzymes acting as oxidases to achieve the reduction of molecular oxygen. The primary criterion used to estimate the Estimated Average Requirement (EAR) for copper is a combination of indicators, including plasma copper and ceruloplasmin concentrations, erythrocyte superoxide dismutase activity, and platelet copper concentration in controlled human depletion/repletion studies. The Recommended Dietary Allowance (RDA) for adult men and women is 900 µg/day. The median intake of copper from food in the United States is approximately 1.0 to 1.6 mg/day for adult men and women. The Tolerable Upper Intake Level (UL) for adults is 10,000 µg/day (10 mg/day), a value based on protection from liver damage as the critical adverse effect.

BACKGROUND INFORMATION

Function

The biochemical role for copper is primarily catalytic, with many copper metalloenzymes acting as oxidases to achieve the reduction of molecular oxygen. Many copper metalloenzymes have been identified in humans (da Silva and Williams, 1991; Harris, 1997).

Amine oxidases participate in important reactions that have markedly different effects. Diamine oxidase inactivates histamine released during allergic reactions. Monoamine oxidase (MAO) is important in serotonin degradation to excretable metabolites and in the metabolism of catecholamines (epinephrine, norepinephrine, and dopamine). MAO inhibitors are used as antidepressant drugs. Lysyl oxidase uses lysine and hydroxylysine found in collagen and elastin as substrates for posttranslational processing to produce cross-linkages needed for the development of connective tissues, including those of bone, lung, and the circulatory system.

Ferroxidases are copper enzymes found in plasma, with a function in ferrous iron oxidation ($Fe^{2+} \rightarrow Fe^{3+}$) that is needed to achieve iron's binding to transferrin (Linder and Hazegh-Azam, 1996). Ferroxidase I, also called ceruloplasmin, is the predominant copper protein in plasma and may also have antioxidant functions. Defects in ceruloplasmin function produce cellular iron accumulation, a result that supports its ferroxidase role (Harris and Gitlin, 1996). Ferroxidase II is found in human plasma, but it may have a role in iron metabolism in specific cellular sites. A transmembrane copper-containing protein (hephaestatin) with ferroxidase activity has been described (Pena et al., 1999; Vulpe et al., 1999). Cytochrome c oxidase is a multisubunit enzyme in mitochondria that catalyzes reduction of O_2 to H_2O. This establishes a high energy proton gradient required for adenosine triphosphate (ATP) synthesis. This copper enzyme is particularly abundant in tissues of greatest metabolic activity including heart, brain, and liver. Dopamine β monooxygenase uses ascorbate, copper, and O_2 to convert dopamine to norepinephrine, a neurotransmitter, produced in neuronal and adrenal gland cells. Dopa, a precursor of dopamine, and metabolites used in melanin formation are oxidatively produced from tyrosine by the copper enzyme tyrosinase. α-Amidating monooxygenase (α-AE), also called peptidylglycine α-AE, uses copper and ascorbate to remove two carbons from a C-terminal glycine of peptides, thus generating an amide. A number of peptide hormones are posttranslationally modified by α-AE (Harris, 1997).

Two forms of superoxide dismutase are expressed in mammalian cells, a mangano and cupro/zinc form (Harris, 1997). Copper/zinc superoxide dismutase (Cu/Zn SOD) uses two copper atoms for conversion of the superoxide anion (O_2^-+) to H_2O_2 and O_2. Zinc atoms have a structural role in the enzyme. The enzyme is localized in the cytosol and, along with the mitochondrial manganese-containing form, provides a defense against oxidative damage from superoxide radicals that, if uncontrolled, can lead to other damaging reactive oxygen species. Mutations in the Cu/Zn SOD gene, which alter the protein's redox behavior, produce amyotrophic lateral sclerosis (Lou Gehrig's disease).

These are the principal copper metalloenzymes found in humans. There is substantial documentation from animal studies that diets low in copper reduce the activities of many of these copper metalloenzymes. Activities of some copper metalloenzymes have been shown to decrease in human copper depletion (Milne, 1994; Turnlund, 1999). Physiologic consequences resulting from copper deficiency include defects in connective tissue that lead to vascular and skeletal problems, anemia associated with defective iron utilization, and possibly specific aspects of central nervous system dysfunction (Harris, 1997; Turnlund, 1999). Some evidence suggests that immune and cardiac dysfunction occurs in experimental copper deficiency and the development of such signs of deficiency has been demonstrated in infants (Graham and Cordano, 1969; Olivares and Uauy, 1996; Turnlund, 1999).

Physiology of Absorption, Metabolism, and Excretion

Metabolism of copper in humans relies on the intestine for control of homeostasis as the capacity for renal copper excretion is limited. Nearly two-thirds of the body copper content is located in skeleton and muscle, but studies with stable isotopes have shown that the liver is a key site in maintaining plasma copper concentrations (Olivares and Uauy, 1996; Turnlund et al., 1998). Copper has a higher binding affinity for proteins than all other divalent trace elements (da Silva and Williams, 1991). Consequently, precise control of intracellular copper trafficking is needed to regulate how it is donated to appropriate sites.

Copper absorption occurs primarily in the small intestine. Some absorption may occur in the stomach where the acidic environment promotes copper solubility by dissociation from copper-containing macromolecules derived from dietary sources (Harris, 1997; Turnlund, 1999). Both saturable-mediated and nonsaturable-nonmediated (possibly paracellular) transepithelial copper movements have been reported. The Menkes P-type ATPase (MNK; ATP7A) is believed to be responsible for copper trafficking to the secretory pathway for efflux from cells, including enterocytes (Harris and Gitlin, 1996). A defective MNK gene causes Menkes' disease, which is characterized by reduced copper absorption and placental copper transport. The extent of copper absorption varies with dietary copper intake (Turnlund, 1998). It ranges from over 50 percent at an intake of less than 1 mg/day to less than 20 percent above 5 mg/day. About

35 percent of a 2 mg/day intake is absorbed and is transported via the portal vein to the liver, bound to albumin, for uptake by liver parenchymal cells.

Biliary copper excretion is adjusted to maintain balance. Copper is released via plasma to extrahepatic sites where up to 95 percent of the copper is bound to ceruloplasmin (Turnlund, 1999). The biological role of ceruloplasmin in copper metabolism has been widely investigated. The autosomal recessive disorder in humans, aceruloplasminemia, does not produce abnormal copper metabolism, thus contradicting a role for the protein in copper delivery to cells. However, this genetic defect results in tissue iron accumulation, supporting the protein's role in cellular iron release. Other P-type ATPases (e.g., Wilson, NND, ATP7B) are responsible for copper trafficking to the secretory pathway for ceruloplasmin synthesis or for endosome formation before transport into the bile (Harris and Gitlin, 1996; Pena et al., 1999). Mutations of this copper-transporting ATPase result in cellular copper accumulation called Wilson's disease. Urinary copper excretion is normally very low (< 0.1 mg/day) over a wide range of dietary intakes (Turnlund, 1999). As with other trace elements, renal dysfunction can lead to increased urinary losses.

Clinical Effects of Inadequate Intake

Frank copper deficiency in humans is rare, but has been found in a number of special conditions. It has been observed in premature infants fed milk formulas, in infants recovering from malnutrition associated with chronic diarrhea and fed cow's milk (Shaw, 1992), and in patients with prolonged total parenteral nutrition (Fujita et al., 1989). In these cases, serum copper and ceruloplasmin concentrations were as low as 0.5 μmol and 35 mg/L, respectively, compared to reported normal ranges of 10 to 25 μmol/L for serum copper concentration and 180 to 400 mg/L for ceruloplasmin concentration (Lentner, 1984). Supplementation with copper resulted in rapid increases in serum copper and ceruloplasmin concentrations.

Symptoms accompanying the copper deficiency included normocytic, hypochromic anemia, leukopenia, and neutropenia (Fujita et al., 1989). Osteoporosis was observed in copper-deficient infants and growing children.

Copper deficiency developed in six severely handicapped patients between the ages of 4 and 24 years who were fed an enteral diet containing 15 μg of copper/100 kcal for 12 to 66 months (Higuchi et al., 1988). Their serum copper concentrations ranged from 0.9 to 7.2 μmol/L and ceruloplasmin concentrations ranged from 30 to 125 mg/L. Two patients had neutropenia, one had macrocytic, normochromic anemia, and some had bone abnormalities including reduced bone density. Neutrophil counts normalized and bone abnormalities improved after copper supplementation. If the copper intake of these patients is extrapolated to adults on the basis of caloric intake, copper deficiency might be expected to develop in adults at an intake of 440 μg/2,900 kcal for men and 290 μg/1,900 kcal for women. This deduction is consistent with a study in which healthy young men who were fed a diet containing 380 μg/day of copper for 42 days had a decline in serum copper and ceruloplasmin concentrations and then an increase with copper repletion (Turnlund et al., 1997). Although serum copper and ceruloplasmin concentrations of these men did not fall to the deficient range in 42 days and clinical symptoms did not appear, these effects might be expected had the low copper diet been continued. In a number of other studies at higher levels of copper intake (i.e., at 600 μg/day and above), serum copper and ceruloplasmin concentrations did not decline significantly (Milne, 1998; Turnlund et al., 1990).

Results of depletion studies in laboratory animals have led to interest in a number of conditions in humans that may be associated with marginal copper intake over a long period. Insufficient data are available at this time to establish whether these conditions are related to dietary copper.

A report of increased blood cholesterol concentrations in one young man consuming 830 μg/day of copper (Klevay et al., 1984) suggested that elevated blood cholesterol concentration may be associated with marginal amounts of dietary copper. This effect was not observed in other subjects or in a number of other studies with this or lower levels of dietary copper. In one study, blood cholesterol concentration decreased with lower dietary copper (Milne and Nielsen, 1996), and in a copper supplementation study investigators found increased blood cholesterol concentrations with supplementation (Medeiros et al., 1991).

Heart beat irregularities were reported in some studies, and investigators linked them to dietary copper intake (Milne, 1998). However, heart beat irregularities are common in normal, healthy people, and other studies with lower copper intake demonstrated that such irregularities, monitored during copper depletion and repletion, were common at all intake levels of dietary copper (Turnlund et al., 1997). Myocardial disease occurs in severely deficient weanling rats, and one investigator has hypothesized that ischemic heart disease is related to marginal copper status (Klevay, 1989). However, the myocardial changes observed in copper-deficient animals are very different from those of ischemic heart disease in humans (Danks, 1988). In severely deficient animals, the myocardium is hypertrophied and may rupture. Coronary artery resistance is decreased in copper-deficient animals, but it is increased in ischemic heart disease.

Several other clinical observations deserve further investigation, but there is insufficient evidence to link them to marginal copper status. Glucose tolerance was lower in two of a group of eight men consuming 80 µg/day of copper than in men consuming higher levels of copper (Klevay et al., 1986), but similar observations have not been reported at lower intakes of copper in other studies. One study reported a negative correlation between ceruloplasmin concentration and blood pressure during a hand grip exercise (Lukaski et al., 1988), but the link between blood pressure and dietary copper has not been investigated further in humans. An index of immune function declined in a depletion study with copper intakes of 380 µg/day that resulted in decreases in indexes of copper status, but other indexes of immune function did not decline and repletion did not result in reversal of the change (Kelley et al., 1995). Changes in blood clotting factors V and VIII were observed in one study with copper intakes of 570 µg/day (Milne and Nielsen, 1996). The role of copper as an antioxidant has led to interest in the possibility that copper deficiency impairs antioxidant status (Johnson et al., 1992). A report of changes in some, but not other, markers of bone metabolism with a dietary copper intake of 700 µg/day deserves further investigation (Baker et al., 1999). Changes in catecholamine metabolism have been investigated, but results are inconsistent (Bhathena et al., 1998).

SELECTION OF INDICATORS FOR ESTIMATING THE REQUIREMENT FOR COPPER

Several indicators are used to diagnose copper deficiency. These indicators—serum or plasma copper concentration, ceruloplasmin concentration, and erythrocyte superoxide dismutase activity—are low with copper deficiency and respond to copper supplementation. However, except when diets are deficient in copper, they do not reflect dietary intake and may not be sensitive to marginal copper status. In addition, serum copper and ceruloplasmin concentrations increase during pregnancy and with a number of diseases, and therefore copper deficiency could be masked under these conditions. Platelet copper concentration and cytochrome *c* oxidase activity may be more sensitive to marginal intakes of dietary copper than plasma copper or ceruloplasmin concentration, but they have been measured in very few studies to date. No single indicator provides an adequate basis on which to estimate the copper requirement.

Serum Copper Concentrations

Serum copper concentration is a reliable indicator of copper deficiency, falling to very low concentrations in copper-deficient individuals. The lower end of the normal range for serum copper concentration is reported to be 10 μmol/L, but serum copper concentrations were considerably lower than this when cases of copper deficiency were discovered. Serum copper concentration returns to normal within a few days of copper supplementation (Danks, 1988). While serum copper concentration is an index of copper deficiency, it does not reflect dietary intake except when intake is below a certain level. Above this level, supplementation with copper does not increase serum copper concentration. Serum copper concentration increases under a number of conditions due to increased concentrations of ceruloplasmin.

Ceruloplasmin Concentration

Ceruloplasmin concentration is also a reliable indicator of copper deficiency. Ceruloplasmin carries between 60 and 95 percent of serum copper, and changes in serum copper concentration usually parallel the ceruloplasmin concentration in the blood. Ceruloplasmin, too, falls to low concentrations with copper deficiency, far below the lower end of the normal range of 180 mg/L, and it responds quickly to repletion (Danks, 1988). Ceruloplasmin does not respond to dietary intake, unless intake is very low. The dietary copper intake at which ceruloplasmin concentration no longer increases in response to increased dietary copper might be considered the copper requirement for ceruloplasmin synthesis. Ceruloplasmin is an acute phase protein and increases markedly with a number of diseases, including liver disease, malignancy, inflammatory diseases, myocardial infarction, and a variety of infectious diseases (Mason, 1979). It also increases with pregnancy and oral contraceptive use. With any of these conditions, copper deficiency might not be diagnosed on the basis of serum copper or ceruloplasmin concentrations.

Erythrocyte Superoxide Dismutase Activity

Erythrocyte superoxide dismutase (SOD) activity, though not as specific as serum copper or ceruloplasmin concentration, may be a reliable indicator of copper status, and some suggest it is more sensitive (Milne, 1998; Uauy et al., 1985). It does not increase with the conditions that increase serum copper and ceruloplasmin concentrations. However, it can increase in situations that produce oxidative stress, and SOD activity is high in some conditions, including alcoholism and Down's syndrome. Methods of analysis are not standardized, and normal ranges for SOD activity are not available. Although SOD activity was measured in fewer studies than were the two indicators above, sufficient data are available to include it as an indicator of change in copper status when it is measured in controlled studies at different levels of dietary copper intake.

Platelet Copper Concentration and Cytochrome c Oxidase Activity

Two studies in women suggest that both platelet copper concentration and platelet cytochrome c oxidase activity may respond more rapidly to low dietary copper than the indicators discussed above. In one study both of these indicators declined when copper intake was 570 µg/day (Milne and Nielsen, 1996). Platelet copper concentration increased after repletion, but platelet cytochrome c oxidase activity did not. In another study, both platelet copper concentration and platelet cytochrome c oxidase activity increased after supplementation of a diet containing 670 µg/day of copper, but baseline measurements were not made, so it is not known whether these parameters declined (Milne et al., 1988). Moreover, an intervening vitamin C supplementation period added another variable to the data interpretation. The fact that serum copper and ceruloplasmin concentrations and SOD activity were not affected at this level of dietary copper suggests the requirement for maintaining serum copper and ceruloplasmin concentration had been met. Therefore, the above research suggests that platelet copper concentration and platelet cytochrome c oxidase activity, when measured in controlled studies, may be more sensitive to changes in copper dietary intake.

Urinary Copper

Urinary copper excretion is extremely low and does not contribute significantly to copper retention, but it has been found to decline when diets are low enough in copper that other indexes of copper status change (Turnlund et al., 1997). Above those levels of dietary intake, urinary copper does not respond to increases in dietary copper. In controlled studies, a decline in urinary copper excretion can be used as supporting evidence for inadequate intake.

Leukocyte Copper Concentration

Leukocyte copper concentration was found to decline along with other indexes of copper status in one study (Turnlund et al., 1997), but it has not been reported in others. Too few data are currently available to use it for establishing dietary recommendations for copper.

Lysyl Oxidase Activity

Lysyl oxidase activity in the skin, which declined with low dietary copper and increased with repletion, is potentially a useful indicator of copper status (Werman et al., 1997). It is not known if lysyl oxidase activity reflects dietary intake at higher levels of dietary copper in humans. Because data are available from only one study, it cannot yet be used as an indicator for estimating copper requirements.

Peptidyl Glycine α-Amidating Monooxygenase Activity

Peptidyl glycine α-amidating monooxygenase (PAM) activity in serum of rats and stimulation of activity are sensitive indicators of copper intake in the rat (Prohaska et al., 1997). Patients with Menkes' disease, who have severe copper deficiency due to a metabolic defect in copper transport, had an increased copper stimulation index of plasma PAM as compared with healthy control subjects. This finding suggests that PAM activity may be a useful indicator of copper status in humans when human dose-response data become available.

Diamine Oxidase Activity

Two copper supplementation studies demonstrated that the activity of serum diamine oxidase (DAO), another cuproenzyme, increases when supplements containing 2 mg (Jones et al., 1997) and 6 mg (Kehoe et al., 2000) of copper were administered daily, a result that suggests the enzyme may be sensitive to increased dietary copper. It has not yet been studied under conditions of copper depletion. Because intestinal damage and a number of conditions also elevate DAO activity, its use as an indicator of copper status is possibly limited.

Copper Balance

Balance studies have been used in the past to estimate dietary recommendations. Numerous copper balance studies in humans have been conducted over a wide range of intakes (Mason, 1979). Unfortunately, there are a number of problems with this approach, as reviewed by Mertz (1987). Copper balance, which can be achieved over a broad range of dietary copper intakes, reflects prior dietary intake; thus long adaptation is required for results to be meaningful. Seldom are studies long enough. Such studies are prone to numerous errors, and data from some studies would suggest that an unacceptable amount of copper would accumulate over time if these levels of retention were continued. In addition, miscellaneous losses, while small, are very difficult to quantify. Therefore, balance studies were not used as an indicator of copper status.

Factorial Analysis

One approach to estimating minimum dietary mineral requirements is by the factorial method. Obligatory losses, the amounts of an element excreted with no dietary intake, are determined, and then the amount needed in the diet to replace these obligatory losses is calculated. Obligatory losses include urinary losses, gastrointestinal losses, sweat, integument, hair, nails, and other miscellaneous losses such as menstrual and semen losses. For copper, as for other elements, reliable values for many of these losses are not available. However, sufficient data are available to make reasonable estimates; therefore, this method can be used in support of estimates of dietary copper requirements made by other methods.

FACTORS AFFECTING THE COPPER REQUIREMENT

The composition of the diet has little effect on the bioavailability of copper, except in unusual circumstances. The bioavailability of copper is influenced markedly by the amount of copper in the diet. Bioavailability ranges from 75 percent of dietary copper absorbed when the diet contains only 400 µg/day to 12 percent absorbed when the diet contains 7.5 mg/day (Turnlund et al., 1989, 1998). The absolute amount of copper absorbed is higher with increasing intake. In addition, excretion of copper into the gastrointestinal tract regulates copper retention. As more copper is absorbed, turnover is faster and more copper is excreted into the gastrointestinal tract (Turnlund et al., 1998). This excretion is probably the primary point of regulation of total body copper. This efficient homeostatic regulation of absorption and retention helps protect against copper deficiency and toxicity.

Zinc

Zinc intakes, well in excess of the amount normally found in the diet, can decrease copper absorption in adults (Turnlund, 1999) (see Table 12-7). In one case report, an infant who was given 16 to 24 mg/day of zinc developed copper deficiency (Botash et al., 1992). Very high doses of zinc have been used to treat patients with Wilson's disease, an inborn error of copper metabolism resulting in copper toxicity (Brewer et al., 1983). This zinc-induced inhibition of copper absorption could be the result of competition for a common, apically oriented transporter or the induction of metallothionein in intestinal cells by zinc. Because this protein has a higher binding affinity for copper than for zinc, copper is retained within enterocytes and its absorption is reduced. This response has been used as a therapy to diminish copper absorption in patients with Wilson's disease (Yuzbasiyan-Gurkan et al., 1992). The interaction could also be responsible for reducing copper absorption during consumption of zinc supplements. When zinc-to-copper ratios of 2:1, 5:1, and 15:1 were fed to humans, there were limited effects on copper absorption (August et al., 1989).

Iron

High iron intakes may interfere with copper absorption in infants. Infants fed a formula containing low concentrations of iron absorbed more copper than infants consuming the same formula with a higher iron concentration (Haschke et al., 1986). Such an interaction has been reported to produce reduced copper status in infants (Lonnerdal and Hernell, 1994; Morais et al., 1994).

Fructose

Studies in rats demonstrated that diets very high in fructose were associated with increased severity of copper deficiency in rats (Fields et al., 1984), but a similar effect was not observed in pigs

(Schoenemann et al., 1990), which have cardiovascular systems and gastrointestinal tracts more similar to those of humans. The effects were inconsistent in humans (Reiser et al., 1985) but did not result in copper depletion, and the extremely high levels of fructose fed (20 percent of energy intake) suggest the effect would not be relevant to normal diets.

FINDINGS BY LIFE STAGE AND GENDER GROUP

Infants Ages 0 through 12 Months

Method Used to Set the Adequate Intake

No functional criteria of copper status have been demonstrated that reflect response to dietary intake in infants. Thus, recommended intakes of copper are based on an Adequate Intake (AI) that reflects the observed mean copper intake of infants principally fed human milk.

Ages 0 through 6 Months. The AI for infants ages 0 through 6 months was based on the usual intake from human milk. The copper content of human milk is highest during early lactation and then declines during the course of lactation. According to a number of reports (Biego et al., 1998; Raiten et al., 1998; Rossipal and Krachler, 1998), the mean copper content of human milk during the first 6 months of lactation is approximately 250 µg/L (Table 7-1). There are no indications that the copper content of human milk is inadequate to maintain copper status. Liver copper stores are high (Widdowson and Dickerson, 1964) and serum copper and ceruloplasmin concentrations are low (Salmenpera et al., 1986) in newborn infants. During the first 6 months of life, liver stores decline and serum copper concentration increases to adult levels, independent of copper intake.

Based on the copper content of human milk and milk consumption (Chapter 2), the AI for infants ages 0 through 6 months is 200 µg/day (250 µg/L × 0.78 L/day) after rounding. For a 7 kg infant (reference weight for 0 through 6 months, Chapter 2), this would be 28 µg/kg/day (200 µg/day/7 kg), rounded up to 30 µg/kg/day.

Ages 7 through 12 Months. One method for estimating the AI for infants receiving human milk, ages 7 through 12 months, is based on the average intake from human milk plus an added increment for complementary foods (Chapter 2). According to the Third

TABLE 7-1 Copper Concentration in Human Milk

Reference	Study Group	Stage of Lactation	Milk Concentration (µg/L)	Estimated Copper Intake of Infants (µg/d)[a]
Picciano and Guthrie, 1976	50 women	6–12 wk	245	190
Vaughan et al., 1979	38 women, 19–42 y	1–3 mo	430	330
		4–6 mo	330	260
		7–9 mo	300	180
		10–12 mo	240	140
		13–18 mo	290	170
		19–31 mo	280	170
Vuori and Kuitunen, 1979	27 women	2 wk	600	470
		20 wk	250	150
Vuori et al., 1980	15 women, 24–35 y	6–8 wk	360	280
		17–22 wk	210	160
Higashi et al., 1982	21 women, 21–35 y	1 mo	450	350
		3 mo	290	230
		5 mo	200	160
Dewey and Lonnerdal, 1983	20 women	1 mo		250
		2 mo		230
		3 mo		220
		4 mo		200
		5 mo		150
		6 mo		200
Fransson and Lonnerdal, 1984	15 milk samples	2–4 mo	320	250
Casey et al., 1985	11 women, 26–39 y	8 d	590	460
		14 d	490	380
		21 d	420	320
		28 d	410	320
Lipsman et al., 1985	7–13 teens	1 mo	350	270
		2 mo	290	230
		3 mo	380	290
		4 mo	280	220
		5 mo	210	160
		6 mo	200	120
		7 mo	190	110

TABLE 7-1 Continued

Reference	Study Group	Stage of Lactation	Milk Concentration (µg/L)	Estimated Copper Intake of Infants (µg/d)[a]
Butte et al., 1987	45 women	1 mo		270
		2 mo		230
		3 mo		210
		4 mo		200
Casey et al., 1989	22 women	7 d	620	480
		5 mo	220	170
Anderson, 1992	7 women	Up to 5 mo	310	240
Anderson, 1993	6 women, 20–30 y		110–380	
Biego et al., 1998	17 milk samples	Mature milk	250	190
Rossipal and Krachler, 1998	46 women	1–3 d	570	440
		12–60 d	230	180
		97–293 d	150	90

NOTE: Maternal intakes were reported in only two studies: in Vaughan et al. (1979), mean intakes (mg/day) were 3.64, 1.90, 2.37, 6.80, and 2.50 at 4–6, 7–9, 10–12, 13–18, and 19–31 months; in Vuori et al. (1980), mean intakes (mg/day) were 1.88 at 6–8 weeks and 1.73 at 17–22 weeks.

[a] Copper intake based on reported data or concentration (µg/L) × 0.78 L/day for 0–6 months postpartum and concentration (µg/L) × 0.6 L/day for 7–12 months postpartum.

National Health and Nutrition Examination Survey, the median copper intake from weaning food for children aged 7 through 12 months is 100 µg/day ($n = 45$). The average copper concentration in human milk declines over time, and between 7 and 12 months postpartum the concentration is 200 µg/L or less (Table 7-1). Based on an average volume of 0.6 L/day of human milk that is secreted, the copper intake from human milk is 120 µg/day (0.6×200). Therefore the total intake of copper from human milk and complementary foods is 220 µg/day ($120 + 100$). For a 9 kg infant (reference weight 7 through 12 months, Chapter 2), this would be 24 µg/kg/day (220 µg/kg ÷ 9 kg).

If the AI were extrapolated from the AI for younger infants by using the calculation in chapter 2, the average intake would be 241 µg/day.

Copper AI Summary, Ages 0 through 12 Months

AI for Infants

0–6 months	200 µg/day of copper	30 µg/kg/day
7–12 months	220 µg/day of copper	24 µg/kg/day

Special Considerations

The concentration of copper in cow milk has been reported to range from 60 to 90 µg/L (Fransson and Lonnerdal, 1983) which is lower than that reported for human milk (Table 7-1). Copper is bound to the fat fraction (15 percent) in cow milk with the remaining bound to casein (King et al., 1959). It has been reported that copper absorption in infants fed human milk is greater than in infants fed a cow milk-based formula (Dorner et al., 1989; Johnson and Canfield, 1989). Copper deficiency has been observed in infants fed cow milk (Cordano et al., 1964; Levy et al., 1985). Dorner and coworkers (1989) showed that 20 percent of children were in negative balance when fed unsupplemented formula, whereas all children were in positive balance when fed either human milk or supplemented formula.

Children and Adolescents Ages 1 through 18 Years

Method Used to Estimate the Average Requirement

No data are available on which to base the Estimated Average Requirement (EAR) for copper for children or adolescents. In the absence of additional information, EARs and Recommended Dietary Allowances (RDAs) for children and adolescents have been estimated by using the method described in Chapter 2, which extrapolates from the adult EAR. Although there are no studies available to indicate that the copper requirement is associated with energy expenditure, metabolic weight ($kg^{0.75}$) was used for extrapolating because of the structural and functional role of copper in a number of enzymes and because using metabolic weight yields an EAR that is higher than when total body weight is used.

Copper EAR and RDA Summary, Ages 1 through 18 Years

EAR for Children

1–3 years	260 µg/day of copper
4–8 years	340 µg/day of copper

EAR for Boys
  9–13 years   540 µg/day of copper
  14–18 years   685 µg/day of copper

EAR for Girls
  9–13 years   540 µg/day of copper
  14–18 years   685 µg/day of copper

The RDA for copper is set by using a coefficient of variation (CV) of 15 percent (see Chapter 1 and the discussion of adult requirements that follows) because information is not available on the standard deviation of the requirement for these age groups. The RDA is defined as equal to the EAR plus twice the CV to cover the needs of 97 to 98 percent of the individuals in the group (therefore, for copper the RDA is 130 percent of the EAR). The calculated RDA is rounded to the nearest 10 µg.

RDA for Children
  1–3 years   340 µg/day of copper
  4–8 years   440 µg/day of copper

RDA for Boys
  9–13 years   700 µg/day of copper
  14–18 years   890 µg/day of copper

RDA for Girls
  9–13 years   700 µg/day of copper
  14–18 years   890 µg/day of copper

Adults Ages 19 Years and Older

Evidence Considered in Estimating the Average Requirement

Biochemical Indicators. No single indicator was judged as sufficient for deriving an EAR for adults. Results for specific indicators vary between studies. To determine the EAR, a combination of indicators was used, including plasma copper concentration, serum ceruloplasmin concentration, erythrocyte superoxide dismutase activity (SOD), and platelet copper concentration in controlled human depletion/repletion studies using specific amounts of copper. If there were significant decreases in serum copper and ceruloplasmin concentrations and SOD activity when the experimental copper diet was fed, and if this decrease was reversed with added copper, then the experimental diet was considered insufficient to maintain status and therefore deficient in copper. If plasma copper and serum ceruloplasmin concentrations did not change significantly when the experimental diet was fed, but platelet copper concentration decreased, then the experimental diet was judged to be marginally adequate in copper. A lack of change in the copper status indicators indicated that the level of copper in the experimental diet was adequate to maintain status. Because of limited data, data from men and women were combined.

Three studies were used to estimate the average requirement on the basis of copper status. These studies are summarized in Table 7-2. Serum copper and ceruloplasmin concentrations and SOD activity declined significantly in eight of 11 young men fed an experimental, depletion diet containing 388 µg/day and increased with repletion (Turnlund et al., 1997). Although these indicators decreased significantly, they did not fall to the deficient range while the deficient diet was fed for 42 days. However, it is expected that they would have fallen to the deficient range over a longer time. Other changes suggesting copper depletion were observed.

When young men were fed 790 µg/day of copper, the above mentioned indicators did not decline significantly (Turnlund et al., 1990). After a decline in copper status, two of the 11 men responded to copper repletion. Therefore, the copper requirement to maintain copper status in half of a group is more than 380 µg/day but less than 790 µg/day. On the basis of these data, a linear model was used to estimate a response curve. The model estimated that half of these men would not maintain copper status at 550 µg/day.

Serum copper and ceruloplasmin concentrations did not decline significantly when ten women were fed 570 µg/day of copper (Milne and Nielsen, 1996). Platelet copper concentration, however, declined significantly for eight of ten women fed 570 µg/day and increased with supplementation. Other indicators did not respond to depletion. Platelet cytochrome *c* oxidase and erythrocyte SOD activity declined but did not respond significantly to repletion. While an EAR based on the first two studies was estimated at 550 µg/day, the latter study suggests that 600 µg/day may be a marginal intake in over half of the population. Therefore, another increment was added to cover half of the population, and the EAR was set at 700 µg/day.

Factorial Analysis. Another approach for estimating the minimum copper requirement is to estimate obligatory losses of copper and calculate the amount of copper required in the diet to replace these

TABLE 7-2 Effects of Copper (Cu) Intake on Copper Status

Reference	Subjects	Duration of Study	Dietary Cu Intake (mg/d)	Results
Turnlund et al., 1990	11 healthy men	90 d	1.68 × 24 d 0.79 × 42 d 7.53 × 24 d	Plasma Cu, ceruloplasmin, superoxide dismutase (SOD), urinary and salivary Cu: no change due to Cu intake Cu sweat losses very low
Milne and Nielsen, 1996	10 post-menopausal women, aged 49–75 y (mean 63 y)	≈ 6 mo	0.57 × 105 d 2.57 × 35 d (2 mg as supple-ment)	Urinary Cu: no change throughout study Plasma Cu and ceruloplasmin: no significant change SOD and platelet cytochrome *c* oxidase: significantly lower after depletion, but no increase during repletion Platelet Cu declined during depletion and increased with repletion
Turnlund et al., 1997	11 healthy men, mean age 26 y	90 d	0.66 × 24 d 0.38 × 42 d 2.49 × 24 d	Plasma Cu, SOD, ceruloplasmin, and urinary Cu declined with depletion and increased with repletion

obligatory losses. This approach provides supporting evidence for the EAR based on copper status estimated above. Endogenous losses, estimated from total parenteral nutrition (TPN) data, were estimated to be 300 µg/day by Shike and coworkers (1981). This estimate was based on gastrointestinal losses from patients without excessive gastrointestinal secretions (less than 0.3 L/day) of 191 µg/day and urinary losses of 90 µg/day, which are higher than urinary losses in normal, healthy adults, and would provide an increment for miscellaneous losses. The TPN patients received no copper orally, but copper from TPN ranged from 250 to 1,850 µg/day.

There are no data on obligatory copper losses in healthy people; therefore the study with the lowest copper intake and data on endogenous losses was used to estimate obligatory losses in healthy people (Turnlund et al., 1997, 1998). When copper intake was 380 µg/day, copper status declined significantly. Endogenous fecal losses were calculated to be 240 µg/day, slightly higher than the estimate from TPN data (Shike et al., 1981), and urinary losses were less than 20 µg/day. A careful study of surface copper losses in men reported that these averaged 42 µg/day (Milne et al., 1991). Other losses, such as hair, nails, semen, or menstrual, have not been measured, and it is assumed they are similar to surface losses. Therefore the amount of absorbed copper needed to replace obligatory losses is 344 µg/day (240 + 20 + 42 + 42). Copper absorption at this level of intake is approximately 75 percent. Therefore, 460 µg/day of dietary copper would be the minimum amount required to replace obligatory losses. Endogenous fecal copper was 50 µg/day higher at 380 µg/day than at 460 µg/day, and so 50 µg/day was added to endogenous fecal losses to account for the increase that occurs between 380 and 460 µg/day. Thus 510 µg/day (460 + 50) of dietary copper is required to replace copper losses from all sources and to achieve zero balance. Estimation of the average requirement based on indicators of copper status is similar to, but slightly higher than, the average requirement determined by the factorial approach. The EAR is based on biochemical indicators of copper status of men and women, and there was no basis for a difference in requirement based on gender. There are no data on which to base an EAR for older adults, and no evidence to suggest that the requirements would be different.

Copper EAR and RDA Summary, Ages 19 Years and Older

EAR for Men
   19–50 years   700 µg/day of copper
   51–70 years   700 µg/day of copper
   > 70 years   700 µg/day of copper

EAR for Women
   19–50 years   700 µg/day of copper
   51–70 years   700 µg/day of copper
   > 70 years   700 µg/day of copper

The data available to set an EAR are limited for men and women, as well as the number of levels of dietary copper in depletion/repletion studies. Thus, a CV of 15 percent is used. The RDA is defined as equal to the EAR plus twice the CV to cover the needs of 97 to 98 percent of individuals in the group (therefore, for copper the RDA is 130 percent of the EAR). The calculated RDA is rounded to the nearest 100 µg.

RDA for Men
19–50 years	900 µg/day of copper
51–70 years	900 µg/day of copper
> 70 years	900 µg/day of copper

RDA for Women
19–50 years	900 µg/day of copper
51–70 years	900 µg/day of copper
> 70 years	900 µg/day of copper

Pregnancy

Evidence Considered in Estimating the Average Requirement

There are no data for establishing an EAR for pregnancy. Therefore, the EAR was based on estimates of the amount of copper that must be accumulated during pregnancy to account for the fetus and products of pregnancy. The full-term fetus contains about 13.7 mg copper (Widdowson and Dickerson, 1964). The copper content of the fetus is high compared to that of adults due to the high concentration of copper in the liver. In addition to the amount of copper accumulated by the fetus, other products that accumulate copper during pregnancy, including placenta amniotic fluid and maternal tissue, should be considered. The concentration of these tissues is lower, about one-third of the concentration of the fetus; therefore another 4.6 mg is added to 13.7 mg for a total of 18 mg copper. Over the course of pregnancy, this additional requirement is approximately 67 µg/day of absorbed copper or 100 µg/day of dietary copper, a value based on 65 to 70 percent bioavailability and rounding. Evidence suggests that copper absorption may be more efficient during pregnancy, and such efficiency could result in absorption of this amount of copper (Turnlund et al., 1983); therefore no additional increment would be required. However, too few data are available to draw this conclusion. Consequently, an additional 100 µg/day was added to the EARs for adolescent girls and women during pregnancy for EARs of 785 and 800 µg/day, respectively.

Copper EAR and RDA Summary, Pregnancy

EAR for Pregnancy
14–18 years	785 µg/day of copper
19–30 years	800 µg/day of copper
31–50 years	800 µg/day of copper

The data available to set an EAR are limited for men and women, as well as the number of levels of dietary copper in the depletion/repletion studies. Thus, a CV of 15 percent is used because information is not available on the standard deviation of the requirement for pregnant women. The RDA is defined as equal to the EAR plus twice the CV to cover the needs of 97 to 98 percent of individuals in the group (therefore, for copper the RDA is 130 percent of the EAR). The calculated RDA is rounded to the nearest 100 µg.

RDA for Pregnancy
14–18 years	1,000 µg/day of copper
19–30 years	1,000 µg/day of copper
31–50 years	1,000 µg/day of copper

Lactation

Evidence Considered in Estimating the Average Requirement

The EAR for lactation is determined on the basis of the copper intake necessary to replace copper secreted daily in human milk plus the EAR for adolescent girls and adult women. The average amount of copper that is secreted in human milk and must be absorbed is approximately 200 µg/day. Copper bioavailability for the adult consuming the EAR for copper is about 65 to 70 percent; therefore an additional 300 µg/day of copper must be consumed to replace the copper secreted in human milk, assuming that there is no increase in the efficiency of copper absorption during lactation. Animal data suggest that maternal absorption of copper increases during lactation and could provide for about half of the added increment, but data are not available for humans on copper absorption during lactation.

Copper EAR and RDA Summary, Lactation

EAR for Lactation

14–18 years	985 µg/day of copper
19–30 years	1,000 µg/day of copper
31–50 years	1,000 µg/day of copper

The data available to set an EAR are limited for men and women, as is the number of levels of dietary copper in the depletion/repletion studies. Thus, a CV of 15 percent is used because information is not available on the standard deviation of the requirement for lactating women. The RDA is defined as equal to the EAR plus twice the CV to cover the needs of 97 to 98 percent of individuals in the group (therefore, for copper the RDA is 130 percent of the EAR). The calculated RDA is rounded to the nearest 100 µg.

RDA for Lactation

14–18 years	1,300 µg/day of copper
19–30 years	1,300 µg/day of copper
31–50 years	1,300 µg/day of copper

INTAKE OF COPPER

Food Sources

Copper is widely distributed in foods. The accumulation of copper in plants is not affected by the copper content of the soil in which they grow. Organ meats, seafood, nuts, and seeds are major contributors of dietary copper (Pennington et al., 1995). Wheat bran cereals and whole grain products are also sources of copper. Foods that contribute substantial amounts of copper to the U.S. diet include those high in copper, such as organ meats, grains, and cocoa products, and those relatively low in copper that are consumed in substantial amounts, such as tea, potatoes, milk, and chicken.

Dietary Intake

Data from nationally representative U.S. surveys are available to estimate copper intakes (Appendix Tables C-15, C-16, D-2, E-3). The median intake of copper for women is approximately 1.0 to 1.1 mg/day, whereas the median intake for men ranges from 1.2 to 1.6 mg/day (Appendix Tables C-15 and D-2).

Intake from Supplements

In 1986, approximately 15 percent of adults in the United States consumed supplements that contained copper (Moss et al., 1989; see Table 2-2). Based on data from the Third National Health and Nutrition Examination Survey provided in Appendix Table C-16, the median dietary plus supplemental copper intake was similar to the intake from food alone. The mean intake of dietary and supplemental copper (1.3 to 2.2 mg/day) was approximately 0.3 to 0.5 mg/day greater for men and women than the mean intake from food (1.0 to 1.7 mg/day).

TOLERABLE UPPER INTAKE LEVELS

The Tolerable Upper Intake Level (UL) is the highest level of daily nutrient intake that is likely to pose no risk of adverse health effects for almost all individuals. Although members of the general population should be advised not to routinely exceed the UL, intake above the UL may be appropriate for investigation within well-controlled clinical trials. Clinical trials of doses above the UL should not be discouraged, as long as subjects participating in these trials have signed informed consent documents regarding possible toxicity and as long as these trials employ appropriate safety monitoring of trial subjects. In addition, the UL is not meant to apply to individuals who are receiving copper under medical supervision.

Hazard Identification

Reviews of the toxicity studies in experimental animals (ATSDR, 1990; EPA, 1987; IPCS, 1998; NRC, 1977) indicate that these studies are not useful for setting a UL for humans. Very few of these studies used chronic exposures, only one or two doses were used, and the reporting of experimental details and results was incomplete. In addition, some studies used routes of exposure that are not relevant to human intake (Toyokuni and Sagripanti, 1994). Finally, animal species vary markedly in their sensitivity to copper (Davis and Mertz, 1987); thus it is difficult to determine the most appropriate model in which to assess human toxicity to copper.

The long-term toxicity of copper is not well studied in humans, but it is rare in normal populations not having some hereditary defect in copper homeostasis (Olivares and Uauy, 1996). Copper homeostasis is affected by the interaction among zinc, copper, iron, and molybdenum. In addition, the level of dietary protein, interacting cations, and sulfate all can influence the absorption and utilization of copper (Davis and Mertz, 1987). Therefore, the derivation of a UL for copper must be made in the context of these interactions. The adverse effects associated with intake of soluble copper salts in supplements and drinking water are reviewed below.

Adverse Effects

Gastrointestinal Effects. There are data from studies of humans indicating gastrointestinal illness including abdominal pain, cramps, nausea, diarrhea, and vomiting from the consumption of beverages or drinking water containing high levels of copper (Berg and Lundh, 1981; Knobeloch et al., 1994; Olivares et al., 1998; Pizarro et al., 1999; Spitalny et al., 1984; Wylie, 1957). Many of these studies had serious experimental design weaknesses and involved very few subjects, or the copper exposures were extremely poorly characterized. Thus they are not suitable for the development of a UL.

In a survey of gastrointestinal effects resulting from high levels of copper in carbonated soft drinks, Donohue (1997) reported adverse effects at copper intakes of 4 mg/L. This concentration is equivalent to approximately 4.8 mg/day based on a mean intake of 1.2 L/day of water (Appendix Table C-27). In a double-blind study, 60 healthy Chilean women were given normal drinking water to which graded concentrations of copper sulfate had been added for 11 weeks (Pizarro et al., 1999). Although the exact threshold could not be determined, the authors reported an increased incidence of nausea and other gastrointestinal effects at copper levels greater than 3 mg/L. The mean consumption of water was 1.6 L/day, and therefore the average copper intake from water was 4.8 mg/day. From these two studies it would appear that the threshold for acute gastrointestinal effects from copper in water is about 4.8 mg/day. However, individuals may be able to adapt to even higher concentrations of copper in drinking water. No adverse gastrointestinal effects were reported in U.S. adults who consumed water containing approximately 8.5 to 8.8 mg/L of copper for over 20 years beginning in childhood (aged 0 through 5 years) (Scheinberg and Sternlieb, 1996). Based on water consumption data from the 1988–1994 Third National Health and Nutrition Examination Survey (NHANES III) (Appendix Table C-27), the mean water consumption for young children is approximately 400 mL, which would be equivalent to 3.5 mg/day of copper.

Liver Damage. Liver damage in humans is observed almost exclusively in patients with Wilson's disease and children with Indian childhood cirrhosis (ICC) and idiopathic copper toxicosis (ICT). ICC and ICT have been associated with high copper intakes. However, familial relationships and genetic factors are required for the expression of liver toxicity from high levels of copper intake (Joshi et al., 1987; Kishore and Prasad, 1993; Pandit and Bhave, 1996; Tanner, 1998). The rarity of ICT and ICC outside of Germany and India and the lack of liver damage noted in children in the United States exposed to levels of copper between 8.5 and 8.8 mg/L in drinking water support the hypothesis that copper is only one factor required for the expression of these diseases (Scheinberg and Sternlieb, 1994).

Further evidence of an underlying hereditary defect in copper homeostasis in ICC comes from Kishore and Prasad (1993). These authors found that one-third of the ICC cases examined have α-1-antitrypsin deficiency. In view of the weight of evidence supporting a genetic basis for the liver damage in Wilson's disease, ICC, and ICT, it is not appropriate to use data from such populations to develop a UL for copper in populations with normal copper homeostatic mechanisms.

Pratt and coworkers (1985) reported no evidence of liver damage or gastrointestinal effects in a double-blind study of seven subjects given 10 mg/day of copper gluconate for a period of 12 weeks. Although from a small study, these results are consistent with the safe upper level of intake of 10 to 12 mg/day of copper proposed by the World Health Organization (WHO, 1996) and the International Programme on Chemical Safety (IPCS, 1998). At higher doses, acute liver failure was reported in one subject, who had no known genetic defect in copper homeostasis, after consuming 30 mg/day of copper from supplements for 2 years, followed by 60 mg/day for an additional but unspecified period of time (O'Donohue et al., 1993).

Other Systemic Effects. Little evidence indicates that chronic exposure to copper results in systemic effects other than liver damage. No association between the level of copper intake and spontaneous abortions has been found, and data are inadequate to assess the reproductive or developmental effects of copper in humans (IPCS, 1998). Also, there is little convincing evidence that copper is causally associated with the development of cancer in humans.

Summary

On the basis of considerations of causality, relevance, and the quality and completeness of the database, liver damage was selected as the critical endpoint on which to base a UL. The selection of gastrointestinal effects as a critical endpoint was considered because of the data involving acute ingestion of soluble (highly ionized) copper salts in drinking water. However, in the United States and Canada, liver damage is a much more relevant endpoint because of the potential for excess intake from food and supplements. Furthermore, extensive evidence from studies in humans and experimental animals indicates that liver damage is the critical endpoint resulting from daily intake of high levels of copper salts (IPCS, 1998).

Dose-Response Assessment

Adults

Data Selection. The human data evaluating liver effects after chronic consumption of copper gluconate appear most relevant to setting a UL. The UL derived below does not apply to individuals at increased risk of adverse effects from excess intake of copper. These subgroups are identified under "Special Considerations."

Identification of a No-Observed-Adverse-Effect Level (NOAEL) and a Lowest-Observed-Adverse-Effect Level (LOAEL). A NOAEL of 10 mg/day of copper was identified on the basis of the results of Pratt and coworkers (1985). In a 12-week, double-blind study, 10 mg of copper as copper gluconate capsules was consumed daily by seven adults. Liver function tests were normal. From a case report, consumption of 30 mg/day as copper tablets for 2 years, followed by 60 mg/day for an additional period of time, resulted in acute liver failure (O'Donohue et al., 1993).

Uncertainty Assessment. The NOAEL of 10 mg/day was considered to be protective of the general population. Therefore, an uncertainty factor (UF) of 1.0 was selected. A larger UF was considered unnecessary in view of the large international database in humans indicating no adverse effects from daily consumption of 10 to 12 mg/day of copper in foods and the rarity of observed liver damage from copper exposures in human populations with normal copper homeostasis.

Derivation of a UL. The NOAEL of 10 mg/day was divided by the UF of 1.0 to obtain a UL of 10 mg/day (10,000 µg/day) of copper intake from food and supplements.

$$UL = \frac{NOAEL}{UF} = \frac{10 \text{ mg/day}}{1.0} = 10 \text{ mg/day}$$

Copper UL Summary, Ages 19 Years and Older

UL for Adults
≥ 19 years   **10 mg/day (10,000 µg/day) of copper**

Other Life Stage Groups

Infants. For infants, the UL was judged not determinable because of insufficient data on adverse effects in this age group and concern about the infant's ability to handle excess amounts of copper. To prevent high levels of copper intake, the only source of intake for infants should be food and formula.

Children and Adolescents. In the general, healthy population there are no reports of liver damage from copper ingestion; however, there are many reports of liver damage in children having defects in copper homeostasis. Given the dearth of information, the UL values for children and adolescents are extrapolated from those established for adults. Thus, the adult UL of 10,000 µg/day of copper was adjusted for children and adolescents on the basis of relative body weight as described in Chapter 2 using reference weights from Chapter 1 (Table 1-1). Values have been rounded down.

Pregnancy and Lactation. No studies involving supplemental copper intake by pregnant or lactating women were found. Given the dearth of information, it is recommended that the UL for pregnant and lactating females be the same as that for the nonpregnant and nonlactating females.

Copper UL Summary, Ages 0 through 18 Years, Pregnancy, Lactation

UL for Infants
0–12 months   **Not possible to establish; source of intake should be from food and formula only**

UL for Children

1–3 years	1 mg/day (1,000 μg/day) of copper
4–8 years	3 mg/day (3,000 μg/day) of copper
9–13 years	5 mg/day (5,000 μg/day) of copper

UL for Adolescents

14–18 years	8 mg/day (8,000 μg/day) of copper

UL for Pregnancy

14–18 years	8 mg/day (8,000 μg/day) of copper
19–50 years	10 mg/day (10,000 μg/day) of copper

UL for Lactation

14–18 years	8 mg/day (8,000 μg/day) of copper
19–50 years	10 mg/day (10,000 μg/day) of copper

Special Considerations

Certain subgroups may be at increased risk of adverse effects from excess intake of copper (Joshi et al., 1987; Kishore and Prasad, 1993; Pandit and Bhave, 1996; Scheinberg and Sternlieb, 1996; Tanner, 1998). These include individuals with Wilson's disease (homozygous), ICT, and ICC. In addition, heterozygotes for Wilson's disease may be at increased risk of adverse effects from excess copper intake.

Intake Assessment

Based on data from NHANES III (Appendix Table C-16), the highest median intake of copper from the diet and supplements for any gender and life stage group was about 1,700 μg/day for men aged 19 through 50 years and about 1,900 μg/day for lactating women. The highest reported intake from food and supplements at the ninety-ninth percentile was 4,700 μg/day in lactating women. The next highest reported intake at the ninety-ninth percentile was 4,600 μg/day in pregnant women and men aged 51 through 70 years.

In situations where drinking water that contains copper at the present U.S. Environmental Protection Agency (EPA) Maximum Contaminant Level Goal is consumed daily, an additional intake of 2,600 μg of copper in adults and 1,000 μg in 1- through 4-year-old children is possible. However, as reported by IPCS (1998), data from the EPA indicate 98 percent of flushed drinking water samples had copper levels of less than 460 μg/L. According to these values, most of the U.S. population receives less than 100 to 900 μg/day of copper from drinking water.

Whether total daily intakes of copper will lead to adverse health effects will depend upon the species of copper in the media of concern, its degree of ionization, and its bioavailability.

Risk Characterization

The risk of adverse effects resulting from excess intake of copper from food, water, and supplements appears to be very low in adults at the highest intakes noted above. However, copper intake data indicate that a small percentage of children aged 1 through 8 years are likely to exceed the UL for their age group. Although members of the general population should be advised not to exceed the UL routinely, intake above the UL may be appropriate for investigation within well-controlled clinical trials. Clinical trials of doses above the UL should not be discouraged, as long as subjects participating in these trials have signed informed consent documents regarding possible toxicity and as long as these trials employ appropriate safety monitoring of trial subjects. In addition, the UL is not meant to apply to individuals who are receiving copper under medical supervision.

RESEARCH RECOMMENDATIONS FOR COPPER

• Determine the specific health risks associated with marginal copper deficiency.

• Define the adverse effects of chronic high copper consumption for establishing upper intake levels and to evaluate the health effects of copper supplements.

• Determine the involvement of low and high copper intakes on neurological and cognitive function.

REFERENCES

Anderson RR. 1992. Comparison of trace elements in milk of four species. *J Dairy Sci* 75:3050–3055.

Anderson RR. 1993. Longitudinal changes of trace elements in human milk during the first 5 months of lactation. *Nutr Res* 13:499–510.

ATSDR (Agency for Toxic Substances and Disease Registry). 1990. *Toxicological Profile for Copper*. Atlanta, GA: U.S. Department of Health and Human Services, Public Health Service.

August D, Janghorbani M, Young VR. 1989. Determination of zinc and copper absorption at three dietary Zn-Cu ratios by using stable isotopic methods in young adult and elderly subjects. *Am J Clin Nutr* 50:1457–1463.

Baker A, Harvey L, Majask-Newman G, Fairweather-Tait S, Flynn A, Cashman K. 1999. Effect of dietary copper intakes on biochemical markers of bone metabolism in healthy adults. *Eur J Clin Nutr* 53:408–412.

Berg R, Lundh S. 1981. Copper contamination of drinking water as a cause of diarrhea in children. *Halsovardskontakt* 1:6–10.

Bhathena SJ, Werman MJ, Turnlund JR. 1998. Opioid peptides, adrenocorticotrophic hormone and dietary copper intake in humans. *Nutr Neurosc* 1:59–67.

Biego GH, Joyeux M, Hartemann P, Debry G. 1998. Determination of mineral contents in different kinds of milk and estimation of dietary intake in infants. *Food Addit Contam* 15:775–781.

Botash AS, Nasca J, Dubowy R, Weinberger HL, Oliphant M. 1992. Zinc-induced copper deficiency in an infant. *Am J Dis Child* 146:709–711.

Brewer GJ, Hill GM, Prasad AS, Cossack ZT, Rabbani P. 1983. Oral zinc therapy for Wilson's disease. *Ann Intern Med* 99:314–319.

Butte NF, Garza C, Smith EO, Wills C, Nichols BL. 1987. Macro- and trace-mineral intakes of exclusively breast-fed infants. *Am J Clin Nutr* 45:42–48.

Casey CE, Hambidge KM, Neville MC. 1985. Studies in human lactation: Zinc, copper, manganese and chromium in human milk in the first month of lactation. *Am J Clin Nutr* 41:1193–1200.

Casey CE, Neville MC, Hambidge KM. 1989. Studies in human lactation: Secretion of zinc, copper, and manganese in human milk. *Am J Clin Nutr* 49:773–785.

Cordano A, Baertl JM, Graham GG. 1964. Copper deficiency in infancy. *Pediatrics* 34:324–336.

Danks DM. 1988. Copper deficiency in humans. *Ann Rev Nutr* 8:235–257.

da Silva FJ, Williams RJ. 1991. Copper: Extracytoplasmic oxidases and matrix formation. In: da Silva FJ, Williams RJ, eds. *The Biological Chemistry of the Elements: The Inorganic Chemistry of Life*. Oxford: Clarendon Press. Pp. 388–399.

Davis GK, Mertz W. 1987. Copper. In: Mertz W, ed. *Trace Elements in Human and Animal Nutrition*, 5th ed. New York: Academic Press. Pp. 301–364.

Dewey KG, Lonnerdal B. 1983. Milk and nutrient intake of breast-fed infants from 1 to 6 months: Relation to growth and fatness. *J Pediatr Gastroenterol Nutr* 2:497–506.

Donohue J. 1997. New ideas after five years of the lead and copper rule: A fresh look at the MCLG for copper. In: Lagos GE, Badilla-Ohlbaum R, eds. *Advances in Risk Assessment of Copper in the Environment*. Santiago, Chile: Catholic University of Chile. Pp. 265–272.

Dorner K, Dziadzka S, Hohn A, Sievers E, Oldigs HD, Schulz-Lell G, Schaub J. 1989. Longitudinal manganese and copper balances in young infants and preterm infants fed on breast-milk and adapted cow's milk formulas. *Br J Nutr* 61:559–572.

EPA (Environmental Protection Agency). 1987. *Summary Review of the Health Effects Associated with Copper. Health Issue Assessment*. EPA/600/8-87/001. Cincinnati, OH: Environmental Criteria and Assessment Office, EPA.

Fields M, Ferretti RJ, Smith JC, Reiser S. 1984. The interaction of type of dietary carbohydrates with copper deficiency. *Am J Clin Nutr* 39:289–295.

Fransson GB, Lonnerdal B. 1983. Distribution of trace elements and minerals in human and cow's milk. *Pediatr Res* 17:912–915.

Fransson GB, Lonnerdal B. 1984. Iron, copper, zinc, calcium, and magnesium in human milk fat. *Am J Clin Nutr* 39:185–189.

Fujita M, Itakura T, Takagi Y, Okada A. 1989. Copper deficiency during total parenteral nutrition: Clinical analysis of three cases. *J Parent Enter Nutr* 13:421–425.

Graham GG, Cordano A. 1969. Copper depletion and deficiency in the malnourished infant. *Johns Hopkins Med J* 124:139–150.

Harris ED. 1997. Copper. In: O'Dell BL, Sunde RA, eds. *Handbook of Nutritionally Essential Mineral Elements*. New York: Marcel Dekker. Pp. 231–273.

Harris ZL, Gitlin JD. 1996. Genetic and molecular basis for copper toxicity. *Am J Clin Nutr* 63:836S–841S.

Haschke F, Ziegler EE, Edwards BB, Foman SJ. 1986. Effect of iron fortification of infant formula on trace mineral absorption. *J Pediatr Gastroenterol Nutr* 5:768–773.

Higashi A, Ikeda T, Uehara I, Matsuda I. 1982. Zinc and copper contents in breast milk of Japanese women. *Tohoku J Exp Med* 137:41–47.

Higuchi S, Higashi A, Nakamura T, Matsuda I. 1988. Nutritional copper deficiency in severely handicapped patients on a low copper enteral diet for a prolonged period: Estimation of the required dose of dietary copper. *J Pediatr Gastroenterol Nutr* 7:583–587.

IPCS (International Programme on Chemical Safety). 1998. *Environmental Health Criteria 200: Copper*. Geneva: World Health Organization.

Johnson PE, Canfield WK. 1989. Stable zinc and copper absorption in free-living infants fed breast milk or formula. *J Trace Elem Exp Med* 2:285–295.

Johnson MA, Fisher JG, Kays SE. 1992. Is copper an antioxidant nutrient? *Crit Rev Food Sci Nutr* 32:1–31.

Jones AA, Di Silvestro RA, Coleman M, Wagner TL. 1997. Copper supplementation of adult men: Effects on blood copper enzyme activities and indicators of cardiovascular disease risk. *Metabolism* 46:1380–1383.

Joshi RM, Kagalwala TY, Bharucha BA, Vaidya VU, Pandya AL, Parikh AP, Kumta NB. 1987. Wilson's disease (a study of 12 cases). *Indian J Gastroenterol* 6:227–228.

Kehoe CA, Turley E, Bonham MP, O'Conner JM, McKeown A, Faughnan MS, Coulter JS, Gilmore WS, Howard AN, Strain JJ. 2000. Response of putative indices of copper status to copper supplementation in human subjects. *Br J Nutr* 84:151–156.

Kelley DS, Daudu PA, Taylor PC, Mackey BE, Turnlund JR. 1995. Effects of low-copper diets on human immune response. *Am J Clin Nutr* 62:412–416.

King RL, Luick JR, Litman II, Jennings WG, Dunkley WL. 1959. Distribution of natural and added copper and iron in milk. *J Dairy Sci* 42:780–790.

Kishore N, Prasad R. 1993. A new concept: Pathogenesis of Indian childhood cirrhosis (ICC)—Hereditary alpha-I-antitrypsin deficiency. *J Trop Pediatr* 39:191–192.

Klevay LM. 1989. Ischemic heart disease as copper deficiency. *Adv Exp Med Biol* 258:197–208.

Klevay LM, Inman L, Johnson LK, Lawler M, Mahalko JR, Milne DB, Lukaski HC, Bolonchuk W, Sandstead HH. 1984. Increased cholesterol in plasma in a young man during experimental copper depletion. *Metabolism* 33:1112–1118.

Klevay LM, Canfield WK, Gallagher SK, Henriksen LK, Lukaski HC, Bolonchuk W, Johnson LK, Milne DB, Sandstead HH. 1986. Decreased glucose tolerance in two men during experimental copper depletion. *Nutr Rep Int* 33:371–382.

Knobeloch L, Ziarnik M, Howard J, Theis B, Farmer D, Anderson H, Proctor M. 1994. Gastrointestinal upsets associated with ingestion of copper-contaminated water. *Environ Health Perspect* 102:958–961.

Lentner C. 1984. *Geigy Scientific Tables. Volume 3: Physical Chemistry of Blood, Hematology, Somatometric Data.* West Caldwell, NJ: CIBA-Geigy.

Levy Y, Zeharia A, Grunebaum M, Nitzan M, Steinherz R. 1985. Copper deficiency in infants fed cow milk. *J Pediatr* 106:786–788.

Linder MC, Hazegh-Azam M. 1996. Copper biochemistry and molecular biology. *Am J Clin Nutr* 63:797S–811S.

Lipsman S, Dewey KG, Lonnerdal B. 1985. Breast-feeding among teenage mothers: Milk composition, infant growth, and maternal dietary intake. *J Pediatr Gastroenterol Nutr* 4:426–434.

Lonnerdal B, Hernell O. 1994. Iron, zinc, copper and selenium status of breast-fed infants and infants fed trace element fortified milk-based infant formula. *Acta Paediatr* 83:367–373.

Lukaski HC, Klevay LM, Milne DB. 1988. Effects of dietary copper on human autonomic cardiovascular function. *Eur J Appl Physiol* 58:74–80.

Mason KE. 1979. A conspectus of research on copper metabolism and requirements of man. *J Nutr* 109:1979–2066.

Medeiros DM, Milton A, Brunett E, Stacy L. 1991. Copper supplementation effects on indicators of copper status and serum cholesterol in adult males. *Biol Trace Elem Res* 30:19–35.

Mertz W. 1987. Use and misuse of balance studies. *J Nutr* 117:1811–1813.

Milne DB. 1994. Assessment of copper nutritional status. *Clin Chem* 40:1479–1484.

Milne DB. 1998. Copper intake and assessment of copper status. *Am J Clin Nutr* 67:1041S–1045S.

Milne DB, Nielsen FH. 1996. Effects of a diet low in copper on copper-status indicators in postmenopausal women. *Am J Clin Nutr* 63:358–364.

Milne DB, Klevay LM, Hunt JR. 1988. Effects of ascorbic acid supplements and a diet marginal in copper on indices of copper nutriture in women. *Nutr Res* 8: 865–873.

Milne DB, Nielsen FH, Lykken GI. 1991. Effects of dietary copper and sulfur amino acids on copper homeostasis and selected indices of copper status in men. *Trace Elem Man Anim* 7 7:5-12–5-13.

Morais MB, Fisberg M, Suzuki HU, Amancio OM, Machado NL.1994. Effects of oral iron therapy on serum copper and serum ceruloplasmin in children. *J Trop Pediatr* 40:51–52.

Moss AJ, Levy AS, Kim I, Park YK. 1989. *Use of Vitamin and Mineral Supplements in the United States: Current Users, Types of Products, and Nutrients.* Advance Data, Vital and Health Statistics of the National Center for Health Statistics, Number 174. Hyattsville, MD: National Center for Health Statistics.

NRC (National Research Council). 1977. *Medical and Biological Effects of Environmental Pollutants: Copper.* Washington, DC: National Academy of Sciences.

O'Donohue J, Reid MA, Varghese A, Portmann B, Williams R. 1993. Micronodular cirrhosis and acute liver failure due to chronic copper self-intoxication. *Eur J Gastroenterol Hepatol* 5:561–562.

Olivares M, Uauy R. 1996. Limits of metabolic tolerance to copper and biological basis for present recommendations and regulations. *Am J Clin Nutr* 63:846S–852S.

Olivares M, Pizarro F, Speisky H, Lonnerdal B, Uauy R. 1998. Copper in infant nutrition: Safety of World Health Organization provisional guideline value for copper content of drinking water. *J Pediatr Gastroenterol Nutr* 26:251–257.

Pandit A, Bhave S. 1996. Present interpretation of the role of copper in Indian childhood cirrhosis. *Am J Clin Nutr* 63:830S–835S.

Pena MM, Lee J, Thiele DJ. 1999. A delicate balance: Homeostatic control of copper uptake and distribution. *J Nutr* 129:1251–1260.

Pennington JA, Schoen SA, Salmon GD, Young B, Johnson RD, Marts RW. 1995. Composition of core foods of the U.S. food supply, 1982–1991. III. Copper, manganese, selenium, and iodine. *J Food Comp Anal* 8:171–217.

Picciano MF, Guthrie HA. 1976. Copper, iron, and zinc contents of mature human milk. *Am J Clin Nutr* 29:242–254.

Pizarro F, Olivares M, Uauy R, Contreras P, Rebelo A, Gidi V. 1999. Acute gastro-intestinal effects of graded levels of copper in drinking water. *Environ Health Perspect* 107:117–121.

Pratt WB, Omdahl JL, Sorenson JR. 1985. Lack of effects of copper gluconate supplementation. *Am J Clin Nutr* 42:681–682.

Prohaska JR, Tamura T, Percy AK, Turnlund JR. 1997. In vitro copper stimulation of plasma peptidylglycine α-amidating monooxygenase in Menkes disease variant with occipital horns. *Pediatr Res* 42:862–865.

Raiten DJ, Talbot JM, Walters JH. 1998. Assessment of nutrient requirements for infant formulas. *J Nutr* 128:2059S–2294S.

Reiser S, Smith JC, Mertz W, Holbrook JT, Scholfield DJ, Powell AS, Canfield WK, Canary JJ. 1985. Indices of copper status in humans consuming a typical American diet containing either fructose or starch. *Am J Clin Nutr* 42:242–251.

Rossipal E, Krachler M. 1998. Pattern of trace elements in human milk during the course of lactation. *Nutr Res* 18:11–24.

Salmenpera L, Perheentupa J, Pakarinen P, Siimes MA. 1986. Cu nutrition in infants during prolonged exclusive breast-feeding: Low intake but rising serum concentrations of Cu and ceruloplasmin. *Am J Clin Nutr* 43:251–257.

Scheinberg IH, Sternlieb I. 1994. Is non-Indian childhood cirrhosis caused by excess dietary copper? *Lancet* 344:1002–1004.

Scheinberg IH, Sternlieb I. 1996. Wilson disease and idiopathic copper toxicosis. *Am J Clin Nutr* 63:842S–845S.

Schoenemann HM, Failla ML, Steele NC. 1990. Consequences of severe copper deficiency are independent of dietary carbohydrate in young pigs. *Am J Clin Nutr* 52:147–154.

Shaw JCL. 1992. Copper deficiency in term and preterm infants. In: Fomon SJ, Zlotkin S, eds. *Nutritional Anemias*. New York: Vevey/Raven Press. Pp. 105–117.

Shike M, Roulet M, Kurian R, Whitwell J, Steward S, Jeejeebhoy KN. 1981. Copper metabolism and requirements in total parenteral nutrition. *Gastroenterology* 81:290–297.

Spitalny KC, Brondum J, Vogt RL, Sargent HE, Kappel S. 1984. Drinking-water-induced copper intoxication in a Vermont family. *Pediatrics* 74:1103–1106.

Tanner MS. 1998. Role of copper in Indian childhood cirrhosis. *Am J Clin Nutr* 67:1074S–1081S.

Toyokuni S, Sagripanti JL. 1994. Increased 8-hydroxydeoxyguanosine in kidney and liver of rats continuously exposed to copper. *Toxicol Appl Pharmacol* 126:91–97.

Turnlund JR. 1998. Human whole-body copper metabolism. *Am J Clin Nutr* 67:960S–964S.

Turnlund JR. 1999. Copper. In: Shils ME, Olson JA, Shike M, Ross AC, eds. *Modern Nutrition in Health and Disease,* 9th ed. Baltimore: Williams & Wilkins. Pp. 241–252.

Turnlund JR, Swanson CA, King JC. 1983. Copper absorption and retention in pregnant women fed diets based on animal and plant proteins. *J Nutr* 113:2346–2352.

Turnlund JR, Keyes WR, Anderson HL, Acord LL. 1989. Copper absorption and retention in young men at three levels of dietary copper by use of the stable isotope ^{65}Cu. *Am J Clin Nutr* 49:870–878.

Turnlund JR, Keen CL, Smith RG. 1990. Copper status and urinary and salivary copper in young men at three levels of dietary copper. *Am J Clin Nutr* 51:658–664.

Turnlund JR, Scott KC, Peiffer GL, Jang AM, Keyes WR, Keen CL, Sakanashi TM. 1997. Copper status of young men consuming a low-copper diet. *Am J Clin Nutr* 65:72–78.

Turnlund JR, Keyes WR, Peiffer GL, Scott KC. 1998. Copper absorption, excretion, and retention by young men consuming low dietary copper determined by using the stable isotope ^{65}Cu. *Am J Clin Nutr* 67:1219–1225.

Uauy R, Castillo-Duran C, Fisberg M, Fernandez N, Valenzuela A. 1985. Red cell superoxide dismutase activity as an index of human copper nutrition. *J Nutr* 115:1650–1655.

Vaughan LA, Weber CW, Kemberling SR. 1979. Longitudinal changes in the mineral content of human milk. *Am J Clin Nutr* 32:2301–2306.

Vulpe CD, Kuo YM, Murphy TL, Cowley L, Askwith C, Libina N, Gitschier J, Anderson GJ. 1999. Hephaestin, a ceruloplasmin homologue implicated in intestinal iron transport, is defective in the sla mouse. *Nat Genet* 21:195–199.

Vuori E, Kuitunen P. 1979. The concentrations of copper and zinc in human milk. A longitudinal study. *Acta Paediatr Scand* 68:33–37.

Vuori E, Makinen SM, Kara R, Kuitunen P. 1980. The effects of the dietary intakes of copper, iron, manganese, and zinc on the trace element content of human milk. *Am J Clin Nutr* 33:227–231.

Werman MJ, Bhathena SJ, Turnlund JR. 1997. Dietary copper intake influences skin lysyl oxidase in young men. *J Nutr Biochem* 8:201–204.

WHO (World Health Organization). 1996. Copper. In: *Trace Elements in Human Nutrition and Health.* Geneva: WHO. Pp. 123–143.

Widdowson EM, Dickerson JWT. 1964. Chemical composition of the body. In: Comar CL, Bronner F, eds. *Mineral Metabolism: An Advanced Treatise,* Vol. II, Part A. New York: Academic Press. Pp. 1–248.

Wylie J. 1957. Copper poisoning at a cocktail party. *Am J Public Health* 47:617.

Yuzbasiyan-Gurkan V, Grider A, Nostrant T, Cousins RJ, Brewer GJ. 1992. Treatment of Wilson's disease with zinc: X. Intestinal metallothionein induction. *J Lab Clin Med* 120:380–386.

8

Iodine

SUMMARY

Iodine is an essential component of the thyroid hormones that are involved in the regulation of various enzymes and metabolic processes. Thyroid iodine accumulation and turnover were used to set the Estimated Average Requirement. The Recommended Dietary Allowance (RDA) for adult men and women is 150 µg/day. The median intake of iodine from food in the United States is approximately 240 to 300 µg/day for men and 190 to 210 µg/day for women. The Tolerable Upper Intake Level (UL) for adults is 1,100 µg/day (1.1 mg/day), a value based on serum thyroptropin concentration in response to varying levels of ingested iodine.

BACKGROUND INFORMATION

Function

Iodine is an essential component of the thyroid hormones, thyroxine (T4) and triiodothyronine (T3), comprising 65 and 59 percent of their respective weights. Thyroid hormones, and therefore iodine, are essential for mammalian life. They regulate many key biochemical reactions, especially protein synthesis and enzymatic activity. Major target organs are the developing brain, muscle, heart, pituitary, and kidney.

Observations in several areas have suggested possible additional roles for iodine. Iodine may have beneficial roles in mammary dysplasia and fibrocystic breast disease (Eskin, 1977; Ghent et al., 1993). In vitro studies show that iodine can work with myeloperoxidase from white cells to inactivate bacteria (Klebanoff, 1967). Other brief reports have suggested that inadequate iodine nutrition impairs immune response and may be associated with an increased incidence of gastric cancer (Venturi et al., 1993). While these other possibilities deserve further investigation, the overwhelming importance of nutritional iodine is as a component of the thyroid hormones.

Physiology of Absorption, Metabolism, and Excretion

Iodine is ingested in a variety of chemical forms. Most ingested iodine is reduced in the gut and absorbed almost completely (Nath et al., 1992). Some iodine-containing compounds (e.g., thyroid hormones and amiodarone) are absorbed intact. The metabolic pathway of iodinated radiocontrast media, such as Lipiodol, is not entirely clear. The oral administration of Lipiodol increases the iodine stores of the organism and has been successfully used in the correction of iodine deficiency (Benmiloud et al., 1994). Iodate, widely used in many countries as an additive to salt, is rapidly reduced to iodide and completely absorbed.

Once in the circulation, iodide is removed principally by the thyroid gland and the kidney. The thyroid selectively concentrates iodide in amounts required for adequate thyroid hormone synthesis, and most of the remaining iodine is excreted in urine. Several other tissues can also concentrate iodine, including salivary glands, breast, choroid plexus, and gastric mucosa. Other than the lactating breast, these are minor pathways of uncertain significance.

A sodium/iodide transporter in the thyroidal basal membrane is responsible for iodine concentration. It transfers iodide from the circulation into the thyroid gland at a concentration gradient of about 20 to 50 times that of the plasma to ensure that the thyroid gland obtains adequate amounts of iodine for hormone synthesis. During iodine deficiency, the thyroid gland concentrates a majority of the iodine available from the plasma (Wayne et al., 1964).

Iodide in the thyroid gland participates in a complex series of reactions to produce thyroid hormones. Thyroglobulin, a large glycoprotein of molecular weight 660,000, is synthesized within the thyroid cell and serves as a vehicle for iodination. Iodide and thyroglobulin meet at the apical surface of the thyroid cell. There thyroperoxidase and hydrogen peroxide promote the oxidation of the iodide and its simultaneous attachment to tyrosyl residues within the thyroglobulin molecule to produce the hormone precursors diiodotyrosine and monoiodotyrosine. Thyroperoxidase further catalyzes the intramolecular coupling of two molecules of diiodotyrosine to produce tetraiodothyronine (T_4). A similar coupling of one monoiodotyrosine and one diiodotyrosine molecule produces triiodothyronine (T_3). Mature iodinated thyroglobulin is stored extracellularly in the lumen of thyroid follicles, each consisting of a central space rimmed by the apical membranes of thyrocytes. Typically, thyroglobulin contains from 0.1 to 1.0 percent of its weight as iodine. About one-third of its iodine is in the form of thyroid hormone, the rest as the precursors. An average adult thyroid in an iodine-sufficient geographic region contains about 15 mg iodine (Fisher and Oddie, 1969b).

Thyroglobulin, which contains the thyroid hormones, is stored in the follicular lumen until needed. Then endosomal and lysosomal proteases digest thyroglobulin and release the hormones into the circulation. About two-thirds of thyroglobulin's iodine is in the form of the inactive precursors, monoiodotyrosine and diiodotyrosine. This iodine is not released into the circulation, but instead is removed from the tyrosine moiety by a specific deiodinase and then recycled within the thyroid gland. This process is an important mechanism for iodine conservation, and individuals with impaired or genetically absent deiodinase activity risk iodine deficiency.

Once in the circulation, T_4 and T_3 rapidly attach to several binding proteins synthesized in the liver, including thyroxine-binding globulin, transthyretin, and albumin. The bound hormone then migrates to target tissues where T_4 is deiodinated to T_3, the metabolically active form. The responsible deiodinase contains selenium, and selenium deficiency may impair T_4 conversion and hormone action. The iodine of T_4 returns to the serum iodine pool and follows again the cycle of iodine or is excreted in the urine.

Thyrotropin (TSH) is the major regulator of thyroid function. The pituitary secretes this protein hormone (molecular weight about 28,000) in response to circulating concentrations of thyroid hormone, with TSH secretion increasing when circulating thyroid hormone decreases. TSH affects several sites within the thyrocyte, the principal actions being to increase thyroidal uptake of iodine and to break down thyroglobulin in order to release thyroid hormone into the circulation. An elevated serum TSH concentration indicates primary hypothyroidism, and a decreased TSH concentration shows hyperthyroidism.

The urine contains the fraction of the serum iodine pool that is not concentrated by the thyroid gland. Typically, urine contains more than 90 percent of all ingested iodine (Nath et al., 1992). Most of the remainder is excreted in feces. A small amount may be in sweat.

Clinical Effects of Inadequate Intake

The so-called iodine deficiency disorders (IDD) include mental retardation, hypothyroidism, goiter, cretinism, and varying degrees of other growth and developmental abnormalities. These result from inadequate thyroid hormone production from lack of sufficient iodine. Most countries in the world currently have some degree of iodine deficiency, including some industrialized countries in Western Europe (Stanbury et al., 1998). Iodine deficiency was a significant problem in the United States and Canada, particularly in the interior, the Great Lakes region, and the Pacific Northwest, during the early part of the 20th century (Trowbridge et al., 1975). The Third National Nutrition and Health Examination Survey study of samples collected from 1988 to 1994 showed a median urinary iodine excretion of 145 μg/L, well above the lower level considered to reflect adequate intake (100 μg/L) (WHO Nutrition Unit, 1994), but this is a decrease from the value of 321 μg/L found in a similar survey in the 1970s (Hollowell et al., 1998). Estimated iodine intakes for Canadians are in excess of 1 mg/day (Fischer and Giroux, 1987). Both countries iodize salt with potassium iodide at 100 ppm (76 mg iodine/kg salt). Iodized salt is mandatory in Canada and used optionally by about 50 percent of the U.S. population.

The most damaging effect of iodine deficiency is on the developing brain. Thyroid hormone is particularly important for myelination of the central nervous system, which is most active in the perinatal period and during fetal and early postnatal development. Numerous population studies have correlated an iodine-deficient diet with increased incidence of mental retardation. A meta-analysis of 18 studies concluded that iodine deficiency alone lowered mean IQ scores by 13.5 points (Bleichrodt and Born, 1994).

The effects of iodine deficiency on brain development are similar to those of hypothyroidism from any other cause. The United States, Canada, and most developed countries have routine screening of all neonates by blood spot for TSH or T_4 to detect among iodine-sufficient children the approximately one in 4,000 who will be hypothyroid, usually from thyroid aplasia. Iodine treatment can reverse cretinism especially when the treatment is begun early (Klein et al., 1972).

Cretinism is an extreme form of neurological damage from fetal hypothyroidism. It occurs in severe iodine deficiency and is characterized by gross mental retardation along with varying degrees of short stature, deaf mutism, and spasticity. As many as one in ten of some populations with very severe iodine deficiency may be cretins. Correction of iodine deficiency in Switzerland completely eliminated the appearance of new cases of cretinism, and a similar experience has occurred in other countries (Stanbury et al., 1998).

Thyroid enlargement (goiter) is usually the earliest clinical feature of iodine deficiency. It reflects an attempt to adapt the thyroid to the increased need, brought on by iodine deficiency, to produce thyroid hormones. Initially, goiters are diffuse but become nodular over time. In later stages they may be associated with hyperthyroidism from autonomous nodules or with thyroid follicular cancer. Goiter can be assessed approximately by palpation and more precisely by field ultrasonography. The International Council for the Control of Iodine Deficiency Disorders (WHO/UNICEF/ICCIDD, 1993) and the World Health Organization (WHO Nutrition Unit, 1994) have recommended surveying schoolchildren for thyroid size as one of the most practical indicators of iodine deficiency, and many reports on iodine nutrition are based primarily on such goiter surveys.

Other consequences of iodine deficiency are impaired reproductive outcome, increased childhood mortality, decreased educability, and economic stagnation. Major international efforts have produced dramatic improvements in the correction of iodine deficiency in the 1990s, mainly through use of iodized salt in iodine-deficient countries.

SELECTION OF INDICATORS FOR ESTIMATING THE REQUIREMENT FOR IODINE

Iodine Accumulation and Turnover

The normal thyroid gland takes up the amount of circulating iodine necessary to make the proper amount of thyroid hormone for the body's needs. The affinity of the thyroid gland for iodine is estimated by the fraction of an orally administered dose of radioactive iodine (^{123}I, ^{131}I) that is concentrated in the thyroid gland (Wayne et al., 1964). The thyroid gland concentrates more radioactive iodine in iodine deficiency and less in iodine excess. Thus, values for euthyroid individuals in Western Europe, where some iodine deficiency exists, are higher than in the iodine-sufficient United States and Canada, where typical values are in the range of 5 to 20 percent at 24 hours. Other factors can influence the radioactive iodine uptake, including thyroidal overproduction of hormone (hyperthyroidism), hypothyroidism, subacute thyroiditis, and many chemical and medicinal products. Assuming iodine equilibrium, the mean daily thyroid iodine accumulation and release are similar. Thus, the average daily uptake and release (turnover) of iodine in the body can be used to estimate the average requirement of iodine, provided that the subjects tested have adequate iodine status and are euthyroid.

Such turnover studies have been conducted in euthyroid adults in the United States (Fisher and Oddie, 1969a, 1969b; Oddie et al., 1964). Turnover studies are based on the intravenous administration of ^{131}I and the calculation of thyroid iodine accumulation from measurements of thyroidal and renal radioiodine clearances, urinary iodine excretion, and fractional thyroidal release rate.

Urinary Iodine

Over 90 percent of dietary iodine eventually appears in the urine (Nath et al., 1992; Vought and London, 1967). Data on urinary iodine excretion are variously expressed as a concentration ($\mu g/L$), in relationship to creatinine excretion (μg iodine/g creatinine), or as 24-hour urine collections ($\mu g/day$). Most studies have used the concentration in casual samples because of the obvious ease of collection. In populations with adequate general nutrition, urinary iodine concentration correlates well with the urine iodine/creatinine ratio. Urinary iodine excretion is recommended by the World Health Organization, the International Council for the Control of Iodine Deficiency Disorders, and the United Nations Children's Fund (WHO Nutrition Unit, 1994) for assessing iodine nutrition worldwide.

In the Third National Health and Nutrition Examination Survey (NHANES III), the urinary iodine concentration ($\mu g/L$) was 1.16 times the urinary iodine excretion expressed as $\mu g/g$ creatinine (Hollowell et al., 1998). In NHANES I, this ratio was 1.09. Some population groups, particularly those with compromised general nutrition, have low creatinine excretion; therefore the urinary iodine to creatinine ratio is misleading (Bourdoux, 1998). The concentration of iodine in 24-hour urine samples correlates well with that in casual samples (Bourdoux, 1998). Information from NHANES III on urinary iodine excretion is provided in Appendix Table G-6. The median urinary iodine excretion was 1.38 to 1.55

μg/L for men and 1.1 to 1.29 μg/L for women. Data are not available on 24-hour urinary excretion of iodine.

Daily iodine intake can be extrapolated from urinary concentration as follows. The median 24-hour urine volume for ages 7 through 15 years is approximately 0.9 mL/hr/kg (or 0.0009 L/hr/kg) (Mattsson and Lindstrom, 1995). The 24-hour urine volume for adults is approximately 1.5 L (Larsson and Victor, 1988), a value in general agreement with an extrapolation of the calculation for children and adolescents. Urine volume among individuals and over time can vary considerably, but these numbers for daily volume appear reasonable for population estimates.

From the above information and assuming an average bioavailability of 92 percent, the daily iodine intake is calculated from urinary iodine concentration by the following formula:

$$\text{Urinary iodine (μg/L)} \div 0.92 \times (0.0009 \text{ L/h/kg} \times 24 \text{ h/d}) \times \text{wt (kg)} = \text{daily iodine intake;}$$

or simplified,

$$\text{Urinary iodine (μg/L)} \times 0.0235 \times \text{wt (kg)} = \text{daily iodine intake.}$$

As an example, urinary iodine excretion of 100 μg/L in a 57-kg girl would indicate a daily iodine intake of 134 μg.

Simple methods for measuring urinary iodine exist (Dunn et al., 1993). Casual samples are easy to collect and have been the mainstay for biological monitoring in global studies of iodine nutrition. The urinary iodine concentration reflects very recent iodine nutrition (days) in contrast to indicators such as thyroid size and serum thyroid stimulating hormone (TSH) and thyroglobulin concentrations.

Thyroid Size

The size of the thyroid gland increases in response to iodine deficiency, mediated at least in part by increased serum TSH concentration. This earliest clinical response to impaired iodine nutrition reflects an adaptation to the threat of hypothyroidism. Excess iodine can also produce goiter because large amounts inhibit intrathyroidal hormone production, again leading to increased TSH stimulation and thyroid growth. Traditionally, goiter was assessed by neck palpation with each lobe of the normal thyroid being regarded as no larger than the terminal phalanx of the subject's thumb. Thyroid size is recommended by WHO/UNICEF/ICCIDD (WHO Nutrition Unit, 1994) for assessing iodine nutrition worldwide. The WHO/UNICEF/ICCIDD classification (WHO Nutrition Unit, 1994) describes grade 1 goiter as palpable but not visible with the neck extended and grade 2 as visible with the neck in the normal position.

Ultrasonography defines thyroid size much more precisely and reliably. The technology—safe, practical, and easily performed in the field—is replacing palpation in most studies. Reference values related to body surface area and to age exist for iodine-sufficient children in the United States (Xu et al., 1999), in Europe (Delange et al., 1993), and in some other countries. Most data come from surveys in school-age children, who are easily available and whose thyroids reflect recent iodine nutrition. Individuals may continue to have thyroid enlargement permanently, even after iodine deficiency has been corrected (Delange and Burgi, 1989; Jooste et al., 2000).

Iodine Balance

Several attempts at iodine balance studies were published in the 1960s (Dworkin et al., 1966; Harrison, 1968; Harrison et al., 1965; Malamos et al., 1967; Vought and London, 1967). Because most iodine in the body is concentrated in the thyroid gland, the ability to determine balance within a short time is more realistic than for most other trace elements. But, as for many trace elements, there are serious limitations for deriving a daily iodine requirement based on balance studies. One limitation is that the baseline iodine intake at the study site and the long-range iodine intake of the subjects before the studies were likely different from current conditions in the United States. This applies particularly to the study of Harrison and coworkers (1965). Second, iodine balance is complicated by the need to consider the thyroidal compartment in addition to iodine intake and excretion (Dworkin et al., 1966). Thus, even in prolonged studies of several months, equilibrium is not clearly established, and in fact negative iodine balance has been reported (Dworkin et al., 1966). Third, techniques for assessment were crude by today's standards and key indicators, such as serum TSH, were not available. A fourth limitation is that while studies such as these try to control intake, iodine appears in many unidentified or unrecognized substances that are ingested; therefore control of iodine intake in these studies would have been limited. Despite the limitations of balance studies, data from them were used for estimating the average requirement for iodine in children.

Serum Thyroid Stimulating Hormone Concentration

Because serum TSH concentration responds to circulating levels of thyroid hormone, which in turn reflect adequate production of thyroid hormone, it is an excellent indicator of altered thyroid function in individuals. Sensitive assays have been widely available for about two decades, and serum TSH concentration is now the preferred test for assessing thyroid function in individuals. It is also used on blood spots by filter paper methodology in most countries for the routine screening of neonates to detect congenital hypothyroidism (WHO Nutrition Unit, 1994). The normal serum TSH concentration range in most assays is approximately 0.5 to 6.0 mU/L, although each individual assay system needs to be standardized for euthyroid subjects. Studies of groups with differing iodine intakes, as reflected in urinary iodine concentrations, show different mean serum TSH concentrations, although they may remain within the normal range. The sensitivity of TSH can be enhanced by previous stimulation with TSH-releasing hormone (TRH) (Jackson, 1982). The latter is a hypothalamic tripeptide that stimulates release of TSH and prolactin. It is used clinically for individuals with borderline or confusing static TSH measurements; an exaggerated response to TRH suggests the threat of inadequate thyroid hormone availability and hypothyroidism. Several studies have shown that the mean serum TSH concentration and its response to TRH are increased in iodine deficiency, although absolute values may remain within the normal range (Benmiloud et al., 1994; Buchinger et al., 1997; Emrich et al., 1982; Moulopoulos et al., 1988).

Serum Thyroglobulin Concentration

Although principally an intrathyroidal and follicular resident, some thyroglobulin (Tg) is normally secreted into the circulation and is detectable by standardized commercially available immunoassays. The largest clinical use of the serum Tg concentration is in detecting metastases of differentiated thyroid cancer, but it is typically elevated in thyroidal hyperplasia from any cause, including the endemic goiter of iodine deficiency. Many studies have shown a correlation between serum Tg concentration and degree of iodine deficiency as shown by urinary iodine excretion or other parameters (Benmiloud et al., 1994; Gutekunst et al., 1986). It is applicable to blood spot filter paper technology (Missler et al., 1994). Individuals with adequate iodine intake have a median serum Tg concentration of 10 ng/mL (WHO Nutrition Unit, 1994; WHO/UNICEF/ICCIDD,

1993). There are insufficient dose-response data on dietary iodine intake and serum Tg concentrations to estimate iodine requirements.

Thyroxine and Triiodothyronine Concentration

Assays for both thyroxine (T_4) and triiodothyronine (T_3) concentrations are standard clinical tools for measuring thyroid function, although they are not as sensitive as TSH. In iodine deficiency, serum T_4 concentration is decreased and serum T_3 concentration is normal or increased, relative to iodine-sufficient controls. This increased T_3 concentration is an adaptive response of the thyroid to iodine deficiency. Fasting and malnutrition are associated with low T_3 concentrations (Croxson et al., 1977; Gardner et al., 1979). However, most changes take place within the normal range, and the overlap with the iodine-sufficient normal population is large enough to make this a relatively insensitive and unreliable means for assessing iodine nutrition.

FACTORS AFFECTING THE IODINE REQUIREMENT

Bioavailability

Under normal conditions, the absorption of dietary iodine is greater than 90 percent (Albert and Keating, 1949; Nath et al., 1992; Vought and London, 1967). The fate of organic compounds of iodine in the intestine is different from that of iodine. When thyroxine is orally administered, the bioavailability is approximately 75 percent (Hays, 1991).

Soya flour has been shown to inhibit iodine absorption (Pinchera et al., 1965), and goiter and hypothyroidism were reported in several infants consuming infant formula containing soya flour (Shepard et al., 1960). If iodine was added to this formula, goiter did not appear.

Goitrogens

Some foods contain goitrogens, that is, substances that interfere with thyroid hormone production or utilization (Gaitan, 1989). Examples include cassava, which may contain linamarin and is metabolized to thiocyanate which in turn can block thyroidal uptake of iodine; millet, some species of which contain goitrogenic substances; water, particularly from shallow or polluted streams and wells, which may contain humic substances that block thyroidal iodination; and crucifera vegetables (e.g., cabbage). Most of these substances are not of major clinical importance unless there is coexisting iodine deficiency. Deficiencies of vitamin A, selenium, or iron can each exacerbate the effects of iodine deficiency.

Other Factors

Many ingested substances contain large amounts of iodine that can interfere with proper thyroid function. These include radio-contrast media, food coloring, certain medicines (e.g., amiodarone), water purification tablets, and skin and dental disinfectants. Erythrosine is a coloring agent widely used in foods, cosmetics, and pharmaceutical products, and contains high amounts of iodine. Data suggest that the increased thyroid stimulating hormone levels found following erythrosine ingestion is related to antithyroid effects of increased serum iodide concentrations, rather than a direct effect of erythrosine on thyroid hormones (Gardner et al., 1987). Similar to erythrosine, amiodarone, a highly effective antiarrhythmic drug that contains high levels of iodine, may alter thyroid gland function (Loh, 2000). Radiographic contrast media, following intravascular administration, results in the formation of iodinated serum proteins, which alter thyroid metabolism (Nilsson et al., 1987).

FINDINGS BY LIFE STAGE AND GENDER GROUP

Infants Ages 0 through 12 Months

Method Used to Set the Adequate Intake

No functional criteria of iodine status have been demonstrated that reflect response to dietary intake in infants. Thus, recommended intakes of iodine are based on an Adequate Intake (AI) that reflects the observed mean iodine intake of infants exclusively fed human milk.

Ages 0 through 6 Months. An AI is used as the recommended intake level for infants as determined by the method described in Chapter 2. The AI reflects the observed mean iodine intake of infants fed human milk. Iodine concentrations in human milk are influenced by maternal iodine intake (Gushurst et al., 1984). The median iodine concentration in human milk of American women who consumed noniodized salt was 113 µg/L, whereas the concentration in breast milk of women who consumed low or high amounts of iodized salt was 143 or 270 µg/L, respectively (Gushurst et al., 1984), and within the range observed by Etling and coworkers (1986) and Johnson and coworkers (1990) (Table 8-1). The median concentration of iodine in human milk for all women was 146 µg/L for 14 days to 3.5 years postpartum. Based on an average milk excretion of 0.78 L/day (Chapter 2) and an average concentration of 146 µg/L, the mean amount of iodine secreted in human milk is 114 µg/day.

Iodine balance studies by Delange and coworkers (1984) showed that for full-term infants, aged 1 month and fed 20 µg/kg/day of iodine, total excretion was 12.7 µg/kg/day and iodine retention was 7.3 µg/kg/day. Thus, if the mean body weight at 6 months is 7 kg, then the infant in positive iodine balance excretes 90 µg/day.

Based on the median intake of iodine consumed from human milk and the average urinary iodine excretion of the infant, the AI for infants ages 0 through 6 months has been set at 110 µg/day.

Ages 7 though 12 Months. The AI for infants ages 7 through 12 months is 130 µg/day as determined by the method described in Chapter 2 to extrapolate from the younger infants. The AI for infants is greater than the Recommended Dietary Allowances (RDAs) for children and adolescents because the latter are based on extrapolation of adult data or on balance data for a specific age group (see "Children and Adolescents Ages 1 through 18 Years").

TABLE 8-1 Iodine Concentration in Human Milk

Reference	Study Group	Stage of Lactation	Milk Iodine Concentration (µg/L)	Estimated Iodine Intakes of Infants (µg/d)[a]
Gushurst et al., 1984	24 women, 21–36 y	14 d–3.5 y	146	114
Etling et al., 1986	23 women, < 34 y		59	46
Johnson et al., 1990	14 women	< 2 mo	247	192
			98	76

NOTE: Maternal intakes were not reported in these studies.

[a] Iodine intake based on reported data or concentration (µg/L) × 0.78 L/day.

Iodine AI Summary, Ages 0 through 12 months

AI for Infants
    0–6 months   **110 µg/day of iodine**
    7–12 months   **130 µg/day of iodine**

Special Considerations

The iodine content in cow milk is dependent on the amount of iodine consumed by the animal (Swanson et al., 1990). As a result, the amount of iodine in cow milk increased by 300 to 500 percent from 1965 to 1980, partly because of the addition of organic iodine to animal feed (Hemken, 1980). There have been no studies in which the bioavailability of iodine in infant formulas and human milk have been compared.

Children and Adolescents Ages 1 through 18 Years

Evidence Considered in Estimating the Average Requirement

Ages 1 through 3 Years. A 4-day balance study was conducted by Ingenbleek and Malvaux (1974) on children aged 1.5 to 2.5 years who were previously malnourished and then nutritionally rehabilitated. The median iodine intake of the seven rehabilitated children was 63.5 µg/day, and the average iodine balance was +19 µg/day. The coefficient of variation (CV) was approximately 20 percent. No other studies assessing iodine requirements for this age group have been conducted. If the Estimated Average Requirement (EAR) for adults is extrapolated down on the basis of body weight (see Chapter 2), the EAR would be 36 µg/day. However, because an average intake of 63.5 µg/day resulted in a positive iodine balance, an EAR of 65 µg/day is set.

Ages 4 through 8 Years. Children 8 years of age who consumed 20 to 40 µg/day of iodine were in negative iodine balance (−23 to −26 µg/day) (Malvaux et al., 1969), indicating that the average minimum requirement is approximately 65 µg/day (40 + 26). If the EAR for adults is extrapolated down on the basis of body weight (see Chapter 2), the EAR would be 47 µg/day. No other studies for assessing iodine requirements for this age group have been conducted; therefore an EAR of 65 µg/day is set, using the higher estimate.

Ages 9 through 13 Years. The prevalence of goiter was estimated in European boys and girls aged 6 to 15 years (Delange et al., 1997). Goiter prevalence in a population increases inversely with iodine intake. Because iodine deficiency is rare in the United States, data from Europe are used to relate goiter, as determined by ultrasound, to urinary iodine excretion. As urinary iodine excretion increases, the goiter prevalence decreases and eventually changes only slightly (Figure 8-1). Although data from this figure are not available for estimating a 50 percent prevalence of goiter, the level of urinary iodine concentration at which there is only a 2 percent prevalence

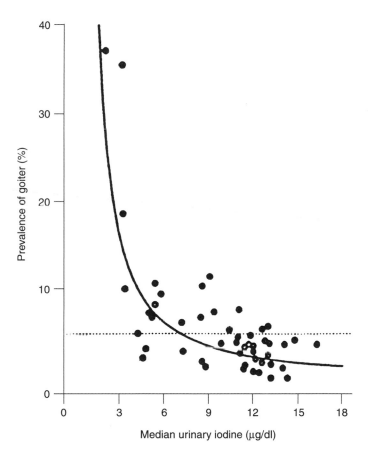

FIGURE 8-1 Inverse relationship between median urinary iodine concentrations and the prevalence of goiter in schoolchildren. The dotted line represents the upper limit of the prevalence of goiter (WHO Nutrition Unit, 1994). Adapted from Delange et al. (1997).

of goiter is approximately 100 µg/L. This approach can be used for estimating the RDA because it estimates the requirement for approximately 98 percent of the population. As described earlier, the daily iodine intake can be estimated from the urinary iodine concentration as follows:

1. Median urine volume is 1.2 mL/hour/kg for a 10-year-old child (the median excretion rate for all children aged 7 to 15 years was 0.9 mL/hour/kg) (Mattsson and Lindstrom, 1995) and the median weight is 40 kg (Chapter 1); therefore the urine volume is about 1.15 L/day (1.2 × 40 × 24 hr).

2. Approximately 92 percent of dietary iodine is excreted in the urine (Nath et al., 1992; Vought and London, 1967).

3. Therefore, for a 10-year-old child weighing 40 kg, the urinary iodine concentration of 100 µg/L approximates a daily iodine intake of 125 µg (1.15 ÷ 0.92 × 100). This value suggests an RDA of approximately 125 µg/day.

Malvaux and coworkers (1969) conducted a balance study on 16 boys and girls (aged 9 to 13 years) in Belgium. The average iodine intake was 31 µg/day, and the average balance was –24 µg/day. This finding would suggest a minimum average requirement of approximately 55 µg/day (31 + 24).

The iodine requirement has not been determined based on energy expenditure; however, the thyroid hormones, which contain iodine, are involved with metabolic rate. Therefore, the EAR is extrapolated from adults by using metabolic body weight ($kg^{0.75}$) and the method described in Chapter 2 to set an EAR at 73 µg/day.

Ages 14 through 18 Years. Malvaux and colleagues (1969) reported that the average iodine balance of 10 children (aged 14 to 16 years) was –24 µg/day when they consumed an average 34 µg/day of iodine, which would give 58 µg/day as an average requirement. No other data are available for estimating an average requirement for this age group. However, extrapolating down from adult data as described in Chapter 2 and using metabolic weight gives an EAR of 95 µg/day, which is used to set the RDA as it is a higher estimate.

Iodine EAR and RDA Summary, Ages 1 through 18 Years

EAR for Children

1–3 years	**65 µg/day of iodine**
4–8 years	**65 µg/day of iodine**

EAR for Boys
9–13 years	73 µg/day of iodine
14–18 years	95 µg/day of iodine

EAR for Girls
9–13 years	73 µg/day of iodine
14–18 years	95 µg/day of iodine

The RDA for iodine is set by using a CV of 20 percent (see "Adults Ages 19 Years and Older"). The RDA is defined as equal to the EAR plus twice the CV to cover the needs of 97 to 98 percent of the individuals in the group (therefore, for iodine the RDA is 140 percent of the EAR). The calculated values for RDAs have been rounded, and are in the range of 125 µg/day for a 10-year-old child as presented on the previous page.

RDA for Children
1–3 years	90 µg/day of iodine
4–8 years	90 µg/day of iodine

RDA for Boys
9–13 years	120 µg/day of iodine
14–18 years	150 µg/day of iodine

RDA for Girls
9–13 years	120 µg/day of iodine
14–18 years	150 µg/day of iodine

Adults Ages 19 Years and Older

Evidence Considered in Estimating the Average Requirement

Thyroid Iodine Accumulation and Turnover. Thyroidal radioiodine accumulation is used to estimate the average requirement. Turnover studies have been conducted in euthyroid adults (Fisher and Oddie, 1969a, 1969b). In one of these studies, the average accumulation of radioiodine by the thyroid gland for 18 men and women aged 21 to 48 years was 96.5 µg/day (Fisher and Oddie, 1969a). The second study involved 274 euthyroid subjects from Arkansas. The calculated uptake and turnover was 91.2 µg/day (Fisher and Oddie, 1969b). The accumulation of radioidine by the thyroid gland correlated well with urinary radioidine excretion. DeGroot (1966) measured iodine turnover in four normal subjects by three methods:

absolute iodine uptake (21 to 97 µg/day) determined by using the method of Riggs (1952), thyroid hormone secretion (69 to 171 µg/day) determined by using the method of Berson and Yalow (1954), and thyroid hormone secretion (49 to 147 µg/day) determined by using the method of Ermans and coworkers (1963). There is no evidence to suggest that the average iodine requirement is altered with aging, or to have differences based on gender in adults.

Supporting Data. Other considerations support an EAR in the general range of 95 µg/day for adults (Delange, 1993; Dunn et al., 1998). A study by Vought and London (1967) demonstrated that the obligatory amount of iodine excreted was 57 µg/day. Despite the methodologic limitations of balance studies, when 100 µg/day of iodine was provided to 13 subjects, an average slight positive balance (13 µg) was observed (Harrison, 1968). In a study of five pregnant and four nonpregnant women, balance was calculated at about 160 µg/day (Dworkin et al., 1966). Given this higher estimate in women, adjusting for smaller body weight in women was not justified.

Iodine EAR and RDA Summary, Ages 19 Years and Older

EAR for Men
19–30 years	**95 µg/day of iodine**
31–50 years	**95 µg/day of iodine**
50–70 years	**95 µg/day of iodine**
> 70 years	**95 µg/day of iodine**

EAR for Women
19–30 years	**95 µg/day of iodine**
31–50 years	**95 µg/day of iodine**
50–70 years	**95 µg/day of iodine**
> 70 years	**95 µg/day of iodine**

The CV was calculated to be 40 percent by using the data of Fisher and Oddie (1969a). Part of this variation is due to the complexity of the experimental design and calculations used to estimate turnover. Assuming that half of the variation is due to experimental design, a CV of 20 percent, rather than 10 percent based on energy (see Chapter 1), is used to set the RDA. The RDA is defined as equal to the EAR plus twice the CV to cover the needs of 97 to 98 percent of the individuals in the group (therefore, for iodine the RDA is 140 percent of the EAR). The calculated values for RDAs were rounded to the nearest 50 µg.

RDA for Men
19–30 years	150 µg/day of iodine
31–50 years	150 µg/day of iodine
50–70 years	150 µg/day of iodine
> 70 years	150 µg/day of iodine

RDA for Women
19–30 years	150 µg/day of iodine
31–50 years	150 µg/day of iodine
50–70 years	150 µg/day of iodine
> 70 years	150 µg/day of iodine

Pregnancy

Evidence Considered in Estimating the Average Requirement

Thyroid Iodine Content of the Newborn. The daily accumulation of iodine by the newborn can be used to estimate the daily fetal iodine uptake. It is estimated that the average iodine content of the newborn thyroid gland is 50 to 100 µg with close to 100 percent being turned over daily (Delange, 1989; Delange and Ermans, 1991). An estimated daily thyroid iodine uptake of approximately 75 µg/day by the fetus and an EAR of 95 µg/day for nonpregnant women would yield an EAR of 170 µg/day during pregnancy.

Iodine Balance. Iodine balance studies by Delange and coworkers (1984) showed that the average iodine retention of full-term infants was 6.7 µg/kg/day. With an average fetal weight of 3 kg, the mean retention of a fully developed fetus would be approximately 22 µg/day. A study demonstrated that pregnant women were at balance when consuming approximately 160 µg/day (Dworkin et al., 1966). Based on balance studies, the EAR ranges from 117 (22 + 95) (Delange et al., 1984) to 160 µg/day (Dworkin et al., 1966).

Iodine Supplementation During Pregnancy. In iodine deficiency, the size of the thyroid gland increases during pregnancy. Studies have measured thyroid volume by ultrasound and correlated it with urinary iodine excretion and the effects of iodine supplementation during pregnancy (Berghout and Wiersinga, 1998). Pregnant women in an iodine-deficient area of Italy were given iodized salt estimated to add 120 to 180 µg/day of iodine (Romano et al., 1991). Their urinary iodine increased from 37 to 154 µg/day during the second trimester and was 100 µg/day during the third trimester. Untreated control subjects showed little change. The initial thyroid volume of 9.8 mL did not change in those treated with iodine, but increased by 16 percent in the controls. Thus, the total daily iodine intake of about 200 µg prevented goiter. In another study from Denmark (Pedersen et al., 1993), 54 pregnant women were given 200 µg/day of iodine as potassium iodide drops beginning the second trimester. Urinary iodine increased from 55 to 105 µg/L, their thyroid volume (initially 9.6 mL) increased by 15.5 percent, and serum thyroid stimulating hormone (TSH) and serum thyroglobulin (Tg) concentrations did not change. Untreated control subjects showed increases of 31 percent in thyroid volume, 75 percent in serum Tg concentration, and 21 percent in serum TSH concentration. Thus, approximately 250 to 280 µg/day of iodine prevented goiter during pregnancy. In a third study (Glinoer, 1998), pregnant women with an initial urinary iodine of 36 µg/L were treated with an additional 100 µg/day. Their median urinary iodine concentration increased to 100 µg/L at 33 weeks, and their thyroid volume increased by 15 percent, compared with 30 percent in control subjects. Thus, a supplement of 100 µg iodine, bringing the total daily iodine intake to about 150 µg/day, was insufficient to prevent increased thyroid size.

On the basis of the above data, the EAR is set at 160 µg/day.

Iodine EAR and RDA Summary, Pregnancy

EAR for Pregnancy

14–18 years	**160 µg/day of iodine**
19–30 years	**160 µg/day of iodine**
31–50 years	**160 µg/day of iodine**

The RDA for iodine is set by using a CV of 20 percent (see "Adults Ages 19 Years and Older"). The RDA is defined as equal to the EAR plus twice the CV to cover the needs of 97 to 98 percent of individuals in the group (therefore, for iodine the RDA is 140 percent of the EAR). The calculated values for RDAs were rounded to the nearest 10 µg.

RDA for Pregnancy

14–18 years	**220 µg/day of iodine**
19–30 years	**220 µg/day of iodine**
31–50 years	**220 µg/day of iodine**

Lactation

Method Used to Estimate the Average Requirement

The EAR during lactation is based on the average requirement of adolescent girls and nonpregnant women plus the average daily loss of iodine in human milk. The EAR for adolescent girls and adult women is 95 µg/day, and the average daily loss of iodine in human milk is approximately 114 µg/day (Gushurst et al., 1984). Therefore, the EAR for lactating women is 209 µg/day.

Iodine EAR and RDA Summary, Lactation

EAR for Lactation
14–18 years	209 µg/day of iodine
19–30 years	209 µg/day of iodine
31–50 years	209 µg/day of iodine

The RDA for iodine is set by using a CV of 20 percent (see "Adults Ages 19 Years and Older"). The RDA is defined as equal to the EAR plus twice the CV to cover the needs of 97 to 98 percent of the individuals in the group (therefore, for iodine the RDA is 140 percent of the EAR). The calculated RDA value is rounded to the nearest 10 µg.

RDA for Lactation
14–18 years	290 µg/day of iodine
19–30 years	290 µg/day of iodine
31–50 years	290 µg/day of iodine

INTAKE OF IODINE

Food Sources

The iodine content in most food sources is low and can be affected by content of soil, irrigation, and fertilizers. Most foods provide 3 to 75 µg per serving. Foods of marine origin have higher concentrations of iodine because marine animals concentrate iodine from seawater. Processed foods may also contain higher levels of iodine due to the addition of iodized salt or additives such as calcium iodate, potassium iodate, potassium iodide, and cuprous iodide.

Dietary Intake

Based on analysis of 234 core foods conducted by the Food and Drug Administration (1982–1991 (Pennington et al., 1995) and analysis of 60 additional core foods and intake data by the U.S. Department of Agriculture Continuing Survey of Food Intakes by Individuals (1994–1996), the median intake of iodine from food in the United States is approximately 240 to 300 μg/day for men and 190 to 210 μg/day for women (Appendix Table E-4). For all life stage and gender groups, less than 25 percent of individuals had intakes below the Estimated Average Requirement.

Intake from Supplements

Information from the Third National Health and Nutrition Examination Survey (NHANES III) on the use of supplements containing iodine is given in Appendix Table C-17. The median intake of iodine from supplements was approximately 140 μg/day for adult men and women. In 1986, approximately 12 percent of men and 15 percent of nonpregnant women took a supplement that contained iodine (Moss et al., 1989; see Table 2-2).

TOLERABLE UPPER INTAKE LEVELS

The Tolerable Upper Intake Level (UL) is the highest level of daily nutrient intake that is likely to pose no risk of adverse health effects in almost all individuals. Although members of the general population should be advised not to routinely exceed the UL, intake above the UL may be appropriate for investigation within well-controlled clinical trials. Clinical trials of doses above the UL should not be discouraged, as long as subjects participating in these trials have signed informed consent documents regarding possible toxicity and as long as these trials employ appropriate safety monitoring of trial subjects. In addition, the UL is not meant to apply to individuals who are receiving iodine under medical supervision.

Hazard Identification

Most people are very tolerant of excess iodine intake from food (Pennington, 1990). Certain subpopulations, such as those with autoimmune thyroid disease and iodine deficiency, respond adversely to intakes considered safe for the general population. For the general population, high iodine intakes from food, water, and supplements have been associated with thyroiditis, goiter, hypo-thyroidism, hyperthyroidism, sensitivity reactions, thyroid papillary cancer, and acute responses in some individuals. There may be other unrecognized sources of iodine that increase the risk of adverse effects. Because of significant species differences in basal metabolic rates and iodine metabolism (Hetzel and Maberly, 1986), animal data were of limited use in setting a UL.

Adverse Effects

Acute Responses. Among human cases of acute iodine poisoning, there are reports of burning of the mouth, throat, and stomach, abdominal pain, fever, nausea, vomiting, diarrhea, weak pulse, cardiac irritability, coma, cyanosis, and other symptoms (Finkelstein and Jacobi, 1937; Tresch et al., 1974; Wexler et al., 1998). These are quite rare and are usually associated with doses of many grams.

Hypothyroidism and Elevated Thyroid Stimulating Hormone (TSH). Clinical hypothyroidism occurs when thyroid hormone production is inadequate. Subclinical hypothyroidism is defined as an elevation in TSH concentration while a normal serum thyroid hormone concentration is maintained. An elevation or increase over baseline (prior to iodine intake) in serum TSH concentration is considered an initial marker for hypothyroidism, although clinical hypothyroidism has not occurred. Laurberg and coworkers (1998) showed that in populations with high iodine intake, impaired thyroid function (i.e., elevated TSH concentration) is increased. Intervention studies looking for the earliest effects in iodine-sufficient populations show an increase in serum TSH concentration, or in TSH response to TSH-releasing hormone (TRH), without the TSH increasing to the abnormal range (Gardner et al., 1988; Paul et al., 1988). A randomized, controlled clinical trial in Wales by Chow and coworkers (1991) showed significantly elevated TSH concentrations associated with total iodide intakes of 750 µg/day or more. The study involved supplemental intake of 500 µg/day of iodide or placebo by 225 adult women (aged 25 to 54 years) for 28 days in addition to the estimated dietary intake of 250 µg/day. The baseline urinary iodide concentrations, however, suggest that many subjects probably had borderline iodine deficiency. Thus their conclusions may not apply to an iodine-sufficient population, such as that of the United States.

Goiter. Excess iodine may produce thyroid enlargement (goiter), mostly from increased TSH stimulation. Evidence of iodine-induced goiter comes from studies involving pharmacological doses (Wolff, 1969) and population groups with high, chronic iodine intakes (50,000 to 80,000 µg/day) in Japan and China (Suzuki and Mashimo, 1973; Suzuki et al., 1965). Wolff (1969) reported that prolonged intakes greater than 18,000 µg/day increased the risk of goiter.

Thyroid Papillary Cancer. Chronic stimulation of the thyroid gland by TSH is known to produce thyroid neoplasms (Money and Rawson, 1950). High iodine intake has also been associated with increased risk of thyroid papillary cancer in humans (Franceschi, 1998; Lind et al., 1998). Such evidence is lacking in experimental animals (Delange and Lecomte, 2000).

Thyroid Effects in Newborn Infants. Iodine goiter and hypothyroidism have been observed in newborns after prenatal exposure to excess iodine (Ayromlooi, 1972; Carswell et al., 1970; LaFranchi et al., 1977; Senior and Chernoff, 1971; Wolff, 1969). Rectal irrigation with povidone-iodine, a topical antiseptic, has been shown to be toxic to infants (Kurt et al., 1996; Means et al., 1990).

Other Adverse Effects. Other adverse effects of excess iodine intake include iodermia, a rare dermatological reaction to iodine intake. These dermatoses may consist of acneiform eruptions, pruritic red rashes, and urticaria (Parsad and Saini, 1998). In its most severe form, iodermia has resulted in death (Sulzberger and Witten, 1952). Iodine-induced hyperthyroidism occurs most frequently with iodine administration to patients with underlying thyroid disease and with iodine supplementation in areas of deficiency (Delange et al., 1999; Stanbury et al., 1998). Seasonal variations in thyrotoxicosis have been related to variations in daily iodine intake from 126 to 195 µg to 236 to 306 µg (Nelson and Phillips, 1985).

Summary

Challenged thyroid function shown by TSH concentrations elevated over baseline is the first effect observed in iodine excess. While an elevated TSH concentration may not be a clinically significant adverse effect, it is an indicator for increased risk of developing clinical hypothyroidism. Therefore, an elevated TSH concentration above baseline was selected as the critical adverse effect on which to base a UL.

Dose-Response Assessment

Adults

Data Selection. The appropriate data for derivation of a UL for adults are those relating intake to thyroid dysfunction shown by elevated TSH concentrations. Studies conducted in countries with a history of inadequate iodine intake were not included in this review because of the altered response of TSH to iodine intake.

Identification of No-Observed-Adverse-Effect Level (NOAEL) and Lowest-Observed-Adverse-Effect Level (LOAEL). Gardner and coworkers (1988) evaluated TSH concentrations in 30 adult men aged 22 to 40 years who received 500, 1,500, or 4,500 µg/day of supplemental iodide for 2 weeks. Baseline urinary iodine excretion was 287 µg/day; therefore baseline iodine intake from food is estimated to be approximately 300 µg/day. The mean basal serum TSH concentration increased significantly in those receiving the two higher doses, although it remained within the normal range. This study shows a LOAEL of 1,500 plus 300 µg/day, for a total of 1,800 µg/day.

In a similar study (Paul et al., 1988), nine men aged 26 to 56 years and 23 women aged 23 to 44 years received iodine supplements of 250, 500, or 1,500 µg/day for 14 days. Baseline urinary iodine excretion was 191 µg/day. Because greater than 90 percent of dietary iodine is excreted in urine (Nath et al., 1992), it was estimated that the baseline iodine intake was approximately 200 µg. Those receiving 1,500 µg/day of iodide showed a significant increase in baseline and TRH-stimulated serum TSH, effects not seen in the two lower doses. No subjects in this study had detectable antithyroid antibodies. The conclusion would be that an iodine intake of about 1,700 µg/day increased TSH secretion. Both of the above studies support a LOAEL between 1,700 and 1,800 µg/day. Thus, the lowest LOAEL of 1,700 µg/day was selected.

Uncertainty Assessment. There is little uncertainty regarding the range of iodine intakes that are likely to induce elevated TSH concentration over baseline. A LOAEL of 1,700 µg/day and a NOAEL of 1,000 to 1,200 µg/day are estimated for adult humans. This results in an uncertainty factor (UF) of 1.5 to derive a NOAEL from a LOAEL. A higher uncertainty factor was not considered because of the mild, reversible nature of elevated TSH over baseline.

Derivation of a UL. The LOAEL of 1,700 µg/day was divided by a UF of 1.5 to obtain a UL of 1,133 µg/day of iodine, which was rounded down to 1,100 µg/day.

$$UL = \frac{LOAEL}{UF} = \frac{1,700 \text{ µg/day}}{1.5} \cong 1,100 \text{ µg/day}$$

Iodine UL Summary, Ages 19 Years and Older

UL for Adults
   ≥ 19 years   **1,100 µg/day of iodine**

Other Life Stage Groups

Infants. For infants, the UL was judged not determinable because of insufficient data on adverse effects in this age group and concern about the infant's ability to handle excess amounts. To prevent high intake, the only source of intake for infants should be from food and formula.

Children and Adolescents. Given the dearth of information, the UL values for children and adolescents are extrapolated from those established for adults. Thus, the adult UL of 1,100 µg/day of iodine was adjusted for children and adolescents on the basis of body weight as described in Chapter 2 and using reference weights from Chapter 1 (Table 1-1). Values have been rounded down.

Pregnancy and Lactation. No altered susceptibility of pregnant or lactating women to excess iodine has been noted. Therefore, the UL for pregnant and lactating females is the same as that for non-pregnant and nonlactating females.

Iodine UL Summary, Ages 0 through 18 Years, Pregnancy, Lactation

UL for Infants
   0–12 months   **Not possible to establish; source of intake should be from food and formula only**

UL for Children
   1–3 years   **200 µg/day of iodine**
   4–8 years   **300 µg/day of iodine**
   9–13 years   **600 µg/day of iodine**

UL for Adolescents
    14–18 years   900 µg/day of iodine

UL for Pregnancy
    14–18 years   900 µg/day of iodine
    19–50 years   1,100 µg/day of iodine

UL for Lactation
    14–18 years   900 µg/day of iodine
    19–50 years   1,100 µg/day of iodine

Special Considerations

Autoimmune thyroid disease (AITD) is common in the U.S. population and particularly in older adult women. Individuals with AITD who are treated for iodine deficiency or nodular goiter (Carnell and Valente, 1998; Foley, 1992; Massoudi et al., 1995) may have increased sensitivity to adverse effects of iodine intake. Some young adults with simple goiter and iodine deficiency who were supplemented with 200 µg/day of iodine developed either mild transient hyperthyroidism or hypothyroidism, positive antibodies, and reversible histological changes of lymphocytic thyroiditis (Kahaly et al., 1997). The sensitivities of these distinct subgroups do not fall within the range of sensitivities expected for the healthy population.

Studies have correlated an increase in the incidence of AITD with a population's higher intake of iodine (Foley, 1992). Additional data provide some correlation between the incidence of circulating antithyroid antibodies (a marker for AITD) and dietary iodine intake (Schuppert et al., 2000). At this time there is not sufficient data to determine a UL for this subpopulation. Therefore, a UL could not be set for individuals with AITD.

Intake Assessment

Iodine is secreted in human and cow's milk and is present in dairy products, marine fish, and a variety of foods grown in iodide-rich soils. It is especially high in some foods, such as certain seaweed. Normal diets are unlikely to supply more than 1 mg/day. Also, a variety of environmental and therapeutic exposures are adventitious sources of iodine (Farwell and Braverman, 1996). Intake of 10 g of 0.001 percent iodized salt results in an intake of 770 µg/day. Based on the Food and Drug Administration Total Diet Study (Appendix Table E-4), the highest intake of dietary iodine for any life stage or gender group at the ninety-fifth percentile was approximately 1.14 mg/day, which is equivalent to the UL for adults. The iodine intake from the diet (Appendix Table E-4) and supplements (Appendix Table C-17) at the ninety-fifth percentile is approximately 1.15 mg/day.

Risk Characterization

For most people, iodine intake from usual foods and supplements is unlikely to exceed the UL. In North America, where much of the iodine consumed is from salt iodized with potassium iodide, symptoms of iodine deficiency are rare. In certain regions of the world where goiter is present, therapeutic doses may exceed the UL. The UL is not meant to apply to individuals who are being treated with iodine under close medical supervision.

RESEARCH RECOMMENDATIONS FOR IODINE

• Correlation of community iodine intake with autoimmune thyroid disease and papillary thyroid cancer.

• Continual monitoring of U.S. urinary iodine by the National Health and Nutrition Examination Survey and inclusion of data on thyroid size in children, determined by ultrasound.

• Role of iodine in fibrocystic breast disease.

• Iodine nutrition and immune response.

• Iodine nutrition in relation to other nutrients, particularly vitamin A, iron, and selenium.

• Effects of iodine concentration in water purification.

• Further standardization of thyroid volume by ultrasound and urinary iodine excretion in areas with different iodine intake.

REFERENCES

Albert A, Keating FR Jr. 1949. Metabolic studies with I^{131} labeled thyroid compounds. *J Clin Endocrinol* 9:1406–1421.

Ayromlooi J. 1972. Congenital goiter due to maternal ingestion of iodides. *Obstet Gynecol* 39:818–822.

Benmiloud M, Chaouki ML, Gutekunst R, Teichert HM, Wood WG, Dunn JT. 1994. Oral iodized oil for correcting iodine deficiency: Optimal dosing and outcome indicator selection. *J Clin Endocrinol Metab* 79:20–24.

Berghout A, Wiersinga W. 1998. Thyroid size and thyroid function during pregnancy: An analysis. *Eur J Endocrinol* 138:536–542.

Berson SA, Yalow RS. 1954. Quantitative aspects of iodine metabolism. The exchangeable organic iodine pool, and the rates of thyroidal secretion, peripheral degradation and fecal excretion of endogenously synthesized organically bound iodine. *J Clin Invest* 1533–1552.

Bleichrodt N, Born MP. 1994. A meta-analysis of research on iodine and its relationship to cognitive development. In: Stanbury JB, ed. *The Damaged Brain of Iodine Deficiency: Cogitive, Behavioral, Neuromotor, Educative Aspects*. NY: Cognizant Communication. Pp. 195–200.

Bourdoux P. 1998. Evaluation of the iodine intake: Problems of the iodine/creatinine ratio—Comparison with iodine excretion and daily fluctuations of iodine concentration. *Exp Clin Endocrinol Diabetes* 106:S17–S20.

Buchinger W, Lorenz-Wawschinek O, Semlitsch G, Langsteger W, Binter G, Bonelli RM, Eber O. 1997. Thyrotropin and thyroglobulin as an index of optimal iodine intake: Correlation with iodine excretion of 39,913 euthyroid patients. *Thyroid* 7:593–597.

Carnell NE, Valente WA. 1998. Thyroid nodules in Graves' disease: Classification, characterization, and response to treatment. *Thyroid* 8:647–652.

Carswell F, Kerr MM, Hutchison JH. 1970. Congenital goitre and hypothyroidism produced by maternal ingestion of iodides. *Lancet* 1:1241–1243.

Chow CC, Phillips DI, Lazarus JH, Parkes AB. 1991. Effect of low dose iodide supplementation on thyroid function in potentially susceptible subjects: Are dietary iodide levels in Britain acceptable? *Clin Endocrinol* 34:413–416.

Croxson MS, Hall TD, Kletzky OA, Jaramillo JE, Nicoloff JT. 1977. Decreased serum thyrotropin induced by fasting. *J Clin Endrocrinol Metab* 45:560–568.

DeGroot LJ. 1966. Kinetic analysis of iodine metabolism. *J Clin Endocrinol Metab* 26:149–173.

Delange F. 1989. Iodine nutrition and congenital hypothyroidism. In: Delange F, Fisher DA, Glinoer D, eds. *Research in Congential Hypothyroidism*. New York: Plenum Press.

Delange F. 1993. Requirements of iodine in humans. In: Delange F, Dunn JT, Glinoer D, eds. *Iodine Deficiency in Europe: A Continuing Concern*. New York: Plenum Press. Pp. 5–13.

Delange F, Burgi H. 1989. Iodine deficiency disorders in Europe. *Bull World Health Organ* 67:317–325.

Delange F, Ermans AM. 1991. Iodine deficiency. In: Braverman LE, Utiger RD, eds. *Werner and Ingbar's the Thyroid: A Fundamental and Clinical Text*, 6th ed. Philadelphia: JD Lippincott.

Delange F, Lecomte P. 2000. Iodine supplementation: Benefits outweigh risks. *Drug Safety* 22:89–95.

Delange F, Bourdoux P, Vo Thi LD, Ermans AM, Senterre J. 1984. Negative iodine balance in preterm infants. *Ann Endocrinol* 45:77.

Delange F, Dunn JT, Glinoer D. 1993. In: *Iodine Deficiency in Europe. A Continuing Concern*. New York: Plenum Press.

Delange F, Benker G, Caron P, Eber O, Ott W, Peter F, Podoba J, Simescu M, Szybinsky Z, Vertongen F, Vitti P, Wiersinga W, Zamrazil V. 1997. Thyroid volume and urinary iodine in European schoolchildren: Standardization of values for assessment of iodine deficiency. *Eur J Endocrinol* 136:180–187.

Delange F, de Benoist B, Alnwick D. 1999. Risks of iodine-induced hyperthyroidism after correction of iodine deficiency by iodized salt. *Thyroid* 9:545–556.

Dunn JT, Crutchfield HE, Gutekunst R, Dunn AD. 1993. Two simple methods for measuring iodine in urine. *Thyroid* 3:119–123.

Dunn JT, Semigran MJ, Delange F. 1998. The prevention and management of iodine-induced hyperthyroidism and its cardiac features. *Thyroid* 8:101–106.

Dworkin HJ, Jacquez JA, Beierwaltes WH. 1966. Relationship of iodine ingestion to iodine excretion in pregnancy. *J Clin Endocrinol Metab* 26:1329–1342.

Emrich D, Karkavitsas N, Facorro U, Schurnbrand P, Schreivogel I, Schicha H, Dirks H. 1982. Influence of increasing iodine intake on thyroid function in euthyroid and hyperthyroid states. *J Clin Endocrinol Metab* 54:1236–1241.

Ermans AM, Dumont JE, Bastenie PA. 1963. Thyroid function in a goiter endemic: I. Impairment of hormone synthesis and secretion in the goitrous gland. *J Clin Endocrinol* 23:539–549.

Eskin BA. 1977. Iodine and mammary cancer. *Adv Exp Med Biol* 91:293–304.

Etling N, Padovani E, Fouque F, Tato L. 1986. First-month variations in total iodine content of human breast milks. *Early Hum Dev* 13:81–85.

Farwell AP, Braverman LE. 1996. Thyroid and Antithyroid Drugs. In: Hardman JG, Limbird LE, Molinoff PB, Ruddon RW, Gilman AG, eds. *Goodman and Gilman's The Pharmacological Basis of Therapeutics,* 9th ed. New York: McGraw-Hill. Pp. 1383–1409.

Finkelstein R, Jacobi M. 1937. Fatal iodine poisoning: A clinicopathologic and experimental study. *Ann Intern Med* 10:1283–1296.

Fischer PW, Giroux A. 1987. Iodine content of a representative Canadian diet. *J Can Diet Assoc* 48:24–27.

Fisher DA, Oddie TH. 1969a. Thyroidal radioiodine clearance and thyroid iodine accumulation: Contrast between random daily variation and population data. *J Clin Endocrinol Metab* 29:111–115.

Fisher DA, Oddie TH. 1969b. Thyroid iodine content and turnover in euthyroid subjects: Validity of estimation of thyroid iodine accumulation from short-term clearance studies. *J Clin Endocrinol Metab* 29:721–727.

Foley TP Jr. 1992. The relationship between autoimmune thyroid disease and iodine intake: A review. *Endokrynol Pol* 43:53–69.

Franceschi S. 1998. Iodine intake and thyroid carcinoma—A potential risk factor. *Exp Clin Endocrinol Diabetes* 106:S38–S44.

Gaitan E. 1989. *Environmental Goitrogenesis.* Boca Raton: CRC Press.

Gardner DF, Kaplan MM, Stanley CA, Utiger RD. 1979. Effect of tri-iodothyronine replacement on the metabolic and pituitary responses to starvation. *N Engl J Med* 300:579–584.

Gardner DF, Utiger RD, Schwartz SL, Witorsch P, Myers B, Braverman LA, Witorsch RJ. 1987. Effects of oral erythrosine (2',4',5',7'-tetraiodofluorescein) on thyroid function in normal men. *Toxicol Appl Pharmacol* 91:299-304.

Gardner DF, Centor RM, Utiger RD. 1988. Effects of low dose oral iodide supplementation on thyroid function in normal men. *Clin Endocrinol* 28:283–288.

Ghent WR, Eskin BA, Low DA, Hill LP. 1993. Iodine replacement in fibrocystic disease of the breast. *Can J Surg* 36:453–460.

Glinoer D. 1998. Iodine supplementation during pregnancy: Importance and biochemical assessment. *Exp Clin Endocrinol Diabetes* 106:S21.

Gushurst CA, Mueller JA, Green JA, Sedor F. 1984. Breast milk iodine: Reassessment in the 1980s. *Pediatrics* 73:354–357.

Gutekunst R, Smolarek H, Hasenpusch U, Stubbe P, Friedrich HJ, Wood WG, Scriba PC. 1986. Goitre epidemiology: Thyroid volume, iodine excretion, thyroglobulin and thyrotropin in Germany and Sweden. *Acta Endocrinol* 112:494–501.

Harrison MT. 1968. Iodine balance in man. *Postgrad Med J* 44:69–71.

Harrison MT, Harden R, Alexander WD, Wayne E. 1965. Iodine balance studies in patients with normal and abnormal thyroid function. *J Clin Endocrinol* 25:1077–1084.

Hays MT. 1991. Localization of human thryoxine absorption. *Thyroid* 1:241–248.

Hemken RW. 1980. Milk and meat iodine content: Relation to human health. *J Am Vet Med Assoc* 176:1119–1121.

Hetzel BS, Maberly GF. 1986. Iodine. In: Mertz W, ed. *Trace Elements in Human and Animal Nutrition,* Vol. 2. Orlando: Academic Press. Pp. 139–208.

Hollowell JG, Staehling NW, Hannon WH, Flanders DW, Gunter EW, Maberly GF, Braverman LE, Pino S, Miller DT, Garbe PL, DeLozier DM, Jackson RJ. 1998. Iodine nutrition in the United States. Trends and public health implications: Iodine excretion data from National Health and Nutrition Examination Surveys I and III (1971–1974 and 1988–1994). *J Clin Endocrinol Metab* 83:3401–3408.

Ingenbleek Y, Malvaux P. 1974. Iodine balance studies in protein-calorie malnutrition. *Arch Dis Child* 49:305–309.

Jackson IM. 1982. Thyrotropin-releasing hormone. *New Engl J Med* 306:145–155.

Johnson LA, Ford HC, Doran J, Richardson VF. 1990. A survey of the iodide concentration of human milk. *N Z Med J* 103:393–394.

Jooste PL, Weight MJ, Lombard CJ. 2000. Short-term effectiveness of mandatory iodization of table salt, at an elevated iodine concentration, on the iodine and goiter status of school children with endemic goiter. *Am J Clin Nutr* 71:75–80.

Kahaly C, Dienes HP, Beyer J, Hommel G. 1997. Randomized, double blind, placebo-controlled trial of low dose iodide in endemic goiter. *J Clin Endocrinol Metab* 82:4049–4053.

Klebanoff SJ. 1967. Iodination of bacteria: A bacterial mechanism. *J Exp Med* 126:1063–1078.

Klein AH, Meltzer S, Kenny FM. 1972. Improved prognosis in congenital hypothyroidism treated before age three months. *J Pediatr* 81:912–915.

Kurt TL, Morgan ML, Hnilica V, Bost R, Petty CS. 1996. Fatal iatrogenic iodine toxicity in a nine-week old infant. *J Toxicol Clin Toxicol* 34:231–234.

LaFranchi SH, Buist NR, Murphey WH, Larsen PR, Foley TP Jr. 1977. Transient neonatal hypothyroidism detected by newborn screening program. *Pediatrics* 60:539–541.

Larsson G, Victor A. 1988. Micturition patterns in a healthy female population, studied with a frequency/volume chart. *Scand J Urol Nephrol* 114:53–57.

Laurberg P, Pedersen KM, Hreidarsson A, Sigfusson N, Iversen E, Knudsen PR. 1998. Iodine intake and the pattern of thyroid disorders: A comparative epidemiological study of thyroid abnormalities in the elderly in Iceland and in Jutland, Denmark. *J Clin Endocrinol Metab* 83:765–769.

Lind P, Langsteger W, Molnar M, Gallowitsch HJ, Mikosch P, Gomez I. 1998. Epidemiology of thyroid diseases in iodine sufficiency. *Thyroid* 8:1179–1183.

Loh KC. 2000. Amiodarone-induced thyroid disorders: A clinical review. *Postgrad Med J* 76:133–140.

Malamos B, Koutras DA, Marketos SG, Rigopoulos GA, Yataganas XA, Binopoulos D, Sfontouris J, Pharmakiotis AD, Vought RL, London WT. 1967. Endemic goiter in Greece: An iodine balance study in the field. *J Clin Endocrinol Metab* 27:1372–1380.

Malvaux P, Beckers C, de Visscher M. 1969. Iodine balance studies in nongoitrous children and in adolescents on low iodine intake. *J Clin Endocrinol Metab* 29:79–84.

Massoudi MS, Meilahn EN, Orchard TJ, Foley TP Jr, Kuller LH, Constantino JP, Buhari AM. 1995. Prevalence of thyroid antibodies among healthy middle-aged women. Findings from the thyroid study in healthy women. *Ann Epidemiol* 5:229–233.

Mattsson S, Lindstrom S. 1995. Diuresis and voiding pattern in healthy schoolchildren. *Br J Urol* 76:783–789.

Means LJ, Rescorla FJ, Grosfeld JL. 1990. Iodine toxicity: An unusual cause of cardiovascular collapse during anesthesia in an infant with Hirschsprung's disease. *J Pediatr Surg* 25:1278–1279.

Missler U, Gutekunst R, Wood WG. 1994. Thyroglobulin is a more sensitive indicator of iodine deficiency than thyrotropin: Development and evaluation of dry blood spot assays for thyrotropin and thyroglobulin in iodine-deficient geographical areas. *Eur J Clin Chem* 32:137–143.

Money WL, Rawson RW. 1950. The experimental production of thyroid tumors in the rat exposed to prolonged treatment with thiouracil. *Cancer* 3:321–335.

Moss AJ, Levy AS, Kim I, Park YK. 1989. *Use of Vitamin and Mineral Supplements in the United States: Current Users, Types of Products, and Nutrients.* Advance Data, Vital and Health Statistics of the National Center for Health Statistics, Number 174. Hyattsville, MD: National Center for Health Statistics.

Moulopoulos DS, Koutras DA, Mantzos J, Souvatzoglou A, Piperingos GD, Karaiskos KS, Makriyannis D, Sfontouris J, Moulopoulos SD. 1988. The relation of serum T4 and TSH with the urinary iodine excretion. *J Endocrinol Invest* 11:437–439.

Nath SK, Moinier B, Thuillier F, Rongier M, Desjeux JF. 1992. Urinary excretion of iodide and fluoride from supplemented food grade salt. *Int J Vitam Nutr Res* 62:66–72.

Nelson M, Phillips DI. 1985. Seasonal variations in dietary iodine intake and thyrotoxicosis. *Hum Nutr Appl Nutr* 39:213–216.

Nilsson R, Ehrenberg L, Fedoresak I. 1987. Formation of potential antigens from radiographic contrast media. *Acta Radiol* 28:473–477.

Oddie TH, Fisher DA, Long JM. 1964. Factors affecting the estimation of iodine entering the normal thyroid gland using short-term clearance studies. *J Clin Endocrinol* 24:924–933.

Parsad D, Saini R. 1998. Acneform eruption with iodized salt. *Int J Dermatol* 37:478.

Paul T, Meyers B, Witorsch RJ, Pino S, Chipkin S, Ingbar SH, Braverman LE. 1988. The effect of small increases in dietary iodine on thyroid function in euthyroid subjects. *Metabolism* 37:121–124.

Pedersen KM, Laurberg P, Iversen E, Knudsen PR, Gregersen HE, Rasmussen OS, Larsen KR, Eriksen GM, Johannesen PL. 1993. Amelioration of some pregnancy-associated variations in thyroid function by iodine supplementation. *J Clin Endocrinol Metab* 77:1078–1083.

Pennington JA. 1990. A review of iodine toxicity reports. *J Am Diet Assoc* 90:1571–1581.

Pennington JAT, Schoen SA, Salmon GD, Young B, Johnson RD, Marts RW. 1995. Composition of core foods in the U.S. food supply, 1982-1991. *J Food Comp and Anal* 8:171-217.

Pinchera A, MacGillivray MH, Crawford JD, Freeman AG. 1965. Thyroid refractoriness in an athyreotic cretin fed soybean formula. *N Engl J Med* 273:83–87.

Riggs DS. 1952. Quantitative aspects of iodine metabolism in man. *Pharmacol Rev* 4:284–370.

Romano R, Jannini EA, Pepe M, Grimaldi A, Olivieri M, Spennati P, Cappa F, D'Armiento M. 1991. The effects of iodoprophylaxis on thyroid size during pregnancy. *Am J Obstet Gynecol* 164:482–485.

Schuppert F, Ehrenthal D, Frilling A, Suzuki K, Napolitano G, Kohn LD. 2000. Increased major histocompatibility complex (MHC) expression in nontoxic goiters is associated with iodine depletion, enhanced ability of the follicular thyroglobulin to increase MHC gene expression, and thyroid antibodies. *J Clin Endocrinol Metab* 85:858–867.

Senior B, Chernoff HL. 1971. Iodide goiter in the newborn. *Pediatrics* 47:510–515.

Shepard TH, Pyne GE, Kirschvink JF, McLean M. 1960. Soybean goiter: Report of three cases. *N Engl J Med* 262:1099–1103.

Stanbury JB, Ermans AE, Bourdoux P, Todd C, Oken E, Tonglet R, Vidor G, Braverman LE, Medeiros-Neto G. 1998. Iodine-induced hyperthyroidism: Occurrence and epidemiology. *Thyroid* 8:83–100.

Sulzberger MB, Witten VH. 1952. Allergic dermatoses due to drugs. *Postgrad Med* 11:549–557.

Suzuki H, Mashimo K. 1973. Further studies of "endemic goiter" in Hokkaido, Japan. In: Mashimo K, Suzuki H, eds. *Iodine Metabolism and Thyroid Function,* Vol. 6. Sapporo, Japan: Hokkaido University School of Medicine. P. 143.

Suzuki H, Higuchi T, Sawa K, Ohtaki S, Horiuchi Y. 1965. "Endemic coast goiter" in Hokkaido, Japan. *Acta Endocrinol* 50:161–176.

Swanson EW, Miller JK, Mueller FJ, Patton CS, Bacon JA, Ramsey N. 1990. Iodine in milk and meat of dairy cows fed different amounts of potassium iodide or ethylenediamine dihydroiodide. *J Dairy Sci* 73:398–405.

Tresch DD, Sweet DL, Keelan MH, Lange RL. 1974. Acute iodide intoxication with cardiac irritability. *Arch Intern Med* 134:760–762.

Trowbridge FL, Hand KE., Nichaman MZ. 1975. Findings relating to goiter and iodine in the Ten-State Nutrition Survey. *Am J Clin Nutr* 28:712–716.

Venturi S, Venturi A, Cimini D, Arduini C, Venturi M, Guidi A. 1993. A new hypothesis: Iodine and gastric cancer. *Eur J Cancer Prev* 2:17–23.

Vought RL, London WT. 1967. Iodine intake, excretion and thyroidal accumulation in healthy subjects. *J Clin Endocrinol Metab* 27:913–919.

Wayne EJ, Koutras DA, Alexander WD. 1964. *Clinical Aspects of Iodine Metabolism.* Oxford: Blackwell Scientific.

Wexler P, Gad SC, Hartung R, Henderson RF, Krenzelok EP, Locey BJ, Mehendale HM, Plaa GL, Pope C, Witschi H. 1998. *Encyclopedia of Toxicology,* Vol. 2. San Diego: Academic Press. Pp. 186–187.

WHO (World Health Organization) Nutrition Unit. 1994. *Indicators for Assessing Iodine Deficiency Disorders and their Control through Salt Iodization.* Geneva: WHO.

WHO/UNICEF/ICCIDD (United Nations Childrens Fund/International Council for Control of Iodine Deficiency Disorders). 1993. *Indicators for Assessing Iodine Deficiency Disorders and their Control Programmes.* Report of a joint WHO/ UNICEF/ICCIDD consultation (review version). Geneva: WHO.

Wolff J. 1969. Iodide goiter and the pharmacologic effects of excess iodide. *Am J Med* 47:101–124.

Xu F, Sullivan K, Houston R, Zhao J, May W, Maberly G. 1999. Thyroid volumes in U.S. and Bangladeshi schoolchildren: Comparison with European schoolchildren. *Eur J Endocrinol* 140: 498–504.

9

Iron

SUMMARY

Iron functions as a component of a number of proteins, including enzymes and hemoglobin, the latter being important for the transport of oxygen to tissues throughout the body for metabolism. Factorial modeling was used to determine the Estimated Average Requirement (EAR) for iron. The components of iron requirement used as factors in the modeling include basal iron losses, menstrual losses, fetal requirements in pregnancy, increased requirement during growth for the expansion of blood volume, and/or increased tissue and storage iron. The Recommended Dietary Allowance (RDA) for all age groups of men and postmenopausal women is 8 mg/day; the RDA for premenopausal women is 18 mg/day. The median dietary intake of iron is approximately 16 to 18 mg/day for men and 12 mg/day for women. The Tolerable Upper Intake Level (UL) for adults is 45 mg/day of iron, a level based on gastrointestinal distress as an adverse effect.

BACKGROUND INFORMATION

Almost two-thirds of iron in the body is found in hemoglobin present in circulating erythrocytes. A readily mobilizable iron store contains another 25 percent. Most of the remaining 15 percent is in the myoglobin of muscle tissue and a variety of enzymes necessary for oxidative metabolism and many other functions in all cells. A 75-kg adult man contains about 4 grams of iron (50 mg/kg) while a

290

menstruating woman has about 40 mg/kg of iron because of her smaller erythrocyte mass and iron store (Bothwell et al., 1979).

Function

Iron can exist in oxidation states ranging from −2 to +6. In biological systems, these oxidation states occur primarily as the ferrous (+2), ferric (+3), and ferryl (+4) states. The interconversion of iron oxidation states is a mechanism whereby iron participates in electron transfer, as well as a mechanism whereby iron can reversibly bind ligands. The common biological ligands for iron are oxygen, nitrogen, and sulfur atoms.

Four major classes of iron-containing proteins exist in the mammalian system: iron-containing heme proteins (hemoglobin, myoglobin, cytochromes), iron-sulfur enzymes (flavoproteins, heme-flavoproteins), proteins for iron storage and transport (transferrin, lactoferrin, ferritin, hemosiderin), and other iron-containing or activated enzymes (sulfur, nonheme enzymes). In iron sulfur enzymes, iron is bound to sulfur in one of four possible arrangements (Fe-S, 2Fe-2S, 4Fe-4S, 3Fe-4S proteins). In heme proteins, iron is bound to porphyrin ring structures with various side chains. In humans, the predominant form of heme is protoporphyrin-IX.

Hemoglobin

The movement of oxygen from the environment to the tissues is one of the key functions of iron. Oxygen is bound to an iron-containing porphyrin ring, either as part of the prosthetic group of hemoglobin within erythrocytes or as part of myoglobin as the facilitator of oxygen diffusion in tissues.

Myoglobin

Myoglobin is located in the cytoplasm of muscle cells and increases the rate of diffusion of oxygen from capillary erythrocytes to the cytoplasm and mitochondria. The concentration of myoglobin in muscle is drastically reduced in tissue iron deficiency, thus limiting the rate of diffusion of oxygen from erythrocytes to mitochondria (Dallman, 1986a).

Cytochromes

The cytochromes contain heme as the active site with the iron-containing porphyrin ring functioning to reduce ferric iron to ferrous iron. Cytochromes act as electron carriers. The 40 different proteins that constitute the respiratory chain contain six different heme proteins, six with iron sulfur centers, two with copper centers, and ubiquinone to connect nicotinamide adenine dinucleotide hydride to oxygen.

Physiology of Absorption, Metabolism, and Excretion

Absorption

The iron content of the body is highly conserved. In the absence of bleeding (including menstruation) or pregnancy, only a small quantity is lost each day (Bothwell et al., 1979). Adult men need to absorb only about 1 mg/day to maintain iron balance. The average requirement for menstruating women is somewhat higher, approximately 1.5 mg/day. There is, however, a marked interindividual variation in menstrual losses, and a small proportion of women must absorb as much as 3.4 mg/day. Towards the end of pregnancy, the absorption of 4 to 5 mg/day is necessary to preserve iron balance. Requirements are also higher in childhood, particularly during periods of rapid growth in early childhood (6 to 24 months), and adolescence.

In the face of these varying requirements, iron balance is maintained by the regulation of absorption in the upper small intestine (Bothwell et al., 1979). There are two pathways for the absorption of iron in humans. One mediates the uptake of the small quantity of heme iron derived primarily from hemoglobin and myoglobin in meat. The other allows for the absorption of nonheme iron, primarily as iron salts, that can be extracted from plant and dairy foods and rendered soluble in the lumen of the stomach and duodenum. Absorption of nonheme iron is enhanced by substances, such as ascorbic acid, that form low molecular weight iron chelates. Most of the iron consumed by humans is in the latter nonheme form.

Heme iron is highly bioavailable and little affected by dietary factors. Nonheme iron absorption depends on the solubilization of predominately ferric food iron in the acid milieu of the stomach (Raja et al., 1987; Wollenberg and Rummel, 1987) and reduction to the ferrous form by compounds such as ascorbic acid or a ferrireductase present at the musosal surfaces of cells in the duodenum (Han et al., 1995; Raja et al., 1993). This bioavailable iron is then absorbed in a three-step process in which the iron is taken up by the enterocytes across the cellular apical membrane by an energy-dependent, carrier-mediated process (Muir and Hopfer, 1985; Simpson et al., 1986), transported intracellularly, and transferred across the basolateral membrane into the plasma.

The duodenal mucosal cells involved in iron absorption are formed in the crypts of Lieberkuhn. They then migrate up the villi becoming functional iron-absorbing cells only when they reach the tips of the villi. After a brief period of functionality, the cells are shed into the lumen together with iron that had entered the cell but had not been transferred to the plasma. In humans, mucosal cell turnover takes between 48 and 72 hours. Cells are programmed to regulate iron absorption when they reach tips of the villi by the amount of iron that they acquire from plasma during their early development. Recent studies by Cannone-Hergaux and coworkers (1999) strongly suggest that a metal transporter (divalent metal transporter [DMT-1] protein), which is a transmembrane protein and an isoform of natural resistance associated macrophage protein (NRAMP2), mediates the uptake of elemental iron into the duodenal cells. The quantity of this transport protein that is formed is inversely proportional to the iron content of the cell; synthesis is regulated by posttranscriptional modification of the DMT-1 messenger ribonucleic acid (mRNA) (Conrad and Umbreit, 2000). The regulatory mechanism involves the cellular iron response proteins (IRP) and the iron response element (IRE) on the mRNA (Eisenstein, 2000).

The mechanism by which iron is transported through the enterocyte has not been completely elucidated. Absorbed iron in the intracellular "labile iron pool" is delivered to the basolateral surface of enterocytes, becomes available for binding onto transferrin, and is then transported via transferrin in the plasma to all body cells. Ceruloplasmin, a copper-containing protein, facilitates the binding of ferric iron to transferrin via ferroxidase activity at the basolateral membrane (Osaki et al., 1966; Wollenberg et al., 1990).

Heme is soluble in an alkaline environment and is less affected by intraluminal factors that influence nonheme iron uptake. Specific transporters exist for heme on the surface of rat enterocytes (Conrad et al., 1967; Grasbeck et al., 1982); however, rats do not absorb heme iron as efficiently as do humans (Weintraub et al., 1965). To date, no specific receptor/transporter for heme has been identified in humans. After binding to its receptor, the heme molecule is internalized and degraded to iron, carbon monoxide, and bilirubin IXa by the enzyme heme oxygenase (Bjorn-Rasmussen et al., 1974; Raffin et al., 1974). This enzyme is induced by iron deficiency (Raffin et al., 1974). It is thought that the iron that is liberated from heme enters the common intracellular (enterocyte) pool of iron before being transported to plasma transferrin.

Transport and Metabolism

Iron movement between cells is primarily conducted via reversible binding of iron to the transport protein, transferrin. One atom of iron can bind to each of two binding sites on transferrin and will then complex with a highly specific transferrin receptor (TfR) located on the plasma membrane surfaces of cells. Internalization of transferrin in clathrin-coated pits results in an endosomal vesicle where acidification to a pH of approximately 5.5 results in the release of the iron from transferrin. The movement of iron from this endosomal space to the cytoplasm is not completely understood at this time, but recent discoveries provide some clues. DMT1 (NRAMP2) has now been identified in endosomal vesicles (Gunshin et al., 1997). Although it is not a specific iron transporter and although it is capable of transporting other divalent metals, recent studies suggest that it may play a primary role in the delivery of iron to the cell. A second transporter, stimulator of iron transport (SFT), has been cloned and characterized as an exclusive iron transporter of both ferric and ferrous iron out of the endosome (Gutierrez et al., 1997).

Iron entering cells may be incorporated into functional compounds, stored as ferritin, or used to regulate future cellular iron metabolism by modifying the activity of the two IRPs. The size of the intracellular iron pool plays a clear regulatory role in the synthesis of iron storage, iron transport, and iron metabolism proteins through an elegant posttranscriptional set of events (see review by Eisenstein and Blemings, 1998).

Storage

Intracellular iron availability is regulated by the increased expression of cellular TfR concentration by iron-deficient cells and increased ferritin production when the iron supply exceeds the cell's functional needs. Iron is stored in the form of ferritin or hemosiderin. The latter is a water-insoluble degradation product of ferritin. The iron content of hemosiderin is variable but generally higher than that of ferritin. While all cells are capable of storing iron, the cells of the liver, spleen, and bone marrow are the primary iron storage sites in humans.

Excretion

In the absence of bleeding (including menstruation) or pregnancy, only a small quantity of iron is lost each day (Bothwell et al., 1979). Body iron is therefore highly conserved. Daily basal iron losses are limited to between 0.90 and 1.02 mg/day in nonmenstruating women (Green et al., 1968). The majority of absorbed iron is lost in the feces. Daily iron losses from urine, gastrointestinal tract, and skin are approximately 0.08, 0.6, and 0.2 to 0.3 mg/day, respectively. These basal losses may drop to 0.5 mg/day in iron deficiency and may be as high as 2 mg/day in iron overload (Bothwell et al., 1979). Menstrual iron losses are quite variable. Studies on Swedish and British women demonstrated a mean iron loss via menses of 0.6 to 0.7 mg/day (Hallberg et al., 1966b).

Clinical Effects of Inadequate Intake

Important subclinical and clinical consequences of iron deficiency are impaired physical work performance, developmental delay, cognitive impairment, and adverse pregnancy outcomes. Several other clinical consequences have also been described. The bulk of experimental and epidemiological evidence in humans suggests that functional consequences of iron deficiency (related both to anemia and tissue iron concentration) occur only when iron deficiency is of a severity sufficient to cause a measurable decrease in hemoglobin concentration.

Once the degree of iron deficiency is sufficiently severe to cause anemia, functional disabilities become evident. It is difficult to determine whether any particular functional abnormality is a specific consequence of the anemia per se, presumably due to impaired oxygen delivery, or the result of concomitant tissue iron deficiency. However, it has been shown that anemia and tissue iron deficiency exert independent effects on skeletal muscle (Davies et al., 1984; Finch et al., 1976). Anemia primarily affects maximal oxygen consumption. Endurance exercise is markedly impaired by intracellular iron deficiency in the muscle cells (Willis et al., 1988). From a practical point of view, the distinction may be relatively unimportant since anemia and tissue iron deficiency develop simultaneously in humans who suffer from nutritional iron deficiency.

Work Performance

Various factors may contribute to impaired work performance

with iron deficiency. It has been shown that anemia and tissue iron deficiency exert independent effects on the function of organs such as skeletal muscle (Davies et al., 1984; Finch et al., 1976). Anemia primarily affects maximal oxygen consumption. Mild anemia reduces performance during brief but intense exercise (Viteri and Torun, 1974) because of the impaired capacity of skeletal muscle for oxidative metabolism. Endurance exercise is more markedly impaired by intracellular iron deficiency in skeletal muscle cells (Willis et al., 1988).

In laboratory animals, the depletion of oxidative enzymes in skeletal muscle occurs more gradually than the development of anemia (Dallman et al., 1982). The significant decrease in myoglobin and other iron-containing proteins in skeletal muscle of laboratory animals contributes significantly to the decline in muscle aerobic capacity in iron-deficiency anemia and may be a more important factor contributing to the limitation in endurance capacity (Dallman, 1986a; Siimes et al., 1980a).

One study used ^{31}P nuclear magnetic resonance spectroscopy to examine the functional state of bioenergetics in iron-deficient and iron-replete rat gastrocnemius muscle at rest and during 10 seconds of contraction (Thompson et al., 1993). Compared to controls, muscle from iron-deficient animals had a marked increase in muscle phosphocreatine breakdown and a decrease in pH and a slower recovery of phosphocreatine and inorganic phosphate concentrations after exercise. During repletion for 2 to 7 days with iron dextran, there was no substantial improvement in these indicators of muscle mitochondrial energetics. These authors concluded that "tissue factors" such as reduced mitochondrial enzyme activity, decreased number of mitochondria, and altered morphology of the mitochondria might be responsible for impaired muscle function.

Cognitive Development and Intellectual Performance

Studies of iron deficiency anemia and behavior in the developing human and in animal models suggest persistent functional changes. Investigators have demonstrated lower mental and motor test scores and behavioral alterations in infants with iron deficiency anemia (Idjradinata and Pollitt, 1993; Lozoff et al., 1982a, 1982b, 1985, 1987, 1996; Nokes et al., 1998; Walter et al., 1989). In studies conducted in Guatemala and Costa Rica, infants with iron deficiency anemia were rated as more wary and hesitant and maintained closer proximity to caregivers (Lozoff et al., 1985, 1986).

Several studies have shown an improvement in either motor or cognitive development according to Bayley's scale of mental development after iron treatment of iron-deficient infants (Idjradinata and Pollitt, 1993; Lozoff et al., 1987; Oski et al., 1983; Walter et al., 1983). Other studies have failed to show an improvement in either motor or cognitive development scores after providing iron supplements to iron-deficient infants (Lozoff et al., 1982a, 1982b, 1987, 1996; Walter et al., 1989). Lower arithmetic and writing scores, poorer motor functioning, and impaired cognitive processes (memory and selective recall) have been documented in children who were anemic during infancy and were treated with iron (Lozoff et al., 1991, 2000).

Specific central nervous system processes (e.g., slower nerve conduction and impaired memory) appear to remain despite correction of the iron deficiency anemia. There is a general lack of specificity of effect and of information about which brain regions are adversely affected. Recent data from Chile showed a decreased nerve conduction velocity in response to an auditory signal in formerly iron-deficient anemic children despite hematologic repletion with oral iron therapy (Roncagliolo et al., 1998). This is strongly suggestive evidence for decreased myelination of nerve fibers, though other explanations could also exist.

Current thinking about the impact of early iron deficiency anemia attributes some role for "functional isolation," a paradigm in which the normal interaction between stimulation and learning from the physical and social environment is altered (Pollitt et al., 1993; Strupp and Levitsky, 1995).

Adverse Pregnancy Outcomes

Increased perinatal maternal mortality is associated with anemia in women when the anemia is severe (hemoglobin < 40 g/L) (Allen, 1997, 2000; WHO, 1992; Williams and Wheby, 1992). However, even moderate anemia (hemoglobin < 80 g/L) has been associated with a two-fold risk of maternal death (Butler and Bonham, 1963). The mechanisms associated with higher mortality of anemic women are not well understood. Heart failure, hemorrhage, and infection have been identified as possible causes (Fleming, 1968; Taylor et al., 1982).

Several large epidemiological studies have demonstrated that maternal anemia is associated with premature delivery, low birth weight, and increased perinatal infant mortality (see Table 9-1) (Allen, 1997; Garn et al., 1981; Klebanoff et al., 1991; Lieberman et al., 1988; Murphy et al., 1986; Williams and Wheby, 1992). Some of

TABLE 9-1 Association of Anemia and Iron Deficiency with Inadequate Weight Gain and Pregnancy Outcome

| Outcome | Anemia[a] | | | |
	Total	Iron Deficiency	Causes Other Than Iron Deficiency	No Anemia
Low birth weight				
Unadjusted, %[b]	17.1	25.9	15.9	12.2
AOR[c]	1.55	3.10	1.34	1.00
95% confidence interval	0.96–2.51	1.16–4.39	0.80–2.22	—
Preterm delivery				
Unadjusted, %	26.2	44.4	23.5	18.4
AOR[c]	1.30	2.66	1.16	1.00
95% confidence interval	0.86–2.24	1.15–6.17	0.76–1.79	—
Small for gestational age				
Unadjusted, %	11.1	8.3	11.5	7.5
AOR[d]	1.66	1.24	1.67	1.00
95% confidence interval	0.90–3.04	0.29–6.94	0.90–3.41	—
Inadequate weight gain				
Unadjusted, %	31.0	40.0	29.9	24.6
AOR[e]	1.62	2.67	1.51	1.00
95% confidence interval	1.10–2.36	1.13–6.30	1.02–2.25	—

[a] Anemia is defined as a hemoglobin concentration < 110 g/L (first trimester), < 105 g/L (second trimester), < 110 g/L (third trimester), and a serum ferritin concentration < 12 µg/L (CDC, 1989; IOM, 1990).
[b] Percent of anemic women at entry into study.
[c] AOR = adjusted odds ratio. Adjusted for maternal age, parity, ethnicity, prior low-birth-weight or preterm delivery, bleeding at entry into study, gestation at initial blood draw taken at entry into study, number of cigarettes smoked per day, and prepregnancy body mass index.
[d] Adjusted for maternal age, parity, prior low-birth-weight delivery, bleeding at entry into study, gestation at initial blood draw taken at entry into study, number of cigarettes smoked per day, and prepregnancy body mass index.
[e] Adjusted for maternal age, parity, ethnicity, bleeding at entry into study, gestation at initial blood draw (entry), and prepregnancy body mass index.
SOURCE: Scholl et al. (1992).

these studies have been criticized because maternal hemoglobin concentration was measured only at the time of delivery. Physiological factors cause the maternal hemoglobin concentration to rise shortly before delivery. Delivery, occurring early because of known or unknown factors unrelated to anemia, could therefore be expected to show an association with a lower hemoglobin concentration even though anemia played no causal role. Other surveys have shown the association to be present even when hemoglobin concentration was measured earlier in pregnancy. In one recent prospective study, only anemia resulting from iron deficiency was associated with premature labor (Scholl et al., 1992). Furthermore, Goepel and coworkers (1988) reported that premature labor was four times more frequent in women with serum ferritin concentrations below 20 μg/L than in those with higher ferritin concentrations, irrespective of hemoglobin concentration.

High hemoglobin concentrations at the time of delivery are also associated with adverse pregnancy outcomes, such as the newborn infant being small for gestational age (Yip, 2000). Therefore, there is a U-shaped relationship between hemoglobin concentration and prematurity, low birth weight, and fetal death, the risk being increased for hemoglobin concentration below 90 g/L or above 130 g/L. The etiological factors are different, however, at each end of the spectrum. Iron deficiency appears to play a causal role in the presence of significant anemia by limiting the expansion of the maternal erythrocyte cell mass. On the other hand, elevated hemoglobin concentration probably reflects a decreased plasma volume associated with maternal hypertension and eclampsia. Both of the latter conditions have an increased risk of poor fetal outcome (Allen, 1993; Hallberg, 1992; Williams and Wheby, 1992).

Fetal requirements for iron appear to be met at the expense of the mother's needs, but the iron supply to the fetus may still be suboptimal. Several studies suggest that severe maternal anemia is associated with lower iron stores in infants evaluated either at the time of delivery by measuring cord blood ferritin concentration or later in infancy. The effect of maternal iron deficiency on infant status has been reviewed extensively by Allen (1997).

While the observations relating iron status of the mother to the size of stores in infants (based on serum ferritin concentration) are important, it should be noted that the total iron endowment in a newborn infant is directly proportional to birth weight (Widdowson and Spray, 1951). Maternal iron deficiency anemia may therefore limit the infant's iron endowment specifically through an association with premature delivery and low birth weight. Preziosi and coworkers (1997) evaluated the effect of iron supplementation during pregnancy on iron status in newborn babies born to women living in Niger. The prevalence of maternal anemia was 65 to 70 percent at 6 months gestation. The iron status of the infants was also evaluated at 3 and 6 months of age. Although there were no differences between the supplemented and unsupplemented women in cord blood iron indexes at both 3 and 6 months of age, the children born to iron-supplemented women had significantly higher serum ferritin concentrations. Furthermore, it was reported that Apgar scores were significantly higher in infants born to supplemented mothers. There were a total of eight fetal or neonatal deaths, seven in the unsupplemented group.

Other Consequences of Iron Deficiency

With use of in vitro tests and animal models, iron deficiency is associated with impaired host defense mechanisms against infection such as cell-mediated immunity and phagocytosis (Cook and Lynch, 1986). The clinical relevance of these findings is uncertain although iron deficiency may be a predisposing factor for chronic mucocutaneous candidiasis (Higgs, 1973). Iron deficiency is also associated with abnormalities of the mucosa of the mouth and gastrointestinal tract leading to angular stomatitis, glossitis, esophageal webs, and chronic gastritis (Jacobs, 1971). Spoon-shaped fingernails (koilonychia) may be present (Hogan and Jones, 1970). The eating of nonfood material (pica) or a craving for ice (pagophagia) are also associated with iron deficiency (Ansell and Wheby, 1972). Finally, temperature regulation may be abnormal in iron deficiency anemia (Brigham and Beard, 1996).

SELECTION OF INDICATORS FOR ESTIMATING THE REQUIREMENT FOR IRON

Functional Indicators

The most important functional indicators of iron deficiency are reduced physical work capacity, delayed psychomotor development in infants, impaired cognitive function, and adverse effects for both the mother and the fetus as discussed above. As indicated earlier, these adverse consequences of iron deficiency are associated with a degree of iron deficiency sufficient to cause measurable anemia.

A specific functional indicator, such as dark adaptation for vitamin A (see Chapter 4), is used to estimate the average requirement for some nutrients. This is done by evaluating the effect on that functional indicator in a group of experimental subjects fed diets containing graded quantities of the nutrient. The effect of different levels of iron intake on the important functional indicators identified above can not be measured in this way because of the difficulty inherent in quantifying abnormalities in these functional indicators, as well as the complexity of the regulation of iron absorption.

Biochemical Indicators

A series of laboratory indicators can be used to characterize iron status precisely and to categorize the severity of iron deficiency. Three levels of iron deficiency are customarily identified:

- depleted iron stores, but where there appears to be no limitation in the supply of iron to the functional compartment;
- early functional iron deficiency (iron-deficient erythropoiesis) where the supply of iron to the functional compartment is suboptimal but not reduced sufficiently to cause measurable anemia; and
- iron deficiency anemia, where there is a measurable deficit in the most accessible functional compartment, the erythrocyte.

Available laboratory tests can be used in combination to identify the evolution of iron deficiency through these three stages (Table 9-2).

Storage Iron Depletion

Serum Ferritin Concentration. Cellular iron that is not immediately needed for functional compounds is stored in the form of ferritin. Small quantities of ferritin also circulate in the blood. The concentration of plasma and serum ferritin is proportional to the size of body iron stores in healthy individuals and those with early iron deficiency. In an adult, each 1 µg/L of serum ferritin indicates the presence of about 8 mg of storage iron (Bothwell et al., 1979). A similar relationship is present in children in that each 1 µg/L of serum ferritin is indicative of an iron store of about 0.14 mg/kg (Finch and Huebers, 1982). When the serum ferritin concentration falls below 12 µg/L, the iron stores are totally depleted.

Based on the Third National Health and Examination Survey (NHANES III), for adults living in the United States the median serum ferritin concentrations were 36 to 40 µg/L in menstruating

TABLE 9-2 Laboratory Measurements Commonly Used in the Evaluation of Iron Status

Stage of Iron Deficiency	Indicator	Diagnostic Range
Depleted stores	Stainable bone marrow iron	Absent
	Total iron binding capacity	> 400 µg/dL
	Serum ferritin concentration	< 12 µg/L
Early functional iron deficiency	Transferrin saturation	< 16%
	Free erythrocyte protoporphyrin	> 70 µg/dL erythrocyte
	Serum transferrin receptor	> 8.5 mg/L
Iron deficiency anemia	Hemoglobin concentration	< 130 g/ (male)
		< 120 g/L (female)
	Mean cell volume	< 80 fL

SOURCE: Ferguson et al. (1992); INACG (1985).

women and 112 to 156 µg/L in men (Appendix Table G-3). The median serum ferritin concentration was 27 µg/L for adolescent girls and 28 µg/L for pregnant women. These concentrations exceed the cut-off concentration of less than 12 µg/L for adolescent girls and pregnant women (IOM, 1990; Table 9-2).

However, direct correlation between the estimation of iron intakes and iron status is low (Appendix Table H-5). Serum ferritin concentrations are known to be affected by factors other than the size of iron stores. Concentrations are increased in the presence of infections, inflammatory disorders, cancers, and liver disease because ferritin is an acute phase protein (Valberg, 1980). Thus, serum ferritin concentration may fall within the normal range in individuals who have no iron stores. Elevated serum ferritin concentrations are also associated with increased ethanol consumption (Leggett et al., 1990; Osler et al., 1998), increasing body mass index (Appendix Table H-3), and elevated plasma glucose concentration (Appendix Table H-4) (Tuomainen et al., 1997). Dinneen and coworkers (1992) reported high serum ferritin concentration in association with newly diagnosed diabetes mellitus. Analysis of the NHANES III database demonstrated a statistically significant direct correlation between body mass index and serum ferritin concentration in non-Hispanic white men over the age of 20 years, non-Hispanic black men and women aged 20 to 49 years, Mexican-American men aged

20 to 49 years, and Mexican-American women over the age of 50 years (Appendix Table H-3). An examination of the NHANES III database also showed that individuals in the highest quartile for plasma glucose concentration had higher serum ferritin concentrations than those in the lowest quartile for all gender and age groups (Appendix Table H-4). Similar findings were reported by Ford and Cogswell (1999). For these reasons and because of the variability in consumption of promoters and inhibitors of iron absorption, iron intake does not necessarily correlate with ferritin status.

Despite the influence of various unrelated factors on serum ferritin concentration, this indicator is the most sensitive indicator of the amount of iron in the storage compartment.

Total Iron-Binding Capacity. Iron is transported in the plasma and extracellular fluid bound to transferrin. This metalloprotein has a very high affinity for iron. Virtually all plasma iron is bound to transferrin. Therefore it is convenient to measure plasma transferrin concentration indirectly by quantifying the total iron-binding capacity (TIBC), which is the total quantity of iron bound to transferrin after the addition of exogenous iron to plasma. TIBC is elevated with storage iron depletion before there is evidence of inadequate delivery of iron to erythropoetic tissue. An increased TIBC (> 400 μg/dL) is therefore indicative of storage iron depletion. It is less precise than the serum ferritin concentration. About 30 to 40 percent of individuals with iron deficiency anemia have TIBCs that are not elevated (Ravel, 1989). TIBC is reduced in infectious, inflammatory, or neoplastic disorders (Konijn, 1994).

Early Iron Deficiency

Early iron deficiency is signaled by evidence indicating that the iron supply to the bone marrow and other tissues is only marginally adequate. A measurable decrease in the hemoglobin concentration is not yet present and therefore there is no anemia.

Serum Transferrin Saturation. As the iron supply decreases, the serum iron concentration falls and the saturation of transferrin is decreased. Levels below 16 percent saturation indicate that the rate of delivery of iron is insufficient to maintain the normal rate of hemoglobin synthesis. Low saturation levels are not specific for iron deficiency and are encountered in other conditions such as anemia of chronic disease (Cook, 1999), which is associated with impaired release of iron from stores.

The median serum transferrin saturation was 26 to 30 percent for men and 21 to 24 percent for women (Appendix Table G-2). The median serum transferrin saturation was 21 percent for pregnant women and 22 percent for adolescent girls. These values exceed the cut-off value of 16 percent (Table 9-2).

Erythrocyte Protoporphyrin Concentration. Heme is formed in developing erythrocytes by the incorporation of iron into protoporphyrin IX by ferrochetalase. If there is insufficient iron for optimal hemoglobin synthesis, erythrocytes accumulate an excess of protoporphyrin, which remains in the cells for the duration of their lifespans (Cook, 1999). An increased erythrocyte protoporphyrin concentration in the blood therefore indicates that the erythrocytes matured at a time when the iron supply was suboptimal. The cut off concentration for erythrocyte protoporphyrin concentration is greater than 70 µg/dL of erythrocytes. Erythrocyte protoporphyrin concentration is again not specific for iron deficiency and is also associated with inadequate iron delivery to developing erythrocytes (e.g., anemia of chronic disease) or impaired heme synthesis (e.g., lead poisoning). In iron deficiency, zinc can be incorporated into protoporphyrin IX, resulting in the formation of zinc protoporphyrin (Braun, 1999). The zinc protoporphyrin:heme ratio is used as an indicator of impaired heme synthesis and is sensitive to an insufficient iron delivery to the erythrocyte (Braun, 1999).

Soluble Serum Transferrin Receptor Concentration. The surfaces of all cells express transferrin receptors in proportion to their requirement for iron. A truncated form of the extracellular component of the transferrin receptor is produced by proteolytic cleavage and released into the plasma in direct proportion to the number of receptors expressed on the surfaces of body tissues. As functional iron depletion occurs, more transferrin receptors appear on cell surfaces. The concentration of proteolytically cleaved extracellular domains, or soluble serum transferrin receptors (sTfR), rises in parallel. The magnitude of the increase is proportional to the functional iron deficit. The sTfR concentration appears to be a specific and sensitive indicator of early iron deficiency (Akesson et al., 1998; Cook et al., 1990). Furthermore, sTfR concentration is not affected by infectious, inflammatory, and neoplastic disorders (Ferguson et al., 1992). Because commercial assays for sTfR have become available only recently, there is a lack of data relating iron intake to sTfR concentration, as well as relating sTfR concentration to functional outcomes. This indicator may prove to be very useful in identifying iron deficiency, especially in patients who have concurrent infections or other inflammatory disorders.

Iron Deficiency Anemia

Anemia is the most easily identifiable indicator of functional iron deficiency. As discussed above, physiological impairment occurs at this stage of iron deficiency both because of inadequate oxygen delivery during exercise and because of abnormal enzyme function in tissues.

Hemoglobin Concentration and Hematocrit. The hemoglobin concentration or hematocrit is neither a sensitive nor a specific indicator of mild yet functionally significant iron deficiency anemia. Iron deficiency anemia is microcytic (reduced mean erythrocyte volume and mean erythrocyte hemoglobin). However, microcytic anemia is characteristic of all anemias in which the primary abnormality is impaired hemoglobin synthesis. Iron deficiency is only one of the potential causal factors. The diagnosis of iron deficiency anemia, based solely on the presence of anemia, can result in misdiagnosis in many cases.

Garby and coworkers (1969) recognized this fundamental problem. After supplemental iron tablets (60 mg/day) or a placebo were provided to a group of women with mild anemia for 3 months, the women were characterized as having iron deficiency anemia based on a change in hemoglobin concentration in response to the iron supplement that was greater than that which occurred with the placebo. There was a significant overlap between the distribution curves for the initial hemoglobin concentration of the responders (iron deficiency anemia) and the nonresponders (no iron deficiency anemia). A single hemoglobin concentration used as a discriminant value for detecting iron deficiency anemia therefore lacks precision.

Based on NHANES III data (Appendix Table G-1), the median hemoglobin concentration for men was 144 to 154 g/L and 132 to 135 g/L for women. The median hemoglobin concentration was 132 g/L for adolescent girls and 121 g/L for pregnant women. The hemoglobin concentration for pregnant women approaches the cutoff concentration of 120 g/L (IOM, 1990).

Erythrocyte Indexes. Iron deficiency leads to the formation of small erythrocytes. Mean corpuscular hemoglobin (MCH) is the amount of hemoglobin in erythrocytes. The mean corpuscular volume (MCV) is the volume of the average erythrocyte. Both MCH and

MCV are reduced in iron deficiency, but their values are not specific for it. They occur in all conditions that cause impaired hemoglobin synthesis, particularly the thalassemias (Chalevelakis et al., 1984).

Surrogate Laboratory Indicators

As discussed earlier, functional abnormalities occur only when iron deficiency is sufficiently severe to cause measurable anemia. Low iron storage does not appear to have functional consequences in most studies. This does not imply that all functional consequences of iron deficiency are mediated by anemia, but rather that cellular enzymes that require iron become depleted in concert with the development of anemia. There is extensive experimental evidence indicating that tissue iron depletion has significant physiological consequences that are independent of the consequences of anemia (Willis et al., 1988).

Early anemia could nevertheless be chosen as the surrogate functional indicator. However, the significant overlap between the iron-sufficient and the iron-deficient segments of a population limit the sensitivity of this indicator. The precision of the laboratory diagnosis of iron deficiency anemia can be improved by combining hemoglobin measurements with one or more indicators of iron status. The Expert Scientific Working Group (1985) described two models or conceptual frameworks. The ferritin model employs a combination of serum ferritin concentration, erythrocyte protoporphyrin concentration, and transferrin saturation. The presence of two or more abnormal indicators of iron status is indicative of iron deficiency. The MCV model uses MCV, transferrin saturation, and erythrocyte protoporphyrin concentration as indicators. Once again, when two or more indicators are abnormal, this is indicative of iron deficiency. The two models give similar results and improve the specificity of the hemoglobin concentration or hematocrit as an indicator of iron deficiency anemia. They were considered as potential surrogate laboratory indicators of functional iron deficiency for use in estimating requirements, but rejected because they were felt to lack sufficient sensitivity to provide an adequate margin of safety in calculating iron requirements.

The sTfR concentration may, in the future, prove to be a sensitive, reliable, and precise indicator of early functional iron deficiency. At present, however, there are insufficient dose-response data to recommend this indicator.

Methods Considered in Estimating the Average Requirement

In light of the rationale developed in the previous section, the calculation of the Estimated Average Requirement (EAR) is based on the need to maintain a normal, functional iron concentration, but only a minimal store (serum ferritin concentration of 15 µg/L) (IOM, 1993). Two methods of calculation were considered—factorial modeling and iron balance.

Factorial Modeling

Because the distribution of iron requirements is skewed, the simple addition of the components of iron requirement (losses and accretion) cannot be done. Instead, the physiological requirement for absorbed iron can be calculated by factorial modeling of each of the components of iron requirement (basal losses, menstrual losses, and accretion). Total need for absorbed iron can be estimated through the summation of the component needs (losses and accretion) (see Chapter 1, "Method for Setting the RDA when Nutrient Requirements Are Not Normally Distributed"). Information about the distribution of values for the components of iron requirement, such as hemoglobin accretion, are modeled on the basis of known physiology. Since the distributions of some components are not normally distributed (i.e., are skewed), simple addition is inappropriate. In this case, Monte Carlo simulation is used to generate a large theoretical population with the characteristics described by the component distributions. When the final distribution representing the convolution of components has been derived, then the median percentile of the distribution can be used directly to estimate the average requirement for absorbed iron and the ninety-seven and one-half percentile can be used for determining the Recommended Dietary Allowance (RDA). The EAR and RDA are then determined from this data set by dividing by the upper limit of iron absorption.

Basal Losses. Basal losses refer to the obligatory loss of iron in the feces, urine, and sweat and from the exfoliation of skin cells. Attempts to quantify these iron losses by measuring the amount of each of individual component have yielded highly variable results because of the technical difficulties encountered in distinguishing between the small quantities of iron lost from the body and contaminant iron in the samples collected. The only reliable quantitative data for basal iron losses in humans are derived from a single study (Green et al., 1968). However, a study by Bothwell and coworkers

(1979) on iron absorption derived from radioiron absorption tests provides collateral support for the accuracy of the measurements made by Green and coworkers (1968).

The observations made by Green and coworkers (1968) were based on earlier experimental data demonstrating that all body iron compartments are in a constant state of flux and that uniform labeling of all body iron could be achieved several months after the injection of a long-lived radiolabelled iron (^{55}Fe, half life 2.6 years). After uniform labeling is achieved, the change in specific activity of a readily accessible iron compartment (circulating hemoglobin) could be used to calculate the physiological rate of iron loss, provided that iron balance is maintained during the period of observation. They also measured individual compartmental losses from skin and in sweat, urine, and feces separately in other volunteers. Results obtained by summing compartmental losses were similar to the whole body excretion studies. They reported an average calculated daily iron loss of 0.9 to 1.0 mg/day ($\approx$14 µg/kg) in three groups of men with normal iron storage status who lived in South Africa, the United States, and Venezuela (Table 9-3). While there is a need for more information associating body weight with basal iron losses, subsequent analyses of the data from South Africa (R. Green, University of Witwatersrand, Johannesburg, South Africa, personal communication, 2000) showed that within the substudy groups, body weight was an important explanatory variable for basal iron loss; the other very important variable was magnitude of iron stores.

TABLE 9-3 Total Body Iron Losses in Adults

Study Site	Ethnic Group	n	Body Weight kg (SD)[a]	Estimated Loss mg/day (SD)
Washington State	Caucasian	12	78.6 (5.9)	0.98 (0.30)
Venezuela	Mestizo	12	67.6 (8.3)	0.90 (0.31)
Durban (S. Africa)	Indian	17	62.3 (9.2)	1.02 (0.22)
Total (non-Bantu)[b]		41	68.6 (8.1)	0.96 (0.27)
Johannesburg (S. Africa)	Bantu	10	79.0 (6.9)	2.42 (1.09)
Durban (S. Africa)	Bantu	9	69.9 (7.5)	2.01 (0.94)

[a] SD = standard deviation.
[b] Bantu not included. They were selected on the basis of phenotypic iron overload.
SOURCE: Green et al. (1968).

Menstrual Losses. Additional iron is lost from the body as a result of menstruation in fertile women. Menstrual iron losses have been estimated in a number of studies (Beaton, 1974) (see review by Hefnawi and Yacout, 1978) and in three large community surveys conducted in Sweden (Hallberg et al., 1966b), England (Cole et al., 1971), and Egypt (Hefnawi et al., 1980). There was a reasonable degree of consistency between the different studies. The median blood volume lost per period reported in the three largest studies was 20.3 mL (Egypt), 26.5 mL (England), and 30.0 mL (Sweden). Losses greater than 80 mL were reported in less than 10 percent of women.

Accretion. The requirement for pregnancy and for growth in children and adolescents can also be estimated from known changes in blood volume, fetal and placental iron concentration, and the increase in total body erythrocyte mass.

Balance Studies

Chemical balance is the classical method for measuring nutrient requirements through the estimation of daily intake and losses. While this direct approach is conceptually appealing, its use in measuring iron requirements presents several major technical obstacles (Hegsted, 1975). For instance, it is difficult to achieve a steady state with nutrients such as iron that are highly conserved in the body. Because the fraction of the dietary intake that is absorbed (and excreted) is very limited, even small errors in the recovery of unabsorbed food iron in the feces invalidate the results.

Thirteen adult balance studies were evaluated (Table 9-4). All of these studies yielded values that exceed the daily iron loss calculated on the basis of the disappearance of a long-lived iron radioisotope after uniform labeling of body iron (Green et al., 1968). One might therefore conclude that all of the subjects were in positive balance during the period of observation. Moreover, the magnitude of estimated positive balance in most cases predicted the relatively rapid accumulation of body iron. Neither of these conclusions is compatible with numerous other experimental observations. Therefore, balance studies were not considered in estimating an average requirement.

TABLE 9-4 Iron Balance Studies in Adults

Reference	Study Group	Duration	Average Iron Intake (mg/d)	Average Balance Data (mg/d)
Kelsay et al., 1979	12 men, 37–58 y	26 d	21.8 (low fiber) 26.4 (high fiber)	3.8 4.6
Johnson et al., 1982	8 men, 21–28 y	40 d	18.8	1.8–2.3
Snedeker et al.,1982	9 men, 24 y	12 d	17.4	0.56
Andersson et al., 1983	5 men and 1 woman, 25–55 y	24 d	14.9 (white bread) 14.2 (brown bread) 14.1 (whole meal)	1.73 0.7 1.56
Mahalko et al., 1983	27 men, 19–64 y	28 d	15.52 16.31	3.42 5.34
Van Dokkum et al., 1983	10 men, 23 y	20 d	14.4 (high fat) 14.8 (low fat)	3.0 3.0
Behall et al., 1987	11 men, 23–62 y	4 wk	16.6	2.5
Hallfrisch et al., 1987	20 men, 23–56 y 19 women, 21–48 y	1 wk duplicate food record	18.93 11.83	3.01 0.13
Holbrook et al., 1989	19 men, 21–57 y	7 wk	14.8–16.3	−0.9–2.3
Hunt et al., 1990	11 women, 22–36 y	5.5 wk	16.3 13.7	6.3 3.9
Turnlund et al., 1991	8 women, 21–30 y	41–21 d	11.5–12.8 (animal protein) 20–23 (plant protein)	2.9 3.7–4.4
Ivaturi and Kies, 1992	24 men and women	14 d	10.59 10.59 (sucrose) 10.59 (fructose) 10.1 11.3 (sucrose) 11.3 (fructose)	0.524 0.677 −1.715 1.02 0.62 0.79
Coudray et al., 1997	9 men, 21 y	28 d	11.6 (control) 11.5 (inulin) 12.3 (beet fiber)	2.52 1.77 2.21

FACTORS AFFECTING THE IRON REQUIREMENT

The proportion of dietary iron absorbed is determined by the iron requirement of the individual. Absorption is regulated by the size of the body iron store in healthy humans (percentage absorption is inversely proportional to serum ferritin concentration) (Cook et al., 1974). There is a several-fold difference in absorption from a meal between an individual who is iron deficient and someone with sizeable iron stores. The calculation of dietary requirements must be based on the maintenance of a well-defined iron status. This has been accomplished by setting the need for the maintenance of a minimal iron store (serum ferritin concentration cutoff of 15 µg/L) as the surrogate indicator of functional adequacy.

The other major factor to take into account when computing dietary iron requirements is iron bioavailability based on the composition of the diet. Iron is present in food as either part of heme, as found in meat, poultry, and fish, or as nonheme iron, present in various forms in all foods. As previously discussed, the absorption mechanisms are different. Heme iron is always well absorbed and is only slightly influenced by dietary factors. The absorption of nonheme iron is strongly influenced by its solubility and interaction with other meal components in the lumen of the upper small intestine.

Gastric Acidity

Decreased stomach acidity, due to overconsumption of antacids, ingestion of alkaline clay, or pathologic conditions such as achlorhydria or partial gastrectomy, may lead to impaired iron absorption (Conrad, 1968; Kelly et al., 1967).

Nutrient-Nutrient Interactions: Enhancers of Nonheme Iron Absorption

Ascorbic Acid. Ascorbic acid strongly enhances the absorption of nonheme iron. In the presence of ascorbic acid, dietary ferric iron is reduced to ferrous iron which forms a soluble iron-ascorbic acid complex in the stomach. Allen and Ahluwalia (1997) reviewed various studies in which ascorbic acid was added to meals consisting of maize, wheat, and rice. They concluded that iron absorption from meals is increased approximately two-fold when 25 mg of ascorbic acid is added and as much as three- to six-fold when 50 mg is added.

There appears to be a linear relation between ascorbic acid intake and iron absorption up to at least 100 mg of ascorbic acid per meal.

Because ascorbic acid improves iron absorption through the release of nonheme iron bound to inhibitors, the enhanced absorption effect is most marked when consumed with foods containing high levels of inhibitors, including phytate and tannins. Ascorbic acid has been shown to improve iron absorption from infant weaning foods by two- to six-fold (Derman et al., 1980; Fairweather-Tait et al., 1995a).

Other Organic Acids. Other organic acids including citric acid, lactic acid, and malic acid have not been studied as thoroughly as ascorbic acid, but they also have some enhancing effects on nonheme iron absorption (Gillooly et al., 1983).

Animal Tissues. Meat, fish, and poultry improve iron nutrition both by providing highly bioavailable heme iron and by enhancing nonheme iron absorption. The mechanism of this enhancing effect on nonheme iron absorption is poorly described though it is likely to involve low molecular weight peptides that are released during digestion (Taylor et al., 1986).

Nutrient:Nutrient Interactions: Inhibitors of Nonheme Iron Absorption

Phytate. Phytic acid (inositol hexaphosphate) is present in legumes, rice, and grains. The inhibition of iron absorption from added iron is related to the level of phytate in a food (Brune et al., 1992; Cook et al., 1997). The absorption of iron was shown to increase four- to five-fold when the phytic acid concentration was reduced from 4.9 to 8.4 mg/g, to less than 0.1 mg/g in soy protein isolate (Hurrell et al., 1992). Genetically modified, low-phytic acid strains of maize have been developed. Iron absorption with consumption of low-phytic acid strains was 49 percent greater than with consumption of wild type strains of maize (Mendoza et al., 1998). Still, the overall availability of iron remained quite low and generally under 8 percent, even for subjects with marginal iron status. The absorption of iron from legumes such as soybeans, black beans, lentils, mung beans, and split peas has been shown to be very low (0.84 to 1.91 percent) and similar to each other (Lynch et al., 1984). Because phytate and iron are concentrated in the aleurone layer and germ of grains, milling to white flour and white rice reduces the content of phytate and iron (Harland and Oberleas, 1987), thereby increasing the bioavailability of the remaining iron (Sandberg, 1991).

Polyphenols. Polyphenols markedly inhibit the absorption of nonheme iron. This was first recognized when tea consumption was shown to inhibit iron absorption (Disler et al., 1975). Iron binds to tannic acid in the intestinal lumen forming an insoluble complex that results in impaired absorption. The inhibitory effects of tannic acid are dose-dependent and reduced by the addition of ascorbic acid (Siegenberg et al., 1991; Tuntawiroon et al., 1991). The response to iron supplementation was shown to be significantly greater for Guatemalan toddlers who did not consume coffee (which contains tannic acid) than for those who did (Dewey et al., 1997). Polyphenols are also found in many grain products, other foods, herbs such as oregano, and red wine (Gillooly et al., 1984).

Vegetable Proteins. Soybean protein has an inhibitory effect on nonheme iron absorption that is not dependent on the phytate effect (Lynch et al., 1994). Bioavailability is improved by fermentation, which leads to protein degradation. The iron bioavailability from other legumes and nuts is also poor.

Calcium. Calcium inhibits the absorption of both heme and nonheme iron (Hallberg et al., 1991). The mechanism is not well understood (Whiting, 1995); however, calcium has been shown to inhibit iron absorption, in part by interfering with the degradation of phytic acid. Furthermore, it has been suggested that calcium inhibits heme and nonheme iron absorption during transfer through the mucosal cell (Hallberg et al., 1993). Calcium has a direct dose-related inhibiting effect on iron absorption such that absorption was reduced by 50 to 60 percent at doses of 300 to 600 mg of calcium added to wheat rolls (Hallberg et al., 1991). Inhibition may be maximal at this level. When preschool children consumed mean calcium intakes of 502 or 1,180 mg/day, no difference was observed in the erythrocyte incorporation of iron (Ames et al., 1999). Despite the significant reduction of iron absorption by calcium in single meals, little effect has been observed on serum ferritin concentrations in supplementation trials with supplement levels ranging from 1,000 to 1,500 mg/day of calcium (Dalton et al., 1997; Minihane and Fairweather-Tait, 1998; Sokoll and Dawson-Hughes, 1992).

Algorithms for Estimating Dietary Iron Bioavailability

Despite the complexity of the food supply, the various inter-actions, and the lack of long-term bioavailability studies, attempts have been made to develop an algorithm for estimating iron bio-availability based on nutrients and food components that improve and inhibit iron bioavailability. Monsen and coworkers (1978) developed a model that was based on the level of dietary meat, fish, or poultry and ascorbic acid.

Most recently, an algorithm has been developed and validated for calculating absorbed heme and nonheme iron by the summation of absorption values derived from single-meal studies to estimate the iron absorption from whole diets (Hallberg and Hulthen, 2000). This algorithm involves estimating iron absorption on the basis of the meal content of phytate, polyphenols, ascorbic acid, calcium, eggs, meat, seafood, soy protein, and alcohol. Reddy and coworkers (2000) have developed another algorithm based on the animal tissue, phytic acid, and ascorbic acid content of meals. It is also important to note that single-meal studies may exaggerate the impact of factors affecting iron bioavailability. Cook and coworkers (1991) compared nonheme iron bioavailability from single meals with that of a diet consumed over a 2-week period. There was a 4.5-fold difference between maximally enhancing and maximally inhibiting single meals. The difference was only two-fold when measured over the 2-week period.

The determination of an Estimated Average Requirement (EAR) depends on a precise assessment of the physiological requirement for absorbed iron and the estimation of the maximum rate of absorption that can be attained by individuals just maintaining the level of iron nutriture considered adequate to ensure normal function. As discussed earlier, normal function is preserved in individuals with a normal functional iron compartment provided that the dietary iron supply is secure and of sufficiently high bioavailability. There appears to be no physiological benefit to maintaining more than a minimal iron store (Siimes et al., 1980a, 1980b). The EAR is therefore set to reflect absorption levels in individuals with a normal complement of functional iron, but only minimal storage iron as indicated by a serum ferritin concentration of 15 µg/L (IOM, 1993). The selection of this criterion for adequate iron balance is critical to determining the EAR because iron absorption is controlled primarily by the size of iron stores. As iron stores rise, the percentage of dietary iron absorption and apparent bioavailability fall (Cook et al., 1974).

The second factor that is critical to determining the EAR is dietary iron bioavailability. Although much is known about the factors that enhance and inhibit iron absorption, the application of specific algorithms based on these factors to complex diets remains imprecise. Based on the general properties of the major dietary enhancers, the FAO/WHO (1988) identified three levels of bioavailability and the associated compositional characteristics of such diets. The typical diversified U.S. and Canadian diets containing generous quantities of flesh foods and ascorbic acid were judged to be 15 percent bioavailable. Constrained vegetarian diets, consisting mainly of cereals and vegetable foods with only small quantities of meat, fish, and ascorbic acid, were judged to be 10 percent bioavailable; very restricted vegetarian diets were judged to be 5 percent bioavailable. These levels of absorption were predicted for individuals who were not anemic, but had no storage iron. A mixed American or Canadian diet would therefore be predicted to allow the absorption of about 15 percent of the dietary iron in an individual whose iron status was selected as a basis for calculating the EAR (serum ferritin concentration of 15 µg/L).

Hallberg and Rossander-Hulten (1991) suggested that the bioavailability of iron in the U.S. diet may be somewhat higher than 15 percent: approximately 17 percent. Some support for this contention was provided by the observation of Cook and coworkers (1991) who measured nonheme iron absorption over a 2-week period in free-living American volunteers eating their customary diets. After correcting nonheme iron values (to a serum ferritin concentration of 15 µg/L), the bioavailability of nonheme iron in self-selected diets was 16.8 percent ([34 µg/L ÷ 15 µg/L] × 7.4 percent). Heme constitutes 10 to 15 percent of iron in the adult diet (Raper et al., 1984) and the diet of children (see Appendix Table I-2) and is always well absorbed. Based on a conservative estimation for overall heme absorption of 25 percent (Hallberg and Rossander-Hulten, 1991) and again a conservative estimate for the proportion of dietary iron that is in the form of heme (10 percent), estimated overall iron bioavailability in the mixed American or Canadian diet is approximately 18 percent:

Overall iron absorption = (Fraction of nonheme iron [0.9] × proportion of nonheme iron absorption [0.168]) + (Fraction of heme iron [0.1] × proportion of heme iron absorption [0.25]) × 100 = 17.6 percent.

For these reasons, 18 percent bioavailability is used to estimate the average requirement of iron for children over the age of 1 year, adolescents, and nonpregnant adults consuming the mixed diet typically consumed in the United States and Canada. The diets of most infants aged 7 through 12 months contain little meat and are rich in cereals and vegetables, a diet that approximates a medium bioavailability of 10 percent (Davidsson et al., 1997; Fairweather-Tait et al., 1995a; FAO/WHO, 1988; Skinner et al., 1997).

FINDINGS BY LIFE STAGE AND GENDER GROUP

Infants Ages 0 through 6 Months

Method Used to Set the Adequate Intake

No functional criteria of iron status have been demonstrated that reflect response to dietary intake in young infants. Thus, recommended intakes of iron are based on an Adequate Intake (AI) that reflects the observed mean iron intake of infants principally fed human milk.

At birth, the normal full-term infant has a considerable endowment of iron and a very high hemoglobin concentration. Because the mobilization of body iron stores is very high, the requirement for exogenous iron is virtually zero. After birth, an active process of shifts in iron compartments takes place. Fetal hemoglobin concentration falls, usually reaching a nadir when the infant is between 4 and 6 months of age, and adult hemoglobin formation begins because hematopoiesis is very active. Some time between 4 and 6 months, exogenous sources of iron are used and after 6 months, it can be assumed that the stores endowed at birth have been utilized and that the physiological norm is to meet iron needs from exogenous rather than endogenous sources as erythropoiesis becomes more active. Thereafter, the hemoglobin concentration rises slowly but continuously (1 to 2 g/L/year) through at least puberty (longer in males) (Beaton et al., 1989). This normal physiological sequence of events complicates the estimation of iron requirements.

It is widely accepted that the iron intake of infants exclusively fed human milk must meet or exceed the actual needs of almost all of these infants and that the described pattern of utilization of iron stores is physiologically normal, not indicative of the beginning of iron deficiency. For this age group, it is assumed that the iron provided by human milk is adequate to meet the iron needs of the infant exclusively fed human milk from birth through 6 months. Therefore, the method described in Chapter 2 is used to set an AI for young infants based on the daily amount of iron secreted in human milk. The average iron concentration in human milk is 0.35 mg/L (Table 9-5). Therefore, the AI is set at 0.27 mg/day (0.78 L/day × 0.35 mg/L).

Since there is strong reason to expect that iron intake and iron requirement are both related to achieved body size and growth rate (milk volume relating to energy demand), it is assumed that a correlation between intake and requirement exists. This allows the group mean intake to be lower than the ninety-seven and one-half percentile of requirements (Recommended Dietary Allowance). Therefore, there should be no expectation that an intake of 0.27 mg/day is adequate to meet the needs of almost all individual infants and therefore should be applied with extreme care.

Iron AI Summary, Ages 0 through 6 Months

AI for Infants
    0–6 months   **0.27 mg/day of iron**

Special Considerations

The iron concentration in cow milk ranges between 0.2 and 0.3 mg/L (Lonnerdal et al., 1981). Although the iron content in human milk is lower, iron is significantly more bioavailable in human milk (45 to 100 percent) compared to infant formula (10 percent) (Fomon et al., 1993; Lonnerdal et al., 1981). Casein is the major iron-binding protein in cow milk (Hegenauer et al., 1979). Because of the poor absorption of iron, in the United States cow milk is not recommended for ingestion by infants until after 1 year of age; in Canada it is not recommended until after 9 months of age. In addition, the ingestion of cow milk by infants, especially in the first 6 months of life, has been associated with small amounts of blood loss in the stool. The cause of the blood loss is not well understood, but is assumed to be an allergic-type reaction between a protein in cow milk and the enterocytes of the gastrointestinal tract. Because the early, inappropriate ingestion of cow milk is associated with a higher risk of iron deficiency anemia, it would be prudent to monitor iron status of any infants ingesting cow milk. If anemia is detected, it should be treated with an appropriate dose of medicinal iron.

The American Academy of Pediatrics (AAP, 1999) and Canadian Paediatric Society (1991) reviewed the role of commercial formulas in infant feeding. Their conclusion was that infants who are not, or only partially, fed human milk should receive an iron-fortified formula.

TABLE 9-5 Iron Concentration in Human Milk

Reference	Study Group	Maternal Intake (mg/d)	Stage of Lactation	Milk Concentration (mg/L)	Estimated Iron Intake of Infants (mg/d)[a]
Picciano and Guthrie, 1976	50 women	Not reported	6–12 wk	0.202	0.15
Vaughan et al., 1979	38 women, 19–42 y	Not reported	1–3 mo	0.49	0.38
		39.3	4–6 mo	0.43	0.34
		47.1	7–9 mo	0.42	0.25
		40.8	10–12 mo	0.38	0.23
		65.5	13–18 mo	0.39	0.23
		16.4	19–31 mo	0.42	0.25
Lemons et al., 1982	7 women	Not reported	1 wk	0.77	0.60
			2 wk	0.98	0.76
			3 wk	0.80	0.62
Mendelson et al., 1982	10 women	Not reported	3–5 d	1.11	0.86
			8–10 d	0.99	0.77
			15–17 d	0.81	0.63
			28–30 d	0.88	0.68
Dewey and Lonnerdal, 1983	20 women	Not reported	1 mo	0.31	0.20
			2 mo	0.22	0.17
			3 mo	0.25	0.21
			4 mo	0.22	0.18
			5 mo	0.20	0.13
			6 mo	0.21	0.13
Garza et al., 1983	6 women, 26–35 y	Not reported	6 mo	0.029	0.02
			7 mo	0.042	0.03
			8 mo	0.050	0.03
Lipsman et al., 1985	7–13 teens	15.0 (mean at 7 mo)	1 mo	0.4	0.31
			2 mo	0.3	0.23
			3 mo	0.4	0.31
			4 mo	0.35	0.27
			5 mo	0.3	0.23
			6 mo	0.25	0.15
			7 mo	0.22	0.13
	12–17 adults	Not reported	1 mo	0.30	0.23
			2 mo	0.22	0.17
			3 mo	0.25	0.19
			4 mo	0.22	0.17
			5 mo	0.20	0.16
			6 mo	0.22	0.17

continued

TABLE 9-5 Continued

Reference	Study Group	Maternal Intake (mg/d)	Stage of Lactation	Milk Concentration (mg/L)	Estimated Iron Intake of Infants (mg/d)[a]
Butte et al., 1987	45 women	16.2	1 mo	Not reported	0.19
		14.1	2 mo		0.15
		13.9	3 mo		0.13
		13.5	4 mo		0.12
Anderson, 1993	7 women	Not reported	Up to 5 mo	0.26	0.20

[a] Iron intake based on reported data or concentration (mg/L) × 0.78 L/day for 0–6 months postpartum and concentration (mg/L) × 0.6 L/day for 7–12 months postpartum.

Infants Ages 7 through 12 Months

Evidence Considered in Estimating the Average Requirement

For older infants the approach to estimation of requirements is parallel to that of other age and gender groups. Although body iron stores decrease during the first 6 months (and this is seen as physiologically normal), it is appropriate to make provision for the maintenance and development of modest iron stores in early life, even though requirements for older children, adolescents, and adults do not make provision for iron storage as a part of requirement.

For infants over the age of 6 months, it becomes both feasible and desirable to model the factorial components of absorbed iron requirements to set the Estimated Average Requirement (EAR) and Recommended Dietary Allowance (RDA) (see "Selection of Indicators for Estimating the Requirement for Iron—Factorial Modeling"). The major components of iron need for older infants are:

• obligatory fecal, urinary, and dermal losses (basal losses);
• increase in hemoglobin mass (increase in blood volume and increase in hemoglobin concentration);
• increase in tissue (nonstorage) iron; and
• increase in storage iron (as noted earlier, building a small reserve in very young children is seen as important).

A number of these component estimates can be linked to achieved size and growth rate. Dibley and coworkers (1987) provided data on both estimates. Median body weights at 6 and 12 months were 7.8 and 10.2 kg for boys and 7.2 and 9.5 kg for girls (Dibley et al., 1987) and the body weight at the midpoint between 7 and 12 months (0.75 years) were 9 and 8.4 kg for male and female infants, respectively. These weights are similar to the reference weights provided in Table 1-1. Approximate normality was assumed and the standard deviation (SD) estimates for infants fed human milk were used as an indicator of likely variability in body size (WHO, 1994). These were taken to present a coefficient of variation (CV) of about 10 percent for this age group.

Basal Losses. The estimated basal loss of iron in infants is taken as 0.03 mg/kg/day (Garby et al., 1964). On the assumption that the variability of these losses is proportional to the variability of weight, the accepted estimates of basal losses at 6 and 12 months are 0.22 ± 0.02 (SD) mg/day at 6 months and 0.31 ± 0.03 (SD) mg/day at 12 months for both genders; the midrange estimate is 0.26 ± 0.03 (SD) mg/day.

Increase in Hemoglobin Mass. The rate of hemoglobin formation, and hence iron needed for that purpose, is a function of rate of growth (weight velocity). The median or average growth rate is estimated as 13 g/day (2,400 g/180 days) for boys and 12.7 g/day (2,300 g/180 days) for girls, suggesting 13.0 g/day (0.39 kg/month) for both genders (Dibley et al., 1987). The World Health Organization Working Group on Infant Growth (WHO, 1994) gathered data on growth velocity from limited longitudinal studies of infants fed human milk. The reported means and SDs for 2-month weight increments at ages 8 to 20 months were 0.27 ± 0.14 kg/month (9 g/day) for boys and 0.26 ± 0.12 kg/month (8.6 g/day) for girls. The observed CV was 45 to 52 percent. Although skewing of the distributions would be expected, no information was provided. For the purposes of this report, the median weight increment is taken as 13 g/day for both genders, and the SD is taken as 6.5 (CV, 50 percent).

If blood volume is estimated to be 70 mL/kg (Hawkins, 1964), the median hemoglobin concentration as 120 g/L, and the iron content of hemoglobin as 3.39 mg/g (Smith and Rios, 1974), then the amount of iron utilized for increase in hemoglobin mass can also be estimated:

Weight gain (0.39 kg/month) × blood volume factor (70 mL/kg) ×
hemoglobin concentration (0.12 mg/mL) ×
iron concentration in hemoglobin (3.39 mg/g) ÷
30 days/month = 0.37 mg/day.

The CV of iron utilization for this function is taken as the CV for weight gain, and thus the estimate becomes 0.37 ± 0.195 (SD) mg/day.

Increase in the Nonstorage Iron Content of Tissues. The nonstorage iron content of tissues has been estimated as 0.7 mg/kg body weight for a 1-year-old child (Smith and Rios, 1974). On the assumption that this estimate can be applied at age 7 months as well, the average tissue iron deposition would be

Weight gain (13.3 g/day) × nonstorage iron content (0.7 mg/kg) =
0.009 mg/day.

Applying the CV accepted for weight gain (50 percent) gives a modeling estimate of tissue iron deposition of 0.009 ± 0.0045 (SD) mg/day.

Increase in Storage Iron. The desired level of iron storage is a matter of judgment rather than physiologically definable need. In this report, it is assumed that body iron storage should approximate 12 percent of total iron deposition (Dallman, 1986b), or

(Increase in hemoglobin iron [0.37 mg/day] +
Increase in nonstorage tissue iron [0.009 mg/day]) ×
(Percent of total tissue iron that is stored [12 percent] ÷
Percent of total iron that is not stored [100 − 12 percent]) =
0.051 mg/day.

The variability would be proportional to the combined variability of hemoglobin deposition and nonstorage iron deposition.

Total Requirement for Absorbed Iron. Median total iron deposition (hemoglobin mass + nonstorage iron + iron storage) is 0.43 mg/day (0.37 + 0.009 + 0.051) and basal iron loss is 0.26 ± 0.03 (SD) mg/day. Therefore, the median total requirement for absorbed iron is 0.69 ± 0.145 (SD) mg/day (Table 9-6).

TABLE 9-6 Summary Illustration of Median Absorbed Iron Requirements for Infants and Young Children

Age (y)	Weight[a] (kg)	Estimated Surface Area[b] (m²)	Estimated Change in Hemoglobin Mass[c] (g/y)	Basal Loss[d] (mg/d)
Infants 6–12 mo[h]	8.7	—	—	0.26
Males				
1.5	11.6	0.5340	30.2	0.29
2.5	13.6	0.6064	19.8	0.33
3.5	15.5	0.6700	22.7	0.36
4.5	17.5	0.7353	21.8	0.39
5.5	19.6	0.7996	26.2	0.43
6.5	21.9	0.8675	26.7	0.47
7.5	24.7	0.9422	29.9	0.51
8.5	26.8	0.9980	35.7	0.54
Females				
1.5	10.8	0.5104	33.5	0.27
2.5	12.8	0.5842	28.4	0.31
3.5	14.7	0.6486	22.5	0.35
4.5	16.8	0.7166	24.4	0.39
5.5	19.0	0.7845	20.7	0.42
6.5	21.3	0.8524	19.7	0.46
7.5	23.8	0.9209	29.9	0.49
8.5	26.9	0.9986	27.0	0.54

[a] Representative anthropometry for modeling, based on Frisancho (1990).
[b] Computed by equation of Haycock et al. (1978).
[c] Derived from Table 9-7.
[d] Based on 0.538 mg/m²/d, extrapolated from Green et al. (1968).
[e] Based on assumed 0.7 g/kg body weight gain (Smith and Rios, 1974).
[f] Calculated as 12 percent of total iron deposition through 3.0 years of age then falling; no provision for storage at 9.0 years of age.

Dietary Iron Bioavailability. During the second 6 months of life, it is assumed that complementary feeding is in place. The primary food introduced at this time is infant cereal, most often fortified with low-bioavailable iron (Davidsson et al., 2000); this cereal is the primary source of iron (see Appendix Table I-1). Feeding with human milk and infant formula (possibly fortified with iron), may continue. Iron absorption averaged 14.8 percent in human milk (Abrams et al., 1997). A study on food intakes of infants showed that by 1 year of age, over half of the infants consumed cereals and fruits, but less

Hemoglobin Iron Deposition (mg/d)	Increase in Tissue Iron[e] (mg/d)	Increase in Storage Iron[f] (mg/d)	Total Iron Need[g]	
			Median (g/d)	97.5th Percentile (g/d)
0.37	0.009	0.051	0.69	1.07
0.28	0.004	0.038	0.62	1.24
0.18	0.004	0.023	0.54	1.23
0.21	0.004	0.025	0.61	1.36
0.20	0.004	0.021	0.63	1.45
0.24	0.004	0.019	0.70	1.60
0.25	0.004	0.015	0.74	1.71
0.28	0.004	0.011	0.81	1.86
0.33	0.004	0.006	0.81	2.01
0.31	0.004	0.038	0.64	1.25
0.26	0.004	0.032	0.63	1.30
0.21	0.004	0.026	0.59	1.32
0.23	0.004	0.023	0.65	1.45
0.19	0.004	0.016	0.64	1.52
0.15	0.004	0.011	0.66	1.61
0.28	0.004	0.011	0.79	1.83
0.25	0.004	0.005	0.80	1.92

[g] Estimates derived from simulated population that take into account impact of skewing and are the basis for the Estimated Average Requirement (EAR) and Recommended Dietary Allowance (RDA).

[h] Requirements for infants and young children were estimated by different methods. Upper limit of absorption for infants and children is 10 and 18 percent, respectively. See text for methods used for infants and children.

than half consumed meat or meat mixtures (Skinner et al., 1997). Only 32 percent of infants consumed beef at 12 months of age. Therefore, a moderate bioavailability of 10 percent is used to set the EAR at 6.9 mg/day (0.69 ÷ 0.1).

Iron EAR and RDA Summary, Ages 7 through 12 Months

The EAR has been set by modeling the components of iron requirements, estimating the requirement for absorbed iron at the fiftieth percentile, with use of an upper limit of 10 percent iron absorption and rounding (see Appendix Table I-3).

EAR for Infants
    7–12 months   **6.9 mg/day of iron**

The RDA has been set by modeling the components of iron requirements, estimating the requirement for absorbed iron at the ninety-seven and one-half percentile, with use of an upper limit of 10 percent iron absorption and rounding (see Appendix Table I-3).

RDA for Infants
    7–12 months   **11 mg/day of iron**

Children Ages 1 through 8 Years

Evidence Considered in Estimating the Average Requirement

The EAR for children 1 through 8 years is determined by factorial modeling of the median components of iron requirements (see "Selection of Indicators for Estimating the Requirement for Iron—Factorial Modeling"). The model is presented for males and females though gender is ignored in deriving the EAR for young children because the gender differences are sufficiently small. The major components of iron need for young children are:

- basal iron losses;
- increase in hemoglobin mass;
- increase in tissue (nonstorage iron); and
- increase in storage iron.

A fundamental influence on body iron accretion is the rate of change of body weight (growth rate). Because variability in body weight is needed for calculating the distribution of basal losses, the reference weights in Table 1-1 were not used. Median change in body weight was estimated as the slope of a linear regression of reported median body weights on age (weight = 7.21 + 2.29 × age, for pooled gender) (Frisancho, 1990) (Table 9-6). The fit was satisfactorily close for the purpose of modeling. Inclusion of gender in the model demonstrated that boys typically weighed more than girls, but the interaction term was insignificant, statistically and biologically. A median rate of weight change of 2.3 kg/year or 6.3 g/day was assumed for both sexes.

For each component discussed above, the data for children 1 through 3.9 years and 4 through 8.9 years were used for modeling the iron needs for children 1.5 through 3.5 years and 4.5 through 8.5 years, respectively. The midpoints for these age ranges are 2.5 and 6.5 years, which were used to estimate the total requirements for absorbed iron.

Basal Losses. Basal iron losses for children, aged 1.5 to 8.5 years, were derived from the total body iron losses directly measured from adult men (Green et al., 1968) (see "Selection of Indicators for Estimating the Requirement for Iron—Factorial Modeling"). Rather than assuming a linear function of body weight, estimated losses were adjusted to the child's body size on the basis of estimated surface area (Haycock et al., 1978). Body surface area was used rather than body weight because it is directly related to dermal iron losses (Bothwell and Finch, 1962) and because it is a predictor of metabolic size. On this basis, the adult male basal loss was computed as 0.538 mg/m^2/day (Green et al., 1968). The derived values are presented in Table 9-6.

Garby and coworkers (1964) found that iron lost from the gastro-intestinal tract alone was 0.03 mg/kg in infants, an amount that would yield higher estimated basal losses than were determined by extrapolating from the data of Green and coworkers (1968). Therefore, the basal losses of children 1 through 8 years of age may be underestimated. Nonetheless, the data of Green coworkers (1968) were used because of the greater number of study subjects ($n = 41$ versus $n = 3$ studied by Garby and coworkers [1964]), as well as the finding that basal losses are related to body size (Bothwell and Finch, 1962; R. Green, University of Witwatersrand, Johannesburg, South Africa, personal communication, 2000).

Increase in Hemoglobin Mass. Median increase in hemoglobin mass was estimated as

$$\text{Hemoglobin mass (g)} = \text{blood volume (mL/kg)} \times \text{hemoglobin concentration (g/L)}.$$

During growth, both blood volume and hemoglobin concentration change with age. Although blood volume is a function of body weight, the actual relationship between blood volume and weight appears to change with age. Hawkins (1964) estimated blood volume at specific ages by averaging estimates obtained by several calculations based on body weight or body surface area. Hawkins' estimates are presented in Table 9-7. Age- and gender-specific hemoglobin concentration is estimated from the equations of Beaton and coworkers (1989) using 119 + 1.4 g/L/year in males and 121 + 1.1 g/L/year in females. Estimated blood volume and hemoglobin mass are shown in Table 9-7. Change in hemoglobin mass was estimated between mass at successive ages (Table 9-6). Iron needs were computed from the estimated change of hemoglobin mass and its expected iron content (3.39 mg/g). Thus, for example, from Table 9-7, the increase in hemoglobin mass between ages 7 and 8 years was 29.9 g (from 231.8 to 261.7). That represents 101.4 mg of iron (29.9 g × 3.39 mg/g) per year or 0.28 mg/day, as shown for increase in hemoglobin mass at 7.5 years in Table 9-6.

TABLE 9-7 Estimates of Blood Volume and Hemoglobin Mass, by Age and Gender

Age (y)	Weight (kg)[a]	Blood Volume (L)[b]	Hemoglobin Concentration (g/L)[c]	Hemoglobin Mass (g)
Males				
1	9.8	0.70	120.4	84.3
2	12.5	0.94	121.8	114.5
3	14.3	1.09	123.2	134.3
4	16.6	1.26	124.6	157.0
5	18.5	1.42	126.0	178.9
6	20.7	1.61	127.4	205.1
7	23.0	1.80	128.8	231.8
8	25.7	2.01	130.2	261.7
9	28.5	2.26	131.6	297.4
Females				
1	9.2	0.66	122.1	80.5
2	11.9	0.92	123.2	113.3
3	13.8	1.06	124.3	131.7
4	16.1	1.23	125.4	154.2
5	18.3	1.41	126.5	178.4
6	20.2	1.56	127.6	199.1
7	22.4	1.70	128.7	218.8
8	25.3	1.91	129.8	247.9
9	27.9	2.10	130.9	274.9

[a] Body weights are estimated by Frisancho (1990).
[b] Blood volume estimates based on Hawkins (1964).
[c] Hemoglobin concentrations estimates from Beaton et al. (1989).

Increase in the Nonstorage Iron Content of Tissues. Iron deposition was derived with use of the estimate of body weight change (0.7 mg/kg) (Smith and Rios, 1974) and the median rate of weight change (2.29 kg/year). The estimated deposition is estimated to be 0.004 mg/day (2.29 kg/year × 0.7 mg/kg ÷ 365 days/year) for all age groups (Table 9-6).

Increase in Storage Iron. Similar to the calculation described for older infants, increase in storage iron was computed as

Increase in hemoglobin mass (mg/day) +
Increase in tissue iron (mg/day) ×
Portion of total tissue iron that is stored (12 percent).

This calculation was used for estimating an increase in iron stores for children up to 3 years old and was based on an estimated 12 percent of iron that enters storage (Dallman, 1986b). Beyond age 3 years, this percent progressively falls to no provision of iron stores by 9 years of age. The iron storage allowance for each age group is shown in Table 9-6

Total Requirement for Absorbed Iron. Total requirement for absorbed iron for children 1 through 8 years is based on the higher estimates derived for males. Median total iron deposition (hemoglobin mass + nonstorage iron + iron storage) is 0.21 mg/day (0.18 + 0.004 + 0.023) and basal iron loss is 0.33 mg/day for children aged 1 through 3 years. Therefore, the median total requirement for absorbed iron is 0.54 mg/day (Table 9-6). The median total iron deposition is 0.27 mg/day (0.25 + 0.004 + 0.015) and basal iron loss is 0.47 mg/day for children 4 through 8 years. Therefore, the median total requirement for absorbed iron is 0.74 mg/day (Table 9-6).

Dietary Iron Bioavailability. Based on a heme iron intake of 11 percent of total iron for children 1 to 8 years old, the upper limit of absorption is 18 percent (see "Factors Affecting the Iron Requirement—Algorithms for Estimating Dietary Iron Bioavailability" and Appendix Table I-2).

The derived estimates of dietary requirements are shown in Table 9-8. Representative values are selected for tabulated EARs and RDAs. The derived distributions of requirements for children 1 year of age and older are skewed and are tabulated in Appendix Table I-3.

Estimation of the Variability of Requirements. For the estimation of

TABLE 9-8 Derived Estimates of the Estimated Average Requirement (EAR) and Recommended Dietary Allowance (RDA) for Young Children

Age (y)	Requirement for Absorbed Iron (mg/d)		Dietary Reference Intakes[a] (mg/d)	
	Median	97.5th Percentile	EAR	RDA
Males				
1.5	0.62	1.24	3.4	6.9
2.5	0.54	1.23	2.9	6.8
3.5	0.61	1.36	3.4	7.6
4.5	0.63	1.45	3.5	7.9
5.5	0.70	1.60	3.9	8.1
6.5	0.74	1.71	4.1	9.5
7.5	0.81	1.86	4.5	10.3
8.5	0.81	2.01	4.5	11.2
Females				
1.5	0.64	1.25	3.4	6.9
2.5	0.63	1.30	2.7	7.2
3.5	0.59	1.32	3.3	7.3
4.5	0.65	1.45	3.4	8.1
5.5	0.64	1.52	3.4	8.4
6.5	0.66	1.61	3.6	8.9
7.5	0.79	1.83	4.3	10.2
8.5	0.80	1.92	4.4	10.7

[a] Based on 18 percent upper limit of absorption.

variability of requirements, it is necessary to have an estimate of the variability of weight velocity. The Infant Growth Study (WHO, 1994) offers an estimate of the variability of 2-month weight gains at 10 to 12 months. The apparent CV was 62.5 percent in boys and 63.6 percent in girls. The report on weight velocity standards for the United Kingdom (Tanner et al., 1966) seems to suggest a CV of 25 to 30 percent for 1-year weight velocities in children in the age group examined at each year of age. Given that the relative variability (CV) increases as the duration of the increment interval decreases, it was judged appropriate to accept a somewhat higher estimate of the variability in biologically meaningful intervals. A CV of 40 percent for weight velocity in boys and girls at ages 1 through 8 years is estimated. In all likelihood, the actual distribution of weight velocities is skewed, but no estimates of the actual distribution characteristics have been identified.

The variabilities of both hemoglobin iron deposition and tissue iron deposition were assigned the CV for weight gain (40 percent). Basal iron loss is estimated on the basis of surface area. The logical variability would be proportional to the variability of surface area. To obtain an estimate of variability of basal losses, these were computed for weights and heights reported in the U.S. Department of Agriculture (USDA) Continuing Survey of Food Intakes by Individuals (CSFII) (self-reported weight and height), and the variability of estimate within 1-year age intervals was examined. CVs of square root-transformed data for individual age-sex groups were examined, as well as the linear scale, and all showed appreciable departure from normality, but the square root transformation was empirically the best fit. CVs for individual age-sex groups ranged from 29 percent in 8-year-old boys to 47.4 percent in 4-year-old boys. With use of a statistical model that took into account age and gender effects, an overall CV of the basal iron loss was estimated as 38 percent. That CV was applied to the square root of the median basal losses shown in Table 9-6.

Iron EAR and RDA Summary, Ages 1 through 8 Years

The EAR has been set by modeling the components of iron requirements, estimating the requirement for absorbed iron at the fiftieth percentile, and with use of an upper limit of 18 percent iron absorption and rounding (see Table 9-8 and Appendix Table I-3).

EAR for Children
1–3 years	3.0 mg/day of iron
4–8 years	4.1 mg/day of iron

The RDA has been set by modeling the components of iron requirements, estimating the requirement for absorbed iron at the ninety-seven and one-half percentile, and with use of an upper limit of 18 percent iron absorption and rounding (see Table 9-8 and Appendix Table I-3).

RDA for Children
1–3 years	7 mg/day of iron
4–8 years	10 mg/day of iron

Children and Adolescents Ages 9 through 18 Years

Evidence Considered in Estimating the Average Requirement

The EAR for children and adolescents ages 9 through 18 years is determined by factorial modeling of the median components of iron requirements (see "Selection of Indicators for Estimating the Requirement for Iron—Factorial Modeling"). The major components of iron need for children are:

- basal iron losses;
- increase in hemoglobin mass;
- increase in tissue (nonstorage iron); and
- menstrual iron losses in adolescent girls (aged 14 through 18 years).

In this model, no provision was made for the development of iron stores after early childhood. It is accepted that all recognized functions of iron are met before significant storage occurs and that stores are a reserve against possible future shortfalls in intake rather than a necessary functional compartment of body iron. Because most individuals in this age group in the United States and Canada are believed to consume iron at levels above their own requirement, it can be assumed that most will accumulate some stores.

The major physiological event occurring in this age group is puberty. The associated physiological processes that have major impacts on iron requirements are the growth spurt in both sexes, menarche in girls, and the major increase in hemoglobin concentrations in boys. Because the growth spurt and menarche are linked to physiological age, the secular age at which these events occur varies among individuals. The factorial model distorts this by using averages. Since the growth spurt and menarche can be detected in the individual, provision is made for adjustments of requirement estimates when counseling specific individuals. These are addressed later under "Special Considerations".

Estimation of the variability of requirements in this age range is complicated because of the physiological changes that occur. In this report, median requirements for absorbed iron are estimated for each year of age, but the variability of requirement and the requirement for absorbed iron at the ninety seven and one-half percentile are estimated at the midpoint for children 9 through 13 years (11 years) and adolescents 14 through 18 years (16 years).

For modeling, the entire age range is treated as a continuum; for description, the conventional age intervals of the DRIs are used. Although requirement estimates have been developed for individual ages, these should be interpreted with care. Unsmoothed data have been used and year-by-year fluctuations may not be meaningful.

In addition to achieved size, it is necessary to estimate growth rates (weight velocities). After fitting linear regressions to median weights for segments of the age range, the regression slopes were taken as estimates of median weight velocities for the age interval. The estimates used are shown in Table 9-9.

Basal Losses. Basal iron loss estimates are based on the study of Green and coworkers (1968) (see "Selection of Indicators for Estimating the Requirement for Iron—Factorial Modeling"). Observations in adult men were extrapolated to adolescents on the basis of 14 mg/kg median weight and the losses for each age group are shown in Table 9-10.

Increase in Hemoglobin Mass. Estimation of the net iron utilization for increasing hemoglobin mass necessitates estimation of the rate of increase in blood volume and estimation of the rate of change in hemoglobin concentration. Blood volume is taken as approximately 75 mL/kg in boys and 66 mL/kg in girls (Hawkins, 1964). The average yearly weight gains for boys and girls are shown in Table 9-9. The rate of change in hemoglobin concentration has been directly estimated as the coefficients of the linear regression models applied to hemoglobin versus age for Nutrition Canada data by Beaton and coworkers (1989). The rate of change in hemoglobin concentration and the average hemoglobin concentrations for boys and girls are shown in Table 9-11. The iron content of hemoglobin is 3.39 mg/g (Smith and Rios, 1974), therefore the daily iron need for increased hemoglobin mass can be calculated as follows:

TABLE 9-9 Growth Velocity for Boys and Girls

Boys		Girls	
Age (y)	(kg/y)	Age (y)	(kg/y)
9–12	4.87	9–11	4.77
13–14	10.43	12–13	7.24
15–17	2.75	14–17	1.63
18	0	18	0

SOURCE: Tanner et al. (1966).

TABLE 9-10 Summary Illustration of Median Absorbed Iron Requirements for Children and Adolescents, Aged 9 through 18 Years[a]

Age (y)	Median Weight[b] (kg)	Components of Iron Needs				
		Change in Hemoglobin Mass (mg/d)	Basal Loss (mg/d)	Tissue Deposit (mg/d)	Storage (mg/d)	Menses (mg/d)[c]
Boys						
9	32.5	0.45	0.48	0.002	0	0
10	36.6	0.50	0.49	0.002	0	0
11	40.0	0.62	0.50	0.002	0	0
12	48.1	0.65	0.51	0.002	0	0
13	52.3	0.75	1.05	0.004	0	0
14	61.2	0.75	1.18	0.004	0	0
15	62.0	0.80	0.43	0.001	0	0
16	66.5	0.78	0.44	0.001	0	0
17	69.9	0.84	0.46	0.001	0	0
18	68.3	0.81	0.16	0	0	0
Girls						
9	31.9	0.45	0.40	0.002	0	0[b]
10	35.8	0.50	0.41	0.002	0	0[b]
11	44.0	0.63	0.42	0.002	0	(0.45)[b]
12	46.3	0.65	0.63	0.003	0	(0.45)[b]
13	53.5	0.75	0.64	0.003	0	(0.45)[b]
14	53.4	0.75	0.14	0.001	0	0.45
15	56.9	0.80	0.14	0.001	0	0.45
16	55.6	0.78	0.14	0.001	0	0.45
17	60.0	0.83	0.15	0.001	0	0.45
18	58.0	0.81	0.10	0	0	0.45

[a] Summation of the median iron components and dividing by 18 percent bioavailability does not yield values that are equivalent to the 50th and 97.5th percentile data shown in Appendix Table I-3. This is because the summation of the median of non-normal distributions (above) do not yield the median of simulation models that represent normalized data.

[b] Third National Health and Nutrition Examination Survey data (not demographically weighted).

[c] The model assumes that all girls are menstruating at age 14.0 years and after; it also assumes that no girls reach menarche before age 14. This is not a valid assumption. In working with individuals, menstrual status can be ascertained and an adjustment can be made.

TABLE 9-11 Equations Used to Estimate Hemoglobin Concentration and Increase in Hemoglobin (Hb) Concentration

Age (y)	Boys	Girls
8–13	Hb^a = 119 + (1.4 × age) ΔHb^b = 1.4	Hb = 121 + (1.1 × age) ΔHb = 1.1
14–18	Hb = 94.3 + (3.4 × age) ΔHb = 3.4	Hb = 131 + (0.28 × age) ΔHb = 0.28

^{a} Hb = g/L.
^{b} ΔHb = g/L/y.
SOURCE: Beaton et al. (1989).

Boys
([Weight (kg) × increase in hemoglobin concentration (kg/L/year)]
+ [Weight gain (kg/year) × hemoglobin concentration (g/L)]) ×
blood volume (0.075 L/kg) × hemoglobin iron (3.39 mg/g) ÷
365 days/year.

Girls
([Weight (kg) × increase in hemoglobin concentration (kg/L/year)]
+ [Weight gain (kg/year) × hemoglobin concentration (g/L)]) ×
blood volume (0.066 L/kg) × hemoglobin iron (3.39 mg/g) ÷
365 days/year.

For example, the medium daily need for increased hemoglobin mass for a 16-year-old girl would be ([55.6 × 0.28] + [1.63 × 135]) × 0.066 × 3.39 ÷ 365, or 0.14 mg/day.

Increase in the Nonstorage Iron Content of Tissues. Nonstorage tissue iron concentration (myoglobin and enzymes) (Table 9-10) can be calculated when the average weight gain for boys and girls and the iron content in muscle tissue are known. The iron deposition is approximately 0.13 mg/kg total weight gain (0.26 mg/kg muscle tissue) (Smith and Rios, 1974). The median need for absorbed iron associated with increase in weight in both sexes is

Tissue iron = Weight gain (kg/year) ×
nonstorage tissue iron (0.13 mg/kg) ÷
365 days/year, or weight gain × 0.00036 mg/day.

For example, the median daily need for nonstorage iron for a 16-year-old boy is 0.001 mg/day (2.75 × 0.13 ÷ 365) after rounding. No provision is made for iron storage after the age of 9 years. It is not a component of requirement though it can be expected to occur when intake exceeds actual requirement.

Menstrual Losses. Iron losses in the menses can be calculated when the average blood loss, the average hemoglobin concentration, and concentration of iron in hemoglobin (3.39 mg/g) (Smith and Rios, 1974) are known. It was deemed appropriate to use the blood losses reported by Hallberg and coworkers (1966a, 1966b) with additional information from Hallberg and Rossander-Hulthen (1991) and, more specifically, to use the blood loss estimates for 15-year-old girls. These losses were lower than those reported for older ages.

Several important features of these and other data related to menstrual blood loss were recognized in developing models to predict requirements:

- Menstrual losses are highly variable among women and the distribution of losses in the population shows major skewing, with some women having losses in excess of three times the median value.
- Menstrual losses are very consistent from one menstrual cycle to the next for an individual woman.
- Once the woman's menstrual pattern is established after her menarche, menstrual losses are essentially unchanged until the onset of menopause in healthy women. Hallberg and coworkers (1966b) found very little difference in blood loss with age. Losses were lower in the 15-year-old group, but incomplete collection might have been a factor. Cole and coworkers (1971) reported a small effect of age that was attributed to two covariates, parity and infant birth weight.
- Contraceptive methods have a major impact on menstrual losses. Bleeding is significantly increased by the use of certain intrauterine devices and significantly decreased in individuals taking oral contraceptives.

Age, body size, and parity were not considered to have an effect of sufficient magnitude on menstrual blood losses to include them as factors in the models for estimating iron requirements in females—except with regard to the lower menstrual loss assumed for adolescents.

The data on menstrual losses reported by Hallberg and coworkers

(1966a, 1966b) were used for all calculations in adolescent and adult females. This data set was selected for the following reasons:

• It is representative of the other survey data quoted above and can be considered generalizable to women living in countries other than that of the study, including the United States and Canada.
• Women were selected to fall into six age groups between 15 and 50 years, thus permitting estimates for all women.
• Although the original data were not available, comprehensive descriptions of the distribution of menstrual losses are available from a series of publications by Hallberg and colleagues.
• The survey was carried out before intrauterine devices and oral contraceptives were widely available. Only one woman in the study was using an oral contraceptive. None of them used an intrauterine device. The measurement can therefore reasonably be assumed to reflect "usual losses".

Blood losses per menstrual cycle were converted into estimated daily iron losses averaged over the whole menstrual cycle. The following assumptions were made:

• Blood loss does not change with mild anemia and is therefore independent of hemoglobin concentration.
• In estimating hemoglobin loss (blood loss × hemoglobin concentration), hemoglobin concentration was taken as a constant (135 ± 9 g/L in adult women and based on age in adolescents) (Hallberg and Rossander-Hulthen, 1991) and variance was ignored.
• The iron content of hemoglobin is 3.39 mg/g (Smith and Rios, 1974).
• The duration of the average menstrual cycle is 28 days. Beaton and coworkers (1970) reported a cycle duration of 27.8 ± 3.6 days in 86 self-selected healthy volunteers.

Since the distribution of menstrual blood losses in the data reported by Hallberg is skewed, it was modeled as described previously (see "Selection of Indicators for Estimating the Requirement for Iron—Factorial Modeling"). Comparison of the observed and modeled values (Table 9-12) provides a way of visualizing the adequacy of the fit of the model. A log-normal distribution was fitted to the reported percentiles of the blood loss distribution (natural log of blood loss = 3.3183 ± 0.6662 [SD]) to result in a median blood loss of 27.6 mL/estrous cycle. Blood losses of greater than 100 mL/estrous cycle are observed at the ninety-fifth percentile (Table 9-12)

TABLE 9-12 Comparison of Reported and Modeled Distributions of Blood Loss Per Menstrual Cycle of Swedish Women

	Blood Loss (mL/estrous cycle)	
Percentile	Observed[a]	Modeled[b]
10	10.4	11.4
25	18.2	18.3
50	30.0	30.9
75	52.4	52.3
90	83.9	83.9
95	118.0	111.4

[a] n = 486. Data from Hallberg et al. (1966a), percentiles 10, 25, 50, 75, 90; Hallberg and Rossander-Hulthen (1991), percentile 95.
[b] The predicted values were estimated from a fitted log normal distribution with mean and standard deviation = -3.4312 ± 0.7783 (see text for methodology).

and the distribution is highly skewed. Although these high menstrual losses were found in apparently healthy women, it would be difficult to exclude unidentified hemostatic disorders (Edlund et al., 1996) or occult uterine disease as possible contributory factors. The investigators considered all the subjects they studied to be free of any condition that might affect menstruation. There are no criteria for identifying a subpopulation at risk for increased menstrual blood loss or for setting an upper limit for "normal" losses. Calculation of the EAR and RDA was therefore based on the complete set of observations.

Regression estimates of hemoglobin concentration and rates of change in hemoglobin concentration by age and gender have been derived by Beaton and coworkers (1989). Estimated hemoglobin concentration for females 14 to 20 years of age was 131 g/L + 0.28 × age (years).

The above data were used to compute median menstrual iron loss as follows:

$$(Blood\ loss\ [27.6\ mL/28\ days]) \times$$
$$(hemoglobin\ concentration\ [131\ g/L] + [0.28 \times age]) \times$$
$$iron\ content\ of\ hemoglobin\ (3.39\ mg/g) \div 1,000.$$

Thus for adolescent girls, the median iron loss would be 0.45 mg/day (Table 9-10). Discussion on menstrual iron losses prior to 14 years is discussed under "Special Considerations." (For a discussion of menstrual iron losses during oral contraceptive use, see the "Special Considerations" section following "Lactation".)

Total Requirement for Absorbed Iron. Because all components (basal iron loss, hemoglobin mass, and nonstorage iron) are not normally distributed (skewed), these components as shown in Table 9-10 can not be summed to accurately determine an EAR and RDA. After summing the components for each individual in the simulated population, the estimated percentiles of distribution were tabulated and are shown in Appendix Tables I-3 and I-4. The modeled distribution of iron requirements are used to set the EAR (fiftieth percentile) and RDA (ninety-seven and one-half percentile) with the assumption of an upper limit of 18 percent for iron absorption.

Dietary Iron Bioavailability. The upper limit of dietary iron absorption was estimated to be 18 percent and used to set the EAR based on the fiftieth percentile of absorbed iron requirements (see "Factors Affecting the Iron Requirement—Algorithms for Estimating Dietary Iron Bioavailability").

Estimation of the Variability of Requirements. While Table 9-10 shows an estimate of median requirement, it is a simple summation and does not reflect the distributions. The distribution of requirements must be modeled using Monte Carlo simulation before the EAR and RDA can be estimated. This necessitates estimation of variability for components of requirements.

Basal or obligatory losses were derived from Green and coworkers (1968) with the assumption of proportionality to body surface area. To derive an estimate of variability of surface area, basal losses were computed with use of heights and weights reported in the USDA CSFII 1994–1996. Various transformations were then tested; a square root transformation approximated normality. The relative variability of surface area in this proxy data set was taken as an estimate of variability of basal iron loss. The observed CVs of proxy basal loss were 22.7 and 8.7 percent for boys aged 11 and 16, respectively, and 19.1 and 13.2 percent for girls aged 11 and 16, respectively. These CVs were applied to the square root of median iron loss, estimated on the basis of weight at ages 11 and 16 years (median loss shown in Table 9-10).

Estimating iron associated with change in hemoglobin mass requires consideration of rate of increase in blood volume and in hemoglobin concentration. Blood volume estimates were based on body size, and estimated median growth velocity is shown in Table 9-9. The algorithm for estimating iron need was presented earlier. For the purpose of modeling, blood volume as a proportion of body weight and rate of hemoglobin change as a function of age were taken as constants. The variability of iron need was attributed to variation in weight and weight velocity.

Based on reported percentiles of body weight in the Third National Health and Nutrition Examination Survey (NHANES III), normal distributions were fitted at 11 and 16 years of age for boys and girls. The fit was approximate only but acceptable for the present purpose. The resultant body weight distributions (kg) were 42.96 ± 12.47 and 70.30 ± 12.70 for boys aged 11 and 16, respectively, and 44.96 ± 9.96 and 61.36 ± 12.88 for girls aged 11 and 16, respectively.

The average weights differ from the median weights shown in Table 9-10. Estimates of weight velocity at ages 11 and 16 years were based on the analyses of longitudinal data reported by Tanner and coworkers (1966) (Table 9-9). Approximation of a normal distribution was assumed. The resultant distributions of weight velocities (kg/year) were used for modeling: 4.87 ± 1.65 and 2.75 ± 2.27 for boys aged 11 and 16, respectively, and 4.77 ± 2.06 and 1.63 ± 1.63 for girls aged 11 and 16, respectively. The variability of tissue iron deposition was based on the variability of body weight.

Values for iron hemoglobin concentration and altered hemoglobin concentration were estimated for these ages from the equations of Beaton and coworkers (1989), and variability in hemoglobin concentration was ignored. Variability arising from menstrual loss was estimated from the fitted regression of blood loss (ln blood loss = 3.3183 ± 0.6662 [SD]).

Iron EAR and RDA Summary, Ages 9 through 18 Years

The EAR has been set by modeling the components of iron requirements, estimating the requirement for absorbed iron at the fiftieth percentile, and with use of an upper limit of 18 percent iron absorption and rounding (see Appendix Tables I-3 and I-4). For the EAR and RDA for girls, it is assumed that girls younger than 14 years do not menstruate and that all girls 14 years and older do menstruate.

EAR for Boys
9–13 years	**5.9 mg/day of iron**
14–18 years	**7.7 mg/day of iron**

EAR for Girls
9–13 years	5.7 mg/day of iron
14–18 years	7.9 mg/day of iron

The RDA has been set by modeling the components of iron requirements, estimating the requirement for absorbed iron at the ninety-seven and one-half percentile, and with use of an upper limit of 18 percent iron absorption and rounding (see Appendix Tables I-3 and I-4).

RDA for Boys
9–13 years	8 mg/day of iron
14–18 years	11 mg/day of iron

RDA for Girls
9–13 years	8 mg/day of iron
14–18 years	15 mg/day of iron

Special Considerations

Adjustment for Growth Spurt. During the growth spurt, median rates of growth of boys might be double those seen in 11-year-olds; for girls the difference is smaller (about a 50 percent increase). The needs for absorbed iron associated with growth (increase in body weight) were estimated as 0.035 mg/g weight gained for boys and 0.030 mg/g weight gained for girls. The additional weight gain in the peak growth spurt years was estimated as the difference between the maximum and average growth rate (Table 9-9), which is 15.2 g/day ([10.43 – 4.87 kg/year] × 1,000 g/kg ÷ 365 day/year) for boys and 6.76 g/day ([7.24 – 4.77 kg/year] × 1,000 g/kg ÷ 365 days/year) for girls. These represent demands of 0.53 mg/day of iron for boys and 0.20 mg/day for girls. Therefore, the increased requirement for dietary iron is 2.9 mg/day for boys identified as currently in the growth spurt, and for girls the increase is approximately 1.1 mg/day.

Menstruation Before Age 14 Years. In the United States, the average age of menarche is about 12.5 years. It is reasonable to assume that by age 14 almost all girls will have started to menstruate, and hence the estimates of iron requirements should include menstrual losses at that time. It would be unreasonable to assume that no girls are menstruating before age 14 years. For girls under age 14 who have started to menstruate, it would be appropriate to consider a median menstrual loss of 0.45 mg/day of iron. Therefore, the requirement is increased by approximately 2.5 mg/day of iron.

Adults Ages 19 Years and Older

Method Used to Estimate the Average Requirement

Factorial modeling was used to calculate the EAR and RDA for adult men and women (see "Selection of Indicators for Estimating the Requirement for Iron—Factorial Modeling"). Requirements for maintaining iron requirements were derived by estimating losses. No provision is made for growth beyond age 19 years, and therefore there is no allowance for deposition of tissue iron.

Men. Basal iron loss was the only component used to estimate total needs for absorbed iron. Basal losses are based on the study by Green and coworkers (1968). Basal iron losses are taken as related to body weight (14 µg/kg/day), and for adult men, the requirement for absorbed iron is equivalent to the basal losses:

$$\text{Basal losses (mg/day)} = \text{Weight (kg)} \times 0.014 \text{ mg/kg/day.} \quad (1)$$

There are insufficient data for estimating variability of basal losses in adult men. Therefore, the median and variability for basal losses were calculated by using the median and variability values for body weight reported in NHANES III. Because variability in body weight is needed for calculating the distribution of basal losses, the reference weights in Table 1-1 were not used. Recorded weights reasonably yield a normal distribution based on the square root of the median weight for men:

$$\text{Weight 77.4 (kg)}^{0.5} = 8.8 \pm 0.84 \text{ kg.} \quad (2)$$

The distribution of basal losses, and therefore requirements in men, was obtained by combining equations (1) and (2). The estimated median daily iron loss in men living in the United States—and therefore the median requirement for absorbed iron—is 1.08 mg/day (77.4 kg × 0.014 mg/kg/day). The ninety-seven and one-half percentile of absorbed iron requirements is 1.53 mg/day.

The upper limit of dietary iron absorption was estimated to be 18 percent (see "Factors Affecting the Iron Requirement—Algorithms for Estimating Dietary Iron Bioavailability"). Using this value, the EAR is 6 mg/day (1.08 mg/day ÷ 0.18).

It is important to note that these calculations ignore the fact that men have higher iron stores than women. Moreover, the calculations assume that this widely recognized observation has no biological importance, but is merely the consequence of a total intake of food energy and associated food iron that is typically higher in men than in women, coupled with a much lower iron need in men. Appendix Table I-3 provides the estimated percentiles of the distribution of iron requirements for adult men.

Menstruating Women. Factorial modeling is again used to estimate the requirement for absorbed iron. Iron requirements for women were estimated by using the customary two-component model:

Iron requirement = basal losses + menstrual losses.

There are no direct measurements of basal iron losses, separated from menstrual iron loss, in women. Values for women have therefore been derived from the observations made in men (Green et al., 1968) (see "Selection of Indicators for Estimating the Iron Requirement—Factorial Modeling") by using a simple linear weight adjustment. The mean and variability in basal losses is based on the distribution of body weights recorded in NHANES III. Because variability in body weight is needed for calculating the distribution of basal losses, the reference weights in Table 1-1 were not used. The square root of reported weights yields a normal distribution reasonably closely:

$$\text{Weight } 64 \text{ (kg)}^{0.5} = 8.0 \pm 1.06 \text{ kg.}$$

Therefore the median basal iron loss was calculated as follows:

$$\text{Basal iron losses (mg/day)} = \text{Median weight (64 kg)} \times 0.014 \text{ mg/kg/day} = 0.896 \text{ mg/day.}$$

The ninety-seven and one-half percentile of the estimated absorbed iron requirement is 1.42 g/day (101.6 kg × 0.014 mg/kg/day). Menstrual blood (iron) losses have been estimated in many small studies (Beaton, 1974) and in two large community surveys, one in Sweden (Hallberg et al., 1966b) and the other in the United Kingdom (Cole et al., 1971). The findings of all of these studies were reasonably consistent. The factors and choice of data selection described for adolescent girls were also used for estimating menstrual losses in premenopausal women. Table 9-12 shows that the modeled median blood lost per menstrual cycle is 30.9 mL. The average concentration of iron in hemoglobin is 3.39 mg/g (Smith and Rios, 1974). As determined by Beaton and coworkers (1989), the average hemoglobin concentration for nonanemic women is 135 g/L. Using the above information, the daily menstrual iron loss can be calculated as follows:

Menstrual iron loss (mg/day) = blood loss/28 days (30.9 mL) × hemoglobin concentration (135 g/L) × iron concentration in hemoglobin (3.39 mg/g) ÷ 28 days = 0.51 mg/day.

The simulated distribution of menstrual losses is shown in Table 9-13. Median total iron needs were derived by summing the component needs (basal loss [0.896] + menstrual losses [0.51] = 1.4 mg/day).

The upper limit of dietary iron absorption was estimated to be 18 percent (see "Factors Affecting the Iron Requirement—Algorithms for Estimating Dietary Iron Bioavailability"). By dividing the sum of absorbed requirements by 18 percent, a distribution of dietary requirements was derived (see Appendix Table I-4). Based on this calculation and rounding, the EAR and RDA are set at 8 and 18

TABLE 9-13 Estimated Distribution of Menstrual Losses and Absorbed and Dietary Iron Needs in Adult Women[a]

Percentile of Women	Basal Iron Losses (mg/d)	Daily Iron Loss (mg/d)[b]	Absorbed Iron Needs (mg/d)[c]	Dietary Iron Requirement (mg/d)[d]
5	0.55	0.14	0.88	4.88
10	0.62	0.19	0.98	5.45
25	0.74	0.30	1.18	6.55
50	0.89	0.51	1.41	8.06
75	1.06	0.86	1.83	10.17
90	1.23	1.38	2.35	13.05
95	1.36	1.83	2.67	14.83
97.5	1.42	2.32	3.15	17.5

[a] Because the distribution of basal and menstrual iron losses are approximated from modeling, the sum of each for a specific percentile will not be equivalent to absorbed iron needs.
[b] Menstrual iron losses, averaged over 28 days.
[c] Menstrual + basal iron losses.
[d] Based on 18 percent bioavailability.

mg/day, respectively, for menstruating women not using oral contraceptives.

Postmenopausal Women. As for men, basal iron loss is the only component of iron needs for postmenopausal women and the physiological iron requirements and the EAR and RDA were derived by factorial modeling using the following equation:

$$\text{Basal losses } (\mu g/day) = \text{weight (kg)} \times 14 \; \mu g/kg.$$

As was the case for men, the median and variability for basal losses was calculated using the median and variability values for body weight reported in NHANES III. Because variability in body weight is needed for calculating the distribution of basal losses, the reference weights in Table 1-1 were not used. Recorded weights approximate a normal distribution based on the square root of weight:

$$\text{Weight 64 (kg)}^{0.5} = 8.0 \pm 1.06 \text{ kg.}$$

The distribution of basal losses, and therefore requirements for postmenopausal women, was obtained by combining the equations relating weight to basal losses and describing the weight distribution as outlined for men (Appendix Table I-3). The estimated median daily iron loss in postmenopausal women living in the United States, and therefore the median requirement for absorbed iron, is 0.896 mg/day (64 kg × 0.014 mg/kg/day). The ninety-seven and one-half percentile of estimated absorbed iron requirement is 1.42 g/day (101.6 kg × 0.014 mg/kg/day).

The upper limit of dietary iron absorption was estimated to be 18 percent (see "Factors Affecting Iron Requirement—Algorithms for Estimating Dietary Iron Bioavailability"). Based on this value, the EAR is set at 5 mg/day (0.896 ÷ 0.18).

It is assumed that basal losses, as a function of lean body mass, are essentially constant with age. Thus with increasing age, the only adjustment made to the EAR was the reduction associated with menopause.

Iron EAR and RDA Summary, Ages 19 Years and Older

The EAR has been set by modeling the components of iron requirements, estimating the requirement for absorbed iron at the fiftieth percentile, and with use of an upper limit of 18 percent iron absorption and rounding (Appendix Tables I-3 and I-4).

EAR for Men
19–30 years	6 mg/day of iron
31–50 years	6 mg/day of iron
51–70 years	6 mg/day of iron
> 70 years	6 mg/day of iron

EAR for Women
19–30 years	8.1 mg/day of iron
31–50 years	8.1 mg/day of iron
51–70 years	5 mg/day of iron
> 70 years	5 mg/day of iron

The RDA has been set by modeling the components of iron requirements, estimating the requirement for absorbed iron at the ninety-seven and one-half percentile, and with use of an upper limit of 18 percent iron absorption and rounding (Appendix Tables I-3 and I-4).

RDA for Men
19–30 years	8 mg/day of iron
31–50 years	8 mg/day of iron
50–70 years	8 mg/day of iron
> 70 years	8 mg/day of iron

RDA for Women
19–30 years	18 mg/day of iron
31–50 years	18 mg/day of iron
51–70 years	8 mg/day of iron
> 70 years	8 mg/day of iron

Pregnancy

Evidence Considered in Estimating the Average Requirement

Factorial modeling is used to estimate median requirements of pregnant women (see "Selection of Indicators for Estimating the Requirement for Iron—Factorial Modeling") with use of the equation:

Requirement for absorbed iron = basal losses +
iron deposited in fetus and related tissues +
iron utilized in expansion of hemoglobin mass.

Basal Losses. Using a body weight of 64 kg for a nonpregnant woman and an average basal loss of 14 µg/kg (Green et al., 1968), basal iron losses were calculated to be 0.896 mg/day (64 kg × 0.014 mg/kg) or approximately 250 mg for the entire pregnancy (280 days).

Fetal and Placental Iron Deposition. Numerous estimates of the iron content of the fetus and placental tissue exist. In the computation of the requirements, an estimate of 315 mg has been used (FAO/WHO, 1988). Bothwell and coworkers (1979) and Bothwell (2000) offered an estimate of 360 mg/pregnancy (270 + 90), whereas Hytten and Leitch (1971) suggested a total of 450 mg/pregnancy (375 + 75) but noted that there were insufficient data to estimate deposition by trimester. Thus, while there is considerable disagreement regarding these estimates, there are no new data to determine which estimate is more accurate. For this reason, the FAO/WHO total of 315 mg of iron partitioned by trimester was used.

Increase in Hemoglobin Mass. Although controversy continues, a general accepted value for iron needed to allow for expansion of hemoglobin mass is approximately 500 mg (FAO/WHO, 1988). Hemoglobin mass changes very little during the first trimester but expands greatly during the second and third trimesters. Information on the precise timing of the increase remains uncertain. For modeling, an equal division between the second and third trimesters is assumed in keeping with FAO/WHO (1988).

The actual magnitude of hemoglobin mass expansion depends on the extent of iron supplementation provided (De Leeuw et al., 1966). Beaton (2000) suggested that for every 10 g/L difference in the final hemoglobin concentration in the last trimester of pregnancy, there would be a difference of about 175 mg in the estimate of need for absorbed iron. It follows from this that the estimate of iron needs in pregnancy is directly dependent upon the cut-off that is used for hemoglobin concentration. In turn, that cut-off may depend on whether one believes that the iron needs of pregnancy can ever be met by diet alone. Evidence is needed concerning the functional significance of using a somewhat lower cut-off for final hemoglobin concentration. In this connection, it is to be recognized that by using a high hemoglobin concentration, the efficiency of dietary iron utilization is being targeted given that iron absorption is strongly affected by body iron status (Beaton, 2000). At this time, the hemoglobin concentration implied by the reference curve portrayed in Figure 9-1 is accepted.

With the above estimates, the total usage of iron throughout pregnancy is 250 mg (basal losses) + 320 mg (fetal and placental deposi-

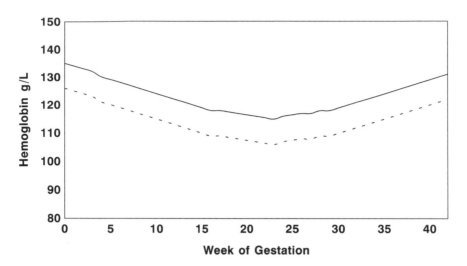

FIGURE 9-1 Hemoglobin concentrations in healthy, iron-supplemented (100–325 mg/day) pregnant women living in industrialized countries. The upper solid line represents the median hemoglobin concentration. The lower dashed curve represents the fifth percentile of hemoglobin concentration.
SOURCE: IOM (1993).

tion) + 500 mg (increase in hemoglobin mass), or 1,070 mg. At delivery, actual loss of iron in blood, including blood trapped in the placenta, may be in the range of 150 to 250 mg. That implies that of the 500 mg allowed for erythrocyte mass expansion during pregnancy, as much as 250 to 350 mg remains in the body to revert to maternal stores. The net cost of pregnancy could then be estimated as approximately 700 to 800 mg of iron (1,070 – [250 to 350]). This amount could be seen as the obligatory need for absorbed iron. Iron is not utilized at a uniform rate during pregnancy. The estimates of deposition of iron in the conceptus by stage of pregnancy are presented in Table 9-14.

Dietary Iron Bioavailability. The upper limit of dietary iron absorption is approximately 25 percent during the second and third trimesters (Barrett et al., 1994). This may be an underestimate of efficiency, coupled perhaps with the acceptance of too high a target for third trimester hemoglobin concentrations.

Table 9-15 presents a summary of the factorial model for estimation of median physiological needs, and Table 9-16 translates this to the median dietary iron requirement for pregnant women for each trimester. The iron requirement for women during the first trimester is less than that for premenopausal women because menstruation has ceased.

TABLE 9-14 Estimated Deposition of Iron in Conceptus by Stage of Pregnancy

Stage of Pregnancy	Fetus (mg)	Umbilicus and Placenta (mg)	Total (mg)
First trimester	25	5	30
Second trimester	75	25	100
Third trimester	145	45	190
Total	245	75	320

SOURCE: Based on Bothwell and Charlton (1981).

TABLE 9-15 Summary of Absorbed Iron Requirements in Pregnant Adult Women

Stage of Gestation	Basal Losses (mg/d)	Erythrocyte Mass mg/d (mg/trimester)	Fetus and Placenta mg/d (mg/trimester)	Total Absorbed Iron Requirement (mg/d)
First trimester	0.896	—	0.27 (25)	1.2
Second trimester	0.896	2.7 (250)	1.1 (100)	4.7
Third trimester	0.896	2.7 (250)	2.0 (190)	5.6

TABLE 9-16 Dietary Iron Requirement During Pregnancy

Stage of Gestation	Absorbed Iron Requirement (mg/d)	Absorption (%)[a]	Requirement (mg/d)
First trimester	1.2	18	6.4
Second trimester	4.7	25	18.8
Third trimester	5.6	25	22.4

[a] Absorption efficiency in the first trimester is as estimated for nonpregnant females; in the second and third trimesters, the efficiency is increased to 25 percent by the increased demand for iron as part of the physiological regulation of iron flux.

Estimation of the Variability of Requirements. Several approaches regarding components of variation could be considered in estimating the CV for iron needs in pregnancy:

• variability of basal requirement based on prepregnancy body weight; this would then need to be matched with the estimates of basal losses in nonpregnant females;
• variability of iron in the fetus based on variation in fetal weight at term; basing variability on birth weight alone would be a conservative (low) approach;
• variability of blood iron based on variation in hemoglobin concentration (SD of about 9 g/L) ignoring variation in blood volume; and
• variation based on the responses to level of iron supplementation.

The most conservative approach is based on variation in basal loss and assumes a CV of body weight of 21 percent (see "Adults Ages 19 Years and Older") and a CV of hemoglobin concentration in iron-supplemented women during the third trimester of about 7 percent (9 g/L/135 g/L) (Beaton et al., 1989). When these assumptions are applied, with basal losses based on prepregnancy weight, the iron need for products of conception is 315 ± 66.2 (SD), and the iron need for hemoglobin mass expansion is 500 ± 35 (SD). For the total pregnancy, this model yielded an estimated requirement of 1,055 mg ± 99.2 (SD) (CV, 9.4 percent). Table 9-16 summarizes the average requirement for absorbed and dietary iron for each trimester.

To estimate the needs of pregnant adolescents, the approach described above was followed with the notable exception that for adolescents the factorial model included basal losses and iron deposition in tissue as computed for adolescents. The fact that birth weights for adolescent mothers tend to be lower than for older women was ignored. In adolescents, the ninety-seven and one-half percentile of requirement was estimated for each trimester from simulation models rather than deriving one CV estimate and applying it to all three trimesters.

Iron EAR and RDA Summary, Pregnancy

The EAR and RDA are established by using estimates for the third trimester to build iron stores during the first trimester of pregnancy.

EAR for Pregnancy

14–18 years	23 mg/day of iron
19–30 years	22 mg/day of iron
31–50 years	22 mg/day of iron

The RDA has been set by modeling the components of iron requirements, estimating the requirement for absorbed iron at the ninety-seven and one-half percentile, and using an upper limit of 25 percent iron absorption and rounding.

RDA for Pregnancy

14–18 years	27 mg/day of iron
19–30 years	27 mg/day of iron
31–50 years	27 mg/day of iron

Lactation

Evidence Considered in Estimating the Average Requirement

Components of Requirement. Until menstruation resumes, assumed to be after 6 months of exclusive breast feeding, median iron needs during lactation are estimated as the sum of iron secretion in human milk and basal iron losses calculated for nonpregnant, nonlactating women (0.896 mg/day). The derived estimate of iron secreted in mature human milk is 0.27 ± 0.089 (SD) mg/day (0.35 mg/L × 0.78 L/day) (Table 9-5 and Chapter 2). Therefore, the median total requirement for absorbed iron is 1.17 mg/day (0.896 mg/day + 0.27 mg/day). For adolescent lactating mothers, the approach was identical to the one above except that in addition to basal losses (0.85 mg/day) and milk secretion (0.27 mg/day), provision was made for the deposition of iron in tissues (0.001 mg/day) and hemoglobin mass (0.14 mg/day) (see Table 9-10) as part of expected growth of the mother. Thus, the median requirement for absorbed iron is 1.26 mg/day (0.85 + 0.27 + 0.001 + 0.14). Again, a simulation model was used to derive the ninety-seven and one-half percentile of need.

Dietary Iron Bioavailability. To estimate the total iron requirement for lactation, iron secreted in milk and basal iron loss must be added by means of simulated distribution. The resultant distribution of iron needs, and assuming 18 percent absorption, results in the EARs and RDAs listed below.

Estimation of the Variability of Requirements. The variability of requirement was based on basal needs modeled as described for non-pregnant, nonlactating women and milk secretion modeled from the above distribution. Large breast-feeding studies suggest CVs between 10 and 40 percent (Dewey and Lonnerdal, 1983; Vaughan et al., 1979). A CV of 30 percent was adopted and iron concentration of mature human milk, for the purpose of modeling, is taken as 0.35 mg/L assuming normality with a CV of 33 percent.

Iron EAR and RDA Summary, Lactation

EAR for Lactation
14–18 years	7 mg/day of iron
19–30 years	6.5 mg/day of iron
31–50 years	6.5 mg/day of iron

The RDA for iron is set by determining the estimate of requirements at the ninety-seven and one-half percentile.

RDA for Lactation
14–18 years	10 mg/day of iron
19–30 years	9 mg/day of iron
31–50 years	9 mg/day of iron

Special Considerations

Use of Oral Contraceptives and Hormone Replacement Therapy

It has been reported that approximately 17 percent of women in the United States use oral contraceptives (Abma et al., 1997), which are known to reduce menstrual blood loss. Although many studies have documented lower menstrual blood losses among women using oral contraceptives, only one study actually allowed estimation of the magnitude of reduction, compared to expected loss. A reanalysis of data from that study (Nilsson and Solvell, 1967) suggested that a reasonable estimate of effect would be the equivalent of a 60 percent reduction from expected loss. Therefore, the requirement at the fiftieth and ninety-seven and one-half percentile for adolescent girls taking oral contraceptives is 6.9 and 11.4 mg/day, respectively and 6.4 and 10.9 mg/day for premenopausal women (see Appendix Table I-4).

Hormone replacement therapy (HRT), which provides estrogen and progesterone, is commonly practiced by postmenopausal women. Some uterine bleeding can occur in some women during HRT, especially during the first year of therapy (Archer et al., 1999; MacLennan et al., 1993; Oosterbaan et al., 1995). Therefore, women on HRT who continue to menstruate may have higher iron requirements than postmenopausal women who are not on HRT.

Vegetarianism

As previously discussed, iron is more bioavailable from meat than from plant-derived foods. Meat and fish also enhance the absorption of nonheme iron. Therefore, nonheme iron absorption is lower for those consuming vegetarian diets than for those eating non-vegetarian diets (Hunt and Roughead, 1999). Serum ferritin concentrations have been observed to be markedly lower in vegetarian men, women, and children than in those consuming a nonvegetarian diet (Alexander et al., 1994; Dwyer et al., 1982; Shaw et al., 1995). For these reasons, individuals who typically consume vegetarian diets may have difficulty consuming adequate intakes of bioavailable iron to meet the EAR. Cook and coworkers (1991) compared iron bioavailability from single meals with that of a diet consumed over a 2-week period. There was a 4.4-fold difference between maximally enhancing and maximally inhibiting single meals, but the difference was only two-fold when measured over the 2-week period. It is therefore estimated that the bioavailability of iron from a vegetarian diet is approximately 10 percent, rather than the 18 percent from a mixed Western diet. Hence the requirement for iron is 1.8 times higher for vegetarians. It is important to emphasize that lower bioavailability diets (approaching 5 percent overall absorption) may be encountered with very strict vegetarianism and in some developing countries where access to a variety of foods is limited.

Intestinal Parasitic Infection

Intestinal parasites infect approximately 1 billion of the world's population. Some of the parasites, particularly hookworm, cause significant intestinal blood loss. These infections are prevalent in developing countries where the intake of bioavailable iron is often inadequate. When possible, the primary intervention should be elimination of the parasitic infection. In addition, an adequate intake of bioavailable dietary iron may be necessary to treat iron deficiency. When bioavailable dietary iron is not available, supplemental iron may be needed. Various regimens are provided for such groups at risk of iron deficiency anemia (Stoltzfus and Dreyfuss, 1998; WHO/UNICEF/UNU, 1998).

Blood Donation

An annual donation of 0.5 L of blood is equivalent to between 200 and 250 mg of iron, which represents approximately 0.6 to 0.7 mg/day. Blood donors have lower serum ferritin concentrations than nondonors (Milman and Kirchhoff, 1991a, 1991b). More frequent donations can be problematic, especially for women, resulting in a need for supplemental iron (Garry et al., 1995).

Increased Iron Losses in Exercise and Intense Endurance Training

Many reviewers of the scientific literature conclude that iron status is marginal or inadequate in a large number of individuals, particularly females, who engage in regular physical exercise (Clarkson and Haymes, 1995; Raunikar and Sabio, 1992; Weaver and Rajaram, 1992). Dietary intake patterns of these individuals are frequently suboptimal with a reduced intake of a number of micronutrients. Weaver and Rajaram (1992) estimated that daily iron losses increase to 1.75 mg/day in male athletes and to 2.3 mg/day in female athletes with prolonged training. This is in contrast to a whole body loss of iron of approximately 1.08 mg/day in males beyond puberty and 1.45 mg/day in menstruating females. Ehn and coworkers (1980) demonstrated that highly trained, long distance runners have a biologic half-life of body iron of only approximately 1,000 days, a significantly shorter time than the 1,300 and 1,200 days, respectively, of male and female nonexercisers. Several reviewers of this topic conclude that increased fecal losses and perhaps sporadic hematuria contribute to depressed iron stores in athletic segments of the population (Siegel et al., 1979; Stewart et al., 1984). There is a notable reduction in hematologic parameters that could be the result of increased intravascular hemolysis of erythrocytes. Many studies have found an increased rate of erythrocyte turnover and fragility in athletes (Lampe et al., 1991; Newhouse and Clement, 1995; Rowland et al., 1991). Thus, several mechanisms by which iron balance could be affected by intense physical exercise have been advanced (Fogelholm, 1995; Magnusson et al., 1984; Weight, 1993), including increased gastrointestinal blood losses after running, and hemoglobinuria as a result of erythrocyte rupture within the foot during running. For the above reasons, and based on the strong whole body iron loss data collected by Ehn and coworkers (1980), the EAR for iron will conservatively be 30 percent greater for those who engage in regular intense exercise. If the estimate of Weaver and Rajaram (1992) is used, the EAR may be as much as 70 percent greater in the subpopulation of athletes.

Validation of Requirement Estimates

The theoretical and operational derivation of iron requirement estimates has been described for each life stage group. Requirements have been based on the estimation of the amount of iron needed to meet body functions with minimal storage. This level of nutriture is marked by a serum ferritin concentration of about 15 µg/L in children, adolescents, and adults and by a somewhat lower concentration (10 to 12 µg/L) in infants. Percentiles of the simulated distributions of requirement are presented in Appendix Tables I-3 and I-4.

The prevalence of apparently inadequate intakes is estimated through an assessment of the estimated distribution of usual intakes and by applying risk tables (Appendix Tables I-5, I-6, I-7) derived from the estimated requirement distributions and compared with the estimated prevalence of inadequate iron status based on serum ferritin concentration (see Table 14-1). The data sets used in this comparison were USDA CSFII 1994–1996 for iron intake and NHANES III for serum ferritin concentration. Statistical procedures were used to derive estimates of the usual iron intake or usual serum ferritin concentration; the data were also adjusted, with use of reported weighting factors, to represent the U.S. population and to compensate for the fact that sampling weights were not identical in the two data sets. Table 9-17 presents the outcome of this comparison. Considering that the dietary data do not include iron ingested as direct supplements and that no adjustment for alleged underreporting has been made, the agreement between apparent dietary inadequacy and apparent biochemical deficiency is reasonable for most age groups.

Children Ages 1 through 8 Years

The estimated prevalence of inadequate intake is lower (less than 5 percent) than the estimated prevalence of inadequate iron status for children (Table 9-17). One reason for the lack of congruence between iron intake and iron status may be the lack of validation of cut-off concentrations for serum ferritin in young children. Although studies have confirmed the correlation between a lack of storage

TABLE 9-17 Comparison of Estimated Prevalence of
Apparently Inadequate Iron Intakes and Serum Ferritin
Concentrations Indicative of Apparent Iron Deficiency, Third
National Health and Nutrition Examination Survey, 1988–1994

Age, Gender	Usual Intake (mean ± standard deviation)	Prevalence Apparently Inadequate Intakes (%)	Prevalence of Biochemical Deficiency (%)	
			Ferritin Concentration < 15 µg/L	Ferritin Concentration < 10 µg/L
1–3 y, both	10.9 ± 4.0	< 5	26	13
4–8 y, both	13.0 ± 3.9	< 5	6	
9–13 y				
Male	17.9 ± 5.7	< 5	< 5	
Female	14.1 ± 4.2	< 5	8	
14–18 y				
Male	20.1 ± 6.9	< 5	< 5	
Female	13.4 ± 5.1	10	15	
19–30 y				
Male	19.6 ± 6.8	< 5	15	
Female	13.2 ± 4.1	< 5	13	
31–50 y				
Male	19.6 ± 6.8	< 5	< 5	
Female	12.7 ± 4.6	15–20	16	
51–70 y				
Male	16.9 ± 6.3	< 5	< 5	
Female	12.3 ± 4.1	< 5	< 5	
71+ y				
Male	16.1 ± 7.1	< 5	< 5	
Female	12.4 ± 4.9	< 5	< 5	

NOTE: Data are limited to individuals who provided complete and reliable Day 1 dietary
intake records. Breastfeeding infants and children were excluded from all analyses. The
intake distributions for children 1–3 years of age are unadjusted. Percentiles for these
groups were computed using SAS PROC UNIVARIATE . For all other groups, data were
adjusted using the Iowa State University method using C-Side.
SOURCE: ENVIRON International Corporation and Iowa State University Department
of Statistics, 2000.

iron and low ferritin concentrations, such studies have not been conducted in children. Thus ferritin concentrations of 10 and 15 μg/L may not be indicative of low iron stores in children.

Children and Adolescents Ages 9 through 18 Years

When the predicted prevalence of inadequate intakes and the reported prevalence of iron deficiency are compared in those aged 9 through 18 years, agreement is not consistent (Table 9-17). For example, in girls aged 9 through 13 years, the prevalence of inadequate intake is less than 5 percent, but the prevalence of low serum ferritin concentration is 8 percent. The lack of congruence of these results is likely due to the fact that a proportion of girls aged 12 and 13 years have reached menarche and have higher iron requirements than those who have not reached menarche. There is better congruence between dietary and biochemical estimates for 14- through 18-year-old girls whose iron requirements include menstrual iron losses. Among boys, the prevalences of inadequate intakes and low serum ferritin concentrations are both less than 5 percent.

Adults Ages 19 Years and Older

There is congruence between the prevalences of inadequate iron intakes and low serum ferritin concentrations for men and for pre- and postmenopausal women (Table 9-17). The prevalence of inadequate iron intakes for premenopausal women is approximately 20 percent and the prevalence of low serum ferritin concentration is 13 to 16 percent, prevalences indicating that the additional iron requirements due to menstrual losses are not being met in this group of women.

The overall pattern offers some degree of reassurance that the general model used to estimate requirements, the specific estimates of components of that model, and the assumed limits to bioavailability of dietary iron are reasonable.

INTAKE OF IRON

Food Sources

The iron content of vegetables, fruits, breads, and pasta varies from 0.1 to 1.4 mg/serving. Because most grain products are fortified with iron, approximately one-half of ingested iron comes from bread and other grain products such as cereals and breakfast bars.

Some fortified cereals contain as much as 24 mg of iron per 1-cup serving. Heme iron represents only 7 to 10 percent of dietary iron of girls and women and only 8 to 12 percent of dietary iron for boys and men (Raper et al., 1984). Human milk provides approximately 0.27 mg/day (Table 9-5).

Dietary Intake

Data from nationally representative U.S. surveys are available to estimate iron intakes (Appendix Tables C-18, C-19, D-3, E-5). Data from these surveys indicate that the median daily intake of dietary iron by men is approximately 16 to 18 mg/day, and the median intake by pre- and postmenopausal women is approximately 12 mg/day. Data from a survey done in two Canadian provinces showed that the dietary intake of iron by both men and women was slightly lower than intakes in the United States (Appendix Table F-2). The median intake of dietary iron by pregnant women was approximately 15 mg/day, which is less than the Estimated Average Requirement (EAR) of 22 mg/day, indicating the need for iron supplementation during pregnancy.

Intake from Supplements

Approximately 21 to 25 percent of women and 16 percent of men were reported to consume a supplement that contains iron (Moss et al., 1989; see Table 2-2). The median intake of iron from supplements is approximately 1 mg/day for men and women, an amount based on the difference in median iron intake from food plus supplements and food alone (Appendix Tables C-18 and C-19). The median iron intake from food plus supplements by pregnant women is approximately 21 mg/day.

TOLERABLE UPPER INTAKE LEVELS

The Tolerable Upper Intake Level (UL) is the highest level of daily nutrient intake that is likely to pose no risk of adverse health effects for almost all individuals. Although members of the general population should be advised not to routinely exceed the UL, intake above the UL may be appropriate for investigation within well-controlled clinical trials. Clinical trials of doses above the UL should not be discouraged, as long as subjects participating in these trials have signed informed consent documents regarding possible toxicity and as long as these trials employ appropriate safety monitoring of trial subjects. In addition, the UL is not meant to apply to individuals who receive iron under medical supervision.

Hazard Identification

Iron is a redox-active transition metal. In health, it is carried from one tissue to another bound to transferrin and stored in cells in the form of ferritin or hemosiderin. These proteins hold iron in the ferric state. Kinetic restrictions prevent the iron from being reduced by cellular reductants, and it is thus shielded from unwanted participation in redox reactions (McCord, 1996). If the transport and storage mechanisms are overwhelmed, the free iron will immediately be chelated by cellular compounds, such as citrate or adenosyl diphosphate, that readily participate in redox reactions catalyzing the formation of highly toxic free radicals or the initiation of lipid peroxidation.

Adverse Effects

Acute Effects. There are reports of acute toxicity resulting from overdoses of medicinal iron, especially in young children (Anderson, 1994; Banner and Tong, 1986; NRC, 1979). Accidental iron overdose is the most common cause of poisoning deaths in children under 6 years of age in the United States (FDA, 1997). Vomiting and diarrhea characterize the initial stages of iron intoxication. With increasing time after ingestion, at least five organ systems can become involved: cardiovascular, central nervous system, kidney, liver, and hematologic (Anderson, 1994). The severity of iron toxicity is related to the amount of elemental iron absorbed. Symptoms occur with doses between 20 and 60 mg/kg with the low end of the range associated primarily with gastrointestinal irritation while systemic toxicity occurs at the high end (McGuigan, 1996). These data, however, are not used because acute intake data are not considered in setting a UL.

Iron-Zinc Interactions. High intakes of iron supplements have been associated with reduced zinc absorption as measured by changes in serum zinc concentrations after dosing (Fung et al., 1997; Meadows et al., 1983; O'Brien et al., 2000; Solomons, 1986; Solomons and Jacob, 1981; Solomons et al., 1983). However, plasma zinc concentrations are not considered to be good indicators of body zinc stores (Whittaker, 1998). Studies using zinc radioisotopes showed reduced zinc absorption when both minerals were administered in the fasting state at an iron-zinc ratio of 25:1 but not at 1:1 or 2.5:1 (Sandstrom et al., 1985). When iron and zinc supplements were given with a meal, however, this effect was not observed. Other investigators have reported similar observations (Davidsson et al., 1995; Fairweather-Tait et al., 1995b; Valberg et al., 1984; Walsh et al., 1994; Yip et al., 1985). A radioisotope-labeling study by Davidsson and coworkers (1995) showed that fortifying foods such as bread, infant formula, and weaning foods with iron had no effect on zinc absorption. In general, the data indicate that large doses of supplemental iron inhibit zinc absorption if both are taken without food, but do not inhibit zinc absorption if they are consumed with food. Because there is no evidence of any clinically significant adverse effect associated with iron-zinc interactions, this effect is not used to determine a UL for iron.

Gastrointestinal Effects. High-dose iron supplements are commonly associated with constipation and other gastrointestinal (GI) effects including nausea, vomiting, and diarrhea (Blot et al., 1981; Brock et al., 1985; Coplin et al., 1991; Frykman et al., 1994; Hallberg et al., 1966c; Liguori, 1993; Lokken and Birkeland, 1979) (Table 9-18). Because GI effects are local, the frequency and severity of the effect depends on the amount of elemental iron released in the stomach (Hallberg et al., 1966c). The adverse effects of supplemental iron appear to be reduced when iron is taken with food (Brock et al., 1985). While most of the observed effects are relatively minor, some individuals have found them severe enough to stop further supplementation (Frykman et al., 1994).

A single-blinded, 8-week study by Brock et al. (1985) reported "moderate to severe" GI effects in 50 percent of subjects taking 50 mg/day of elemental iron as ferrous sulfate. This finding is supported by other better-controlled, prospective studies showing GI effects at similar doses (Coplin et al., 1991; Frykman et al., 1994; Lokken and Birkeland, 1979). These data suggest a definite causal relation between high iron intake and GI effects.

Secondary Iron Overload. Secondary iron overload occurs when the body iron stores are increased as a consequence of parenteral iron administration, repeated blood transfusions, or hematological disorders that increase the rate of iron absorption. Although the iron in patients with secondary iron overload tends to be stored initially in macrophages where it is less damaging, the typical pathological consequences of iron overload that are characteristic of hereditary hemochromatosis may eventually occur.

Whether an excessive iron intake alone can lead to secondary iron overload and associated organ damage is unknown. Some individuals appear to control their rates of iron acquisition very effectively in the face of a high iron intake, but as yet there has been no study with a large number of experimental subjects and a sufficient duration to be certain of this conclusion. Individuals who are heterozygous for hemochromatosis manifest minor phenotypic expression, usually a slight to moderate increase in serum ferritin concentrations and transferrin saturation (Bulaj et al., 1996). Iron stores are modestly increased but do not continue to rise significantly with increasing age, and the pathological features of homozygous hemochromatosis do not occur.

There is only one clear example of dietary iron overload. The high prevalence of iron overload in South African and Zimbabwean blacks is associated with the consumption of traditional beer with an average iron content of 80 mg/L (Bothwell et al., 1964). The iron is highly bioavailable and some people may consume several liters of the beer per day. Iron overload does not occur in members of the population who are not consuming large quantities of beer or iron. There is therefore little doubt that the high iron intake plays a major role in the pathogenesis of sub-Saharan iron overload. However, intake may not be the only factor. Gordeuk and coworkers (1992) collected evidence to suggest that there is also a genetic component involving a gene different from the HFE gene-linked hereditary hemochromatosis (Feder, 1999).

Cardiovascular Disease. Sullivan (1981) first hypothesized that increased body iron plays a role in the development of coronary heart disease (CHD). This hypothesis was based on the difference in the prevalence of ischemic heart disease between men and postmenopausal women, on one hand, and between men and premenopausal women on the other. According to Sullivan's hypothesis, the prevalence of CHD is higher in men and increases after menopause in women as a result of higher body iron stores.

Epidemiological support for this hypothesis was provided by Salonen and coworkers (1992). In a cohort study, they demonstrated a significant association between high serum ferritin concentrations and the risk of myocardial infarction (MI) among middle-aged men in Finland. Men with serum ferritin concentrations greater than 200 µg/L had a 2.2-fold greater risk of acute MI than men with levels less than 200 µg/L. The association was even stronger in those with high cholesterol concentrations. Their original conclusions were confirmed by a reanalysis of the same group of subjects after a

TABLE 9-18 Iron and Gastrointestinal (GI) Adverse Effects, by Increasing Dose

Reference	Form of Iron (Fe) Sample Size	Study Group
Coplin et al., 1991 Randomized double-blind, cross-over trial	Ferrous sulfate n = 38 women	18–40 y nonpregnant women
	Bis-glycino Fe II (chelated Fe)[b] n = 38 women	18–40 y nonpregnant women
Brock et al., 1985 Single-blind, parallel group study	Ferrous sulfate n = 272 women and men[c]	18–39 y nonpregnant women
	Ferrous sulfate in wax matrix prep (control group) n = 271 women and men[c]	18–39 y nonpregnant women
Critical Study Frykman et al., 1994	n = 97 (total)	Blood donors
Controlled, double-blind crossover study	Placebo n = 46 men n = 51 women	34–48 y 35–52 y
	Ferrous fumarate n = 23 men n = 25 women	34–45 y 40–52 y

Dose of Supplemental Iron (mg/d)	When Taken	Duration	Results/Comments
50	Before breakfast	2 wk	25/38 GI problems[a] 7 abdominal pain 10 bloating 13 constipation 9 diarrhea 12 nausea
50		2 wk	23/38 GI problems 9 abdominal pain 9 bloating 13 constipation 7 diarrhea 9 nausea No placebo control
50	Before breakfast	8 wk	53 abdominal discomfort[d] 26 nausea[d] 5 vomiting 47 constipation[d] 26 diarrhea[d]
50	Before breakfast	8 wk	25 abdominal discomfort 11 nausea 3 vomiting 18 constipation 13 diarrhea Wax matrix coating was used to help minimize GI distress
	Not indicated	4 wk	GI side effects 14% all GI side effects[d] 4% nausea 10% gastric pain 20% constipation[d] 19% diarrhea
60	Not indicated	4 wk	GI side effects 25% all GI side effects[d] 6% nausea 19% gastric pain 35% constipation[d] 37% diarrhea

continued

TABLE 9-18 Continued

Reference	Form of Iron (Fe) Sample Size	Study Group
Liguori, 1993 Double-blind, randomized, multicenter study	ITF 282 (iron protein succinylate) $n = 549$ (64 men; 485 women)	15–85 y
	Ferrous sulfate-controlled release $n = 546$ (55 men; 491 women)	15–88 y nonpregnant
Blot et al., 1981	Elemental iron $n = 132$ pregnant women	27.5 ± 4.5 y
Lokken and Birkeland, 1979 Double-blind, cross-over	Ferrous fumarate $n = 19$	18–28 y
Hallberg et al., 1966c (I)	Placebo $n = 195$	Blood donors
	Ferrous sulfate $n = 198$	Blood donors
Hallberg et al., 1966c (II)	Placebo $n = 119$	Blood donors
	Ferrous sulfate $n = 120$	Blood donors
	Ferrous fumarate $n = 118$	Blood donors
	Ferrous gluconate $n = 120$	Blood donors

Dose of Supplemental Iron (mg/d)	When Taken	Duration	Results/Comments
120 (60 mg 2× per day)	Before breakfast and before dinner	8.5 wk	63/546 (11%) GI side effects 31 epigastric pain 23 constipation 32 abdominal pain 14 nausea 25 heartburn
105	Before breakfast	8.5 wk	127/549 (26%) GI side effects[d] 23 constipation 31 abdominal pain 14 nausea 33 heartburn No placebo control
105		90 d	14% had severe alimentary side effects No placebo control
120		8 wk	5/19 GI distress 1 diarrhea 1 epigastric pain 3 constipation 2/19 GI distress (placebo) 2 epigastric pain and constipation
		14 d	GI side effects 14% (6 men, 17 women)
222		14 d	GI side effects 23% (6 men, 34 women[d])
		14 d	GI side effects 14% (2 men, 16 women)
222		14 d	GI side effects 28% (5 men, 26 women[d])
222		14 d	GI side effects 26% (4 men, 25 women[d])
222		14 d	GI side effects 31% (8 men, 27 women[d])

continued

TABLE 9-18 Continued

Reference	Form of Iron (Fe) Sample Size	Study Group
Hallberg et al., 1966c (III)	Placebo $n = 200$	Blood donors
	Ferrous sulfate $n = 195$	Blood donors
	Ferrous glycine sulfonate $n = 200$	Blood donors
	Ferrous gluconate	Blood donors

[a] Coplin et al. (1991) observed no statistically significant difference in frequency of side effects for the different preparations.

[b] The iron glycine chelate has been shown to be more bioavailable than the sulfate.

5-year follow-up (Salonen et al., 1994). Another prospective cohort study reported an association between high serum ferritin concentrations and carotid vascular disease (Kiechl et al., 1997). However, several other large prospective cohort studies failed to demonstrate a significant relationship between serum ferritin concentrations and increased risk for CHD (Aronow and Ahn, 1996; Frey and Krider, 1994; Magnusson et al., 1994; Manttari et al., 1994; Stampfer et al., 1993) (Table 9-19).

The relationships between various other measures of iron status (e.g., serum transferrin saturation, serum iron concentration, and total iron-binding capacity) and CHD severity, incidence, or mortality have been examined in other prospective cohort studies. Investigators reported that transferrin saturation (Liao et al., 1994), serum iron concentrations (Liao et al., 1994; Morrison et al., 1994; Reunanen et al., 1995), and total iron-binding capacity (Magnusson et al., 1994) were related to CHD (Tables 9-19 through 9-22). However, some of these same studies and several other large prospective cohort studies failed to demonstrate any relationship with transferrin saturation (Baer et al., 1994; Reunanen et al., 1995; Sempos et al., 1994; Van Asperen et al., 1995) or total iron-binding capacity (Liao et al., 1994; Reunanen et al., 1995; Van Asperen et al., 1995).

Dose of Supplemental Iron (mg/d)	When Taken	Duration	Results/Comments
		14 d	GI side effects 12% (6 men, 16 women)
180		14 d	GI side effects 26% (15 men, 30 women)
180		14 d	GI side effects 24% (11 men, 33 women)
			GI side effects 27% (9 men, 39 women)

[c] The 543 subjects evaluated in this study comprised 484 nonpregnant, premenopausal women and 59 men, aged 18 to 39 years.

[d] Statistically significant difference ($p < 0.05$) in frequency of side-effects between the iron and the placebo group.

Danesh and Appleby (1999) recently conducted a systematic assessment of 12 prospective epidemiological studies of iron status and CHD. They concluded that these studies do not support a strong association between iron status and CHD.

There was no association between CHD and heterozygosity in two studies (Franco et al., 1998; Nassar et al., 1998). Two subsequent surveys from Europe demonstrated a two-fold increase in acute MI in heterozygous men (Tuomainen et al., 1999) and a 1.6-fold increase in overall CHD mortality in heterozygous women (Roest et al., 1999). In summary, the currently available data do not provide convincing support for an association between high body iron stores and increased risk for CHD.

Taken as a whole, this body of evidence does not provide convincing support for a causal relationship between the level of dietary iron intake and the risk for CHD. However, it is also important to note that the evidence is insufficient to definitively exclude iron as a risk factor. Several studies suggest that the serum ferritin concentration is directly correlated with the risk for CHD. However, serum ferritin concentrations are affected by several factors other than dietary iron intake. The significance of the high serum ferritin concentrations that have been observed in population surveys and the

TABLE 9-19 Serum Ferritin Concentration and
Cardiovascular Disease

Study	Type of Study	Follow-up	Subjects[a]	Disease Outcome[b]
Salonen et al., 1992	Prospective cohort	3 y	51 M (42, 48, 54, or 60 y)	MI
Stampfer et al., 1993	Nested case-control[e]	About 10 y	238 M w/MI 238 M controls (40–84 y)	MI
Frey and Krider, 1994	Prospective cohort	1–10 y (mean 5 y)	298 M (42–60 y)[g]	MI (in 32 of 298 M)
Magnusson et al., 1994	Prospective cohort	8.5 y	81 M 18 W (25–74 y)	MI
Manttari et al., 1994	Nested case-control	5 y	136 cases (M, 49 y) 132 controls (M, 47 y)	CHD
Salonen et al., 1994	Prospective cohort	5 y	83 M	MI
Aronow and Ahn, 1996	Prospective cohort	3 y	171 M 406 W (62–100 y)	New CHD events
Kiechl et al., 1997	Prospective cohort	5 y	826 M/W (40–79 y)	Carotid athero-sclerosis

[a] M = men, W = women.
[b] MI = myocardial infarction, CHD = coronary heart disease.
[c] S = smoking, ECG = echocardiogram, BP = blood pressure, G = blood glucose, HDL = high density lipoprotein, TG = triglyceride concentration, AB = apolipoprotein B, L = blood leukocyte count, Fe = serum iron, Ch = total cholesterol, BM = body mass, Hb = hemoglobin concentration, Alc = alcohol intake, AA-1 = Apolipoprotein A-1, Hyp = hypertension.
[d] Amount provided as mean concentrations.
[e] The blood samples were collected in 1982 from 14,916 men aged 40–84 years without prior MI or stroke.

Other Risk Factors Assessed[c]	Ferritin Concentration ($\mu g/L$)[d]	Association
Age, exam year, S, ischemic ECG test, BP, G, HDL, TG, AB, L	> 200	Elevated ferritin concentration was a strong risk factor for acute MI (relative risk [RR] = 2.2) compared to men with lower ferritin levels
S, age, other coronary risk factors	250 cases 222 controls ($p = 0.08$)[f]	No association was observed between serum ferritin concentration and risk of myocardial infarction
Reviewed med. charts for Ch, G, L, lipid profile	156 all 148 cases	No association of serum ferritin with risk of MI
Age, other Fe parameters, BP, S, Ch, HDL	198 (M) 91 (W)	No association between serum ferritin and MI, RR = 0.99
Age, BM, BP, Ch, Hb, HDL, TG, L, S	84 cases 85 control	No association between serum ferritin concentration and risk of CHD
	≥ 200	Elevated ferritin concentration was a strong risk factor for acute MI compared to men with lower ferritin levels[h]
Age, sex, S, prior CHD	143 M-CHD 146 M-no new events 122 W-CHD 128 W-no new events	No association with new CHD events
Age, S, Ch, BP, G, Alc, Hb, AB, AA-1, Hyp	185 with athero- sclerosis 114 no athero- sclerosis	Serum ferritin was a strong predictor of atherosclerosis

[f] After adjusting for other coronary risk factors (aside from age and smoking), men with levels ≥ 200 $\mu g/L$ had a relative risk of 1.1 compared with those having lower levels.

[g] These patients were from two southern West Virginia counties with a high number of mine workers who had been exposed to mine dust.

[h] This association remained statistically significant when the following risk factors were added to the model individually and together: systolic blood pressure, height, weight, body mass index, serum apolipoprotein B concentration, concentrations of triglycerides and HDL2 subfraction of high-density lipoprotein cholesterol, plasma fibrinogen concentration, ischemia on exercise testing, maximal oxygen uptake, energy, and saturated fat intake.

TABLE 9-20 Transferrin Saturation and Coronary Heart Disease

Study	Type of Study	Follow-up (y)	Subjects[a]	Disease Outcome[b]
Baer et al., 1994	Retrospective cohort	14	46,932 (≥ 30 y)	MI
Liao et al., 1994	Follow-up	13	4,237 (40–74 y)	MI, CHD
Sempos et al., 1994	Cohort	13	4,518 (47–74 y)	CHD, MI
Reunanen et al., 1995	Prospective cohort	14	6,086 M 6,102 W (45–64 y)	Mortality from CHD
Van Asperen et al., 1995	Cohort	17	129 M 131 W (64–87 y)	Mortality from IHD

[a] M = men, W = women.
[b] MI = myocardial infarction, CHD = coronary heart disease, IHD = ischemic heart disease.

TABLE 9-21 Serum Iron Concentration and Cardiovascular Disease

Study	Type of Study	Follow-up Period (y)	Subjects[a]	Disease Outcome[b]
Liao et al., 1994	Prospective cohort	13	1,827 M 2,410 W (40–74 y at baseline)	MI, CHD
Morrison et al., 1994	Cohort	15	10,000	MI
Reunanen et al., 1995	Prospective cohort	15	6,086 M 6,102 W	CHD

[a] M = men, W = women.
[b] MI = myocardial infarction, CHD = coronary heart disease.
[c] BP = blood pressure, Ch = total cholesterol, S = smoking.

Adjusted for These Factors[c]	Intake Values	Association
Age, race, S, Alc, education, family history of CAD and diabetes, G, Ch, BMI, systolic BP	Not provided	Relative risk = 1.3 The relative risk for subjects with increased iron stores (TS ≥ 62%) was not statistically significant
Age, S, Ch, systolic BP, education	Not provided	Transferrin saturation inversely related to CHD; not related to MI
Age, diabetes, BP, S, Ch, education	Not provided	Transferrin saturation is not related to CHD or MI risk in men or women
S, BP, BMI, diabetes, history of heart disease	Mean Fe intakes: 17 mg (M) 13 mg (W)	Transferrin saturation was inversely but not significantly associated with CHD mortality
Age, S, Alc, systolic BP, Ch, BMI, history of diabetes and IHD	Not provided	No significant association between transferrin saturation and ischemic heart disease

[c] S = smoking, Alc = alcohol intake, CAD = coronary artery disease, G = blood glucose, Ch = total cholesterol, BMI = body mass index, BP = blood pressure.

Adjusted for These Factors[c]	Relative Risk and Associations
Age, systolic BP, Ch, S, education	Inversely associated with MI and CHD in women (0.82 and 0.86; $p < 0.01$) Inversely associated with CHD in men (0.92, $p = 0.065$)
Age, S, BP, Ch, diabetes status	Serum iron significantly associated with risk of MI, rate ratio = 2.18 (men); 5.53 (women) No association between risk of acute MI and dietary or supplemental iron intake
Age, Ch, BP, S, diabetes, obesity	Risk for CHD mortality was highest in the lowest serum iron quartile

TABLE 9-22 Total Iron-binding Capacity and Cardiovascular Disease

Study	Type of Study	Follow-up Period (y)	Subjects[a]	Disease Outcome[b]
Liao et al., 1994	Cohort	13	1,827 M 2,410 W	CHD, MI
Magnusson et al., 1994	Prospective cohort	8.5	2,036 M/W (25–74 y)	MI incidence
Reunanen et al., 1995	Prospective cohort	14	6,086 M 6,102 F (45–64 y at baseline)	CHD mortality
Van Asperen et al., 1995	Prospective cohort	17	129 M 131 W (64–87 y)	IHD mortality

[a] M = men, W = women.

[b] CHD = coronary heart disease, MI = myocardial infarction, IHD = ischemic heart disease.

nature of the relationship between serum ferritin concentration and CHD risk remain to be determined.

Cancer. The increased risk for hepatocellular carcinoma in individuals with hereditary hemochromatosis and cirrhosis is well established (Powell, 1970). The evidence for an association between advanced hereditary hemochromatosis and other types of cancer is less certain. One large controlled study failed to demonstrate an increased incidence of extrahepatic malignancies (Niederau et al., 1985) whereas others have reported higher risk (Bomford and Williams, 1976; Hsing et al., 1995).

Several epidemiological studies have reported a positive correlation between measures of iron status and cancer in the general population. Stevens and coworkers (1988) reported serum transferrin saturation to be significantly higher among men who had cancer than among men who remained free of cancer. Further anal-

Adjusted for These Factors[c]	Association
Age, systolic BP, Ch, education, S	Total iron binding capacity not related to MI or CHD
Age, sex, Ch, HDL, triglycerides, BP, serum ferritin, log (ferritin), Fe, Hb, leukocyte count	Total iron binding capacity was a significant ($p = 0.007$) independent negative risk factor for CHD
S, BP, BMI, diabetes, history of heart disease	No relationship between total iron binding capacity and CHD mortality in men; an inverse (nonsignificant) association found in women
Age, S, Alc, systolic BP, Ch, BMI, prevalence of diabetes, IHD	No clear association between total iron binding capacity and IHD

[c] BP = blood pressure, Ch = total cholesterol, S = smoking, HDL – high density lipo-protein cholesterol, Fe = serum iron, Hb = hemoglobin concentration, BMI = body mass index, Alc = alcohol intake.

ysis of these data showed a significant positive correlation between transferrin saturation and cancer risk for both men and women (Stevens et al., 1994). However, these findings were not confirmed when follow-up was extended to 17 years and upon reanalysis of the data (Sempos et al., 1994).

Selby and Friedman (1988) found a lower incidence of cancer in iron-depleted women, but the possible confounding effect of ciga-rette smoking was not eliminated in this study. Another prospective study found significantly higher serum iron concentrations in indi-viduals with colorectal cancer than in control subjects (Wurzelmann et al., 1996), but the differences in the serum iron concentrations were small and well within the normal range for the general popu-lation. The biological relevance of this finding is therefore ques-tionable.

Nelson and coworkers (1994) reported an apparent association between serum ferritin concentrations and adenoma of the colon in a case-control study of 264 men and 98 women. This association was independent of other risk factors including smoking, gender, and alcohol consumption. In a later study in heterozygous carriers of the gene for hemochromatosis, Nelson and coworkers (1995) found a small, but statistically significant increase in the apparent relative risk for colorectal cancer, hematological malignancy, colonic adenomas, and stomach cancer.

There is no doubt that iron accumulation in the liver is a risk factor for hepatocellular carcinoma in patients with hemochromatosis. However, the evidence for a relationship between dietary iron intake and cancer, particularly colon cancer, in the general population is inconclusive.

Identification of Distinct and Highly Sensitive Subpopulations

Between 1 in 200 and 1 in 400 individuals of northern European descent are affected by an autosomal, recessive disorder known as hereditary hemochromatosis (Bacon et al., 1999). In populations of Celtic extraction, a single missense mutation of the hemochromatosis (HFE) gene (C282Y) is found in over 90 percent of affected individuals. A few patients with hemochromatosis are compound heterozygotes for C282Y and a second mutation, H63D, which is relatively common in the general population (Beutler et al., 2000), but on its own does not appear to cause iron overload (Worwood, 1999). The remaining patients lack an identified mutation suggesting evidence of other undiscovered genetic disorders. The clinical disorder is characterized by excessive absorption of food iron associated with the failure to store the additional iron in reticuloendothelial cells. The iron intake of these individuals is in the normal range. Iron accumulation occurs at a rate of about 2 mg/day with the development of clinical manifestations between the fourth and sixth decades of life. At this stage, the total body iron burden may reach 20 to 30 g. The additional iron is stored preferentially in parenchymal cells. Extensive organ damage is the result. If untreated, the disorder results in cirrhosis of the liver, primary liver cancer, myocardial injury with congestive cardiopathy and heart failure, and damage to endocrine organs, particularly the pancreatic islets and the anterior pituitary gland, with resultant diabetes and impotence or amenorrhea (Bothwell and MacPhail, 1998; Walker et al., 1998). Arthritis and increased pigmentation of the skin are also characteristic findings (Bothwell et al., 1979; Olynyk et al., 1999). Individuals with hereditary hemochromatosis as described above (i.e., homozygotes for the HFE gene) are considered distinct and exceptionally sensitive to the effects of iron overload; therefore, they were not considered in deriving a UL for the general healthy population. Effective and widespread screening for early detection of hemochromatosis is needed so that studies investigating the adverse effects of dietary iron in individuals with this disorder will be useful in setting a UL for this subpopulation.

Summary

Gastrointestinal side effects were selected as the critical adverse effects on which to base the UL for iron. Although gastrointestinal distress is not a serious side effect when compared with the possible risk for vascular disease and cancer, the other side effects considered (impaired zinc absorption, increased risk for vascular disease and cancer, and systemic iron overload) did not permit the determination of a UL. Gastrointestinal distress is primarily observed in individuals who have consumed high levels of supplemental iron on an empty stomach. Large doses of iron supplements may inhibit zinc absorption when both are consumed in the fasting state, but zinc absorption is not impaired when supplementary iron is taken with meals. The relationship between iron intake and both vascular disease and cancer is unclear at the present time. With the possible exception of individuals living in Southern Africa who suffer from sub-Saharan iron overload, iron overload has not been shown to result solely from a high dietary iron intake. Moreover, no differences were found in the serum ferritin concentrations between individuals who fell in the lower and upper quartiles for total dietary iron intake in the Third National Health and Nutrition Examination Survey (NHANES III) (Appendix Table H-5). Heterozygous carriers of the C282Y mutation most commonly associated with hereditary hemochromatosis could be at increased risk for accumulating harmful amounts of iron, but there are no direct observations to confirm this suspicion. Homozygotes and individuals with other iron-loading disorders may not be protected by the UL and are addressed under "Special Considerations".

Dose-Response Assessment

Adults

Data Selection. The data on GI effects following supplemental intakes of iron salts were used to derive a UL for iron for apparently healthy adults.

Identification of a No-Observed-Adverse-Effect Level (NOAEL) and a Lowest-Observed-Adverse-Effect Level (LOAEL). A LOAEL of 60 mg/day of supplemental iron salts was identified on the basis of a controlled, double-blind study by Frykman and coworkers (1994). They evaluated GI effects in 97 Swedish adult men and women after intake of either a nonheme iron supplement (60 mg/day as iron fumarate), a supplement containing both heme iron and nonheme iron (18 mg/day, 2 mg from porcine blood and 16 mg as iron fumarate), or a placebo. The groups were similar with respect to gender, age, and basic iron status. The frequency of constipation and the total incidence of all side effects were significantly higher among those receiving nonheme iron than among those receiving either the combination of heme and nonheme iron or the placebo (Table 9-18). Although most of the reported GI effects were minor, five individuals found them to be severe enough to stop taking the medication. Four of these withdrawals occurred during the nonheme-containing iron treatment and one occurred just after changing from the nonheme-containing iron treatment to the placebo.

To estimate a LOAEL for total iron intake, the LOAEL for supplemental ferrous fumarate intake of 60 mg/day for Swedish men and women was added to 11 mg/day, the estimated mean iron intake from food in women from six European countries (Van de Vijver et al., 1999) and in men from Denmark (Bro et al., 1990). The LOAEL for total intake is therefore approximately 70 mg/day (11 + 60). It was not possible to identify a NOAEL based on the data on GI effects. Therefore, the LOAEL of 70 mg/day was used to derive a UL. There is supportive evidence for a LOAEL of 50 to 120 mg/day of supplemental iron salts from several other prospective studies (Brock et al., 1985; Coplin et al., 1991; Liguori, 1993; Lokken and Birkeland, 1979). However, these studies either failed to include a placebo control or contained fewer subjects than the study by Frykman and coworkers (1994).

Uncertainty Assessment. An uncertainty factor (UF) of 1.5 was selected to account for extrapolation from a LOAEL to a NOAEL. Because of the self-limiting nature of the observed GI effects, a higher UF was not justified.

Derivation of a UL. The LOAEL of 70 mg/day was divided by a UF of 1.5 to obtain a LOAEL and UL value of 45 mg/day of iron, after rounding.

$$UL = \frac{LOAEL}{UF} = \frac{70 \text{ mg/day}}{1.5} \cong 45 \text{ mg/day}$$

Iron UL Summary, Ages 19 Years and Older

UL for Adults
    ≥ 19 years   45 mg/day of iron

Pregnancy and Lactation

Data are limited on GI effects in pregnant and lactating women. Rybo and Solvell (1971) compared the side effects of ferrous sulfate, sustained release iron, and placebo in pregnant women. They found that the frequency of severe nausea or vomiting, or both, was significantly higher when 200 mg/day of elemental iron as ferrous sulfate was given than when placebo was given. The lack of data involving doses less than 100 mg/day in pregnant women presents uncertainty as to what dose constitutes a NOAEL for pregnant women. In the absence of data from studies involving lower doses, the UL for nonpregnant and nonlactating adult women (45 mg/day) was specified for pregnant and lactating women as well.

Iron UL Summary, Pregnancy and Lactation

UL for Pregnancy
    14–18 years   45 mg/day of iron
    19–50 years   45 mg/day of iron

UL for Lactation
    14–18 years   45 mg/day of iron
    19–50 years   45 mg/day of iron

Infants, Children, and Adolescents

Data Selection. Data from several studies in infants and young children (Burman, 1972; Farquhar, 1963; Fuerth, 1972; Reeves and Yip, 1985) were judged appropriate for use in deriving a UL for infants and children, and in aggregate they define a dose-response relationship.

Identification of a NOAEL and a LOAEL. No adverse GI effects were reported when 1-month-old infants were supplemented with 5 mg/day of nonheme iron for up to 1 year (Farquhar, 1963) and when 3-

month-old infants were supplemented with 10 mg/day of nonheme iron for up to 21 months (Burman, 1972) (i.e., no adverse effects as compared with infants supplemented with a placebo). Using a higher dose of supplemental nonheme iron (30 mg/day) for 18 months, Farquhar (1963) reported no adverse GI effects in 132 infants. Similarly, no significant adverse GI effects were reported when 124 infants 11 to 14 months of age were supplemented with 3 mg/kg body weight/day (approximately 30 mg/day) of nonheme iron for 3 months (Reeves and Yip, 1985). The median intake of iron for infants, aged 11 to 14 months, is approximately 10 mg/day. Thus, the above human data suggest that an intake of 40 mg/day would be a NOAEL for infants and young children.

Uncertainty Assessment. There is little uncertainty regarding the range of intakes that is likely to induce GI effects in infants and young children. Therefore a UF of 1 is specified.

Derivation of a UL. The NOAEL of 40 mg/day was divided by a UF of 1, resulting in a UL of 40 mg/day of supplemental nonheme iron for infants and young children. Because the safety of excess supplemental nonheme iron in children aged 4 through 18 years has not been studied, a UL of 40 mg/day is recommended for children 4 through 13 years of age, and the adult UL of 45 mg/day is recommended for adolescents.

Iron UL Summary, Ages 0 through 18 Years

UL for Infants
    0–12 months   **40 mg/day of iron**

UL for Children
    1–3 years   **40 mg/day of iron**
    4–8 years   **40 mg/day of iron**
    9–13 years   **40 mg/day of iron**

UL for Adolescents
    14–18 years   **45 mg/day of iron**

Special Considerations

Individuals with the following conditions are susceptible to the adverse effects of excess iron intake: hereditary hemochromatosis; chronic alcoholism, alcoholic cirrhosis, and other liver diseases;

iron-loading abnormalities, particularly thalassemias; congenital atransferrinemia; and aceruloplasminemia (Fairbanks, 1999). These individuals may not be protected by the UL for iron. A UL for subpopulations such as persons with hereditary hemochromatosis can not be determined until information on the relationship between iron intake and the risk of adverse effects from excess iron stores becomes available.

A body of experimental evidence suggests that intermittent dosing (once or twice per week) of iron supplements may be an effective means of controlling iron deficiency in developing countries (Beaton and McCabe, 1999). Under these circumstances, individuals receiving intermittent doses of iron supplements may exceed the UL. The effects of intermittent dosing on gastrointestinal side effects has not been studied adequately.

Intake Assessment

Based on distribution data from NHANES III (Appendix Table C-19), the highest median reported intake of iron from food and supplements for all life stage and gender groups, excluding pregnancy and lactation, was approximately 19 mg/day. This was the median intake reported by men 31 through 50 years of age. The highest intake from food and supplements at the ninetieth percentile reported for any life stage and gender group, excluding pregnancy and lactation, was approximately 34 mg/day for men 51 years of age and older. This value is below the UL of 45 mg/day. Between 50 and 75 percent of pregnant and lactating women consumed iron from food and supplements at a level greater than 45 mg/day, but iron supplementation is usually supervised in pre- and postnatal care programs.

Risk Characterization

Based on a UL of 45 mg/day of iron for adults, the risk of adverse effects from dietary sources appears to be low. Gastrointestinal distress does not occur from consuming a diet containing naturally occurring or fortified iron. Individuals taking iron salts at a level above the UL may encounter gastrointestinal side effects, especially when taken on an empty stomach. Twenty-five percent of men aged 31 to 50 years in the United States have ferritin concentrations greater than 200 µg/L (Appendix Table G-3), which may be a risk factor for cardiovascular disease (Sullivan, 1981). This prevalence is higher in men older than 50 years. However, the significance of these high ferritin concentrations and their relationship to dietary iron intake is uncertain. Nevertheless, the association between a high iron intake and iron overload in sub-Saharan Africa makes it prudent to recommend that men and postmenopausal women avoid iron supplements and highly fortified foods. Currently, doses equal to or greater than the UL are used for the treatment of iron deficiency anemia. The UL is not meant to apply to individuals who are being treated with iron under close medical supervision.

RESEARCH RECOMMENDATIONS FOR IRON

- Determination of the significance of high ferritin concentration.
- Investigation of the effect of iron absorption and dietary iron on phenotypic expressions in individuals with hereditary hemochromatosis.
- Research to distinguish between hereditary hemochromatosis and iron overload.
- Study of the effect of limited iron intake during pregnancy on infant iron status during the first 6 months of life.
- Bioavailability of supplemental iron.
- Concurrence on valid indicators for assessing the effect of iron deficiency anemia on cognitive development and function.
- The risk of cardiovascular disease for those with high stores of body iron.
- The relationship between high iron stores in men and the bioavailability of dietary iron and impaired regulation of iron balance.
- The relationship between iron consumption and oxidative cellular damage.
- Integrative mechanisms of iron transporter proteins that influence gastrointestinal absorption in various dietary conditions and physiologic states.

REFERENCES

AAP (American Academy of Pediatrics). 1999. Iron fortification of infant formulas. *Pediatrics* 104:119–123.

Abma JC, Chandra A, Mosher WD, Peterson LS, Piccinino LJ. 1997. Fertility, family planning, and women's health: New data from the 1995 National Survey of Family Growth. *Vital Health Stat* 23:1–114.

Abrams SA, Wen J, Stuff JE. 1997. Absorption of calcium, zinc, and iron from breast milk by five- to seven-month-old infants. *Pediatr Res* 41:384–390.

Akesson A, Bjellerup P, Berglund M, Bremme K, Vahter M. 1998. Serum transferrin receptor: A specific marker of iron deficiency in pregnancy. *Am J Clin Nutr* 68:1241–1246.

Alexander D, Ball MJ, Mann J. 1994. Nutrient intake and haematological status of vegetarians and age-sex matched omnivores. *Eur J Clin Nutr* 48:538–546.

Allen LH. 1993. Iron-deficiency anemia increases risk of preterm delivery. *Nutr Rev* 51:49–52.

Allen LH. 1997. Pregnancy and iron deficiency: Unresolved issues. *Nutr Rev* 55:91–101.

Allen LH. 2000. Anemia and iron deficiency: Effects on pregnancy outcome. *Am J Clin Nutr* 71:1280S–1284S.

Allen LH, Ahluwalia N. 1997. *Improving Iron Status through Diet. The Appilcation of Knowledge Concerning Dietary Iron Bioavailability in Human Populations.* OMNI Technical Papers, No. 8. Arlington, VA: John Snow International.

Ames SK, Gorham BM, Abrams SA. 1999. Effects of high compared with low calcium intake on calcium absorption and incorpration of iron by red blood cells in small children. *Am J Clin Nutr* 70:44–48.

Anderson AC. 1994. Iron poisoning in children. *Curr Opin Pediatr* 6:289 294.

Anderson RR. 1993. Longitudinal changes of trace elements in human milk during the first 5 months of lactation. *Nutr Res* 13:499–510.

Andersson H, Navert B, Bingham SA, Englyst HN, Cummings JH. 1983. The effects of breads containing similar amounts of phytate but different amounts of wheat bran on calcium, zinc and iron balance in man. *Br J Nutr* 50:503–510.

Ansell JE, Wheby MS. 1972. Pica: Its relation to iron deficiency, A review of the recent literature. *Va Med Mon* 99:951–954.

Archer DF, Dorin MH, Heine W, Nanavati N, Arce JC. 1999. Uterine bleeding in postmenopausal women on continuous therapy with estradiol and norethindrone acetate. *Obstet Gynecol* 94:323–329.

Aronow WS, Ahn C. 1996. Three-year follow-up shows no association of serum ferritin levels with incidence of new coronary events in 577 persons aged ≥ 62 years. *Am J Cardiol* 78:678–679.

Bacon BR, Olynyk JK, Brunt EM, Britton RS, Wolff RK. 1999. HFE genotype in patients with hemochromatosis and other liver diseases. *Ann Intern Med* 130:953–962.

Baer DM, Tekawa IS, Hurley LB. 1994. Iron stores are not associated with acute myocardial infarction. *Circulation* 89:2915–2918.

Banner W Jr, Tong TG. 1986. Iron poisoning. *Pediatr Clin North Am* 33:393–409.

Barrett JF, Whittaker PG, Williams JG, Lind T. 1994. Absorption of non-haem iron from food during normal pregnancy. *Br Med J* 309:79–82.

Beaton GH. 1974. Epidemiology of iron deficiency. In: Jacobs A, Worwood M, eds. *Iron in Biochemistry and Medicine.* London: Academic Press. Pp. 477–528.

Beaton GH. 2000. Iron needs during pregnancy: Do we need to rethink our targets? *Am J Clin Nutr* 72:265S–271S.

Beaton GH, McCabe GP. 1999. *Efficacy of Intermittent Iron Supplementation in the Control of Iron Deficiency Anemia in Developing Countries: An Analysis of Experience.* Report to the Micronutrient Initiative and the Canadian International Development Agency. Ottawa: International Development Research Centre.

Beaton GH, Thein M, Milne H, Veen MJ. 1970. Iron requirements of menstruating women. *Am J Clin Nutr* 23:275–283.

Beaton GH, Corey PN, Steeles C. 1989. Conceptual and methodological issues regarding the epidemiology of iron deficiency and their implications for studies of the functional consequences of iron deficiency. *Am J Clin Nutr* 50:575–588.

Behall KM, Scholfield DJ, Lee K, Powell AS, Moser PB. 1987. Mineral balance in adult men: Effect of four refined fibers. *Am J Clin Nutr* 46:307–314.

Beutler E, Felitti V, Gelbart T, Ngoc H. 2000. The effect of HFE genotypes on measurements of iron overload in patients attending a health appraisal clinic. *Ann Intern Med* 133:329-337.

Bjorn-Rasmussen E, Hallberg L, Isaksson B, Arvidsson B. 1974. Food iron absorption in man. Applications of the two-pool extrinsic tag method to measure heme and non-heme iron absorption from the whole diet. *J Clin Invest* 53:247–255.

Blot I, Papiernik E, Kaltwasser JP, Werner E, Tchernia G. 1981. Influence of routine administration of folic acid and iron during pregnancy. *Gynecol Obstet Invest* 12:294–304.

Bomford A, Williams R. 1976. Long term results of venesection therapy in idiopathic haemochromatosis. *Q J Med* 45:611–623.

Bothwell TH. 2000. Iron requirements in pregnancy and strategies to meet them. *Am J Clin Nutr* 72:257S–264S.

Bothwell TH, Charlton RW. 1981. *Iron Deficiency in Women.* Washington, DC: The Nutrition Foundation. Pp. 7–9.

Bothwell TH, Finch CA. 1962. *Iron Metabolism.* Boston: Little, Brown.

Bothwell TH, MacPhail AP. 1998. Hereditary hemochromatosis: Etiologic, pathologic, and clinical aspects. *Semin Hematol* 35:55–71.

Bothwell TH, Seftel H, Jacobs P, Torrance JD, Baumslag N. 1964. Iron overload in Bantu subjects. Studies on the availability of iron in Bantu beer. *Am J Clin Nutr* 14:47–51.

Bothwell TH, Charlton RW, Cook JD, Finch CA. 1979. *Iron Metabolism in Man.* Oxford: Blackwell Scientific.

Braun J. 1999. Erythrocyte zinc protoporphyrin. *Kidney Int Suppl* 69:S57–S60.

Brigham D, Beard J. 1996. Iron and thermoregulation: A review. *Crit Rev Food Sci Nutr* 36:747–763.

Bro S, Sandstrom B, Heydorn K. 1990. Intake of essential and toxic trace elements in a random sample of Danish men as determined by the duplicate portion sampling technique. *J Trace Elem Electrolytes Health Dis* 4:147–155.

Brock C, Curry H, Hanna C, Knipfer M, Taylor L. 1985. Adverse effects of iron supplementation: A comparative trial of wax-matrix iron preparation and conventional ferrous sulfate tablets. *Clin Ther* 7:568–573.

Brune M, Rossander-Hulten L, Hallberg L, Gleerup A, Sandberg AS. 1992. Iron absorption from bread in humans: Inhibiting effects of cereal fiber, phytate and inositol phosphates with different numbers of phosphate groups. *J Nutr* 122:442–449.

Bulaj ZJ, Griffen LM, Jorde LB, Edwards CQ, Kushner JP. 1996. Clinical and biochemical abnormalities in people heterozygous for hemochromatosis. *N Engl J Med* 335:1799–1805.

Burman D. 1972. Haemoglobin levels in normal infants aged 3 to 24 months, and the effect of iron. *Arch Dis Child* 47:261–271.

Butler NR, Bonham DB. 1963. *Perinatal Mortality.* The first report of the 1958 British Perinatal Mortality Survey. Edinburgh: Livingstone.

Butte NF, Garza C, Smith EO, Wills C, Nichols BL. 1987. Macro- and trace-mineral intakes of exclusively breast-fed infants. *Am J Clin Nutr* 45:42–48.

Canadian Paediatric Society. 1991. Meeting the iron needs of infants and young children: An update. *Canadian Med Assoc J* 144:1451–1454.

Cannone-Hergaux F, Gruenheid S, Ponka P, Gros P. 1999. Cellular and subcellular localization of the Nramp2 iron transporter in the intestinal brush border and regulation by dietary iron. *Blood* 93:4406–4417.

CDC (Centers for Disease Control). 1989. CDC criteria for anemia in children and childbearing-aged women. *Morbid Mortal Weekly Rpt* 38:400–404.

Chalevelakis G, Tsiroyannis K, Hatziioannou J, Arapakis G. 1984. Screening for thalassaemia and/or iron deficiency: Evaluation of some discrimination functions. *Scan J Clin Lab Invest* 44:1–6.

Clarkson PM, Haymes EM. 1995. Exercise and mineral status of athletes: Calcium, magnesium, phosphorous, and iron. *Med Sci Sports Exerc* 27:831–843.

Cole SK, Billewicz WZ, Thomson AM. 1971. Sources of variation in menstrual blood loss. *J Obstet Gynaecol Br Commonw* 78:933–939.

Conrad ME. 1968. Intraluminal factors affecting iron absorption. *Isr J Med Sci* 4:917–931.

Conrad ME, Umbreit JN. 2000. Iron absorption and transport—An update. *Am J Hematol* 64:287–298.

Conrad ME, Benjamin B, Williams H, Foy A. 1967. Human absorption of hemoglobin-iron. *Gastroenterology* 53:5–10.

Cook J. 1999. The nutritional assessment of iron status. *Arch Latinoam Nutr* 49:11S–14S.

Cook JD, Lynch SR. 1986. The liabilities of iron deficiency. *Blood* 68:803–809.

Cook JD, Lipschitz DA, Miles LE, Finch CA. 1974. Serum ferritin as a measure of iron stores in normal subjects. *Am J Clin Nutr* 27:681–687.

Cook JD, Dassenko S, Skikne BS. 1990. Serum transferrin receptor as an index of iron absorption. *Br J Haematol* 75:603–609.

Cook JD, Dassenko SA, Lynch SR. 1991. Assessment of the role of nonheme-iron availability in iron balance. *Am J Clin Nutr* 54:717–722.

Cook JD, Reddy MB, Burri J, Juillerat MA, Hurrell RF. 1997. The influence of different cereal grains on iron absorption from infant cereal foods. *Am J Clin Nutr* 65:964–969.

Coplin M, Schuette S, Leichtmann G, Lashner B. 1991. Tolerability of iron: A comparison of bis-glycino iron II and ferrous sulfate. *Clin Ther* 13:606–612.

Coudray C, Bellanger J, Castiglia-Delavaud C, Remesy C, Vermorel M, Rayssignuier Y. 1997. Effect of soluble or partly soluble dietary fibres supplementation on absorption and balance of calcium, magnesium, iron and zinc in healthy young men. *Eur J Clin Nutr* 51:375–380.

Dallman PR. 1986a. Biochemical basis for the manifestations of iron deficiency. *Annu Rev Nutr* 6:13–40.

Dallman PR. 1986b. Iron deficiency in the weanling: A nutritional problem on the way to resolution. *Acta Paediatr Scand Suppl* 323:59–67.

Dallman PR, Refino CA, Yland MJ. 1982. Sequence of development of iron deficiency in the rat. *Am J Clin Nutr* 35:671–677.

Dalton MA, Sargent JD, O'Connor GT, Olmstead EM, Klein RZ. 1997. Calcium and phosphorous supplementation of iron-fortified infant formula: No effect on iron status of healthy full-term infants. *Am J Clin Nutr* 65:921–926.

Danesh J, Appleby P. 1999. Coronary heart disease and iron status: Meta-analyses of prospective studies. *Circulation* 99:852–854.

Davidsson L, Almgren A, Sandstrom B, Hurrell RF. 1995. Zinc absorption in adult humans: The effect of iron fortification. *Br J Nutr* 74:417–425.

Davidsson L, Galan P, Cherouvrier F, Kastenmayer P, Juillerat MA, Hercberg S, Hurrell RF. 1997. Bioavailability in infants of iron from infant cerals: Effect of dephytinization. *Am J Clin Nutr* 65:916–920.

Davidsson L, Kastenmayer P, Szajewska H, Hurrell RF, Barclay D. 2000. Iron bioavailability in infants from an infant cereal fortified with ferric pyrophosphate or ferrous fumarate. *Am J Clin Nutr* 71:1597–1602.

Davies KJ, Donovan CM, Refino CJ, Brooks GA, Packer L, Dallman PR. 1984. Distinguishing effects of anemia and muscle iron deficiency on exercise bioenergetics in the rat. *Am J Physiol* 246:E535–E543.

De Leeuw NK, Lowenstein L, Hsieh YS. 1966. Iron deficiency and hydremia in normal pregnancy. *Medicine* 45:291–315.

Derman DP, Bothwell TH, MacPhail AP, Torrance JD, Bezwoda WR, Charlton RW, Mayet FG. 1980. Importance of ascorbic acid in the absorption of iron from infant foods. *Scand J Haematol* 25:193–201.

Dewey KG, Lonnerdal B. 1983. Milk and nutrient intake of breast-fed infants from 1 to 6 months: Relation to growth and fatness. *J Pediatr Gasteroenterol Nutr* 2:497–506.

Dewey KG, Romero-Abal ME, Quan de Serrano J, Bulux J, Peerson JM, Engle P, Solomons NW. 1997. A randomized intervention study of the effects of discontinuing coffee intake on growth and morbidity of iron-deficient Guatemalan toddlers. *J Nutr* 127:306–313.

Dibley MJ, Goldsby JB, Staehling NW, Trowbridge FL. 1987. Development of normalized curves for the international growth reference: Historical and technical considerations. *Am J Clin Nutr* 46:736–748.

Dinneen SF, O'Mahony MS, O'Brien T, Cronin CC, Murray DM, O'Sullivan DJ. 1992. Serum ferritin in newly diagnosed and poorly controlled diabetes mellitus. *Ir J Med Sci* 161:636–638.

Disler PB, Lynch SR, Charlton RW, Torrance JD, Bothwell TH, Walker RB, Mayet F. 1975. The effect of tea on iron absorption. *Gut* 16:193–200.

Dwyer JT, Dietz WH, Andrews EM, Suskind RM. 1982. Nutritional status of vegetarian children. *Am J Clin Nutr* 35:204–216.

Edlund M, Blomback M, von Schoultz B, Andersson O. 1996. On the value of menorrhagia as a predictor for coagulation disorders. *Am J Hematol* 53:234–238.

Ehn L, Carlmark B, Hoglund S. 1980. Iron status in athletes involved in intense physical activity. *Med Sci Sports Exerc* 12:61–64.

Eisenstein RS. 2000. Iron regulatory proteins and the molecular control of mammalian iron metabolism. *Annu Rev Nutr* 20:627–662.

Eisenstein RS, Blemings KP. 1998. Iron regulatory proteins, iron responsive elements and iron homeostasis. *J Nutr* 128:2295–2298.

Expert Scientific Working Group. 1985. Summary of a report on assessment of the iron nutritional status of the United States population. *Am J Clin Nutr* 42:1318–1330.

Fairbanks VF. 1999. Iron in medicine and nutrition. In: Shils ME, Olson JA, Shike M, Ross AC, eds. *Modern Nutrition in Health and Disease,* 9th ed. Baltimore: Williams & Wilkins. Pp. 193–221.

Fairweather-Tait S, Fox T, Wharf SG, Eagles J. 1995a. The bioavailability of iron in different weaning foods and the enhancing effect of a fruit drink containing ascorbic acid. *Pediatr Res* 37:389–394.

Fairweather-Tait S, Wharf SG, Fox TE. 1995b. Zinc absorption in infants fed iron-fortified weaning food. *Am J Clin Nutr* 62:785–789.

FAO/WHO (Food and Agriculture Organization of the United Nations/World Health Organization). 1988. *Requirements of Vitamin A, Iron, Folate and Vitamin B_{12}*. FAO Food and Nutrition Series No. 23. Rome: FAO. Pp. 33–50.

Farquhar JD. 1963. Iron supplementation during first year of life. *Am J Dis Child* 106:201–206.

FDA (Food and Drug Administration). 1997. *Preventing Iron Poisoning in Children.* FDA Backgrounder. [Online]. Available: http://www.fda.gov/opacom/backgrounders/ironbg.html [accessed July 1999].

Feder JN. 1999. The hereditary hemochromatosis gene (HFE): A MHC class I-like gene that functions in the regulation of iron homeostasis. *Immunol Res* 20:175–185.

Ferguson BJ, Skikne BS, Simpson KM, Baynes RD, Cook JD. 1992. Serum transferrin receptor distinguishes the anemia of chronic disease from iron deficiency anemia. *J Lab Clin Med* 119:385–390.

Finch CA, Huebers H. 1982. Perspectives in iron metabolism. *N Engl J Med* 306:1520–1528.

Finch CA, Miller LR, Inamdar AR, Person R, Seiler K, Mackler B. 1976. Iron deficiency in the rat. Physiological and biochemical studies of muscle dysfunction. *J Clin Invest* 58:447–453.

Fleming AF. 1968. Hypoplastic anaemia in pregnancy. *J Obstet Gynaecol Br Commonw* 75:138–141.

Fogelholm M. 1995. Inadequate iron status in athletes: An exaggerated problem? In: Kies CV, Driskell JA, eds. *Sports Nutrition: Minerals and Electrolytes.* Boca Raton: CRC Press. Pp. 81–95.

Fomon SJ, Ziegler EE, Nelson SE. 1993. Erythrocyte incorporation of ingested ^{58}Fe by 56-day-old breast-fed and formula-fed infants. *Pediatr Res* 33:573–576.

Ford ES, Cogswell ME. 1999. Diabetes and serum ferritin concentration among U.S. adults. *Diabetes Care* 22:1978-1983.

Franco RF, Zago MA, Trip MD, ten Cate H, van den Ende A, Prins MH, Kastelein JJ, Reitsma PH. 1998. Prevalence of hereditary haemochromatosis in premature atherosclerotic vascular disease. *Br J Haematol* 102:1172–1175.

Frey GH, Krider DW. 1994. Serum ferritin and myocardial infarct. *WV Med J* 90:13–15.

Frisancho AR. 1990. *Anthropometric Standards for the Assessment of Growth and Nutritional Status.* Ann Arbor: University of Michigan Press.

Frykman E, Bystrom M, Jansson U, Edberg A, Hansen T. 1994. Side effects of iron supplements in blood donors: Superior tolerance of heme iron. *J Lab Clin Med* 123:561–564.

Fuerth JH. 1972. Iron supplementation of the diet in full-term infants: A controlled study. *J Pediatr* 80:974–979.

Fung EB, Ritchie LD, Woodhouse LR, Roehl R, King JC. 1997. Zinc absorption in women during pregnancy and lactation: A longitudinal study. *Am J Clin Nutr* 66:80–88.

Garby L, Sjolin S, Vuille JC. 1964. Studies on erythro-kinetics in infancy. IV. The long-term behaviour of radioiron in circulating foetal and adult haemoglobin and its faecal excretion. *Acta Paediatr Scand* 53:33–41.

Garby L, Irnell L, Werner I. 1969. Iron deficiency in women of fertile age in a Swedish community. II. Efficiency of several laboratory tests to predict the response to iron supplementation. *Acta Med Scand* 185:107–111.

Garn SM, Ridella SA, Petzold AS, Falkner F. 1981. Maternal hematologic levels and pregnancy outcomes. *Sem Perinatol* 5:155–162.

Garry P, Koehler KM, Simon TL. 1995. Iron stores and iron absorption: Effects of repeated blood donations. *Am J Clin Nutr* 62:611–620.

Garza C, Johnson CA, Smith EO, Nichols BL. 1983. Changes in the nutrient composition of human milk during gradual weaning. *Am J Clin Nutr* 37:61–65.

Gillooly M, Bothwell TH, Torrance JD, MacPhail AP, Derman DP, Bezwoda WR, Mills W, Charlton RW, Mayet F. 1983. The effects of organic acids, phytates and polyphenols on the absorption of iron from vegetables. *Br J Nutr* 49:331–342.

Gillooly M, Bothwell TH, Charlton RW, Torrance JD, Bezwoda WR, MacPhail AP, Derman DP, Novelli L, Morrall P, Mayet F. 1984. Factors affecting the absorption of iron from cereals. *Br J Nutr* 51:37–46.

Goepel E, Ulmer HU, Neth RD. 1988. Premature labor contractions and the value of serum ferritin during pregnancy. *Gynecol Obstet Invest* 26:265–273.

Gordeuk V, Mukiibi J, Hasstedt SJ, Samowitz W, Edwards CQ, West G, Ndambire S, Emmanual J, Nkanza N, Chapanduka Z, Randall M, Boone P, Romano P, Martell RW, Yamashita T, Effler P, Brittenham G. 1992. Iron overload in Africa. Interaction between a gene and dietary iron content. *N Engl J Med* 326:95–100.

Grasbeck R, Majuri R, Kouvonen I, Tenhunen R. 1982. Spectral and other studies on the intestinal haem receptor of the pig. *Biochim Biophys Acta* 700:137–142.

Green R, Charlton R, Seftel H, Bothwell T, Mayet F, Adams B, Finch C, Layrisse M. 1968. Body iron excretion in man. *Am J Med* 45:336–353.

Gunshin H, Mackenzie B, Berger UV, Gunshin Y, Romero MF, Boron WF, Nussberger S, Gollan JL, Hediger MA. 1997. Cloning and characterization of a mammalian proton-coupled metal-ion transporter. *Nature* 388:482–488.

Gutierrez JA, Yu J, Rivera S, Wessling-Resnick M. 1997. Functional expression cloning and characterization of SFT, a stimulator of Fe transport. *J Cell Biol* 139:895–905.

Hallberg L. 1992. Iron balance in pregnancy and lactation. In: Fomon SJ, Zlotkin S, eds. *Nutritional Anemias*. Nestle Nutrition Workshop Series, Vol. 30. New York: Raven Press. Pp. 13–28.

Hallberg L, Hulthen L. 2000. Prediction of dietary iron absorption: An algorithm for calculating absorption and bioavailability of dietary iron. *Am J Clin Nutr* 71:1147–1160.

Hallberg L, Rossander-Hulthen L. 1991. Iron requirements in menstruating women. *Am J Clin Nutr* 54:1047–1058.

Hallberg L, Hogdahl AM, Nilsson L, Rybo G. 1966a. Menstrual blood loss and iron deficiency. *Acta Med Scand* 180:639–650.

Hallberg L, Hogdahl AM, Nilsson L, Rybo G. 1966b. Menstrual blood loss: A population study. Variation at different ages and attempts to define normality *Acta Obstet Gynecol Scand* 45:320–351.

Hallberg L, Ryttinger L, Solvell L. 1966c. Side-effects of oral iron therapy. A double-blind study of different iron compounds in tablet form. *Acta Med Scand Suppl* 459:3–10.

Hallberg L, Brune M, Erlandsson M, Sandberg AS, Rossander-Hulthen L. 1991. Calcium: Effect of different amounts of nonheme- and heme-iron absorption in humans. *Am J Clin Nutr* 53:112–119.

Hallberg L, Rossander-Hulthen L, Brune M, Gleerup A. 1993. Inhibition of haem-iron absorption in man by calcium. *Br J Nutr* 69:533–540.

Hallfrisch J, Powell A, Carafelli C, Reiser S, Prather ES. 1987. Mineral balances of men and women consuming high fiber diets with complex or simple carbohydrate. *J Nutr* 117:48–55.

Han O, Failla ML, Hill AD, Morris ER, Smith JC. 1995. Reduction of Fe(III) is required for uptake of nonheme iron by Caco-2 cells. *J Nutr* 125:1291–1299.

Harland BF, Oberleas D. 1987. Phytate in foods. *World Rev Nutr Diet* 52:235–259.

Hawkins WW. 1964. Iron, copper and cobalt. In: Beaton GH, McHenry EW, eds. *Nutrition: A Comprehensive Treatise*. New York: Academic Press. Pp. 309–372.

Haycock GB, Schwartz GJ, Wisotsky DH. 1978. Geometric method for measuring body surface area: A height-weight formula validated in infants, children, and adults. *J Pediatr* 93:62–66.

Hefnawi F, Yacout MM. 1978. Intrauterine contraception in developing countries. In: Ludwig H, Tauber PF, eds. *Human Fertilization*. Stuttgart: Georg Thieme. Pp. 249–253.

Hefnawi F, el-Zayat AF, Yacout MM. 1980. Physiologic studies of menstrual blood loss. *Int J Gynaecol Obstet* 17:348–352.

Hegenauer J, Saltman P, Ludwig D, Ripley L, Ley A. 1979. Iron-supplemented cow milk. Identification and spectral properties of iron bound to casein micelles. *J Agric Food Chem* 27:1294–1301.

Hegsted DM. 1975. Balance studies. *J Nutr* 106:307–311.

Higgs JM. 1973. Chronic mucocutaneous candidiasis: Iron deficiency and the effects of iron therapy. *Proc R Soc Med* 66:802–804.

Hogan GR, Jones B. 1970. The relationship of koilonychia and iron deficiency in infants. *J Pediatr* 77.1051 1057.

Holbrook JT, Smith JC, Reiser S. 1989. Dietary fructose or starch: Effects on copper, zinc, iron, manganese, calcium, and magnesium balances in humans. *Am J Clin Nutr* 49:1290–1294.

Hsing AW, McLaughlin JK, Olsen JH, Mellemkjar L, Wacholder S, Fraumeni JF. 1995. Cancer risk following primary hemochromatosis: A population-based cohort study in Denmark. *Int J Cancer* 60:160–162.

Hunt JR, Roughead ZK. 1999. Nonheme-iron absorption, fecal ferritin excretion, and blood indexes of iron status in women consuming controlled lactoovovegetarian diets for 8 weeks. *Am J Clin Nutr* 69:944–952.

Hunt JR, Mullen LM, Lykken GI, Gallagher SK, Nielsen FH. 1990. Ascorbic acid: Effect on ongoing iron absorption and status in iron-depleted young women. *Am J Clin Nutr* 51:649–655.

Hurrell RF, Juillerat MA, Reddy MB, Lynch SR, Dassenko SA, Cook JD. 1992. Soy protein, phytate and iron absorption in humans. *Am J Clin Nutr* 56:573–578.

Hytten FE, Leitch I. 1971. *The Physiology of Human Pregnancy*, 2nd ed. Oxford: Blackwell Scientific.

Idjradinata P, Pollitt E. 1993. Reversal of developmental delays in iron-deficient anaemic infants treated with iron. *Lancet* 341:1–4.

INACG (International Nutritional Anemia Consultative Group). 1985. *Measurements of Iron Status*. Washington, DC: Nutrition Foundation.

IOM (Institute of Medicine). 1990. *Nutrition During Pregnancy*. Washington, DC: National Academy Press.

IOM. 1993. *Iron Deficiency Anemia: Recommended Guidelines for the Prevention, Detection, and Management Among U.S. Children and Women of Childbearing Age*. Washington, DC: National Academy Press.

Ivaturi R, Kies C. 1992. Mineral balances in humans as affected by fructose, high fructose corn syrup and sucrose. *Plant Foods Hum Nutr* 42:143–151.

Jacobs A. 1971. The effect of iron deficiency on the tissues. *Gerontol Clin (Basel)* 13:61–68.

Johnson MA, Baier MJ, Greger JL. 1982. Effects of dietary tin on zinc, copper, iron, manganese, and magnesium metabolism of adult males. *Am J Clin Nutr* 35:1332–1338.

Kelly KA, Turnbull A, Cammock EE, Bombeck CT, Nyhus LM, Finch CA. 1967. Iron absorption after gastrectomy: An experimental study in the dog. *Surgery* 62:356–360.

Kelsay JL, Behall KM, Prather ES. 1979. Effect of fiber from fruits and vegetables on metabolic responses of human subjects. *Am J Clin Nutr* 32:1876–1880.

Kiechl S, Willeit J, Egger G, Poewe W, Oberhollenzer F. 1997. Body iron stores and the risk of carotid atherosclerosis: Prospective results from the Bruneck Study. *Circulation* 96:3300–3307.

Klebanoff MA, Shiono PH, Selby JV, Trachtenberg AI, Graubard BI. 1991. Anemia and spontaneous preterm birth. *Am J Obstet Gynecol* 164:59–63.

Konijn AM. 1994. Iron metabolism in inflammation. *Baillieres Clin Haematol* 7:829–849.

Lampe JW, Slavin JL, Apple FS. 1991. Iron status of active women and the effect of running a marathon on bowel function and gastrointestinal blood loss. *Int J Sports Med* 12:173–179.

Leggett BA, Brown NN, Bryant SJ, Duplock L, Powell LW, Halliday JW. 1990. Factors affecting the concentrations of ferritin in serum in a healthy Australian population. *Clin Chem* 36:1350–1355.

Lemons JA, Moye L, Hall D, Simmons M. 1982. Differences in the composition of preterm and term human milk during early lactation. *Pediatr Res* 16:113–117.

Liao Y, Cooper RS, McGee DL. 1994. Iron status and coronary heart disease: Negative findings from the NHANES I Epidemiologic Follow-Up Study. *Am J Epidemiol* 139:704–712.

Lieberman E, Ryan KJ, Monson RR, Schoenbaum SC. 1988. Association of maternal hematocrit with premature labor. *Am J Obstet Gynecol* 159:107–114.

Liguori L. 1993. Iron protein succinylate in the treatment of iron deficiency: Controlled, double-blind, multicenter clinical trial on over 1,000 patients. *Int J Clin Pharmacol Ther Toxicol* 31:103–123.

Lipsman S, Dewey KG, Lonnerdal B. 1985. Breast-feeding among teenage mothers: Milk composition, infant growth, and maternal dietary intake. *J Pediatr Gastroenterol Nutr* 4:426–434.

Lokken P, Birkeland JM. 1979. Dental discolorations and side effects with iron and placebo tablets. *Scand J Dent Res* 87:275–278.

Lonnerdal B, Keen CL, Hurley LS. 1981. Iron, copper, zinc and maganese in milk. *Ann Rev Nutr* 1:149–174.

Lozoff B, Brittenham G, Viteri FE, Wolf AW, Urrutia JJ. 1982a. Developmental deficits in iron-deficient infants: Effects of age and severity of iron lack. *J Pediatr* 101:948–952.

Lozoff B, Brittenham G, Viteri FE, Wolf AW, Urrutia JJ. 1982b. The effects of short-term oral iron therapy on developmental deficits in iron-deficient anemic infants. *J Pediatr* 100:351–357.

Lozoff B, Wolf AW, Urrutia JJ, Viteri FE. 1985. Abnormal behavior and low developmental test scores in iron-deficient anemic infants. *J Dev Behav Pediatr* 6:69–75.

Lozoff B, Klein NK, Prabucki KM. 1986. Iron-deficient anemic infants at play. *J Dev Behav Pediatr* 7:152–158.

Lozoff B, Brittenham G, Wolf AW, McClish DK, Kuhnert PM, Jimenez E, Jimenez R, Mora LA, Gomez I, Krauskoph D. 1987. Iron deficiency anemia and iron therapy effects on infant developmental test performance. *Pediatrics* 79:981–995.

Lozoff B, Jimenez E, Wolf AW. 1991. Long-term developmental outcome of infants with iron deficiency. *N Engl J Med* 325:687–694.

Lozoff B, Wolf AW, Jimenez E. 1996. Iron-deficiency anemia and infant development: Effects of extended oral iron therapy. *J Pediatr* 129:382–389.

Lozoff B, Jimenez E, Hagen J, Mollen E, Wolf AW. 2000. Poorer behavioral and developmental outcome more than 10 years after treatment for iron deficiency in infancy. *Pediatrics* 105:E51.

Lynch SR, Beard JL, Dassenko SA, Cook JD. 1984. Iron absorption from legumes in humans. *Am J Clin Nutr* 40:42–47.

Lynch SR, Dassenko SA, Cook JD, Juillerat MA, Hurrell RF. 1994. Inhibitory effect of a soybean-protein—Related moiety on iron absorption in humans. *Am J Clin Nutr* 60:567–572.

MacLennan AH, MacLennan A, Wenzel S, Chambers HM, Eckert K. 1993. Continuous low-dose oestrogen and progestogen hormone replacement therapy: A randomised trial. *Med J Aust* 159:102–106.

Magnusson B, Hallberg L, Rossander L, Swolin B. 1984. Iron metabolism and "sports anemia". II. A hematological comparison of elite runners and control subjects. *Acta Med Scand* 216:157–164.

Magnusson MK, Sigfusson N, Sigvaldason H, Johannesson GM, Magnusson S, Thorgeirsson G. 1994. Low iron-binding capacity as a risk factor for myocardial infarction. *Circulation* 89:102–108.

Mahalko JR, Sandstead HH, Johnson L, Milne DB. 1983. Effect of moderate increase in dietary protein on the retention and excretion of Ca, Cu, Fe, Mg, P, and Zn by adult males. *Am J Clin Nutr* 37:8–14.

Manttari M, Manninen V, Huttunen JK, Palosuo T, Ehnholm C, Heinonen OP, Frick MH. 1994. Serum ferritin and ceruloplasmin as coronary risk factors. *Eur Heart J* 15:1599–1603.

McCord JM. 1996. Effects of positive iron status at a cellular level. *Nutr Rev* 54:85–88.

McGuigan MA. 1996. Acute iron poisoning. *Pediatr Ann* 25:33–38.

Meadows NJ, Grainger SL, Ruse W, Keeling PW, Thompson RP. 1983. Oral iron and the bioavailability of zinc. *Br Med J* 287:1013–1014.

Mendelson RA, Anderson GH, Bryan MH. 1982. Zinc, copper and iron content of milk from mothers of preterm and full-term infants. *Early Hum Dev* 6:145–151.

Mendoza C, Viteri FE, Lonnerdal B, Young KA, Raboy V, Brown KH. 1998. Effect of genetically modified, low-phytic acid maize on absorption of iron from tortillas. *Am J Clin Nutr* 68:1123–1127.

Milman N, Kirchhoff M. 1991a. Iron stores in 1433, 30- to 60-year-old Danish males. Evaluation by serum ferritin and haemoglobin. *Scand J Clin Lab Invest* 51:635–641.

Milman N, Kirchhoff M. 1991b. The influence of blood donation on iron stores assessed by serum ferritin and hemoglobin in a population survey of 1,359 Danish women. *Ann Hematol* 63:27–32.

Minihane AM, Fairweather-Tait SJ. 1998. Effect of calcium supplementation on daily nonheme-iron absorption and long-term iron status. *Am J Clin Nutr* 68:96–102.

Monsen ER, Hallberg L, Layrisse M, Hegsted DM, Cook JD, Mertz W, Finch CA. 1978. Estimation of available dietary iron. *Am J Clin Nutr* 31:134–141.

Morrison HI, Semenciw RM, Mao Y, Wigle DT. 1994. Serum iron and risk of fatal acute myocardial infarction. *Epidemiology* 5:243–246.

Moss AJ, Levy AS, Kim I, Park YK. 1989. *Use of Vitamin and Mineral Supplements in the United States: Current Users, Types of Products, and Nutrients.* Advance Data, Vital and Health Statistics of the National Center for Health Statistics, Number 174. Hyattsville, MD: National Center for Health Statistics.

Muir A, Hopfer U. 1985. Regional specificity of iron uptake by small intestinal brush-border membranes from normal and iron-deficient mice. *Am J Physiol* 248:G376–G379.

Murphy JF, O'Riordan J, Newcombe RG, Coles EC, Pearson JF. 1986. Relation of haemoglobin levels in first and second trimesters to outcome of pregnancy. *Lancet* 1:992–995.

Nassar BA, Zayed EM, Title LM, O'Neill BJ, Bata IR, Kirkland SA, Dunn J, Dempsey GI, Tan MH, Johnstone DE. 1998. Relation of HFE gene mutations, high iron stores and early onset coronary artery disease. *Can J Cardiol* 14:215–220.

Nelson RL, Davis FG, Sutter E, Sobin LH, Kikendall JW, Bowen P. 1994. Body iron stores and risk of colonic neoplasia. *J Natl Cancer Inst* 86:455–460.

Nelson RL, Davis FG, Persky V, Becker E. 1995. Risk of neoplastic and other diseases among people with heterozygosity for hereditary hemochromatosis. *Cancer* 76:875–879.

Newhouse IJ, Clement DB. 1995. The efficacy of iron supplementation in iron depleted women. In: Kies CV, Driskell JA, eds. *Sports Nutrition: Minerals and Electrolytes.* Boca Raton: CRC Press. Pp. 47–57.

Niederau C, Fischer R, Sonnenberg A, Stremmel W, Trampisch HJ, Strohmeyer G. 1985. Survival and causes of death in cirrhotic and in noncirrhotic patients with primary hemochromatosis. *N Engl J Med* 313:1256–1262.

Nilsson L, Solvell L. 1967. Clinical studies on oral contraceptives—A randomized, doubleblind, crossover study of 4 different preparations (Anovlar mite, Lyndiol mite, Ovulen, and Volidan). *Acta Obstet Gynecol Scand* 46:1–31.

Nokes C, van den Bosch C, Bundy DAP. 1998. *The Effects of Iron Deficiency and Anemia on Mental and Motor Performance, Educational Acheivement, and Behavior in Children.* The International Nutritional Anemia Consultative Group. Washington, DC: ILSI Press.

NRC (National Research Council). 1979. *Iron.* Baltimore: University Park Press. Pp. 248.

O'Brien KO, Zavaleta N, Caulfield LE, Wen J, Abrams SA. 2000. Prenatal iron supplements impair zinc absorption in pregnant Peruvian women. *J Nutr* 130:2251–2255.

Olynyk JK, Cullen DJ, Aquilia S, Rossi E, Summerville L, Powell LW. 1999. A population-based study of the clinical expression of the hemochromatosis gene. *N Engl J Med* 341:718–724.

Oosterbaan HP, van Buuren AH, Schram JH, van Kempen PJ, Ubachs JM, van Leusden HA, Beyer GP. 1995. The effects of continuous combined transdermal oestrogen-progestogen treatment on bleeding patterns and the endometrium in postmenopausal women. *Maturitas* 21:211–219.

Osaki S, Johnson DA, Frieden E. 1966. The possible significance of the ferrous oxidase activity of ceruloplasmin in normal human serum. *J Biol Chem* 241:2746–2751.

Oski FA, Honig AS, Helu B, Howanitz P. 1983. Effect of iron therapy on behavior performance in nonanemic, iron-deficient infants. *Pediatrics* 71:877–880.

Osler M, Milman N, Heitmann BL. 1998. Dietary and non-dietary factors associated with iron status in a cohort of Danish adults followed for six years. *Eur J Clin Nutr* 52:459–463.

Picciano MF, Guthrie HA. 1976. Copper, iron, and zinc contents of mature human milk. *Am J Clin Nutr* 29:242–254.

Pollitt E, Gorman KS, Engle PL, Martorell R, Rivera J. 1993. Early supplemental feeding and cognition: Effects over two decades. *Monogr Soc Res Child Dev* 58:1–99.

Powell LW. 1970. Tissue damage in haemochromatosis: An analysis of the roles of iron and alcoholism. *Gut* 11:980.

Preziosi P, Prual A, Galan P, Daouda H, Boureima H, Hercberg S. 1997. Effect of iron supplementation on the iron status of pregnant women: Consequences for newborns. *Am J Clin Nutr* 66:1178–1182.

Raffin SB, Woo CH, Roost KT, Price DC, Schmid R. 1974. Intestinal absorption of hemoglobin iron-heme cleavage by mucosal heme oxygenase. *J Clin Invest* 54:1344–1352.

Raja KB, Simpson RJ, Peters TJ. 1987. Comparison of $^{59}Fe^{3+}$ uptake in vitro and in vivo by mouse duodenum. *Biochim Biophys Acta* 901:52–60.

Raja KB, Simpson RJ, Peters TJ. 1993. Investigation of a role for reduction in ferric iron uptake by mouse duodenum. *Biochim Biophys Acta* 1135:141–146.

Raper NR, Rosenthal JC, Woteki CE. 1984. Estimates of available iron in diets of individuals 1 year old and older in the Nationwide Food Consumption Survey. *J Am Diet Assoc* 84:783–787.

Raunikar RA, Sabio H. 1992. Anemia in the adolescent athelete. *Am J Dis Child* 146:1201–1205.

Ravel R. 1989. *Clinical Laboratory Medicine: Clinical Application of Laboratory Data.* Chicago: Year Book Medical Publishers.

Reddy MB, Hurrell RF, Cook JD. 2000. Estimation of nonheme-iron bioavailability from meal composition. *Am J Clin Nutr* 71:937–943.

Reeves JD, Yip R. 1985. Lack of adverse side effects of oral ferrous sulfate therapy in 1-year-old infants. *Pediatrics* 75:352–355.

Reunanen A, Takkunen H, Knekt P, Seppanen R, Aromaa A. 1995. Body iron stores, dietary iron intake and coronary heart disease mortality. *J Intern Med* 238:223–230.

Roest M, van der Schouw YT, de Valk B, Marx JJ, Tempelman MJ, de Groot PG, Sixma JJ, Banga JD. 1999. Heterozygosity for a hereditary hemochromatosis gene is associated with cardiovascular death in women. *Circulation* 100:1268–1273.

Roncagliolo M, Garrido M, Walter T, Peirano P, Lozoff B. 1998. Evidence of altered central nervous system development in infants with iron deficiency anemia at 6 months: Delayed maturation of auditory brainstem responses. *Am J Clin Nutr* 68:683–690.

Rowland TW, Stagg L, Kelleher JF. 1991. Iron deficiency in adolescent girls. Are athletes at risk? *J Adolesc Health* 12:22–25.

Rybo G, Solvell L. 1971. Side-effect studies on a new sustained release iron preparation. *Scand J Haematol* 8:257–264.

Salonen JT, Nyyssonen K, Korpela H, Tuomilehto J, Seppanen R, Salonen R. 1992. High stored iron levels are associated with excess risk of myocardial infarction in eastern Finnish men. *Circulation* 86:803–811.

Salonen JT, Nyyssonen K, Salonen R. 1994. Body iron stores and the risk of coronary heart disease. *N Engl J Med* 331:1159.

Sandberg AS. 1991. The effect of food processing on phytate hydrolysis and availability of iron and zinc. *Adv Exp Med Biol* 289:499–508.

Sandstrom B, Davidsson L, Cederblad A, Lonnerdal B. 1985. Oral iron, dietary ligands and zinc absorption. *J Nutr* 115:411–414.

Scholl TO, Hediger ML, Fischer RL, Shearer JW. 1992. Anemia vs iron deficiency: Increased risk of preterm delivery in a prospective study. *Am J Clin Nutr* 55:985–988.

Selby JV, Friedman GD. 1988. Epidemiologic evidence of an association between body iron stores and risk of cancer. *Int J Cancer* 41:677–682.

Sempos CT, Looker AC, Gillum RF, Makuc DM. 1994. Body iron stores and the risk of coronary heart disease. *N Engl J Med* 330:1119–1124.

Shaw NS, Chin CJ, Pan WH. 1995. A vegetarian diet rich in soybean products compromises iron status in young students. *J Nutr* 125:212–219.

Siegel AJ, Hennekens CH, Solomon HS, Van Boeckel B. 1979. Exercise-related hematuria. Findings in a group of marathon runners. *J Am Med Assoc* 241:391–392.

Siegenberg D, Baynes RD, Bothwell TH, Macfarlane BJ, Lamparelli RD, Car NG, MacPhail P, Schmidt U, Tal A, Mayet F. 1991. Ascorbic acid prevents the dose-dependent inhibitory effects of polyphenols and phytates on nonheme-iron absorption. *Am J Clin Nutr* 53:537–541.

Siimes MA, Refino C, Dallman P. 1980a. Manifestation of iron deficiency at various levels of dietary iron intake. *Am J Clin Nutr* 33:570–574.

Siimes MA, Refino C, Dallman P. 1980b. Physiological anemia of early development in the rat: Characterization of the iron-responsive component. *Am J Clin Nutr* 33:2601–2608.

Simpson RJ, Raja KB, Peters TJ. 1986. Fe2+ uptake by mouse intestinal musosa in vivo and by isolated intestinal brush-border membrane vesicles. *Biochim Biophys Acta* 860:229–235.

Skinner JD, Carruth BR, Houck KS, Coletta F, Cotter R, Ott D, McLeod M. 1997. Longitudinal study of nutrient and food intakes of infants aged 2 to 24 months. *J Am Diet Assoc* 97:496–504.

Smith NJ, Rios E. 1974. Iron metabolism and iron deficiency in infancy and childhood. *Adv Pediatr* 21:239–280.

Snedeker SM, Smith SA, Greger JL. 1982. Effect of dietary calcium and phosphorus levels on the utilization of iron, copper, and zinc by adult males. *J Nutr* 112:136–143.

Sokoll LJ, Dawson-Hughes B. 1992. Calcium supplementation and plasma ferritin concentrations in premenopausal women. *Am J Clin Nutr* 56:1045–1048.

Solomons NW. 1986. Competitive interaction of iron and zinc in the diet: Consequences for human nutrition. *J Nutr* 116:927–935.

Solomons NW, Jacob RA. 1981. Studies on the bioavailability of zinc in humans: Effects of heme and nonheme iron on the absorption of zinc. *Am J Clin Nutr* 34:475–482.

Solomons NW, Pineda O, Viteri F, Sandstead H. 1983. Studies on the bioavailability of zinc in humans: Mechanism of the intestinal interaction of nonheme iron and zinc. *J Nutr* 113:337–349.

Stampfer MJ, Grodstein F, Rosenberg I, Willett W, Hennekens C. 1993. A prospective study of plasma ferritin and risk of myocardial infarction in US physicians. *Circulation* 87:688.

Stevens RG, Jones DY, Micozzi MS, Taylor PR. 1988. Body iron stores and the risk of cancer. *N Engl J Med* 319:1047–1052.

Stevens RG, Graubard BI, Micozzi MS, Neriishi K, Blumberg BS. 1994. Moderate elevation of body iron level and increased risk of cancer occurrence and death. *Int J Cancer* 56:364–369.

Stewart JG, Ahlquist DA, McGill DB, Ilstrup DM, Schwartz S, Owen RA. 1984. Gastrointestinal blood loss and anemia in runners. *Ann Intern Med* 100:843–845.

Stoltzfus R, Dreyfuss M. 1998. *Guidelines for the Use of Iron Supplements to Prevent and Treat Iron Deficiency Anemia.* Washington, DC: ILSI Press.

Strupp BJ, Levitsky DA. 1995. Enduring cognitive effects of early malnutrition: A theoretical reappraisal. *J Nutr* 125:2221S–2232S.

Sullivan JL. 1981. Iron and the sex difference in heart disease risk. *Lancet* 1:1293–1294.

Tanner JM, Whitehouse RH, Takaishi M. 1966. Standards from birth to maturity for height, weight, height velocity and weight velocity: British children, 1965. Part II. *Arch Dis Child* 41:613–635.

Taylor D, Mallen C, McDougall N, Lind T. 1982. Effect of iron supplementation on serum ferritin levels during and after pregnancy. *Br J Obstet Gynecol* 89:1011–1017.

Taylor PG, Martinz-Torres C, Romano EL, Layrisse M. 1986. The effect of cysteine-containing peptides released during meat digestion on iron absorption in humans. *Am J Clin Nutr* 43:68–71.

Thompson CH, Green YS, Ledingham JG, Radda GK, Rajagopalan B. 1993. The effect of iron deficiency on skeletal muscle metabolism of the rat. *Acta Physiol Scand* 147:85–90.

Tuntawiroon M, Sritongkul N, Brune M, Rossander-Hulten L, Pleehachinda R, Suwanik R, Hallberg L. 1991. Dose-dependent inhibitory effect of phenolic compounds in foods on nonheme-iron absorption in men. *Am J Clin Nutr* 53:554–557.

Tuomainen TP, Nyyssonen K, Salonen R, Tervahauta A, Korpela H, Lakka T, Kaplan GA, Salonen JT. 1997. Body iron stores are associated with serum insulin and blood glucose concentrations. Population study in 1,013 eastern Finnish men. *Diabetes Care* 20:426–428.

Tuomainen TP, Kontula K, Nyyssonsen K, Lakka TA, Helio T, Salonen JT. 1999. Increased risk of acute myocardial infarction in carriers of the hemochromatosis gene Cys282Tyr mutation: A prospective cohort study in men in eastern Finland. *Circulation* 100:1274–1279.

Turnlund JR, Keyes WR, Hudson CA, Betschart AA, Kretsch MJ, Sauberlich HE. 1991. A stable-isotope study of zinc, copper, and iron absorption and retention by young women fed vitamin B-6-deficient diets. *Am J Clin Nutr* 54:1059–1064.

Valberg LS. 1980. Plasma ferritin concentration: Their clinical significance and relevance to patient care. *Can Med Assoc* 122:1240–1248.

Valberg LS, Flanagan PR, Chamberlain MJ. 1984. Effects of iron, tin, and copper on zinc absorption in humans. *Am J Clin Nutr* 40:536–541.

Van Asperen IA, Feskens EJ, Bowles CH, Kromhout D. 1995. Body iron stores and mortality due to cancer and ischaemic heart disease: A 17-year follow-up study of elderly men and women. *Int J Epidemiol* 24:665–670.

Van de Vijver LP, Kardinaal AF, Charzewska J, Rotily M, Charles P, Maggiolini M, Ando S, Vaananen K, Wajszczyk B, Heikkinen J, Deloraine A, Schaafsma G. 1999. Calcium intake is weakly but consistently negatively associated with iron status in girls and women in six European countries. *J Nutr* 129:963–968.

Van Dokkum W, Cloughley FA, Hulshof KF, Oosterveen LA. 1983. Effect of variations in fat and linoleic acid intake on the calcium, magnesium and iron balance of young men. *Ann Nutr Metab* 27:361–369.

Vaughan LA, Weber CW, Kemberling SR. 1979. Longitudinal changes in the mineral content of human milk. *Am J Clin Nutr* 32:2301–2306.

Viteri FE, Torun B. 1974. Anaemia and physical work capacity. *Clin Haematol* 3:609–626.

Walker EM, Wolfe MD, Norton ML, Walker SM, Jones MM. 1998. Herditary hemochromatosis. *Ann Clin Lab Sci* 28:300–312.

Walsh CT, Sandstead HH, Prasad AS, Newberne PM, Fraker PJ. 1994. Zinc: Health effects and research priorities for the 1990s. *Environ Health Perspect* 102:5–46.

Walter T, Kovalskys J, Stekel A. 1983. Effect of mild iron deficiency on infant mental developmental scores. *J Pediatr* 102:519–522.

Walter T, de Andraca I, Chadud P, Perales CG. 1989. Iron deficiency anemia: Adverse effects on infant psychomotor development. *Pediatrics* 84:7–17.

Weaver CM, Rajaram S. 1992. Exercise and iron status. *J Nutr* 122:782–787.

Weight LM. 1993. Sports anemia. Does it exist? *Sports Med* 16:1–4.

Weintraub LR, Conrad ME, Crosby WH. 1965. Absorption of hemoglobin iron by the rat. *Proc Soc Exp Biol Med* 120:840–843.

Whiting SJ. 1995. The inhibitory effect of dietary calcium on iron bioavailability: A cause for concern? *Nutr Rev* 53:77–80.

Whittaker P. 1998. Iron and zinc interactions in humans. *Am J Clin Nutr* 68:442S–446S.

WHO (World Health Organization). 1992. *The Prevalence of Anaemia in Women. A Tabulation of Available Information.* Geneva: WHO.

WHO. 1994. *An Evaluation of Infant Growth. A Summary of Analyses Performed in Preparation for the WHO Expert Committee on Physical Status: The Use and Interpretation of Anthropometry.* WHO Working Group on Infant Growth. WHO/NUT/94.8. Geneva: WHO.

WHO/UNICEF/UNU (United Nations Children Fund/United Nations University). 1998. *IDA: Prevention, Assessment and Control.* Report of a joint WHO/UNICEF/UNU consultation. Geneva: WHO.

Widdowson EM, Spray CM. 1951. Chemical development in utero. *Arch Dis Child* 26:205–214.

Williams MD, Wheby MS. 1992. Anemia in pregnancy. *Med Clin North Am* 76:631–647.

Willis WT, Dallman PR, Brooks GA. 1988. Physiological and biochemical correlates of increased work in trained iron-deficient rats. *J Appl Physiol* 65:256–263.

Wollenberg P, Rummel W. 1987. Dependence of intestinal iron absorption on the valency state of iron. *Naunyn Schmiedebergs Arch Pharmacol* 336:578–582.

Wollenberg P, Mahlberg R, Rummel W. 1990. The valency state of absorbed iron appearing in the portal blood and ceruloplasmin substitution. *Biometals* 3:1–7.

Worwood M. 1999. Inborn errors of metabolism: Iron. *Br Med Bull* 55:556–567.

Wurzelmann JI, Sliver A, Schreinemachers DM, Sandler RS, Everson RB. 1996. Iron intake and the risk of colorectal cancer. *Cancer Epidemiol Biomarkers Prev* 5:503–507.

Yip R. 2000. Significance of an abnormally low or high hemoglobin concentration during pregnancy: Special consideration of iron nutrition. *Am J Clin Nutr* 72:272S–279S.

Yip R, Reeves JD, Lonnerdal B, Keen CL, Dallman PR. 1985. Does iron supplementation compromise zinc nutrition in healthy infants? *Am J Clin Nutr* 42:683–687.

10

Manganese

SUMMARY

Manganese is involved in the formation of bone and in amino acid, lipid, and carbohydrate metabolism. There were insufficient data to set an Estimated Average Requirement (EAR) for manganese. An Adequate Intake (AI) was set based on median intakes reported from the Food and Drug Administration Total Diet Study. The AI for adult men and women is 2.3 and 1.8 mg/day, respectively. A Tolerable Upper Intake Level (UL) of 11 mg/day was set for adults based on a no-observed-adverse-effect level for Western diets.

BACKGROUND INFORMATION

Function

Manganese is an essential nutrient involved in the formation of bone and in amino acid, cholesterol, and carbohydrate metabolism. Manganese metalloenzymes include arginase, glutamine synthetase, phosphoenolpyruvate decarboxylase, and manganese superoxide dismutase. Glycosyltransferases and xylosyltransferases, which are important in proteoglycan synthesis and thus bone formation, are sensitive to manganese status in animals. Several other manganese-activated enzymes, including pyruvate carboxylase, can also be activated by other ions, such as magnesium.

394

Physiology of Absorption, Metabolism, and Excretion

Only a small percentage of dietary manganese is absorbed. Absorbed manganese is excreted very rapidly into the gut via bile (Britton and Cotzias, 1966; Davis et al., 1993). Most estimates of absorption have been based on whole body retention curves at approximately 10 to 20 days after dosing with [54]Mn. Using this method, Finley and coworkers (1994) estimated absorption from a test meal containing 1 mg manganese to be 1.35 ± 0.51 percent (standard deviation [SD]) for men and 3.55 ± 2.11 percent (SD) for women. From a test meal containing 0.3 to 0.34 mg of manganese, Davidsson and coworkers (1988) found the retention of [54]Mn to be 5.0 ± 3.1 percent (SD) 10 days after administration to young adult women. Turnover of orally administered [54]Mn was much more rapid after oral administration than after intravenous administration (Davidsson et al., 1989b; Sandstrom et al., 1986). Furthermore, absorption of manganese after 30 weeks of supplementation was 30 to 50 percent lower than had been observed in nonsupplemented subjects (Sandstrom et al., 1990). Some studies indicate that manganese is absorbed through an active transport mechanism (Garcia-Aranda et al., 1983), but passive diffusion has been suggested on the basis of studies indicating that manganese absorption occurs by a nonsaturable process (Bell et al., 1989).

Manganese is taken up from the blood by the liver and transported to extrahepatic tissues by transferrin (Davidsson et al., 1989c) and possibly α_2-macroglobulin (Rabin et al., 1993) and albumin (Davis et al., 1992). Manganese inhibited iron absorption, both from a solution and from a hamburger meal (Rossander-Hulten et al., 1991). [54]Mn has a longer half-life in men than in women (Finley et al., 1994). A significant negative association between manganese absorption and plasma ferritin concentrations has recently been reported (Finley, 1999). Serum ferritin concentrations differ in men and women (Appendix Table G-3); therefore, a major factor in establishing manganese requirements may be gender.

Manganese is excreted primarily in feces. Urinary excretion of manganese is low and has not been found to be sensitive to dietary manganese intake (Davis and Greger, 1992). Urinary excretion in a balance study of five healthy men varied from 0.04 to 0.14 percent of their intake, and absolute amounts in the urine decreased during the depletion phases of the study (Freeland-Graves et al., 1988). Therefore, potential risk for manganese toxicity is highest when bile excretion is low, such as in the neonate or in liver disease (Hauser et al., 1994). Plasma manganese concentrations can become elevated in infants with choleostatic liver disease given supplemental manganese in total parenteral nutrition solutions (Kelly, 1998). It is not certain at what age human infants can maintain manganese homeostasis. Neonatal mice were unable to maintain manganese homeostasis until 17 to 18 days of age (Fechter, 1999).

Clinical Effects of Inadequate Intake

Manganese deficiency has been observed in various species of animals with the signs of deficiency, including impaired growth, impaired reproductive function, impaired glucose tolerance, and alterations in carbohydrate and lipid metabolism. Furthermore, manganese deficiency interferes with normal skeletal development in various animal species (Freeland-Graves, 1994; Hurley and Keen, 1987; Keen et al., 1994). Although a manganese deficiency may contribute to one or more clinical symptoms, a clinical deficiency has not been clearly associated with poor dietary intakes of healthy individuals. One man was depleted of vitamin K and inadvertently of manganese when fed a diet containing only 0.34 mg/day of manganese for 6.5 months. Symptoms included hypocholesterolemia, scaly dermatitis, hair depigmentation, and reduced vitamin K-dependent clotting proteins. Symptoms were not reversed with vitamin K supplementation but gradually disappeared after the study ended (Doisy, 1973).

In a manganese depletion study, seven young men were fed a purified diet containing 0.01 mg/day of manganese for 10 days and 0.11 mg/day of manganese for 30 days after a 3-week baseline period when they consumed 2.59 mg/day (Friedman et al., 1987). After 35 days, five of the seven subjects developed a finely scaling, minimally erythematous rash that primarily covered the upper torso and was diagnosed as *Miliaria crystallina*. After two days of repletion, the blisters disappeared and the affected areas became scaly and then cleared. Plasma cholesterol concentrations declined during the depletion period, perhaps because manganese is required at several sites in the biosynthetic pathway of cholesterol (Krishna et al., 1966).

Decreased plasma manganese concentrations have been reported in osteoporotic women. Furthermore, bone mineral density was improved when trace minerals, including manganese, were included with calcium in their diets or supplements (Freeland-Graves and Turnlund, 1996; Strause and Saltman, 1987; Strause et al., 1986, 1987).

Penland and Johnson (1993) reported that diets containing only 1 mg/day of manganese altered mood and increased pain during the premenstrual phase of the estrous cycle in young women.

SELECTION OF INDICATORS FOR ESTIMATING THE REQUIREMENT FOR MANGANESE

Balance and Depletion Studies

Interindividual variations in manganese retention can be large (Davidsson et al., 1989b). Ten days after giving [54]Mn in an infant formula to 14 healthy men and women, manganese retention ranged from 0.6 to 9.2 percent. Mean retention in these subjects was 2.9 ± 1.8 percent (standard deviation [SD]). Intraindividual variation was not as large, and retention values of 2.3 ± 1.1, 3.3 ± 3.1, and 2.4 ± 1.4 percent (SD) were observed for three repeated doses in six subjects (Davidsson et al., 1989b).

In one study, seven healthy men, aged 19 to 22 years, were fed a purified low-protein diet containing 0.01 mg/day of manganese for days 1 to 10, followed by a protein-adequate diet containing 0.11 mg/day of manganese until day 39. Using a factorial method, the authors estimated that the minimum requirement for manganese was 0.74 mg/day and estimated on the basis of the percentage of manganese retention that 2.11 mg/day would be required (Friedman et al., 1987). Subsequently, five young men were fed a diet of ordinary foods (1.21 mg/day of manganese) supplemented with manganese sulfate or placebo at the evening meal to create five different levels of manganese intake (Freeland-Graves et al., 1988). Total manganese intakes were 2.89 mg/day for days 1 to 21, 2.06 mg/day for days 22 to 42, 1.21 mg/day for days 43 to 80, 3.79 mg/day for days 81 to 91 (repletion), and 2.65 mg/day for days 92 to 105. The mean manganese balances for the corresponding days were 0.083, -0.018, -0.088, +0.657, and +0.0136 mg/day, respectively.

An 8-week balance study conducted by Hunt and coworkers (1998) showed that women, aged 20 to 42 years, were in slightly positive mean balance when consuming 2.5 mg/day of manganese.

Some adolescent girls were observed to be in negative or slightly positive balance when consuming 3 mg/day of manganese (Greger et al., 1978a, 1978b).

Balance studies are problematic for investigation of manganese requirement because of the rapid excretion of manganese into bile and because manganese balances during short- and moderate-term studies do not appear to be proportional to manganese intakes (Greger, 1998, 1999). For these reasons, a number of studies have achieved balance over a wide range of manganese intakes (Table 10-1). Therefore, balance data were not used for estimating an average requirement for manganese.

TABLE 10-1 Manganese Balance Studies in Adults

Reference	Study Group	Duration	Diet (mg/d)	Balance Data (mg/d)
McLeod and Robinson, 1972	4 women, 19–22 y	27 d	2.78	0.32
Spencer et al., 1979	9 men, 41–63 y	18–24 d	2.23	−0.28
Johnson et al., 1982	8 men, 21–28 y	40 d	3.28	−10 to −21
Patterson et al., 1984	28 men and women, 20–53 y	7d	2.8 3.0 2.9 3.2	−0.16 −0.16 −0.21 −0.12
Behall et al., 1987	11 men, 23–62 y	4 wk	5.5	−0.4
Friedman et al., 1987	7 men, 29–22 y	39 d 5 d 5 d	0.11 1.53 2.55	−0.02 0.84 1.02
Hallfrisch et al., 1987	20 men, 23–56 y 19 women, 21–48 y	1 wk duplicate food record	5.35 6.14	1.65 3.19
Freeland-Graves et al., 1988	5 young men	21 d 20 d 37 d 10 d 13 d	2.89 2.06 1.21 3.79 2.65	0.083 0.018 −0.088 0.657 0.0136
Holbrook et al., 1989	19 men, 21–57 y	7 wk	2.4 to 2.9	−0.6 to 0.4
Johnson and Lykken, 1991	14 women, 27 y	39 d	5.66 5.52 0.95 0.94 0.16	0.1 0.3 −0.01 0.06 0.46

continued

TABLE 10-1 Continued

Reference	Study Group	Duration	Diet (mg/d)	Balance Data (mg/d)
Ivaturi and Kies, 1992	24 men and women	14 d	3.21	0.3
			3.92	0.3
			3.13	–0.2
			2.64	0.23
			3.13	0.51
			3.15	0.32
Finley et al., 1994	20 men and 20 women, 18–40 y	14 d	5.43 (men)	0.27
			4.01 (women)	–0.12
Hunt et al., 1998	21 women, 20–42 y	8 wk	2.5 (non-vegetarian)	0.1
			5.9 (lacto-ovo-vegetarian)	0.6

Serum and Plasma Manganese Concentration

Several studies reported that serum or plasma manganese concentrations respond to dietary intake. Serum manganese concentration of women consuming 1.7 mg/day of manganese was lower than that of women ingesting 15 mg/day of supplemental manganese for more than 20 days (Davis and Greger, 1992). In a depletion trial (Freeland-Graves and Turnlund, 1996), plasma manganese concentration was 1.28 µg/L at baseline. Concentrations were significantly lower during the second (0.95 µg/L) and third (0.80 µg/L) dietary periods with manganese intakes of 2.06 and 1.21 mg/day, respectively. Values increased significantly to 1.11 ± 0.35 µg/L when the diet was repleted with 3.8 mg/day of manganese. During the final dietary periods, manganese intake was 2.65 mg/day, and plasma manganese concentration was 0.97 ± 0.33 µg/L. Plasma manganese concentration was not significantly correlated with manganese intake levels.

In a study in which 10 men consumed 0.52 to 5.33 mg/day of manganese, serum manganese concentration did not respond to varied dietary intakes (Greger et al., 1990). Individual serum manganese concentrations varied from 0.4 to 2.12 µg/L with an average of 1.04 µg/L. However, serum manganese concentrations of four of five subjects who consumed 15 mg of chelated manganese as a dietary supplement for 5 days were 27 nmol/L (1.48 µg/L), whereas unsupplemented control subjects had a mean serum concentration of 20 nmol/L (1.1 µg/L).

Serum or plasma manganese concentrations appear to be somewhat sensitive to large variations in manganese intake, but longer studies are needed to evaluate the usefulness of serum manganese concentrations as indicators of manganese status.

Blood Manganese Concentration

An advantage of whole blood manganese concentration over plasma or serum manganese concentration as an indicator is that slight hemolysis of samples can markedly increase plasma or serum manganese concentrations. Whole blood manganese seems to be extremely variable, however, which may preclude it as a viable status indicator. In a manganese depletion study, manganese concentration in whole blood was 9.57 µg/L (range 5.40 to 17.1) at the end of the baseline period and 6.01 µg/L (4.43 to 7.57) at the end of the 39-day depletion period, but there was not a significant difference between these values (Friedman et al., 1987). With 10 days of manganese repletion, whole blood manganese concentration increased to 6.99 µg/L (3.93 to 18.3).

Urinary Manganese

Urinary manganese is responsive to severe manganese depletion. After a patient spent 7 days on a depletion diet containing 0.11 mg/day of manganese, the patient's urinary manganese excretion significantly decreased from 8.64 to 2.45 µg/day, and it continued to decrease to as low as 0.39 µg/day after 35 days (Friedman et al., 1987). In a second manganese depletion trial, urinary manganese decreased significantly as manganese intake decreased from 2.9 to 2.1 to 1.2 mg/day (Freeland-Graves et al., 1988). After repletion with 3.8 mg/day, urinary manganese excretion increased then decreased following an intake of 2.65 mg/day.

In contrast to the above findings, when ten men consumed 0.52 to 5.33 mg/day, urinary excretion of manganese did not correspond with manganese intake (Greger et al., 1990). Urinary losses of manganese averaged 0.38 µg/g creatinine. Also, Davis and Greger (1992) could not demonstrate that women given 15 mg/day of manganese during a 125-day supplementation period excreted more manganese in urine than women consuming 1.7 mg/day in food. Thus, there is controversy on the use of urinary manganese for assessment of status when typical amounts of manganese are consumed.

Arginase Activity

Arginase is depressed in the livers of manganese-deficient rats (Paynter, 1980). Brock and coworkers (1994) noted that manganese-deficient rats also had depressed plasma urea and elevated plasma ammonia concentrations. Arginase is affected by a variety of factors, however, including high protein diet and liver disease (Morris, 1992).

Manganese-Superoxide Dismutase Activity

Manganese-deficient animals have low manganese-superoxide dismutase (MnSOD) activity (Davis et al., 1992; Malecki et al., 1994; Zidenberg-Cherr et al., 1983). Davis and Greger (1992) demonstrated that lymphocyte MnSOD activity was elevated in 47 women supplemented with 15 mg/day of manganese for more than 90 days. However, other factors like ethanol (Dreosti et al., 1982) and dietary polyunsaturated fatty acids (Davis et al., 1990) may affect MnSOD activity. A fairly large blood sample is required to measure lymphocyte MnSOD.

FACTORS AFFECTING THE MANGANESE REQUIREMENT

Bioavailability

Prior intakes of manganese and of other elements, such as calcium, iron, and phosphorus, have been found by some investigators to affect manganese retention (Freeland-Graves and Lin, 1991; Greger, 1998; Lutz et al., 1993). Adding calcium to human milk significantly reduced the absorption of ^{54}Mn from 4.9 to 3.0 percent (Davidsson et al., 1991). Low ferritin concentrations are associated with increased manganese absorption, therefore having a gender effect on manganese bioavailability (Finley, 1999).

Sandstrom and coworkers (1990) gave a multimineral supplement that included 18 mg of iron, 15 mg of zinc, and 2.5 mg of manganese for a minimum of 30 weeks. Neither whole blood manganese concentration nor superoxide dismutase activity was increased significantly from baseline with supplementation. Seven healthy volunteers subsequently consumed a tracer dose containing ^{54}Mn, ^{75}Se, and ^{65}Zn. Manganese absorption was only 1 percent of the oral dose. Sandstrom and coworkers (1987) reported a higher rate of absorption from this dose in subjects without prior consumption of a supplement, but high interindividual variability of manganese absorption and other potential confounders would require a study specifically designed to test the effect of prior supplementation on ^{54}Mn absorption.

Davidsson and coworkers (1995) administered ^{54}Mn in either a soy-based infant formula or a similar dephytinized formula to eight men and women. The geometric mean manganese absorption was 0.7 percent for the native formula and 1.6 percent for the dephytinized formula. Therefore, the presence of phytate reduced the efficiency of absorption of manganese.

Johnson and colleagues (1991) reported that manganese absorption did not significantly differ between plant foods that were extrinsically or intrinsically labeled with ^{54}MnCl$_2$. Absorption of ^{54}Mn from a meal, extrinsically labeled with ^{54}MnCl$_2$, was significantly higher (8.9 percent) than the absorption of ^{54}Mn from lettuce (5.2 percent), spinach (3.8 percent), wheat (2.2 percent), or sunflower seeds (1.7 percent). Absorption of ^{54}MnCl$_2$ did not differ whether the dose was 0.53 or 1.24 mg (7 to 10 percent).

Gender

Finley and coworkers (1994) reported that men absorbed significantly less manganese than women and that this difference may be related to iron status. A subsequent study specifically demonstrated that high ferritin concentrations were associated with reduced ^{54}Mn absorption (Finley, 1999). Serum ferritin concentrations are higher in men (Appendix Table G-3) and therefore may affect, in part, the lower bioavailability of manganese observed in men.

FINDINGS BY LIFE STAGE AND GENDER GROUP

Infants Ages 0 through 12 Months

Method Used to Set the Adequate Intake

No functional criteria of manganese status have been demonstrated that reflect response to dietary intake in infants. Thus, recommended intakes of manganese are based on an Adequate Intake (AI) that reflects the observed mean manganese intake of infants principally fed human milk.

Ages 0 through 6 Months. On the basis of the method described in Chapter 2 and the manganese concentration of milk produced by well-nourished mothers, the AI reflects the observed mean manganese intake of infants exclusively fed human milk during their first 6 months. There are no reports of full-term infants exclusively and freely fed human milk by U.S. or Canadian mothers who manifested any signs of manganese deficiency (Davidsson et al., 1989a). Mean manganese concentrations of human milk at 1 month were approximately 4.0 µg/L (Aquilio et al., 1996; Casey et al., 1985, 1989) and declined to 1.87 µg/L by 3 months postpartum (Casey et al., 1989) (Table 10-2). Total manganese secretion in human milk averaged 1.9 µg/day over the first 3 months and 1.6 µg/day over the second 3 months (Casey et al., 1989). Based on the above data, the AI is set according to average milk volume consumption (0.78 L/day) × the average manganese concentration in human milk (3.5 µg/L), or 3 µg/day, after rounding (see Chapter 2).

TABLE 10-2 Manganese Concentration in Human Milk

Reference	Study Group	Stage of Lactation	Milk Concentration (µg/L)	Estimated Manganese Intake of Infants (µg/d)[a]
Stastny et al., 1984	24 women	4 wk	6.6	5.2
		8 wk	4.8	3.7
		12 wk	3.5	2.7
Casey et al., 1985	11 women, 26–39 y	8 d	3.7	2.9
		14 d	3.8	2.9
		21 d	3.2	2.5
		28 d	4.1	3.2
Casey et al., 1989	22 women	1 mo	3.5	2.7
		3 mo	1.87	1.5
Anderson, 1992	10 women	Up to 5 mo	6.97	5.4
Aquilio et al., 1996	14 women	2–6 d	3.9	3.0
		12–16 d	3.9	3.0
		21 d	4.1	3.2

NOTE: Maternal intakes were not reported in these studies.

[a] Manganese intake based on reported data or concentration (µg/L) × 0.78 L/day.

Ages 7 through 12 Months. With the introduction of complementary foods, it has been estimated that the average consumption of manganese by 6- and 12-month-old infants is 71 and 80 μg/kg, respectively (Gibson and De Wolfe, 1980). Based on reference weights of 7 and 9 kg for these two ages, the total manganese intake would be 500 and 720 μg/day.

Using the reference body weight method described in Chapter 2 to extrapolate from adults, the average intake is 567 μg/day. Based on these two approaches, the AI is set at 600 μg/day for older infants. The AI for older infants is markedly greater than the AI for younger infants because the concentration of manganese is higher in foods than in human milk.

Manganese AI Summary, Ages 0 through 12 Months

AI for Infants
  0–6 months   **0.003 mg/day (3 μg/day) of manganese**
  7–12 months   **0.6 mg/day of manganese**

Special Considerations

The manganese concentration in cow milk has been reported to range from 20 to 50 μg/L (Lonnerdal et al., 1981), which is significantly greater than the concentration in human milk (Table 10-2). Manganese is partly present in the fat globule membrane in cow milk (Murthy, 1974). Davidsson and coworkers (1989a) reported that the fractional manganese absorption from human milk (8.2 percent) was higher than from soy formula (0.7 percent) and whey-preponderant cow's milk formula (3.1 percent).

Children and Adolescents Ages 1 through 18 Years

Method Used to Set the Adequate Intake

Ages 1 through 3 Years. There are insufficient data to set an Estimated Average Requirement (EAR) for manganese for children ages 1 through 3 years. Therefore, median intake data were used to set the AI. Data from the Food and Drug Administration Total Diet Study indicate a median intake of 1.22 mg/day of manganese for children aged 1 through 3 years (Appendix Table E-6).

Ages 4 through 13 Years. There have been a few manganese balance studies with children and all are subject to the caveats previously discussed. Therefore, they were not considered in setting an EAR. The Total Diet Study indicates a median intake of 1.48 mg/day for children aged 4 through 8 years. Median intakes for girls and boys, ages 9 through 13 years, were 1.57 and 1.91 mg/day, respectively (Appendix Table E-6).

Ages 14 through 18 Years. A few studies have been conducted to assess the manganese requirement in adolescent girls. Adolescent girls were observed to be in negative (Greger et al., 1978a) or slight positive balance (Greger et al., 1978b) when consuming 3 mg/day of manganese. These varied findings in adolescent girls may be due to a variation in iron status given that a significant negative association between manganese absorption and plasma ferritin concentrations has been reported recently (Finley, 1999). Because of the limitations of balance data, as previously discussed, these data were not used to set the EAR.

The Total Diet Study indicates that the median manganese intake for adolescent girls and boys was 1.55 and 2.17 mg/day, respectively (Appendix Table E-6). Because clear associations between low manganese intake and clinical symptoms of a manganese deficiency have not been observed, the AI is based on median intakes for each of the age groups.

Manganese AI Summary, Ages 1 through 18 Years

AI for Children
1–3 years	**1.2 mg/day of manganese**
4–8 years	**1.5 mg/day of manganese**

AI for Boys
9–13 years	**1.9 mg/day of manganese**
14–18 years	**2.2 mg/day of manganese**

AI for Girls
9–13 years	**1.6 mg/day of manganese**
14–18 years	**1.6 mg/day of manganese**

Adults Ages 19 Years and Older

Method Used to Set the Adequate Intake

Because a wide range of manganese intakes can result in manganese balance, balance data could not be used to set an EAR. Several balance studies have collectively concluded that manganese balance can be achieved at around 2.1 to 2.5 mg/day (Freeland-Graves et al., 1988; Friedman et al., 1987; Hunt et al., 1998). Based on a coefficient of variation of 10 percent, balance data would yield a Recommended Dietary Allowance (RDA) of 2.5 to 3 mg/day. Based on the Total Diet Study (Appendix Table E-6), the median manganese intake for men was 2.1 to 2.3 mg/day, and the median intake for women was 1.6 to 1.8 mg/day. Because overt symptoms of a manganese deficiency are not apparent in North America, an RDA based on balance data most likely overestimates the requirement for most North American individuals. Therefore, intake data are used to set an AI for manganese. Because dietary intake assessment methods tend to underestimate the actual daily intake of foods, the highest intake value reported for the four adult age groups was used to set the AI for each gender.

Manganese AI Summary, Ages 19 Years and Older

AI for Men
19–30 years	2.3 mg/day of manganese
31–50 years	2.3 mg/day of manganese
51–70 years	2.3 mg/day of manganese
> 70 years	2.3 mg/day of manganese

AI for Women
19–30 years	1.8 mg/day of manganese
31–50 years	1.8 mg/day of manganese
51–70 years	1.8 mg/day of manganese
> 70 years	1.8 mg/day of manganese

Pregnancy

Method Used to Set the Adequate Intake

There are limited data, such as fetal manganese concentration, on which to base an EAR specific to pregnancy. Casey and Robinson (1978) reported that manganese concentrations in fetal tissues ranged from 0.35 to 9.27 µg/g dry weight. In animals, manganese deficiency in utero produces ataxia and impaired otolith development, but these defects have not been reported in humans.

The additional manganese requirement during pregnancy is determined by extrapolating up from adolescent girls and adult women as described in Chapter 2. Carmichael and coworkers (1997) reported that the median weight gain of 7,002 women who had good pregnancy outcomes was 16 kg. No consistent relationship between maternal age and weight gain was observed in six studies of U.S. women (IOM, 1990). Therefore, 16 kg is added to the reference weight for adolescent girls and adult women for extrapolation. The AI for pregnant adolescent girls and women is 2 mg/day after rounding. This value is similar to dietary manganese intake data obtained from the Total Diet Study (Appendix Table E-6).

Manganese AI Summary, Pregnancy

AI for Pregnancy
14–18 years	**2 mg/day of manganese**
19–30 years	**2 mg/day of manganese**
31–50 years	**2 mg/day of manganese**

Lactation

Method Used to Set the Adequate Intake

There are no data available that directly assess the manganese requirement in lactating women. Approximately 3 µg/day of manganese is secreted in human milk. Even though the requirement during lactation does not appear to be greater than the requirement for nonlactating women, the median intake of 2.56 mg/day of manganese is greater during lactation (Appendix Table E-6). Because a manganese deficiency has not been observed in North American lactating women, the AI is based on the median intake and rounding to 2.6 mg/day.

Manganese AI Summary, Lactation

AI for Lactation
14–18 years	**2.6 mg/day of manganese**
19–30 years	**2.6 mg/day of manganese**
31–50 years	**2.6 mg/day of manganese**

INTAKE OF MANGANESE

Food Sources

Based on the Total Diet Study, grain products contributed 37 percent of dietary manganese, while beverages (tea) and vegetables contributed 20 and 18 percent, respectively, to the adult male diet (Pennington and Young, 1991).

Dietary Intake

Patterson and coworkers (1984) analyzed manganese intakes for 7 days during each of the four seasons for 28 healthy adults living at home. The mean nutrient density for all subjects was 1.6 mg/1,000 kcal. Mean manganese intake for men was 3.4 mg/day and for women, 2.7 mg/day. Greger and coworkers (1990) analyzed duplicate portions of all foods and beverages consumed for ten men. With unrestricted diets, the mean manganese intake was 2.8 mg/day. Daily intakes of manganese throughout the study varied from 0.52 to 5.33 mg/day. Based on the Total Diet Study (Appendix Table E-6), median intakes for women and men ranged from 1.6 to 2.3 mg/day. In various surveys, average manganese intakes of adults eating Western-type and vegetarian diets ranged from 0.7 to 10.9 mg/day (Freeland-Graves, 1994; Gibson, 1994).

Intake from Supplements

Approximately 12 percent of the adult U.S. population consumed supplements containing manganese in 1986 (Moss et al., 1989; Table 2-2). Based on the Third National Health and Nutrition Examination Survey data, the median supplemental intake of manganese by adults who take supplements was approximately 2.4 mg/day, an amount similar to the dietary intake of manganese (Appendix Table C-20).

TOLERABLE UPPER INTAKE LEVELS

The Tolerable Upper Intake Level (UL) is the highest level of daily nutrient intake that is likely to pose no risk of adverse health effects in almost all individuals. Although members of the general population should be advised not to exceed the UL routinely, intake above the UL may be appropriate for investigation within well-controlled clinical trials. Clinical trials of doses above the UL should not be discouraged, as long as subjects participating in these trials have signed informed consent documents regarding possible toxicity and as long as these trials employ appropriate safety monitoring of trial subjects. In addition, the UL is not meant to apply to individuals who are receiving manganese under medical supervision.

Hazard Identification

Adverse Effects

Manganese toxicity in humans is a well-recognized occupational hazard for people who inhale manganese dust. The most prominent effect is central nervous system pathology, especially in the extra-pyramidal motor system. The lesions and symptoms are similar to those of Parkinson's disease (Barceloux, 1999; Keen et al., 1994). Manganese is probably transported into the brain via transferrin (Aschner et al., 1999). These authors hypothesize that the greater vulnerability of the extrapyramidal system (globus pallidus and substantia nigra) for manganese accumulation could be due to the fact that these are areas that are efferent to areas of high transferrin receptor density. These same efferent areas are also regions of high iron content.

Neurotoxicity of orally ingested manganese at relatively low doses is more controversial. However, several lines of evidence suggest this possibility. The data on manganese neurotoxicity are reviewed below.

Elevated Blood Manganese and Neurotoxicity. People with chronic liver disease have neurological pathology and behavioral signs of manganese neurotoxicity, probably because elimination of manganese in bile is impaired (Butterworth et al., 1995; Hauser et al., 1994; Spahr et al., 1996). This impairment results in higher circulating concentrations of manganese, which then has access to the brain via transferrin. Hauser and coworkers (1994) reported whole blood manganese concentrations of 18.8 to 45 µg/L in three patients with chronic liver disease, as compared to a normal range of 4.2 to 14.3 µg/L. Spahr and coworkers (1996) reported blood manganese concentrations of 124.7 nmol/L (6.85 µg/L) in control subjects versus 331.4 nmol/L (18.2 µg/L) in patients with cirrhosis. High concentrations of circulating manganese as a result of total parenteral nutrition have also been associated with manganese toxicity (Keen et al., 1999). Davis and Greger (1992) reported that women who ingested 15 mg/day of supplemental manganese had serum manganese concentrations that increased gradually throughout the 125-day study; significant differences were reported after 25 days of supplementation.

Neurotoxicity in Laboratory Animals. High subchronic or chronic doses of manganese given to animals in food or water result in central nervous system pathology and behavioral changes, although these changes are not necessarily identical to those seen in humans. A review by Newland (1999) suggests that manganese toxicity occurs at progressively lower doses when manganese is administered in food, in water, or by injection, respectively. Differences in toxic potency by route of administration may be an order of magnitude or more. The lowest dose study of manganese administered in food identified by Newland (1999) was by Komura and Sakamoto (1992). They fed male mice diets high in manganese (2 g/kg food) for 12 months (either as $MnCl_2$, manganese acetate, $MnCO_3$, or MnO_2). Thus, a 30-gram mouse eating 4 g/day of food would have ingested about 266 mg/kg/day of manganese. Changes in brain regional biogenic amines and decreases in locomotor activity were observed, but changes were somewhat different for each salt. In general, manganese dioxide was found to be more toxic than other forms, and manganese chloride was least toxic.

Several studies have examined neurotoxic effects of manganese in drinking water or administered by gavage. The two lowest dose studies are reviewed here. Bonilla (1984) gave male rats 0.1 or 5.0 mg/mL of manganese in drinking water for 8 months and measured locomotor activity throughout this period. A significant increase in activity during the first month was found at both doses. Activity returned to normal for months 2 through 6, but in the seventh and eighth months, activity was less than that of control subjects in both groups. In a related study, Bonilla and Prasad (1984) gave rats 0.1 or 1.0 mg/L of manganese in drinking water for 8 months. They observed decreases of norepinephrine in striatum and pons of rats treated with the lower dose. Increases in the dopamine metabolite dihydroxyphenylacetic acid were found in striatum and hypothalamus at both doses. Homovanillic acid (another dopamine metabolite) decreased in striatum of the lower dose group. Changes in serotonin and its metabolite, 5-hydroxyindole acetic acid, were seen in some brain regions in the high dose group. As with the Komura and Sakamoto (1992) study, the actual doses of manganese in this study can only be approximated. Assuming that a 300 g rat ingests about 30 mL/day of water, then the daily dose of manganese in this study was about 10 mg/kg/day.

Senturk and Oner (1996) exposed rats to 0.357 to 0.714 mg/kg/day of manganese (as $MnCl_2$) by gavage in distilled water for 39 days. Manganese levels in brain regions were elevated, and learning in a T-maze task was retarded. The learning impairment was associated with hypercholesterolemia, and the impairment was not seen when rats were co-administered mevilonin (a cholesterol biosynthesis inhibitor). The doses used in this study were very low.

While no animal data exist showing that the neonate exhibits neurotoxic effects at lower doses of manganese than do adults, effects could be more severe in the developing brain. Pappas and colleagues (1997) exposed dams and litters to 2 or 10 mg/mL of manganese (as $MnCl_2$) in drinking water from conception until postnatal day 20. Thinning of the cerebral cortex was observed in neonates exposed to both low and high doses.

Keen and colleagues (1994) and Fechter (1999) suggested that the developing neonatal brain of animals may be more sensitive to high intakes of manganese. This sensitivity could be due to the greater expression of transferrin receptors in developing neurons or to an immature liver bile elimination system (Cotzias et al., 1976). Transfer of manganese to the fetus appears to be limited by the placenta (Fechter, 1999); therefore, the lack of development of manganese transport and elimination mechanisms is probably insignificant in the fetus.

Ecological Studies in Humans. There is some indication that high manganese intake in drinking water is associated with neuromotor deficits similar to Parkinson's disease. Kondakis and coworkers (1989) studied people 50 years of age or older in three villages in Greece exposed to 3.6 to 14.6 µg/L of manganese in drinking water ($n = 62$), 81.6 to 252.6 µg/L ($n = 49$), or 1,800 to 2,300 µg/L ($n = 77$). People drinking the water with the highest concentration of manganese had signs and symptoms of motor deficits. Kawamura and coworkers (1941) reported severe neurological symptoms in 25 people who drank water contaminated with manganese from dry cell batteries for 2 to 3 months. The concentration of manganese in the water was between 14 and 28 mg/L. Vieregge and coworkers (1995) found no evidence of toxicity in people living in northern Germany (mean age of 57.5 years) drinking water with a manganese concentration between 300 and 2,160 µg/L ($n = 41$); they were compared with people drinking water with less than 50 µg/L of manganese.

None of these studies measured dietary intakes of manganese, and so total intake is not known. However, it is possible that manganese in drinking water is more bioavailable than manganese in food (Velazquez and Du, 1994), and it is also possible that manganese in drinking water could be more toxic in people who already consume large amounts of dietary manganese from diets high in plant products.

Summary

Elevated blood manganese concentrations and neurotoxicity were selected as the critical adverse effects on which to base a UL for manganese. The totality of evidence in animals and humans supports a causal association.

Dose-Response Assessment

Adults

Data Selection. Human data, even if sparse, provide a better basis for determination of a UL than animal data. The low-dose animal studies do not establish a no-observed-adverse-effect level (NOAEL). Also, in the animal studies in which manganese was administered in food or water (Bonilla and Prasad, 1984; Komura and Sakamoto, 1992), only approximate doses or average doses can be established. A conservative approach was followed in order to protect against manganese neurotoxicity.

Identification of NOAEL and Lowest-Observed-Adverse-Effect Level (LOAEL). A NOAEL of 11 mg/day of manganese from food was identified based on the data presented by Greger (1999). Greger (1999) reviewed information indicating that people eating Western-type and vegetarian diets may have intakes as high as 10.9 mg/day of manganese. Schroeder and coworkers (1966) reported that a manganese-rich vegetarian diet could contain 13 to 20 mg/day of manganese. Because no adverse effects due to manganese intake have been noted, at least in people consuming Western diets, 11 mg/day is a reasonable NOAEL from food. A LOAEL of 15 mg/day can be identified on the basis of an earlier study by Davis and Greger (1992). At this dose, there were significant increases in serum manganese concentrations after 25 days of supplementation and in lymphocyte manganese-dependent superoxide dismutase activity after 90 days of supplementation.

Uncertainty Assessment. Because of the lack of evidence of human toxicity from doses less than 11 mg/day of manganese from food, an uncertainty factor (UF) of 1.0 was selected.

Derivation of a UL. The NOAEL of 11 mg/day was divided by a UF of 1.0 to obtain a UL of 11 mg/day of total manganese intake from food, water, and supplements for an adult.

$$UL = \frac{NOAEL}{UF} = \frac{11 \text{ mg/day}}{1.0} = 11 \text{ mg/day}$$

Manganese UL Summary, Ages 19 Years and Older

UL for Adults
  ≥ 19 years   **11 mg/day of manganese**

Other Life Stage Groups

Infants. For infants, the UL was judged not determinable because of lack of data on adverse effects in this age group and concern about the infant's ability to handle excess amounts. To prevent high levels of manganese intake, the only source of intake for infants should be from food or formula.

Children and Adolescents. There are no reports of manganese toxicity in children and adolescents. Given the dearth of information, the UL values for children and adolescents are extrapolated from those established for adults. Thus, the adult UL of 11 mg/day was adjusted on the basis of relative body weight as described in Chapter 2 using reference weights from Chapter 1 (Table 1-1).

Pregnancy and Lactation. There are no data showing increased susceptibility of pregnant or lactating women to manganese intake. Therefore, the ULs for pregnant and lactating women are the same as those for the nonpregnant and nonlactating women.

Manganese UL Summary, Ages 0 through 18 Years, Pregnancy, Lactation

UL for Infants
  0–12 months   **Not possible to establish; source of intake should be from food and formula only**

UL for Children
  1–3 years   **2 mg/day of manganese**
  4–8 years   **3 mg/day of manganese**
  9–13 years   **6 mg/day of manganese**

UL for Adolescents
  14–18 years   **9 mg/day of manganese**

UL for Pregnancy
> 14–18 years   9 mg/day of manganese
> 19–50 years   11 mg/day of manganese

UL for Lactation
> 14–18 years   9 mg/day of manganese
> 19–50 years   11 mg/day of manganese

Special Considerations

Because manganese in drinking water and supplements may be more bioavailable than manganese from food, caution should be taken when using manganese supplements, especially among those persons already consuming large amounts of manganese from diets high in plant products. In addition, a review of the literature revealed that individuals with liver disease may be distinctly susceptible to the adverse effects of excess manganese intake.

Intake Assessment

Based on the Total Diet Study (Appendix Table E-6), the highest dietary manganese intake at the ninety-fifth percentile was 6.3 mg/day, which was the level consumed by men aged 31 to 50 years. Data from the Third National Health and Nutrition Examination Survey indicate that the highest supplemental intake of manganese at the ninety-fifth percentile was approximately 5 mg/day, which was consumed by men and women aged 19 years and older and pregnant women (Appendix Table C-20).

Risk Characterization

The risk of an adverse effect resulting from excess intake of manganese from food and supplements appears to be low at the highest intakes noted above.

RESEARCH RECOMMENDATIONS FOR MANGANESE

- Identification of functional indicators for manganese.
- Analysis of effects of graded levels of dietary manganese intake on leukocyte superoxide dismutase activity or another appropriate functional indicator to provide an appropriate basis for setting an Estimated Average Requirement.

REFERENCES

Anderson RR. 1992. Comparison of trace elements in milk of four species. *J Dairy Sci* 75:3050–3055.

Aquilio E, Spagnoli R, Seri S, Bottone G, Spennati G. 1996. Trace element content in human milk during lactation of preterm newborns. *Biol Trace Elem Res* 51:63–70.

Aschner M, Vrana KE, Zheng W. 1999. Manganese uptake and distribution in the central nervous system (CNS). *Neurotoxicology* 20:173–180.

Barceloux DG. 1999. Manganese. *J Toxicol Clin Toxicol* 37:293–307.

Behall KM, Scholfield DJ, Lee K, Powell AS, Moser PB. 1987. Mineral balance in adult men: Effect of four refined fibers. *Am J Clin Nutr* 46:307–314.

Bell JG, Keen CL, Lonnerdal BJ. 1989. Higher retention of manganese in suckling than in adult rats is not due to maturational differences in manganese uptake by rat small intestine. *J Toxicol Environ Health* 26:387–398.

Bonilla E. 1984. Chronic manganese intake induces changes in the motor activity of rats. *Exp Neurol* 84:696–700.

Bonilla E, Prasad ALN. 1984. Effects of chronic manganese intake on the levels of biogenic amines in rat brain regions. *Neurobehav Toxicol Teratol* 6:341–344.

Britton AA, Cotzias GC. 1966. Dependence of manganese turnover on intake. *Am J Physiol* 211:203–206.

Brock AA, Chapman SA, Ulman EA, Wu G. 1994. Dietary manganese deficiency decreases rat hepatic arginase activity. *J Nutr* 124:340–344.

Butterworth RF, Spahr L, Fontaine S, Layrargues GP. 1995. Manganese toxicity, dopaminergic dysfunction and hepatic encephalopathy. *Metab Brain Dis* 10:259–267.

Carmichael S, Abrams B, Selvin S. 1997. The pattern of maternal weight gain in women with good pregnancy outcomes. *Am J Public Health* 87:1984–1988.

Casey CE, Robinson MF. 1978. Copper, manganese, zinc, nickel, cadmium and lead in human foetal tissues. *Br J Nutr* 39:639–646.

Casey CE, Hambidge KM, Neville MC. 1985. Studies in human lactation: Zinc, copper, manganese and chromium in human milk in the first month of lactation. *Am J Clin Nutr* 41:1193–1200.

Casey CE, Neville MC, Hambidge KM. 1989. Studies in human lactation: Secretion of zinc, copper, and manganese in human milk. *Am J Clin Nutr* 49:773–785.

Cotzias GC, Miller ST, Papavasiliou PS, Tang LC. 1976. Interactions between manganese and brain dopamine. *Med Clin North Am* 60:729–738.

Davidsson L, Cederblad A, Hagebo E, Lonnerdal B, Sandstrom B. 1988. Intrinsic and extrinsic labeling for studies of manganese absorption in humans. *J Nutr* 118:1517–1521.

Davidsson L, Cederblad A, Lonnerdal B, Sandstrom B. 1989a. Manganese absorption from human milk, cow's milk, and infant formulas in humans. *Am J Dis Child* 143:823–827.

Davidsson L, Cederblad A, Lonnerdal B, Sandstrom B. 1989b. Manganese retention in man: A method for estimating manganese absorption in man. *Am J Clin Nutr* 49:170–179.

Davidsson L, Lonnerdal B, Sandstrom B, Kunz C, Keen CL. 1989c. Identification of transferrin as the major plasma carrier protein for manganese introduced orally or intravenously or after in vitro addition in the rat. *J Nutr* 119:1461–1464.

Davidsson L, Cederblad A, Lonnerdal B, Sandstrom B. 1991. The effect of individual dietary components on manganese absorption in humans. *Am J Clin Nutr* 54:1065–1070.

Davidsson L, Almgren A, Juillerat MA, Hurrell RF. 1995. Manganese absorption in humans: The effect of phytic acid and ascorbic acid in soy formula. *Am J Clin Nutr* 62:984–987.

Davis CD, Greger JL. 1992. Longitudinal changes of manganese-dependent superoxide dismutase and other indexes of manganese and iron status in women. *Am J Clin Nutr* 55:747–752.

Davis CD, Ney DM, Greger JL. 1990. Manganese, iron and lipid interactions in rats. *J Nutr* 120:507–513.

Davis CD, Wolf TL, Greger JL. 1992. Varying levels of manganese and iron affect absorption and gut endogenous losses of manganese by rats. *J Nutr* 122:1300–1308.

Davis CD, Zech L, Greger JL. 1993. Manganese metabolism in rats: An improved methodology for assessing gut endogenous losses. *Proc Soc Exp Biol Med* 202:103–108.

Doisy EA Jr. 1973. Micronutrient controls on biosynthesis of clotting proteins and cholesterol. In: Hemphill DD, ed. *Trace Substances in Environmental Health*, VI. Columbia, MO: University of Missouri. Pp. 193–199.

Dreosti IE, Manuel SJ, Buckley RA. 1982. Superoxide dismutase (EC 1.15.1.1), manganese and the effect of ethanol in adult and foetal rats. *Br J Nutr* 48:205–210.

Fechter LD. 1999. Distribution of manganese in development. *Neurotoxicology* 20:197–201.

Finley JW. 1999. Manganese absorption and retention by young women is associated with serum ferritin concentration. *Am J Clin Nutr* 70:37–43.

Finley JW, Johnson PE, Johnson LK. 1994. Sex affects manganese absorption and retention by humans from a diet adequate in manganese. *Am J Clin Nutr* 60:949–955.

Freeland-Graves J. 1994. Derivation of manganese estimated safe and adequate daily dietary intakes. In: Mertz W, Abernathy CO, Olin SS, eds. *Risk Assessment of Essential Elements*. Washington, DC: ILSI Press. Pp. 237–252.

Freeland-Graves J, Lin PH. 1991. Plasma uptake of manganese as affected by oral loads of manganese, calcium, milk, phosphorous, copper and zinc. *J Am Coll Nutr* 10:38–43.

Freeland-Graves J, Turnlund JR. 1996. Deliberations and evaluations of the approaches, endpoints and paradigms for manganese and molybdenum dietary recommendations. *J Nutr* 126:2435S–2440S.

Freeland-Graves J, Behmardi F, Bales CW, Dougherty V, Lin PH, Crosby JB, Trickett PC. 1988. Metabolic balance of manganese in young men consuming diets containing five levels of dietary manganese. *J Nutr* 118:764–773.

Friedman BJ, Freeland-Graves JH, Bales CW, Behmardi F, Shorey-Kutschke RL, Willis RA, Crosby JB, Trickett PC, Houston SD. 1987. Manganese balance and clinical observations in young men fed a manganese-deficient diet. *J Nutr* 117:133–143.

Garcia-Aranda JA, Wapnir RA, Lifshitz F. 1983. In vivo intestinal absorption of manganese in the rat. *J Nutr* 113:2601–2607.

Gibson RS. 1994. Content and bioavailability of trace elements in vegetarian diets. *Am J Clin Nutr* 59:1223S–1232S.

Gibson RS, De Wolfe MS. 1980. The dietary trace metal intake of some Canadian full-term and low birthweight infants during the first twelve months of infancy. *J Can Diet Assoc* 41:206–215.

Greger JL. 1998. Dietary standards for manganese: Overlap between nutritional and toxicological studies. *J Nutr* 128:368S–371S.

Greger JL. 1999. Nutrition versus toxicology of manganese in humans: Evaluation of potential biomarkers. *Neurotoxicology* 20:205–212.

Greger JL, Baligar P, Abernathy RP, Bennett OA, Peterson T. 1978a. Calcium, magnesium, phosphorous, copper, and manganese balance in adolescent females. *Am J Clin Nutr* 31:117–121.

Greger JL, Zaikis SC, Abernathy RP, Bennett OA, Huffman J. 1978b. Zinc, nitrogen, copper, iron, and manganese balance in adolescent females fed two levels of zinc. *J Nutr* 108:1449–1456.

Greger JL, Davis CD, Suttie JW, Lyle BJ. 1990. Intake, serum concentrations, and urinary excretion of manganese by adult males. *Am J Clin Nutr* 51:457–461.

Hallfrisch J, Powell A, Carafelli C, Reiser S, Prather ES. 1987. Mineral balances of men and women consuming high fiber diets with complex or simple carbohydrate. *J Nutr* 117:48–55.

Hauser RA, Zesiewicz TA, Rosemurgy AS, Martinez C, Olanow CW. 1994. Manganese intoxication and chronic liver failure. *Ann Neurol* 36:871–875.

Holbrook JT, Smith JC Jr, Reiser S. 1989. Dietary fructose or starch: Effects on copper, zinc, iron, manganese, calcium, and magnesium balances in humans. *Am J Clin Nutr* 49:1290–1294.

Hunt JR, Matthys LA, Johnson LK. 1998. Zinc absorption, mineral balance, and blood lipids in women consuming controlled lactoovovegetarian and omnivorous diets for 8 weeks. *Am J Clin Nutr* 67:421–430.

Hurley LS, Keen CL. 1987. Manganese. In: Mertz W, ed. *Trace Elements in Human and Animal Nutrition,* 5th ed. San Diego: Academic Press. Pp. 185–223.

IOM (Institute of Medicine) 1990. *Nutrition During Pregnancy.* Washington, DC: National Academy Press.

Ivaturi R, Kies C. 1992. Mineral balances in humans as affected by fructose, high fructose corn syrup and sucrose. *Plant Foods Hum Nutr* 42:143–151.

Johnson MA, Baier MJ, Greger JL. 1982. Effects of dietary tin on zinc, copper, iron, manganese, and magnesium metabolism of adult males. *Am J Clin Nutr* 35:1332–1338.

Johnson P, Lykken G. 1991. Manganese and calcium absorption and balance in young women fed diets with varying amounts of manganese and calcium. *J Trace Elem Exp Med* 4:19–35.

Johnson PE, Lykken GI, Korynta ED. 1991. Absorption and biological half-life in humans of intrinsic and extrinsic ^{54}Mn tracers from foods of plant origin. *J Nutr* 121:711–717.

Kawamura R, Ikuta H, Fukuzumi S, Yamada R, Tsubaki S, Kodama T, Kurata S. 1941. Intoxication by manganese in well water. *Kitasato Arch Exp Med* 18:145–169.

Keen CL, Zidenberg-Cherr S, Lonnerdal B. 1994. Nutritional and toxicological aspects of manganese intake: An overview. In: Mertz W, Abernathy CO, Olin SS, eds. *Risk Assessment of Essential Elements.* Washington, DC: ILSI Press. Pp. 221–235.

Keen CL, Ensunsa JL, Watson MH, Baly DL, Donovan SM, Monaco MH, Clegg MS. 1999. Nutritional aspects of manganese from experimental studies. *Neurotoxicology* 20:213–223.

Kelly DA. 1998. Liver complications of pediatric parenteral nutrition—epidemiology. *Nutrition* 14:153–157.

Komura J, Sakamoto M. 1992. Effects of manganese forms on biogenic amines in the brain and behavioral alterations in the mouse: Long-term oral administration of several manganese compounds. *Environ Res* 57:34–44.

Kondakis XG, Makris N, Leotsinidis M, Prinou M, Papapetropoulos T. 1989. Possible health effects of high manganese concentration in drinking water. *Arch Environ Health* 44:175–178.

Krishna G, Whitlock HW Jr, Feldbruegge DH, Porter JW. 1966. Enzymatic conversion of farnesyl pyrophosphate to squalene. *Arch Biochem Biophys* 114: 200–215.

Lonnerdal B, Keen CL, Hurley LS. 1981. Iron, copper, zinc and manganese in milk. *Ann Rev Nutr* 1:149–174.

Lutz TA, Schroff A, Scharrer E. 1993. Effects of calcium and sugars on intestinal manganese absorption. *Biol Trace Elem Res* 39:221–227.

Malecki EA, Huttner DL, Greger JL. 1994. Manganese status, gut endogenous losses of manganese, and antioxidant enzyme activity in rats fed varying levels of manganese and fat. *Biol Trace Elem Res* 42:17–29.

McLeod BE, Robinson MF. 1972. Metabolic balance of manganese in young women. *Br J Nutr* 27:221–227.

Morris SM Jr. 1992. Regulation of enzymes of urea and arginine synthesis. *Ann Rev Nutr* 12:81–101.

Moss AJ, Levy AS, Kim I, Park YK. 1989. *Use of Vitamin and Mineral Supplements in the United States: Current Users, Types of Products, and Nutrients.* Advance Data, Vital and Health Statistics of the National Center for Health Statistics, Number 174. Hyattsville, MD: National Center for Health Statistics.

Murthy GK. 1974. Trace elements in milk. *Crit Rev Environ Control* 4:1–38.

Newland MC. 1999. Animal models of manganese's neurotoxicity. *Neurotoxicology* 20:415–432.

Pappas BA, Zhang D, Davidson CM, Crowder T, Park GAS, Fortin T. 1997. Perinatal manganese exposure: Behavioral, neurochemical, and histopathological effects in the rat. *Neurotoxicol Teratol* 19:17–25.

Patterson KY, Holbrook JT, Bodner JE, Kelsay JL, Smith JC Jr, Veillon C. 1984. Zinc, copper, and manganese intake and balance for adults consuming self-selected diets. *Am J Clin Nutr* 40:1397–1403.

Paynter DI. 1980. Changes in activity of the manganese superoxide dismutase enzyme in tissues of the rat with changes in dietary manganese. *J Nutr* 110:437–447.

Penland JG, Johnson PE. 1993. Dietary calcium and manganese effects on menstrual cycle symptoms. *Am J Obstet Gynecol* 168:1417–1423.

Pennington JA, Young BE. 1991. Total Diet Study nutritional elements, 1982–1989. *J Am Diet Assoc* 91:179–183.

Rabin O, Hegedus L, Bourre JM, Smith QR. 1993. Rapid brain uptake of manganese (II) across the blood-brain barrier. *J Neurochem* 61:509–517.

Rossander-Hulten L, Brune M, Sandstrom B, Lonnerdal B, Hallberg L. 1991. Competitive inhibition of iron absorption by manganese and zinc in humans. *Am J Clin Nutr* 54:152–156.

Sandstrom B, Davidsson L, Cederblad A, Eriksson R, Lonnerdal B. 1986. Manganese absorption and metabolism in man. *Acta Pharmacol Toxicol* 59:60–62.

Sandstrom B, Davidsson L, Eriksson R, Alpsten M, Bogentoft C. 1987. Retention of selenium (75Se), Zinc (65Zn) and manganese (54Mn) in humans after intake of a labelled vitamin and mineral supplement. *J Trace Elem Electrolytes Health Dis* 1:33–38.

Sandstrom B, Davidsson L, Erickson RA, Alpsten M. 1990. Effects of long-term trace element supplementation on blood trace element levels and absorption of (75Se), (54Mn), and (65Zn). *J Trace Elem Electrolytes Health Dis* 4:65–72.

Schroeder HA, Balassa JJ, Tipton IH. 1966. Essential trace metals in man: Manganese. A study in homeostasis. *J Chron Dis* 19:545–571.

Senturk UK, Oner G. 1996. The effect of manganese-induced hypercholesterolemia on learning in rats. *Biol Trace Elem Res* 51:249–257.

Spahr L, Butterworth RF, Fontaine S, Bui L, Therrien G, Milette PC, Lebrun LH, Zayed J, LeBlanc A, Pomier-Layrargues G. 1996. Increased blood manganese in cirrhotic patients: Relationship to pallidal magnetic resonance signal hyperintensity and neurological symptoms. *Hepatology* 24:1116–1120.

Spencer H, Asmussen CR, Holtzman RB, Kramer L. 1979. Metabolic balances of cadmium, copper, manganese, and zinc in man. *Am J Clin Nutr* 32:1867–1875.

Stastny D, Vogel RS, Picciano MF. 1984. Manganese intake and serum manganese concentration of human milk-fed and formula-fed infants. *Am J Clin Nutr* 39:872–878.

Strause L, Saltman P. 1987. Role of manganese in bone metabolism. In: Kies C, ed. *Nutritional Bioavailability of Manganese.* Washington, DC: American Chemical Society. Pp. 46–55.

Strause L, Hegenauer J, Saltman P, Cone R, Resnick D. 1986. Effects of long-term dietary manganese and copper deficiency on rat skeleton. *J Nutr* 116:135–141.

Strause L, Saltman P, Glowacki J. 1987. The effect of deficiencies of manganese and copper on osteoinduction and on resorption of bone particles in rats. *Calcif Tissue Int* 41:145–150.

Velazquez SF, Du JT. 1994. Derivation of the reference dose for manganese. In: Mertz W, Abernathy CO, Olin SS, eds. *Risk Assessment of Essential Elements.* Washington, DC: ILSI Press. Pp. 253–266.

Vieregge P, Heinzow B, Korf G, Teichert HM, Schleifenbaum P, Mosinger HU. 1995. Long term exposure to manganese in rural well water has no neurological effects. *Can J Neurol Sci* 22:286–289.

Zidenberg-Cherr S, Keen CL, Lonnerdal B, Hurley LS. 1983. Superoxide dismutase activity and lipid peroxidation in the rat: Developmental correlations affected by manganese deficiency. *J Nutr* 113:2498–2504.

11

Molybdenum

SUMMARY

Molybdenum functions as a cofactor for a limited number of enzymes in humans. The primary criterion used to set an Estimated Average Requirement (EAR) is molybdenum balance in controlled studies with specific amounts of molybdenum consumed. Adjustments are made for the bioavailability of molybdenum. The Recommended Dietary Allowance (RDA) for adult men and women is 45 µg/day. The average dietary intake of molybdenum by adult men and women is 109 and 76 µg/day, respectively. The Tolerable Upper Intake Level (UL) is 2 mg/day, a level based on impaired reproduction and growth in animals.

BACKGROUND INFORMATION

Function

Molybdenum has been shown to act as a cofactor for a limited number of enzymes in humans: sulfite oxidase, which is believed to be most important for health, xanthine oxidase, and aldehyde oxidase. In all mammalian molybdoenzymes, functional molybdenum is present as an organic component called molybdopterin (Rajagopalan, 1988). These enzymes are involved in catabolism of sulfur amino acids and heterocyclic compounds, including purines and pyridines. A clear molybdenum deficiency syndrome producing physiological signs of molybdenum restriction has not been achieved in animals, despite major reduction in the activity of these molybdoenzymes. Rather, molybdenum essentiality is based on a genetic defect that prevents sulfite oxidase synthesis. Because sulfite is not oxidized to sulfate, severe neurological damage leading to early death occurs with this inborn error of metabolism (Johnson, 1997). Further support for an essential metabolic role for molybdenum relates to amino acid intolerance in a patient who received long-term total parenteral nutrition without molybdenum (Abumrad et al., 1981). The intolerance, which was probably due to abnormal sulfur amino acid metabolism, was reversed with intravenous repletion of ammonium molybdate.

Physiology of Absorption, Metabolism, and Excretion

The high efficiency of molybdenum absorption over an extensive range of intakes suggests that molybdenum absorption is a passive (nonmediated) process. The competitive inhibition of molybdenum uptake by sulfate that has been observed in rat intestines suggests a carrier may be involved. The mechanism of molybdenum absorption (transcellular or paracellular transport) and the location(s) within the gastrointestinal tract responsible for absorption have not been studied (Nielsen, 1999). Molybdenum concentrations in whole blood vary widely but average about 5 nmol/L (Versieck et al., 1978). Protein-bound molybdenum constitutes between 83 and 97 percent of the total molybdenum in erythrocytes. Potential plasma molybdenum transport proteins include α-macroglobulin. Molybdenum retention may be conserved in part through formation of the molybdopterin complex. Urinary excretion is a direct reflection of the dietary molybdenum intake level (Turnlund et al., 1995a, 1995b). Stable isotope studies showing molybdenum retention at low molybdenum intakes and rapid excretion at high intakes suggest that the kidney is the primary site of molybdenum homeostatic regulation. However, widely different oral test doses of molybdenum, between 22 and 1,490 µg/day, resulted in only a small difference in absorption of 88 and 93 percent, respectively. The source of fecal molybdenum is not clear, but could include biliary molybdenum (Nielsen, 1999).

Clinical Effects of Inadequate Intake

Molybdenum deficiency has not been observed in healthy people. A severe metabolic defect, molybdenum cofactor deficiency, had been identified in 47 patients by 1993. The disease results in deficiency in the three molybdoenzymes known to occur in humans: sulfite oxidase, xanthine dehydrogenase, and aldehyde oxidase. Few infants with these defects survive the first days of life (Johnson et al., 1993), and those who survive have severe neurological abnormalities and a variety of other abnormalities. Only one case of molybdenum deficiency that might be considered a dietary deficiency has been reported in humans (Abumrad et al., 1981). A man with Crohn's disease who was on total parenteral nutrition (TPN) for the last 18 months of his life developed symptoms of tachycardia, headache, night blindness, and other symptoms during the final 6 months of TPN. Biochemical changes included elevated plasma methionine concentration, low serum uric acid concentration, high urinary thiosulfate, and low urinary uric acid and sulfate. After administration of ammonium molybdate, the biochemical abnormalities were reversed.

SELECTION OF INDICATORS FOR ESTIMATING THE REQUIREMENT FOR MOLYBDENUM

Plasma and Serum Molybdenum Concentration

Plasma and serum molybdenum concentrations are very low in humans and are difficult to measure. As a consequence, there are few reports on plasma or serum molybdenum concentrations. The concentration in plasma increases with dietary intake, peaks about an hour after meals, and then returns to basal levels (Cantone et al., 1995; Versieck et al., 1978). Infused tracers of molybdenum disappear rapidly from the blood, with only 2.5 to 5 percent remaining after 1 hour (Cantone et al., 1995; Rosoff and Spencer, 1964). Therefore, plasma concentrations do not reflect molybdenum status and cannot be used as an indicator for estimating requirements.

Urinary Molybdenum

The primary route of molybdenum excretion is the urine (Rosoff and Spencer, 1964; Turnlund et al., 1995a, 1995b). Urinary molybdenum reflects dietary intake, increasing as dietary intake increases. When molybdenum intake is low, about 60 percent of ingested molybdenum is excreted in the urine, but when molybdenum intake is high, over 90 percent is excreted in the urine (Turnlund et al., 1995a, 1995b). In the United States, the average concentration of urinary molybdenum is 69 µg/L (Paschal et al., 1998). Although related to dietary intake, urinary molybdenum alone does not reflect status.

Biochemical Indicators

Several biochemical changes have been observed in special situations. In molybdenum cofactor deficiency and in the one case of molybdenum deficiency reported, urinary sulfate was low and urinary sulfite was present. Serum uric acid concentrations were low, urinary xanthine and hypoxanthine increased, and plasma methionine was increased (Abumrad et al., 1981; Johnson et al., 1993). However, these observations have not been associated with molybdenum intakes in normal, healthy people and cannot be used as indicators for estimating the molybdenum requirement.

Molybdenum Balance

Balance studies are used to establish whether homeostasis is maintained and whether body stores are being depleted or increased. Ideally, sufficient time (at least 12 days or longer) is allowed for the body to adapt to each dietary intake before collecting balance data, diets are constant, and conditions are controlled to assure food consumption and sample collections are complete. Two balance studies have been conducted in adult men (Turnlund et al., 1995a, 1995b). These studies provided adaptation periods and were conducted in metabolic research facilities. Diets were controlled and molybdenum intake was constant at each amount. Balance in these studies could be achieved over a broad range of intakes. In one study, five levels of molybdenum ranging from 22 to 1,490 µg/day were provided for 24 days each (Turnlund et al., 1995a). In another study, a low molybdenum diet (22 µg/day) was provided for 102 days, followed by a higher molybdenum diet (467 µg/day) (Turnlund et al., 1995b). Miscellaneous losses, such as sweat and integument, were too low to measure and were not accounted for. The minimum requirement was estimated to be approximately 25 µg/day. Balance studies were conducted among preadolescent girls between 1956 and 1962 for 6 to 56 days (Engel et al., 1967). They demonstrated that balance was positive (3 to 33 µg/day) in all of 36 girls between the ages of 6 and 10 years when intake ranged from 43 to 80 µg/day.

FACTORS AFFECTING THE MOLYBDENUM REQUIREMENT

Interactions

Molybdenum:Tungsten Ratio

Tungsten and molybdenum are both Group 6B elements and thus have similar atomic size and valence states. Tungsten has been used as an antagonist of molybdenum absorption in animal studies to produce molybdenum deficiency as measured by molybdoenzyme activity (Rajagopalan, 1988). Major effects of such treatment have not been observed in humans. The interaction is not considered significant in human nutrition.

Molybdenum:Copper and Sulfate Ratios

Excess molybdenum intake has been documented to produce copper deficiency in ruminants and is a potential practical feeding problem in some areas of the world (Bremner, 1979). The mechanism could be an interaction that involves formation of a thiomolybdate complex with copper. The interaction is not considered to be of significance to humans.

There is one report of increased urinary copper excretion with molybdenum intake from sorghum with molybdenum intakes of 500 and 1,500 µg (Deosthale and Gopalan, 1974). The effect was not confirmed in a controlled study at those levels of dietary molybdenum (Turnlund and Keyes, 2000).

Bioavailability

Little is known about the bioavailability of molybdenum from different food sources, but one study among men and another among women demonstrated that it is less efficiently absorbed from soy, which contains relatively high amounts (Turnlund et al., 1999). Bioavailability of other minerals is also lower from soy than from many other dietary sources (Hurrell et al., 1992; O'Dell, 1989). In one study with 12 young women, the absorption of stable isotopically labeled molybdenum was 87.5 percent from extrinsic molybdenum, 86.1 percent from kale, and 56.7 percent from soy (Turnlund et al., 1999). A study in young men with higher (300 µg) molybdenum intakes demonstrated that molybdenum absorption was 92.8 percent from foods extrinsically labeled with molybdenum and 58.3 percent from soy (Turnlund et al., 1999). The absorption of molybdenum was 35 and 37 percent less from soy than from an extrinsic source of molybdenum and from the molybdenum in kale. Utilization of absorbed molybdenum was similar regardless of source. It is unlikely that molybdenum in other commonly consumed foods would be less available than the molybdenum in soy.

FINDINGS BY LIFE STAGE AND GENDER GROUP

Infants Ages 0 through 12 Months

Method Used to Set the Adequate Intake

No functional criteria of molybdenum status have been demonstrated that reflect response to dietary intake in infants. Thus, recommended intakes of molybdenum are based on an Adequate Intake (AI) that reflects the observed mean molybdenum intake of infants principally fed human milk.

Ages 0 through 6 Months. With use of the method described in Chapter 2, the AI for young infants is based on mean intake data from infants fed human milk as the principal food during their first 6 months, and it uses the molybdenum concentration of milk produced by well-nourished mothers. There are no reports of full-term infants exclusively and freely fed human milk from U.S. and Canadian mothers who manifested any signs of a molybdenum deficiency. Friel and coworkers (1999) found that the molybdenum concentration of human milk of mothers of premature infants ranged from 2.1 to 23 µg/L with a median concentration of 5 µg/L. Studies by Bougle and coworkers (1988) found that the molybdenum concentration of human milk decreases rapidly from 15 µg/L on day 1, to 4.8 µg/L at 7 to 10 days postpartum, and 2.6 µg/L by 1 month (Table 11-1). Rossipal and Krachler (1998) found human milk to contain 1.42 µg/L at 42 to 60 days postpartum and 1.78 µg/L at 97 to 293 days postpartum. Biego and coworkers (1998) reported an average molybdenum concentration of 4 µg/L in human milk with stage of lactation not reported and much higher concentrations of molybdenum in cow's milk and infant formula. With an average molybdenum concentration of 2 µg/L, an average milk volume of 0.78 L/day (Chapter 2), and rounding, the AI is 2 µg/day.

Ages 7 through 12 months. One method of estimating the AI for infants receiving human milk from 7 through 12 months of age is based on the average breast milk content and 0.6 L/day, the aver-

TABLE 11-1 Molybdenum Concentration in Human Milk

Reference	Study Group	Stage of Lactation	Milk Concentration (µg/L)	Estimated Molybdenum Intake of Infants (µg/d)[a]
Casey and Neville, 1987	13 women	5 d	Not reported	5.1
		14 d		3.0
		21 d		2.4
		28 d		1.6
		35 d		2.1
Bougle et al., 1988	6 women	1 d	15	11.7
		3–5 d	10.2	7.9
		7–10 d	4.8	3.7
		14 d	1.5	1.2
		1 mo	2.6	2.0
		2 mo	0.2	0.15
Anderson, 1992	7 women	Up to 5 mo	17.0	13.2
Aquilio et al., 1996	14 women	21 d	4.1	3.2
Biego et al., 1998	17 milk samples	Mature milk	4	3.1
Krachler et al., 1998	46 women	Up to 293 d	3.6	2.8
Rossipal and Krachler, 1998		42–60 d	1.42	1.1
		97–293 d	1.78	1.1

NOTE: Maternal intakes were not reported in these studies.

[a] Molybdenum intake based on reported data or concentration (µg/L) × 0.78 L/day for 0–6 months postpartum and concentration (µg/L) × 0.6 L/day for 7–12 months postpartum.

age volume of milk consumed in this age group, plus an added increment for complementary food (see Chapter 2). However, data on molybdenum content of weaning foods are not available. By using the reference weight ratio method described in Chapter 2 to extrapolate from the AI for infants ages 0 through 6 months, the AI is 3 µg/day after rounding.

Molybdenum AI Summary, Ages 0 through 12 Months

AI for Infants

0–6 months	**2 µg/day of molybdenum**	**0.3 µg/kg/day**
7–12 months	**3 µg/day of molybdenum**	**0.3 µg/kg/day**

Special Considerations

Cow milk contains considerably more molybdenum (50 µg/L) than human milk, as does soymilk (Tsongas et al., 1980). Data on the bioavailability of molybdenum in cow milk and infant formulas are not available.

Children and Adolescents Ages 1 through 18 Years

Evidence Considered in Estimating the Average Requirement

No data are available on which to base an Estimated Average Requirement (EAR) for children or adolescents. EARs for these groups were extrapolated from adult EARs by the method described in Chapter 2. Although there are no studies available to indicate that the molybdenum requirement is associated with energy expenditure, metabolic weight ($kg^{0.75}$) was used for extrapolating because of the functional role of molybdenum in a select number of enzymes, and because using metabolic weight yields an EAR that is higher than when total body weight is used.

Molybdenum EAR and RDA Summary, Ages 1 through 18 years

EAR for Children

1–3 years	**13 µg/day of molybdenum**
4–8 years	**17 µg/day of molybdenum**

EAR for Boys

9–13 years	**26 µg/day of molybdenum**
14–18 years	**33 µg/day of molybdenum**

EAR for Girls

9–13 years	**26 µg/day of molybdenum**
14–18 years	**33 µg/day of molybdenum**

The Recommended Dietary Allowance (RDA) for molybdenum is set by using a coefficient of variation (CV) of 15 percent (see "Adults

Ages 19 Years and Older"). The RDA is defined as equal to the EAR plus twice the CV to cover the needs of 97 to 98 percent of individuals in the group (therefore, for molybdenum the RDA is 130 percent of the EAR). The calculated RDA is rounded to the nearest 1 µg.

RDA for Children
       1–3 years   **17 µg/day of molybdenum**
       4–8 years   **22 µg/day of molybdenum**

RDA for Boys
       9–13 years   **34 µg/day of molybdenum**
       14–18 years   **43 µg/day of molybdenum**

RDA for Girls
       9–13 years   **34 µg/day of molybdenum**
       14–18 years   **43 µg/day of molybdenum**

Adults Ages 19 Years and Older

Evidence Considered in Estimating the Average Requirement

The basis for an EAR for molybdenum was molybdenum balance in controlled studies with specific amounts of molybdenum consumed. Average balance achieved in four young men with an intake of 22 µg/day is shown in 6-day intervals in Figure 11-1 (Turnlund et al., 1995b). From day 1 to day 48, average balance was negative. Beginning at day 49, balance became slightly positive; through day 102, the average balance was positive in six of nine 6-day periods and negative in the other three 6-day periods. Over that entire period, average balance was near 0 (0.2 µg/day). Sixteen of the 36 individual 6-day balance periods were negative and 20 were positive. The average standard deviation of the nine 6-day balance periods was 2.6 µg/day with a range of 1.2 to 4.3 µg/day. The variability in balance for the 54-day balance period was 1.5 µg/day, or 7 percent of the dietary intake. The variability in the nine 6-day balance periods averaged 2.6 µg/day, or 12 percent.

The balance data suggest that 22 µg/day is near the minimum requirement. No clinical signs of deficiency were observed and biochemical changes associated with molybdenum deficiency were not found. Another group of four young men showed a similar balance pattern with negative balance during the first 6 days and becoming less negative over a 24-day period (Turnlund et al., 1995a). Twenty-

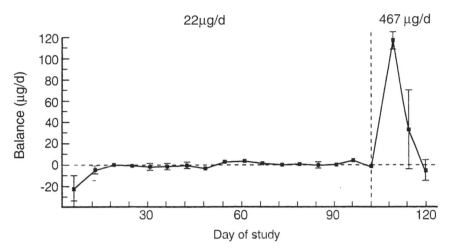

FIGURE 11-1 Molybdenum balance of four individuals who consumed 22 and 467 µg/day. Mean ± standard deviation.
SOURCE: Reprinted with permission from Turnlund et al. (1995b). Copyright 1995 by the *American Journal of Clinical Nutrition.*

four days was not sufficiently long to adapt to the dietary molybdenum intake.

On the basis of balance data and lack of molybdenum deficiency, the average minimum molybdenum requirement for maintaining adequate molybdenum status is estimated to be 22 µg/day plus an increment for miscellaneous losses. There are no data on sweat and integumentary losses of molybdenum, and they are too low to measure with current technology. Data from other minerals suggest that these losses amount to a small fraction of dietary intake. An additional 3 µg/day was added to allow for miscellaneous losses. The minimum requirement of 25 µg/day is consistent with estimates of the minimum molybdenum requirement of several species of animals (Anke et al., 1985; WHO, 1996).

Because some diets contain foods, such as soy, with a lower bioavailability (58 percent) than that (more than 85 percent) of foods provided by Turnlund and coworkers (1995a, 1995b), an average bioavailability of 75 percent was used to set an EAR of 34 µg/day. There are no data on which to base an EAR for women or older adults, and no evidence to suggest that requirements would be different. Therefore, the values are the same for women and older adults.

Molybdenum EAR and RDA Summary, Ages 19 Years and Older

EAR for Men
19–50 years	34 µg/day of molybdenum
51–70 years	34 µg/day of molybdenum
> 70 years	34 µg/day of molybdenum

EAR for Women
19–50 years	34 µg/day of molybdenum
51–70 years	34 µg/day of molybdenum
> 70 years	34 µg/day of molybdenum

The number of molybdenum levels in the adult depletion/repletion study was very limited, and the number of subjects was low. Thus, a CV of 15 percent is used; the RDA is defined as the EAR plus twice the CV to cover the needs of 97 to 98 percent of the individuals in the group (therefore, for molybdenum the RDA is set at 130 percent of the EAR). The calculated RDA was rounded up.

RDA for Men
19–50 years	45 µg/day of molybdenum
51–70 years	45 µg/day of molybdenum
> 70 years	45 µg/day of molybdenum

RDA for Women
19–50 years	45 µg/day of molybdenum
51–70 years	45 µg/day of molybdenum
> 70 years	45 µg/day of molybdenum

Pregnancy

Evidence Considered in Estimating the Average Requirement

No direct data are available for determining the additional daily requirement for molybdenum during pregnancy. The additional molybdenum requirement during pregnancy is determined by extrapolating up from adolescent and adult women as described in Chapter 2. Carmichael and coworkers (1997) reported that the median weight gain of 7,002 women who had good pregnancy outcomes was 16 kg. No consistent relationship between maternal age and weight gain was observed in six studies of U.S. women (IOM, 1990). Therefore, 16 kg is added to the reference weight for adolescent girls and adult women for extrapolation.

Molybdenum EAR and RDA Summary, Pregnancy

EAR for Pregnancy
  14–18 years   40 µg/day of molybdenum
  19–30 years   40 µg/day of molybdenum
  31–50 years   40 µg/day of molybdenum

The RDA for molybdenum is set by using a CV of 15 percent (see "Adults Ages 19 Years and Older"). The RDA is defined as the EAR plus twice the CV to cover the needs of 97 to 98 percent of the individuals in the group (therefore, for molybdenum the RDA is set at 130 percent of the EAR). The calculated RDA is rounded to the nearest 10 µg.

RDA for Pregnancy
  14–18 years   50 µg/day of molybdenum
  19–30 years   50 µg/day of molybdenum
  31–50 years   50 µg/day of molybdenum

Lactation

Evidence Considered in Estimating the Average Requirement

The EAR for lactation is estimated as the sum of the molybdenum intake necessary to replace the molybdenum secreted daily in human milk and the EAR for adolescent girls and women. Based on a daily excretion of 2 µg/day, the EAR for molybdenum is set at 35 and 36 µg/day for lactating adolescents and adults, respectively.

Molybdenum EAR and RDA Summary, Lactation

EAR for Lactation
  14–18 years   35 µg/day of molybdenum
  19–30 years   36 µg/day of molybdenum
  31–50 years   36 µg/day of molybdenum

The RDA for molybdenum is set by using a CV of 15 percent (see "Adults Ages 19 Years and Older"). The RDA is defined as the EAR plus twice the CV to cover the needs of 97 to 98 percent of the individuals in the group (therefore, for molybdenum the RDA is set at 130 percent of the EAR). The calculated RDA is rounded to the nearest 10 µg.

RDA for Lactation
14–18 years	**50 µg/day of molybdenum**
19–30 years	**50 µg/day of molybdenum**
31–50 years	**50 µg/day of molybdenum**

INTAKE OF MOLYBDENUM

Food Sources

The molybdenum content of plant foods varies depending upon the soil content in which they are grown. Legumes are major contributors of molybdenum in the diet, as well as grain products and nuts (Pennington and Jones, 1987; Tsongas et al., 1980). Animal products, fruits, and many vegetables are generally low in molybdenum.

Dietary Intake

Information on dietary intake of molybdenum is limited because of lack of a simple, reliable analytical method for determining molybdenum. One U.S. study reported intakes ranging from 120 to 240 µg/day, with an average intake of 180 µg/day (Tsongas et al., 1980). Data from the Total Diet Study indicate an average molybdenum intake of 76 µg/day for women and 109 µg/day for men (Pennington and Jones, 1987). Reports of molybdenum intake from other countries vary widely, probably because of differences in analytical methods and differences in the molybdenum content of soils in which foods are grown. Usual intake is well above the dietary molybdenum requirement.

Intake from Supplements

Based on data from Third National Health and Nutrition Examination Survey (Appendix Table C-21), the median intake of molybdenum from supplements was approximately 23 and 24 µg/day for men and women who took supplements, respectively.

TOLERABLE UPPER INTAKE LEVELS

The Tolerable Upper Intake Level (UL) is the highest level of daily nutrient intake that is likely to pose no risk of adverse health effects for almost all individuals. Although members of the general population should be advised not to routinely exceed the UL, intake above the UL may be appropriate for investigation within well-controlled clinical trials. Clinical trials of doses above the UL should not be discouraged, as long as subjects participating in these trials have signed informed consent documents regarding possible toxicity, and as long as these trials employ appropriate safety monitoring of trial subjects. In addition, the UL is not meant to apply to individuals who are receiving molybdenum under medical supervision.

Hazard Identification

Adverse Effects

Molybdenum compounds appear to have low toxicity in humans. More soluble forms of molybdenum have greater toxicity than insoluble or less soluble forms. The UL applies to all forms of molybdenum.

There are limited toxicity data for molybdenum in humans; most of the toxicity data are for animals, especially ruminants. Ruminants are more sensitive to molybdenum than monogastric animals, but the basis for the toxicity of molybdenum in ruminants is not relevant for humans. In monogastric laboratory animals, molybdenum has been associated with reduced growth or weight loss, renal failure, skeletal abnormalities, infertility, anemia, diarrhea, and thyroid injury (Vyskocil and Viau, 1999). Since none of these effects have been observed in humans, it is impossible to determine which ones might be considered most relevant to humans.

Molybdenum toxicity in animals varies according to age, species, sex, and duration of exposure (Vyskocil and Viau, 1999). In ruminants, the relative amounts of copper and sulfur in the diet are also important determinants of toxicity (Rajagopalan, 1988), but the effect of molybdenum on copper metabolism in humans is not significant (Turnlund and Keyes, 2000). The data on adverse effects of molybdenum intake are summarized below.

Renal Failure. Mild renal failure has been observed in rats after subchronic ingestion (by gastric intubation) at 80 mg/kg/day but not at 40 mg/kg/day of a molybdenum salt (Bompart et al., 1990).

There is weak evidence of diuresis and proteinuria after high dose molybdenum intake in animals (Bompart et al., 1990). Asmangulyan (1965) evaluated the effects of molybdenum in rabbits receiving four different oral doses (0.025, 0.5, 5, and 50 mg/kg/day) for 6 months. At a dose of 5 mg/kg/day, histological changes were observed in kidney and liver along with body weight loss. No effects were observed at lower molybdenum dosage levels.

Increased Uric Acid in Plasma and Urine. Key human studies on this endpoint include Chappell and coworkers (1979), Deosthale and Gopalan (1974), and Kovalsky and coworkers (1961). Kovalsky and coworkers (1961) observed hyperuricemia and arthralgias in Armenians who consumed 10 to 15 mg/day of molybdenum from food. Serum molybdenum concentration was positively correlated with serum uric acid concentration. Elevations in blood molybdenum concentrations were accompanied by decreases in blood copper concentrations. However, serious methodological difficulties are noted with this particular study including possible analytical problems in the assessment of blood and urinary copper levels and the very small size of the control group in contrast to the molybdenum-exposed group.

Other studies in humans do not support the existence of this particular adverse manifestation in association with elevated dietary intakes of molybdenum. For example, Chappell and coworkers (1979) reported reduced uric acid concentrations in serum after molybdenum intakes of greater than 7 µg/kg/day from drinking water. Deosthale and Gopalan (1974) reported no change in uric acid excretion at intakes up to 1.5 mg/day in four volunteers.

Impaired Copper Utilization. Impaired utilization of copper has been observed in ruminants (Mills and Davis, 1987) and is based on an interaction between molybdenum, copper, and sulfur that occurs in ruminants but not in humans. A human study involving doses up to 1.5 mg/day showed no adverse effects on copper utilization (Turnlund and Keyes, 2000).

Reproductive Effects. The administration of supplemental dietary molybdenum was associated with a prolonged estrus cycle, decreased gestational weight gain of the pups, and several adverse effects on embryogenesis in female Sprague-Dawley rats (Fungwe et al., 1990). These effects were not observed at 0.9 mg/kg/day, but were observed at doses of 1.6 mg/kg/day (based on a gestational weight of 100 g). Schroeder and Mitchener (1971) evaluated the effect of molybdate in drinking water (10 mg/L) on the reproduction of mice over three generations. Because water consumption was not reported in the publication, daily molybdenum intake can only be estimated. Vyskocil and Viau (1999) estimated that a 20-mg mouse's consumption of 3 mL of water (10 mg/L) daily would result in a dose of 1.5 mg/kg/day of molybdenum. At this dose, Schroeder and Mitchener (1971) reported some early deaths of offspring, dead litters, maternal deaths, and failure to breed.

Other Endpoints. There is no evidence that molybdenum causes cancer in humans or animals (Vyskocil and Viau, 1999). There are consistent findings of decreased hemoglobin concentration and hematocrit in rabbits (Arrington and Davis, 1953; McCarter et al., 1962; Ostrom et al., 1961; Valli et al., 1969). These effects were seen at doses of 25 mg/kg/day or more.

Growth depression has been noted in several studies with mono-gastric laboratory animals (Arthur, 1965; Jeter and Davis, 1954; Miller et al., 1956). In the study by Jeter and Davis (1954), rats were administered four different doses of molybdenum (20, 80, 140, and 700 mg/kg of diet) for 13 weeks. Growth depression was noted in female rats fed 80 mg/kg, which according to Vyskocil and Viau (1999), corresponds to 8 mg/kg/day of molybdenum. Miller and coworkers (1956) observed body weight loss and bone deformities in rats fed 75 and 300 mg/kg of diet molybdenum for 6 weeks. The lowest dose corresponds to 7.5 mg/kg/day according to Vyskocil and Viau (1999). Arthur (1965) fed guinea pigs diets containing various levels of molybdenum for 8 weeks. At the lowest dose (estimated to be 75 mg/kg/day), growth depression, loss of copper, and achromotrichia were observed.

Bioavailability and Toxicokinetics. Possible reasons for the presumed low toxicity of molybdenum include its rapid excretion in the urine, especially at higher intake levels (Miller et al., 1956; Turnlund et al., 1995b).

Summary

Because of the deficiencies in the study conducted in Armenia (Kovalsky et al., 1961), inadequate data exist to identify a causal association between excess molybdenum intake in normal, apparently healthy individuals and any adverse health outcomes. In addition, studies have identified levels of dietary molybdenum intake that appear to be associated with no harm (Deosthale and Gopalan,

1974; Turnlund and Keyes, 2000). Thus, reproductive effects in rats were selected as the most definitive toxicological indices.

Dose-Response Assessment

Adults

Data Selection. In the absence of adequate human studies, animal studies were evaluated. Rats, mice, and rabbits appear to be more sensitive than guinea pigs to the adverse effects of dietary molybdenum. The effects of molybdenum on reproduction and fetal development in rats and mice were found to be the most sensitive and therefore were used to set the UL.

Identification of a No-Observed-Adverse-Effect Level (NOAEL) and Lowest-Observed-Adverse-Effect Level (LOAEL). The study of Fungwe and co-workers (1990) provides a dose-response relationship for adverse reproductive effects in female rats. The NOAEL from this study was 0.9 mg/kg/day and the LOAEL was 1.6 mg/kg/day of molybdenum. This study is supported by observations of reproductive effects in mice in a three-generation study at a single dose of 1.5 mg/kg/day (Schroeder and Mitchener, 1971). Since only one level was used in this study, it is difficult to use this study independently to determine a LOAEL. In addition, Jeter and Davis (1954) noted decreased fertility in male rats after 13 weeks of exposure to 8 mg/kg/day of molybdenum. The NOAEL from that study was 2 mg/kg/day. Taken together, these observations suggest that numerous adverse reproductive effects were encountered in rats and mice at dietary molybdenum levels exceeding the NOAEL of 0.9 mg/kg/day established from the study of Fungwe and coworkers (1990).

Uncertainty Assessment. There do not appear to be sufficient data to justify lowering the degree of uncertainty from the usual uncertainty factor (UF) for extrapolating from experimental animals to humans. Thus, the usual value of 10 was selected. A UF of 3 for intraspecies variation was based on the expected similarity in pharmokinetics of molybdenum among humans. Although Vyskocil and Viau (1999) have argued for a larger UF for intraspecies differences, they have based their concerns on possible interactions with copper and concerns about copper-deficient humans. Recent information suggests that molybdenum does not have any effect on copper metabolism in humans (Turnlund and Keyes, 2000). Thus, these two UFs are multiplied to yield a UF of 30.

Derivation of a UL. The NOAEL of 0.9 mg/kg/day was divided by the overall UF of 30 to obtain a UL of 30 µg/kg/day for humans. The value of 30 µg/kg/day was multiplied by the average of the reference body weights for adult women, 61 kg, from Chapter 1 (Table 1-1). The resulting UL for adults is rounded to 2 mg/day (2,000 µg/day).

$$UL = \frac{NOAEL}{UF} = \frac{0.9 \text{ mg/kg/day}}{30} = 30 \text{ µg/kg/day} \times 68.5 \text{ kg} \cong$$

$$2 \text{ mg/day (2,000 µg/day)}$$

Although adult men and women have different reference body weights, the uncertainties in the estimation of the UL were considerable and distinction of separate ULs for men and women was therefore not attempted. This level is supported by limited human data from Deosthale and Gopalan (1974) who demonstrated no effect on uric acid or copper excretion in humans exposed to 22 µg/kg/day or 1.5 mg/day for an adult. Only four subjects were included in that study and no LOAEL was established. In addition, Turnlund and Keyes (2000) demonstrated no effect of 1.5 mg/day on copper metabolism in humans.

Molybdenum UL Summary, Ages 19 Years and Older

UL for Adults
≥ 19 years   **2 mg/day (2,000 µg/day) of molybdenum**

Other Life Stage Groups

Infants. For infants, the UL was judged not determinable because of insufficient data on adverse effects in this age group and concern about the infant's ability to handle excess amounts. To prevent high levels of intake, the only source of intake for infants should be from food and formula.

Children and Adolescents. There are no reports of molybdenum toxicity in children and adolescents. Given the dearth of information, the UL values for children and adolescents are extrapolated from those established for adults. Thus, the adult UL of 2 mg/day of molybdenum was adjusted for children and adolescents on the basis of relative body weight as described in Chapter 2 with use of reference weights from Chapter 1 (Table 1-1). Values have been rounded down.

Pregnancy and Lactation. Because the UL is based on adverse reproductive effects in animals and because there are no reports of molybdenum toxicity in lactating women, the UL for pregnant and lactating women is the same as that for the nonpregnant and nonlactating female.

Molybdenum UL Summary, Ages 0 through 18 Years, Pregnancy, Lactation

UL for Infants
    0–12 months   Not possible to establish; source of intake should be from food and formula only

UL for Children
    1–3 years   0.3 mg/day (300 µg/day) of molybdenum
    4–8 years   0.6 mg/day (600 µg/day) of molybdenum
    9–13 years   1.1 mg/day (1,100 µg/day) of molybdenum

UL for Adolescents
    14–18 years   1.7 mg/day (1,700 µg/day) of molybdenum

UL for Pregnancy
    14–18 years   1.7 mg/day (1,700 µg/day) of molybdenum
    19–50 years   2.0 mg/day (2,000 µg/day) of molybdenum

UL for Lactation
    14–18 years   1.7 mg/day (1,700 µg/day) of molybdenum
    19–50 years   2.0 mg/day (2,000 µg/day) of molybdenum

Special Considerations

Individuals who are deficient in dietary copper intake or have some dysfunction in copper metabolism that makes them copper-deficient could be at increased risk of molybdenum toxicity. However, the effect of molybdenum intake on copper status in humans remains to be clearly established.

Intake Assessment

National surveys do not provide percentile data on the dietary intake of molybdenum. Data available from the 1988–1994 Third National Health and Nutrition Examination Survey (Appendix Table C-21) indicate that the average U.S. intake of molybdenum from supplements at the ninety-fifth percentile was 80 and 84 µg/day for men and women, respectively.

Risk Characterization

Because there is no information from national surveys on percentile distribution of molybdenum intakes, the risk of adverse effects cannot be characterized.

RESEARCH RECOMMENDATIONS FOR MOLYBDENUM

- Bioavailability of molybdenum.
- Further data to estimate an average requirement for molybdenum.

REFERENCES

Abumrad NN, Schneider AJ, Steel D, Rogers LS. 1981. Amino acid intolerance during prolonged total parenteral nutrition reversed by molybdate therapy. *Am J Clin Nutr* 34:2551–2559.

Anderson RR. 1992. Comparison of trace elements in milk of four species. *J Dairy Sci* 75:3050–3055.

Anke M, Groppel B, Kronemann H, Grun M. 1985. Molybdenum supply and status in animals and human beings. *Nutr Res* 1:S180–S186.

Aquilio E, Spagnoli R, Seri S, Bottone G, Spennati G. 1996. Trace element content in human milk during lactation of preterm newborns. *Biol Trace Elem Res* 51:63–70.

Arrington LR, Davis GK. 1953. Molybdenum toxicity in the rabbit. *J Nutr* 51:295–304.

Arthur D. 1965. Interrelationships of molybdenum and copper in the diet of the guinea pig. *J Nutr* 87:69–76.

Asmangulyan TA. 1965. The maximum permissible concentration of molybdenum in the water of surface water basins. *Gig Sanit* 30:6–11.

Biego GH, Joyeux M, Hartemann P, Debry G. 1998. Determination of mineral contents in different kinds of milk and estimation of dietary intake in infants. *Food Addit Contam* 15:775–781.

Bompart G, Pecher C, Prevot D, Girolami JP. 1990. Mild renal failure induced by subchronic exposure to molybdenum: Urinary kallikrein excretion as a marker of distal tubular effect. *Toxicol Lett* 52:293–300.

Bougle D, Bureau F, Foucault P, Duhamel J-F, Muller G, Drosdowsky M. 1988. Molybdenum content of term and preterm human milk during the first 2 months of lactation. *Am J Clin Nutr* 48:652–654.

Bremner I. 1979. The toxicity of cadmium, zinc and molybdenum and their effects on copper metabolism. *Proc Nutr Soc* 38:235–242.

Cantone MC, de Bartolo D, Gambarini G, Giussani A, Ottolenghi A, Pirola L. 1995. Proton activation analysis of stable isotopes for a molybdenum biokinetics study in humans. *Med Phys* 22:1293–1298.

Carmichael S, Abrams B, Selvin S. 1997. The pattern of maternal weight gain in women with good pregnancy outcomes. *Am J Public Health* 87:1984–1988.

Casey CE, Neville MC. 1987. Studies in human lactation 3: Molybdenum and nickel in human milk during the first month of lactation. *Am J Clin Nutr* 45:921–926.

Chappell WR, Meglen RR, Moure-Eraso R, Solomons CC, Tsongas TA, Walravens PA, Winston PW. 1979. *Human Health Effects of Molybdenum in Drinking Water.* EPA-600/1-79-006. Cincinnati, OH: U.S. Environmental Protection Agency, Health Effects Research Laboratory.

Deosthale YG, Gopalan C. 1974. The effect of molybdenum levels in sorghum (Sorghum vulgare Pers.) on uric acid and copper excretion in man. *Br J Nutr* 31:351–355.

Engel RW, Price NO, Miller RF. 1967. Copper, manganese, cobalt, and molybdenum balance in preadolescent girls. *J Nutr* 92:197–204.

Friel JK, MacDonald AC, Mercer CN, Belkhode SL, Downton G, Kwa PG, Aziz K, Andrews WL. 1999. Molybdenum requirements in low-birth-weight infants receiving parenteral and enteral nutrition. *J Parenter Enteral Nutr* 23:155–159.

Fungwe TV, Buddingh F, Demick DS, Lox CD, Yang MT, Yang SP. 1990. The role of dietary molybdenum on estrous activity, fertility, reproduction and molybdenum and copper enzyme activities of female rats. *Nutr Res* 10:515–524.

Hurrell RF, Juillerat MA, Reddy MB, Lynch SR, Dassenko SA, Cook JD. 1992. Soy protein, phytate and iron absorption in humans. *Am J Clin Nutr* 56:573–578.

IOM (Institute of Medicine). 1990. *Nutrition During Pregnancy.* Washington, DC: National Academy Press.

Jeter MA, Davis GK. 1954. The effect of dietary molybdenum upon growth, hemoglobin, reproduction and lactation of rats. *J Nutr* 54:215–220.

Johnson JL. 1997. Molybdenum. In: O'Dell BL, Sunde RA, eds. *Handbook of Nutritionally Essential Mineral Elements. Clinical Nutrition in Health and Disease.* New York: Marcel Dekker. Pp. 413–438.

Johnson JL, Rajagopalan KV, Wadman SK. 1993. Human molybdenum cofactor deficiency. In: Ayling JE, Nair GM, Baugh CM, eds. *Chemistry and Biology of Pteridines and Folates.* New York: Plenum Press. Pp. 373–378.

Kovalsky VV, Yarovaya GA, Shmavonyan DM. 1961. The change in purine metabolism of humans and animals under the conditions of molybdenum biogeochemical provinces. *Zh Obshch Biol* 22:179–191.

Krachler M, Li FS, Rossipal E, Irgolic KJ. 1998. Changes in the concentrations of trace elements in human milk during lactation. *J Trace Elem Med Biol* 12:159–176.

McCarter A, Riddell PE, Robinson GA. 1962. Molybdenosis induced in laboratory rabbits. *Can J Biochem Physiol* 40:1415–1425.

Miller RF, Price NO, Engel RW. 1956. Added dietary inorganic sulfate and its effect upon rats fed molybdenum. *J Nutr* 60:539–547.

Mills CF, Davis GK. 1987. Molybdenum. In: Mertz W, ed. *Trace Elements in Human and Animal Nutrition,* Vol. 1. San Diego: Academic Press. Pp. 429–463.

Nielsen FH. 1999. Ultratrace minerals. In: Shils ME, Olson JA, Shike M, Ross AC, eds. *Modern Nutrition in Health and Disease,* 9th ed. Baltimore: Williams & Wilkins. Pp. 283–303.

O'Dell BL. 1989. Mineral interactions relevant to nutrient requirements. *J Nutr* 119:1832–1838.

Ostrom CA, Van Reen R, Miller CW. 1961. Changes in the connective tissue of rats fed toxic diets containing molybdenum salts. *J Dent Res* 40:520–528.

Paschal DC, Ting BG, Morrow JC, Pirkle JL, Jackson RJ, Sampson EJ, Miller DT, Caldwell KL. 1998. Trace metals of United States residents: reference range concentrations. *Environ Res* 76:53-59.

Pennington JAT, Jones JW. 1987. Molybdenum, nickel, cobalt, vanadium, and strontium in total diets. *J Am Diet Assoc* 87:1644–1650.

Rajagopalan KV. 1988. Molybdenum: An essential trace element in human nutrition. *Ann Rev Nutr* 8:401–427.

Rosoff B, Spencer H. 1964. Fate of molybdenum-99 in man. *Nature* 202:410–411.

Rossipal E, Krachler M. 1998. Pattern of trace elements in human milk during the course of lactation. *Nutr Res* 18:11–24.

Schroeder HA, Mitchener M. 1971. Toxic effects of trace elements on the reproduction of mice and rats. *Arch Environ Health* 23:102–106.

Tsongas TA, Meglen RR, Walravens PA, Chappell WR. 1980. Molybdenum in the diet: An estimate of average daily intake in the United States. *Am J Clin Nutr* 33:1103–1107.

Turnlund JR, Keyes WR. 2000. Dietary molybdenum: Effect on copper absorption, excretion, and status in young men. In: Roussel AM, Anderson RA, Favier A, eds. *Trace Elements in Man and Animals 10.* New York: Kluwer Academic.

Turnlund JR, Keyes WR, Peiffer GL. 1995a. Molybdenum absorption, excretion, and retention studied with stable isotopes in young men at five intakes of dietary molybdenum. *Am J Clin Nutr* 62:790–796.

Turnlund JR, Keyes WR, Peiffer GL, Chiang G. 1995b. Molybdenum absorption, excretion, and retention studied with stable isotopes in young men during depletion and repletion. *Am J Clin Nutr* 61:1102–1109.

Turnlund JR, Weaver CM, Kim SK, Keyes WR, Gizaw Y, Thompson KH, Peiffer GL. 1999. Molybdenum absorption and utilization in humans from soy and kale intrinsically labeled with stable isotopes of molybdenum. *Am J Clin Nutr* 69:1217–1223.

Valli VE, McCarter A, McSherry BJ, Robinson GA. 1969. Hematopoiesis and epiphyseal growth zones in rabbits with molybdenosis. *Am J Vet Res* 30:435–445.

Versieck J, Hoste J, Barbier F, Vanballenberghe L, De Rudder J, Cornelis R. 1978. Determination of molybdenum in human serum by neutron activation analysis. *Clin Chim Acta* 87:135–140.

Vyskocil A, Viau C. 1999. Assessment of molybdenum toxicity in humans. *J Appl Toxicol* 19:185–192.

WHO (World Health Organization). 1996. *Trace Elements in Human Nutrition and Health.* Geneva: WHO. Pp. 144–154.

12
Zinc

SUMMARY

Zinc functions as a component of various enzymes in the maintenance of the structural integrity of proteins and in the regulation of gene expression. Overt human zinc deficiency in North America is not common, and the symptoms of a mild deficiency are diverse due to zinc's ubiquitous involvement in metabolic processes. Factorial analysis was used to set the Estimated Average Requirement (EAR). The Recommended Dietary Allowance (RDA) for adults is 8 mg/day for women and 11 mg/day for men. Recently, the median intake from food in the United States was approximately 9 mg/day for women and 14 mg/day for men. The Tolerable Upper Intake Level (UL) for adults is 40 mg/day, a value based on reduction in erythrocyte copper-zinc superoxide dismutase activity.

BACKGROUND INFORMATION

Function

Zinc has been shown to be essential for microorganisms, plants, and animals. Deprivation of zinc arrests growth and development and produces system dysfunction in these organisms. The biological functions of zinc can be divided into three categories: catalytic, structural, and regulatory (Cousins, 1996). There is extensive evidence in support of each of these functions, and there may be some overlap.

442

Nearly 100 specific enzymes (e.g., EC 1.1.1.1 alcohol dehydrogenase) depend on zinc for catalytic activity. Zinc removal results in loss of activity, and reconstitution of the holoenzyme with zinc usually restores activity. Examples of zinc metalloenzymes can be found in all six enzyme classes (Vallee and Galdes, 1984). Well-studied zinc metalloenzymes include the ribonucleic acid (RNA) polymerases, alcohol dehydrogenase, carbonic anhydrase, and alkaline phosphatase. Zinc is defined as a Lewis acid, and its action as an electron acceptor contributes to its catalytic activity in many of these enzymes. Changes in activity of zinc metalloenzymes during dietary zinc restriction or excess have not been consistent in experimental studies with humans or animals.

The structural role of zinc involves proteins that form domains capable of zinc coordination, which facilitates protein folding to produce biologically active molecules. The vast majority of such proteins form a "zinc finger-like" structure created by chelation centers, including cysteine and histidine residues (Klug and Schwabe, 1995). Some of these proteins have roles in gene regulation as dioxyribonucleic acid binding transcription factors. Examples include nonspecific factors such as Sp1 and specific factors such as retinoic acid receptors and vitamin D receptors. These structural motifs are found throughout biology and include the zinc-containing nucleocapside proteins of viruses such as the human immunodeficiency virus (Berg and Shi, 1996). The relationship of zinc finger protein bioactivity to zinc in the diet has not received extensive study. Zinc also provides a structural function for some enzymes; copper-zinc superoxide dismutase is the most notable example. In this instance, copper provides catalytic activity, whereas zinc's role is structural. Also of potential relevance as a structural role is the essentiality of zinc for intracellular binding of tyrosine kinase to T-cell receptors, CD4 and CD8α, which are required for T-lymphocyte development and activation (Huse et al., 1998; Lin et al., 1998).

The role of zinc as a regulator of gene expression has received less attention than its other functions. Metallothionein expression is regulated by a mechanism that involves zinc's binding to the transcription factor, metal response element transcription factor (MTF1), which activates gene transcription (Cousins, 1994; Dalton et al., 1997). The number of genes that are activated by this type of mechanism is not known, however, because a null mutation for MTF1 is lethal during fetal development of mice, suggesting some critical genes must be regulated by MTF1 (Günes et al., 1998). Zinc transporter proteins associated with cellular zinc accumulation and release may be among the metal response element-regulated family of genes (McMahon and Cousins, 1998). Zinc has been shown to influence both apoptosis and protein kinase C activity (McCabe et al., 1993; Telford and Fraker, 1995; Zalewski et al., 1994), which is within the regulatory function. The relationship of zinc to normal synaptic signaling processes also falls within the regulatory role (Cole et al., 1999). The most widely studied MTF-regulated gene is the metallothionein gene. An unequivocal function has not been established, but this metalloprotein appears to act as a zinc trafficking molecule for maintaining cellular zinc concentrations (Cousins, 1996) and perhaps as part of a cellular redox system for zinc donation to zinc finger proteins (Jacob et al., 1998; Roesijadi et al., 1998). Upregulation of metallothionein by specific cytokines and some hormones suggests a function that is critical to a stress response. Induction of metallothionein by changes in dietary zinc intake has received considerable attention in experiments with both animals and humans (reviewed in Chesters, 1997; Cousins, 1994). Erythrocyte metallothionein concentrations decreased rapidly in humans fed a phytate-containing diet of very low zinc content (Grider et al., 1990). Erythrocyte metallothionein concentration appears to be a measure of severe zinc depletion, and the extent of a change in concentration can distinguish between low and adequate levels of zinc intake under experimental conditions (Thomas et al., 1992). Erythrocyte metallothionein and monocyte metallothionein messenger RNA concentrations increase with elevated zinc intake levels such as those encountered with dietary supplements (Grider et al., 1990; Sullivan et al., 1998). Studies of metallothionein concentration in blood cells or plasma during large human dietary trials have not been undertaken. Consequently, the use of metallothionein as a static or functional indicator of zinc status needs further study.

While knowledge of the biochemical and molecular genetics of zinc function is well developed and expanding, neither the relationship of these genetics to zinc deficiency or toxicity nor the function(s) for which zinc is particularly critical have been established. For example, explanations for depressed growth, immune dysfunction, diarrhea, altered cognition, host defense properties, defects in carbohydrate utilization, reproductive teratogenesis, and numerous other clinical outcomes of mild and severe zinc deficiency (Hambidge, 1989; King and Keen, 1999) have not been conclusively established.

Physiology of Absorption, Metabolism, and Excretion

Zinc is widely distributed in foods. Because virtually none of it is present as the free ion, bioavailability is a function of the extent of digestion. Digestion produces the opportunity for zinc to bind to exogenous and endogenous constituents in the intestinal lumen, including peptides, amino acids, nucleic acids, and other organic acids and inorganic anions such as phosphate. The vast majority of zinc is absorbed by the small intestine through a transcellular process with the jejunum being the site with the greatest transport rate (Cousins, 1989b; Lee et al., 1989; Lonnerdal, 1989).

Absorption kinetics appear to be saturable, and there is an increase in transport velocity with zinc depletion. Paracellular transport may occur at high zinc intakes. Transit time also influences the extent of absorption to an extent that, in malabsorption syndromes, zinc absorption is reduced. Transfer from the intestine is via the portal system with most newly absorbed zinc bound to albumin.

Considerable amounts of zinc enter the intestine from endogenous sources. Homeostatic regulation of zinc metabolism is achieved principally through a balance of absorption and secretion of endogenous reserves involving adaptive mechanisms programmed by dietary zinc intake (King and Keen, 1999). Zinc depletion in humans is accompanied by reduced endogenous zinc loss on the order of 1.3 to 4.6 mg/day, derived from both pancreatic and intestinal cell secretions. Strong evidence suggests zinc transporter proteins in the various tissues act in concert to obtain such adaptation, but evidence is lacking in humans (McMahon and Cousins, 1998).

Measurement of true absorption, which eliminates the contribution of endogenous zinc from calculations, shows that zinc depletion increases the efficiency of intestinal zinc absorption. Regulation of absorption may provide a "coarse control" of body zinc, whereas endogenous zinc release provides "fine control" to maintain balance (King and Keen, 1999). An autosomal recessive trait, acrodermatitis enteropathica, is a zinc malabsorption problem of undetermined genetic basis. The mutation causes severe skin lesions and cognitive dysfunction (Aggett, 1989). The genetic defect suggests that one gene has a major influence on zinc absorption.

Tracer studies have shown that zinc is metabolically very active with initial uptake by liver representing a rapid phase of zinc turnover. Over 85 percent of the total body zinc is found in skeletal muscle and bone (King and Keen, 1999). While plasma zinc is only 0.1 percent of this total, its concentration is tightly regulated at about 10 to 15 µmol/L. Stress, acute trauma, and infection cause changes in hormones (e.g., cortisol) and cytokines (e.g., interleukin 6) that lower plasma concentration. Small changes in tissue pools could cause the decrease. In humans, plasma zinc concentrations are maintained without notable change when zinc intake is restricted or increased unless these changes in intake are severe and prolonged (Cousins, 1989a). Preliminary kinetic data indicate that the combined size of readily exchangeable zinc pools (i.e., those that exchange with zinc in plasma within 72 hours) decreases with dietary zinc restriction (Miller et al., 1994). Fasting results in increased plasma zinc concentration, an outcome that possibly reflects catabolic changes in muscle protein. Cyclic postprandial changes in plasma zinc concentration have been documented (King et al., 1994). In both cases, hormonally regulated events are the biochemical basis for the changes. Albumin is the principal zinc-binding protein in plasma from which most metabolic zinc flux occurs. Functional aspects of zinc tightly bound to α-2-macroglobulin have not been described. Plasma amino acids bind some zinc and could be an important source of zinc excretion.

Zinc secretion into and excretion from the intestine provides the major route of endogenous zinc excretion. It is derived partially from pancreatic secretions, which are stimulated after a meal. Biliary secretion of zinc is limited, but intestinal cell secretions also contribute to fecal loss (Lonnerdal, 1989). These losses may range from less than 1 mg/day with a zinc-poor diet to greater than 5 mg/day with a zinc-rich diet, a difference that reflects the regulatory role that the intestinal tract serves in zinc homeostasis. Urinary zinc losses are only a fraction (less than 10 percent) of normal fecal losses (King and Keen, 1999). Zinc transporter activity may account for renal zinc reabsorption (McMahon and Cousins, 1998), and glucagon may help regulate it. Increases in urinary losses are concomitant with increases in muscle protein catabolism due to starvation or trauma. The increase in plasma amino acids, which constitute a potentially filterable zinc pool, is at least partially responsible. Zinc loss from the body is also attributed to epithelial cell desquamation, sweat, semen, hair, and the menstrual cycle.

Clinical Effects of Inadequate Intake

Individuals with malabsorption syndromes including sprue, Crohn's disease, and short bowel syndrome are at risk of zinc deficiency due to malabsorption of zinc and increased urinary zinc losses (Pironi et al., 1987; Valberg et al., 1986). In mild human zinc deficiency states, the detectable features and laboratory/functional abnormalities of mild zinc deficiency are diverse. This diversity is not altogether surprising in view of the biochemistry of zinc and the ubiquity of this metal in biology with its participation in an extraordinarily wide range of vital metabolic processes. Impaired growth velocity is a primary clinical feature of mild zinc deficiency and can be corrected with zinc supplementation (Hambidge et al., 1979b; Walravens et al., 1989). Other functions that respond to zinc supplementation include pregnancy outcome (Goldenberg et al., 1995) and immune function (Bogden et al., 1987). Evidence of the efficacy of zinc lozenges in reducing the duration of common colds is still unclear (Jackson et al., 2000).

Severe zinc deficiency has been documented in patients fed intravenously without the addition of adequate zinc to the infusates (Chen et al., 1991) and in cases of the autosomal recessively inherited disease acrodermatitis enteropathica (Walling et al., 1989). Because of the ubiquity of zinc and the involvement of this micronutrient in so many core areas of metabolism, it is not surprising that the features of zinc deficiency are frequently quite basic and nonspecific, including growth retardation, alopecia, diarrhea, delayed sexual maturation and impotence, eye and skin lesions, and impaired appetite. Clinical features and laboratory criteria are not always consistent. This inconsistency poses a major difficulty in the quest to validate reliable, sensitive clinical or functional indicators of zinc status that apply to a range of otherwise potentially useful laboratory indicators such as alkaline phosphatase activity.

A further major conundrum is posed by the impressive, yet apparently imperfect, homeostatic mechanisms that maintain a narrow range of zinc concentrations within the body in spite of widely diverse dietary intakes of this metal and in spite of differences in bioavailability. This situation applies, for example, to circulating zinc in the plasma, which consequently provides only an insensitive index of zinc status (King, 1990). Therefore, it has become increasingly apparent that homeostatic mechanisms fall short of perfection and that clinically important features of zinc deficiency can occur with only modest degrees of dietary zinc restriction while circulating zinc concentrations are indistinguishable from normal.

SELECTION OF INDICATORS FOR ESTIMATING THE REQUIREMENT FOR ZINC

Principal Indicator

The selection of zinc absorption (more specifically, the minimal quantity of absorbed zinc necessary to match total daily excretion of endogenous zinc) as the principal indicator for adult Estimated Average Requirements (EAR) has been based on the evaluation of a factorial approach to determining zinc requirements. Details of this approach are discussed under "Findings by Life Stage and Gender Group—Adults Ages 19 Years and Older". A sufficient number of metabolic studies of zinc homeostasis have been reported to permit an estimation of dietary zinc requirements in adults.

The first step in this approach is to calculate nonintestinal losses of endogenous zinc, that is, losses via the kidney and integument with smaller quantities in semen and menstrual losses. Although urinary zinc excretion decreases markedly with severe dietary zinc restriction (Baer and King, 1984), extensive data indicate that excretion by this route is unrelated to dietary zinc intake over a wide range (4 to 25 mg/day) that is certain to encompass the dietary zinc requirements for adults. Data regarding this lack of relation between intake and integumental and semen losses of zinc are more limited. Therefore, nonintestinal losses of endogenous zinc have been treated as a constant in response to varied zinc intake.

In contrast to excretion of zinc via other routes, excretion of endogenous zinc via the intestine is a major variable in the maintenance of zinc homeostasis and is strongly correlated with absorbed zinc. The second step in estimating dietary zinc requirements is to define this relationship (Figure 12-1). After it has been defined and adjusted by the constant for other endogenous losses, one can calculate the minimum quantity of absorbed zinc necessary to offset endogenous zinc losses (Figure 12-1).

The dietary zinc intake corresponding to this average minimum quantity of absorbed zinc is the EAR. This value has been determined from the plot of the asymptotic regression analysis of absorbed zinc versus ingested zinc (Figure 12-2).

Theoretically, given the results described in detail for adults below, balance could also be used as an indicator. However, review of all published data on zinc balance (and net [apparent] absorption) studies in young adult men (excluding those studies that have included tracer data and are being utilized for the current factorial calculations) collectively revealed no correlation with dietary zinc. Presumably this lack of correlation reflects the vagaries of balance studies. The factorial calculations for adults are based on tracer/metabolic studies in which participants were fed diets from which the bioavailability of zinc was likely to be representative of typical diets in North America or, in some instances, possibly greater than average.

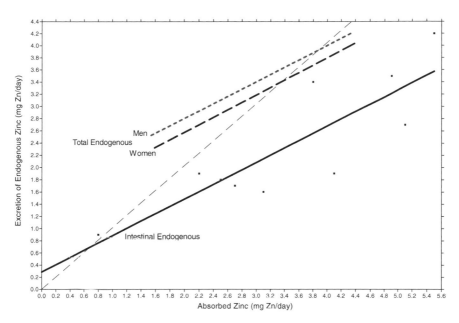

FIGURE 12-1 The relationship between endogenous zinc excretion and absorbed zinc. Heavy line represents the linear regression of intestinal excretion of endogenous zinc (mg/day) versus absorbed zinc (mg/day) from means of ten data sets for healthy men ages 19 through 50 years. The bold dashed lines above and parallel to the regression line represent the total endogenous zinc losses for men and women in relation to zinc absorption. The faint dashed line is the line of perfect agreement or equality of endogenous zinc and absorbed zinc. The intersect of this line with that of total endogenous zinc excretion indicates the average minimum quantity of absorbed zinc necessary to match endogenous losses for men and women. SOURCE: Hunt JR et al. (1992), Jackson et al. (1984), Lee et al. (1993), Taylor et al. (1991), Turnlund et al. (1984, 1986), Wada et al. (1985).

Secondary Indicators

Physical Growth Response to Zinc Supplementation

In contrast to studies on the effects of low-dose zinc supplements on clinical features (e.g., pneumonia, diarrhea [Bhutta et al., 1999]) and on nonspecific laboratory functional tests of zinc status (e.g., tests of neuro-cognitive function [Sandstead et al., 1998]) or immune status (Shankar and Prasad, 1998), studies of the effects of zinc supplementation on physical growth velocity in children are useful in evaluating dietary zinc requirements for several reasons.

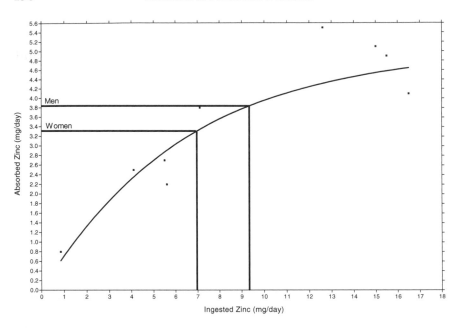

FIGURE 12-2 Asymptotic regression of absorbed zinc and ingested zinc. Individual points are means for the same data sets in Figure 12-1. SOURCE: Hunt JR et al. (1992), Jackson et al. (1984), Lee et al. (1993), Taylor et al. (1991), Turnlund et al. (1984, 1986), Wada et al. (1985).

First, confirmation of the effect of zinc supplements on growth velocity (linear growth and weight) in children with varying degrees of growth retardation has been shown in a number of studies from many countries (Brown et al., 1998; Umeta et al., 2000). Second, because a sufficient number of these studies have been undertaken in North America, growth is applicable as a functional/clinical indicator of zinc requirement in North American children (Gibson et al., 1989; Walravens and Hambidge, 1976; Walravens et al., 1983, 1989). Third, baseline dietary data typically included in these studies are adequate to use for group analyses.

Size and Turnover Rates of Zinc Pools

Strong positive correlations have been observed between dietary zinc content, especially the amount of absorbed zinc, and estimates of the size of the combined pools of zinc that exchange with zinc in plasma (Miller et al., 1994; Sian et al., 1996). Once links to clinical, biochemical, or molecular effects of zinc deficiency have been achieved and appropriate cut-off levels for different age groups and gender have been defined, pool size and turnover measurements may be of value in future refinements of EARs. Even simpler models involving the measurement of plasma zinc clearance may be useful in assessing zinc deficiency, but dietary data derived by such a method are not available at this time (Kaji et al., 1998; Nakamura et al., 1993; Yokoi et al., 1994). More detailed model-based compartmental analyses, when specifically applied to the evaluation of dietary requirements, also have the potential to contribute to a more precise understanding of zinc requirements (Miller et al., 1998; Wastney et al., 1986).

Plasma and Serum Zinc Concentration

While both plasma zinc concentration and serum zinc concentration are used as indicators of zinc status, plasma zinc concentration is preferable because of the lack of contamination of zinc from the erythrocyte. Homeostatic mechanisms are effective in maintaining plasma zinc concentrations for many weeks of even severe dietary zinc restriction (Johnson et al., 1993; Wada et al., 1985). A number of studies have reported no association between dietary zinc intake and plasma or serum zinc concentration (Artacho et al., 1997; Kant et al., 1989; Neggers et al., 1997; Thomas et al., 1988). Payette and Gray-Donald (1991) did observe a significant correlation between dietary zinc intake and serum zinc concentration in noninstitutionalized elderly; however, the correlation was positive for men and negative for women. Discernible relationships have been reported between plasma zinc concentration and habitual dietary zinc intake, even within the range typically occurring in North America. These relationships are of some utility in providing a supportive indicator of zinc requirements. For example, serum zinc concentrations of Canadian adolescent girls aged 14 to 19 years vary inversely with phytate:zinc molar ratios, and a greater percentage of lacto-ovo-vegetarians have serum zinc values below 70 µg/dL than do omnivores (Donovan and Gibson, 1995). Cut-off concentrations for lower limits have been established and depend on the time of day at which collections are made because of the substantial and cumulative effects of meals in lowering concentrations (King et al., 1994). The cut-off concentrations for prebreakfast samples is 70 µg/dL. Different cut-off concentrations are not considered necessary for different age groups or genders.

Insufficient and inconsistent data exist for plasma or serum zinc concentrations in apparently normal subjects whose habitual dietary zinc intakes straddle the vicinity of the average requirement, and therefore use of those concentrations for estimating an average requirement is limited. Furthermore, plasma and serum zinc concentrations do not seem to be sufficiently sensitive to serve as a subsidiary indicator.

Zinc Concentration in Erythrocytes

Erythrocyte zinc concentration is depressed at moderately severe levels of dietary zinc restriction (Thomas et al., 1992), but the sensitivity of this assay is inadequate to provide more than a secondary supportive indicator of dietary zinc requirements. Sample preparation may account for some of the lack of sensitivity. Results from experimental depletion studies (Baer and King, 1984; Bales et al., 1994; Grider et al., 1990; Ruz et al., 1992; Thomas et al., 1992) have been mixed, and the value of erythrocyte zinc concentrations as an indicator of zinc nutritional status is not well defined.

Zinc Concentration in Hair

Associations between low zinc concentration in hair and poor growth have been documented (Ferguson et al., 1993; Gibson et al., 1989; Hambidge et al., 1972; Walravens et al., 1983). In three of these studies, low zinc concentration in hair was used as a criterion for zinc supplementation in children and resulted in increased growth velocity. Low zinc concentrations in hair have been reported in Canadian children with low meat consumption (Smit-Vanderkooy and Gibson, 1987). Subjects whose habitual diets are high in phytate or who have very high phytate:zinc molar ratios have also been noted to have relatively low zinc concentrations in hair. However, there is a lack of uniformity in apparently low zinc concentrations in hair, and no lower cut-off values have been defined clearly for any age group or either gender. The use of zinc in hair as a supportive indicator for establishing zinc requirements needs further research.

Activity of Zinc-Dependent Enzymes

With the large number of zinc-dependent enzymes that have been identified, it is perhaps remarkable that no single zinc-dependent enzyme has found broad acceptance as an indicator of zinc status or requirement. This state of affairs is attributable to a number of factors, including the homeostatic processes that maintain zinc occupancy of the catalytic sites of these enzymes and the lack of consistency in findings between studies. Other factors include a lack of sensitivity, the inaccessibility of optimal tissues to assay, or, simply, inadequate research. The lack of baseline dietary data also negates the potential value of some reports. Given these limitations, limited dose-response data, and inconsistent responses to dietary zinc (Bales et al., 1994; Davis et al., 2000; Paik et al., 1999; Ruz et al., 1992; Samman et al., 1996), the activities of zinc-dependent enzymes, including alkaline phosphatase, copper-zinc superoxide dismutase, and lymphocyte 5'-nucleotidase, can at most serve as supportive indicators of dietary zinc requirements at this time. Although it is not consistently responsive to zinc intake, the activity of plasma 5'-nucleotidase (Beck et al., 1997a), which is derived from the CD73 cell surface markers of B and T cells, merits specific recognition as a potential marker of zinc status (Failla, 1999).

Metallothionein and Zinc-Regulated Gene Markers

Erythrocyte metallothionein concentrations have been reported to be responsive to both increased and restricted dietary zinc (Grider et al., 1990; Thomas et al., 1992), but the sensitivity and precision of this index has not been thoroughly evaluated. Monocyte metallothionein messenger RNA responds rapidly to in vivo zinc supplementation (Sullivan et al., 1998) and merits additional research. Moreover, this approach points the way for future exploration of molecular markers of zinc status including, for example, a whole family of zinc transporters that are now being identified (Failla, 1999; McMahon and Cousins, 1998).

Indexes of Immune Status

Zinc is essential for the integrity of the immune system, and inadequate zinc intake has many adverse effects (Shankar and Prasad, 1998). Though the immune system, which is thought to underlie several of the most important sequelae of mild zinc deficiency, is sensitive to even mild zinc deficiency, the effects on functional indexes of zinc status are not specific. At this time, therefore, changes in indexes of immune status with manipulation of dietary zinc can serve only as a limited indicator for dietary zinc requirements.

Hormones

The biology of zinc is linked extensively to hormone metabolism. Notable examples are the zinc finger motifs of regulatory proteins required for hormonal signals to regulate gene transcription (Cousins, 1994; Klug and Schwabe, 1995). Zinc has been reported to have roles in the synthesis, transport, and peripheral action of hormones. Low dietary zinc status has been associated with low circulating concentrations of several hormones including testosterone (Prasad et al., 1996), free T4 (Wada and King, 1986), and IGF-1 (Ninh et al., 1996). Zinc supplementation has been associated with an increase in both circulating IGF-1 concentration and growth velocity (Ninh et al., 1996). However, no studies have directly related hormone concentrations to decreases or increases in zinc intake.

Circulating Hepatic Proteins

Reductions in retinol binding protein, albumin, and pre-albumin concentrations have been reported with moderate dietary zinc restriction (Wada and King, 1986). Serum zinc and retinol binding protein concentrations are significantly correlated in zinc-deficient Thai children (Udomkesmalee et al., 1990). Changes in circulating concentrations of these proteins with changes in dietary zinc may serve as minor supportive indicators. The relationship of such indicators to general malnutrition or to dietary deficiency that is not related to zinc status supports their being minor indicators for zinc requirements.

FACTORS AFFECTING THE ZINC REQUIREMENT

Bioavailability

Bioavailability of zinc can be affected by many factors at many sites. The intestine is the major organ in which variations in bioavailability affect dietary zinc requirements. These effects occur through two key regulatory processes: absorption of exogenous zinc and reabsorption of endogenous zinc. Dietary factors that affect bioavailability can have an impact on each of these processes (Cousins, 1989b; Lonnerdal, 1989).

Zinc absorption from foods and supplements has received extensive study. The environment within the gastrointestinal tract drastically influences zinc solubility and absorptive efficiency. The propensity of zinc to bind tenaciously to ligands provided by dietary constituents is accentuated at the near neutral pH in the intestinal lumen. The exact nature of the form in which zinc is needed for uptake has not been established. Some transporters responsible for transcellular zinc movement may require the free ion, but cotransport with small peptides and nucleotides has not been ruled out. Absorption of zinc, when consumed as a chelate, has not been investigated extensively. The option for zinc to be absorbed by the paracellular route adds to the lack of a unified form or path of zinc absorption from foods. Furthermore, the methods used to assess zinc absorption have varied widely, including balance studies, intestinal perfusion, responses of plasma zinc to single meals or aqueous doses, and tracer studies with intrinsically or extrinsically stable or radioactive zinc isotopes (Sandstrom and Lonnerdal, 1989).

Nutrient-Nutrient Interactions

Iron

Daily intake of iron at levels such as those found in some supplements could decrease zinc absorption (O'Brien et al., 2000; Solomons and Jacob, 1981; Valberg et al., 1984). This relationship is of some concern in management of iron supplementation during pregnancy and lactation (Fung et al., 1997). Recent studies of the mechanism of nonheme iron absorption suggest that upregulation of an iron transport protein occurs in iron deficiency (Gunshin et al., 1997). The comparable affinity of this transporter for zinc suggests that, during low iron intake, zinc absorption may be stimulated and suggests one possible locus for a zinc-iron interaction. The influence of heme iron on zinc absorption has not received much attention. The activity of other divalent metal transporters may also affect zinc absorption.

Calcium and Phosphorus

The importance of calcium in the diet and the mass of the element that must be consumed daily to maintain maximum bone density suggest that special attention should be given to its potential inhibitory effect on zinc absorption. Nutrition experiments with swine have shown conclusively that excess dietary calcium produces a decrease in zinc absorption, which leads to a skin condition called parakeratosis. Experiments in humans have been equivocal, with calcium phosphate (1,360 mg/day of calcium) decreasing zinc absorption (Wood and Zheng, 1997) and calcium as the citrate-malate complex (1,000 mg/day of calcium) having no statistically significant effect on zinc absorption (McKenna et al., 1997). Differences could be related to the calcium sources, techniques used, and the extent of luminal zinc solubility. At present, data suggest consumption of a calcium-rich diet does not have a major effect on zinc absorption at an adequate intake level of the nutrient. Calcium effects at low dietary zinc intakes have not been adequately investigated. Dietary phosphorus-containing salts over an extensive intake range have not been shown to influence zinc balance (Greger and Snedeker, 1980; Spencer et al., 1984). Other dietary sources of phosphorus include phytate and phosphorus-rich proteins, for example, milk casein and nucleic acids, all of which bind zinc tenaciously and decrease zinc absorption.

Copper

Large-scale studies on the influence of dietary copper intake on zinc absorption and utilization have not been carried out with human subjects. Various experimental approaches with animals have not revealed a uniform influence of copper on intestinal zinc uptake (Cousins, 1985; Sandstrom and Lonnerdal, 1989). Rather, evidence for an interaction derives from the therapeutic effect of zinc in reducing copper absorption in patients with Wilson's disease (Yuzbasiyan-Gurkan et al., 1992). This action includes the induction of intestinal metallothionein by zinc and the subsequent binding of excess copper by this metalloprotein, which may limit transcellular copper absorption. The relationship may have relevance in situations where zinc supplements are consumed with marginal dietary copper intake.

Folate

Folate bioavailability is enhanced when polyglutamate folate is hydrolyzed by the zinc-dependent enzyme, polyglutamate hydrolase, to the monoglutamate. This occurrence suggests a possible point of interaction. Some studies have shown a relationship between folate and zinc (Milne et al., 1984), with low zinc intake decreasing folate absorption/status. More recent evidence does not support any effect of low zinc intake on folate utilization and shows that folate supplementation does not adversely affect zinc status (Kauwell et al., 1995). Extensive studies on this potential relationship have not been carried out in women. Given that these nutrients have important functions in both fetal and postnatal development, the relationship requires further study.

Protein

Zinc binds tenaciously to proteins at near neutral pH. Consequently, the amount of protein in the diet is a factor contributing to the efficiency of zinc absorption. As protein digestion proceeds, zinc becomes more accessible for zinc transport mechanisms of intestinal cells. The relative abundance of zinc as small molecular weight complexes of low binding affinity enhances the process. Small changes in protein digestion may produce significant changes in zinc absorption (Sandstrom and Lonnerdal, 1989). These changes in absorption may explain the correlation between zinc deficiency symptoms and certain malabsorption disorders (Cousins, 1996). The markedly greater bioavailability of zinc from human milk than from cow's milk is an example of how protein digestibility, which is much lower in casein-rich cow's milk than in human milk, influences zinc absorption (Roth and Kirchgessner, 1985). In general, zinc absorption from a diet high in animal protein will be greater than from a diet rich in proteins of plant origin such as soy (King and Keen, 1999).

Other Food Components

Phytic Acid

Plants contain phytic acid (myo-inositol hexaphosphate) for use as a storage form of phosphorus. Consequently, plant-based foods, particularly grains and legumes, have a significant phytic acid content. Enzymatic action of yeast during the leavening of bread and other fermentations reduce phytate levels, whereas extrusion processes (used in preparation of some breakfast cereals), may not (Williams and Erdman, 1999). In Caco-2 cells, the metal binding property of phytic acid decreases proportionally as fewer than six phosphate groups are bound to each inositol molecule (Han et al., 1994). Phytate binding of zinc has been demonstrated as a contributing factor for the zinc deficiency related to consumption of unleavened bread seen in certain population groups in the Middle East (Prasad, 1991). The overall effect of phytate is to reduce zinc absorption from the gastrointestinal tract through complexation and precipitation (Oberleas et al., 1966). These chemical effects appear to be enhanced by simultaneous binding of calcium. Phytate binding in the intestinal lumen includes zinc of both food origin and endogenous origin. Since zinc homeostasis is controlled in part by endogenous secretions, consumption of phytate-rich foods may be of practical importance as a factor that limits absorption and maintenance of zinc balance. While high-fiber-containing foods tend also to be phytate-rich, fiber alone may not have a major effect on zinc absorption.

Picolinic Acid

A metabolite of tryptophan metabolism, picolinic acid has a high metal binding affinity. Picolinate complexes of zinc and chromium are not formed in nature in appreciable amounts, but are sold commercially as dietary supplements. Zinc picolinate as a zinc source for humans has not received extensive investigation. In an animal model, picolinic acid supplementation promoted negative zinc balance (Seal and Heaton, 1985), presumably by promoting urinary excretion.

Algorithms

To date, a useful algorithm for establishing dietary zinc requirements based on the presence of other nutrients and food components has not been established, and much information is still needed to develop one that can predict zinc bioavailability (Hunt, 1996). Algorithms for estimating dietary zinc bioavailability will need to include the dietary content of phytic acid, protein, zinc, and possibly calcium, iron, and copper. The World Health Organization (WHO, 1996) developed zinc requirements from low, medium, and high bioavailability diets on the basis of estimates of fractional absorption on single test meals with varying zinc and phytate content. The results of single test meals for measuring zinc absorption, however, may be different from the long-term response of zinc absorption, as has been shown to be the case for iron (see Chapter 9).

FINDINGS BY LIFE STAGE AND GENDER GROUP

Infants Ages 0 through 6 Months

No functional criteria of zinc status have been demonstrated that reflect response to dietary intake in infants. Thus, recommended intakes of zinc are based on an Adequate Intake (AI) that reflects the observed mean zinc intake of infants exclusively fed human milk.

Method Used to Set the Adequate Intake

Using the method described in Chapter 2, an AI has been used as the goal for intake during the first 6 months of life. The AI is based on the maternal zinc supply to the infant exclusively fed human milk.

There is an unusually rapid physiologic decline in the zinc concentration of human milk and consequently in the zinc supplied to infants fed human milk during the first 6 months of lactation (Krebs et al., 1985, 1994, 1995; Moser and Reynolds, 1983) (Figure 12-3). Concentrations of zinc in human milk decline from approximately 4 mg/L at 2 weeks to 3 mg/L at 1 month, 2 mg/L at 2 months, 1.5 mg/L at 3 months, and 1.2 mg/L at 6 months postpartum (Krebs et al., 1995; see Table 12-1). With a standard volume of intake of 0.78 L/day (Chapter 2), calculated zinc intakes are 2.15 mg/day at 1 month, 1.56 mg/day at 2 months, 1.15 mg/day at 3 months, and 0.94 mg/day at 6 months (Table 12-1). Measured zinc intake of infants fed human milk was 2.3 mg/day at 2 weeks and 1 mg/day at 3 months (Krebs et al., 1994).

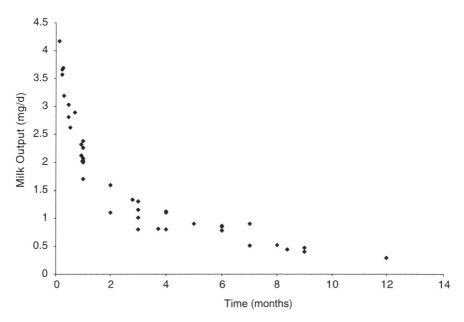

FIGURE 12-3 Average zinc consumption from human milk during the first 12 months of lactation.
SOURCE: Table 12-1.

TABLE 12-1 Zinc Concentration in Human Milk

Reference	Study Group	Maternal Intake (mg/d)
Picciano and Guthrie, 1976	50 women	Not reported
Johnson and Evans, 1978	10 women	Not reported
Vuori et al., 1980	15 women, 24–35 y	13.7 ± 2.7 mg/d 12.8 ± 2.8 mg/d
Fransson and Lonnerdal, 1982	23 women	Not reported
Moser and Reynolds, 1983	23 women, 30 y	9.4 12.8 9.6
Casey et al., 1985	11 women, 26–39 y	Not reported
Casey et al., 1989	22 women	10.9
Sievers et al., 1992	10 women	Not reported
Anderson, 1993	6 women, 20–30 y	Not reported
Krebs et al., 1995	71 women, 30 y	13–25.7
Aquilio et al., 1996	14 women, 21–29 y	Not reported
Biego et al., 1998	17 milk samples	Not reported

[a] Zinc intake based on reported data or concentration (mg/L) × 0.78 L/day for 0–6 months postpartum and concentration (mg/L) × 0.6 L/day for 7–12 months postpartum.

Stage of Lactation	Milk Concentration (mg/L)	Estimated Zinc Intake of Infants (mg/d)[a]
6–12 wk	1.7	1.33
2 mo–2 y	1.8	1.40
6–8 wk	1.89	1.47
17–22 wk	0.72	0.56
Various stages	1.1	0.86
1 mo	2.6	2.03
3 mo	1.3	1.01
6 mo	1.1	0.86
8 d	4.74	3.69
14 d	3.88	3.03
21 d	3.71	2.89
28 d	2.98	2.32
7 d	4.7	3.66
1 mo	2.9	2.26
12 mo	0.5	0.39
17 d	3.6	2.81
35 d	2.6	2.03
56 d	1.7	1.33
85 d	1.3	1.01
117 d	1.2	0.94
Up to 5 mo	1.1–3.4	0.86–2.65
0.5 mo	4	3.12
1 mo	2.75	2.15
2 mo	2	1.56
3 mo	1.5	1.17
4 mo	1.4	1.09
5 mo	1.2	0.94
6 mo	1.2	0.94
7 mo	0.8	0.48
8 mo	0.9	0.52
9 mo	0.8	0.48
2–6 d	2.2	1.72
12–16 d	2.3	1.79
21 d	2.3	1.79
Mature milk	2	1.6

In order to match the zinc intake of the infant in early weeks (Figure 12-3), the AI is set at 2.0 mg/day (2.5 mg/L × 0.78 L/day). This amount appears to be generous at ages 4 to 6 months when evaluated by zinc intake from human milk at this age, and human milk has been shown to result in weight gain and body lengths similar to those of infants provided complementary foods at 4 to 6 months (Dewey et al., 1999). A positive association between zinc content of human milk at 5 months and changes in the weight-for-age Z scores for the 5- to 7-month interval have, however, been documented (Krebs et al., 1994). There is also some evidence, however, that growth-limiting zinc deficiency can occur in infants principally fed human milk after the age of 4 months (Walravens et al., 1992).

Factorial estimates of requirements (i.e., 2.1 mg/day at 1 month and 1.54 mg/day at 5 months) are consistent with this AI for infants ages 0 through 6 months. These factorial estimates are based on measurements of zinc intake of infants fed human milk, fractional absorption, and endogenous losses (Krebs et al., 1996). Integumental and urine losses are from published calculations (Krebs and Hambidge, 1986). Also consistent with this AI is an earlier report that physical growth of male infants fed a zinc-fortified cow milk formula (5.8 mg/L) was greater than that of infants receiving the same formula but with a zinc concentration of 1.8 mg/L, which provided about 1.4 mg/day of zinc (Walravens and Hambidge, 1976).

Zinc AI Summary, Ages 0 through 6 Months

AI for Infants
    0–6 months   **2.0 mg/day of zinc**

Special Considerations

The zinc concentration in cow milk ranges from 3 to 5 mg/L (Lonnerdal et al., 1981) which is greater than the average concentration in human milk (Table 12-1). Singh and coworkers (1989) reported that approximately 32 percent of zinc in cow milk is bound to casein and the majority of the remaining zinc (63 percent) is bound to colloidal calcium phosphate. The absorption of zinc from human milk is higher than from cow milk-based infant formula and cow milk (Lonnerdal et al., 1988; Sandstrom et al., 1983). The zinc bioavailability from soy formulas is significantly lower than from milk-based formulas (Lonnerdal et al., 1988; Sandstrom et al., 1983).

Infants and Children Ages 7 Months through 3 Years

Evidence Considered in Estimating the Average Requirement

Intake from Human Milk. Zinc nutriture in later infancy is quite different from that in the younger infant. It is likely that neonatal hepatic stores, which may contribute to metabolically usable zinc pools in early postnatal life, have been dissipated (Zlotkin and Cherian, 1988). Human milk provides only 0.5 mg/day of zinc by 7 months postpartum (Krebs et al., 1994), and the concentration declines even further by 12 months (Casey et al., 1989). It is apparent, therefore, that human milk alone is an inadequate source of zinc after the first 6 months. As a result, extrapolation from human milk intake during the 0 through 6 months postpartum period, which yields 2.4 mg/day, does not reflect adequate zinc intake during the second 6 months.

Intake from Human Milk and Complementary Foods. Data from the Third National Health and Nutrition Examination Survey indicate that the median intake of zinc from complementary foods is 1.48 mg/day ($n = 45$) for older infants consuming human milk. Thus, the average zinc intake from human milk and complementary foods is estimated to be approximately 2 mg/day (0.5 + 1.48).

Factorial Analysis. Excretion of endogenous zinc is used to estimate the physiological requirement of zinc in older infants and young children. The Estimated Average Requirement (EAR) for zinc is determined by dividing the physiological requirement by the fractional zinc absorption. Apart from some data on excretion of zinc in the urine (Alexander et al., 1974; Cheek et al., 1968; Ziegler et al., 1978), direct measurements of endogenous zinc excretion are not available for older infants, children, or adolescents. These endogenous zinc losses (intestinal, urinary, and integumental), therefore, are estimated by extrapolation from measured values for either adults (see "Adults Ages 19 Years and Older") or younger infants. These extrapolations have been based on a reference weight.

Intestinal losses vary directly with the quantity of zinc absorbed (see "Adults Ages 19 Years and Older"). The average intestinal excretion of endogenous zinc in infants aged 2 to 4 months who receive human milk is approximately 50 µg/kg/day (Krebs et al., 1996). There is a "critical" level of intestinal excretion of endogenous zinc in adults at which the quantity of absorbed zinc is equal to the total endogenous zinc losses. This critical level, derived from all available sets of data for adult men, yields an average excretion of 34 μg/kg/ day of zinc and is used for children beyond 1 year of age and adolescents. Therefore, 50 μg/kg/day is used for older infants and 34 μg/ kg/day for children aged 1 through 3 years. It is recognized that this is an approximation, not only because of the extrapolation of values but also because intestinal excretion of endogenous zinc is strongly correlated with zinc absorption.

Urinary losses of zinc are approximately 7.5 μg/kg/day for both men and women (see "Adults Ages 19 Years and Older"). After early infancy, excretion rates for children on a body weight basis seem to differ very little from adult values (Krebs and Hambidge, 1986). No data are available on the *integumental losses* in children, so estimates for children are derived from data in adult men (Johnson et al., 1993), which provide an estimate of 14 μg/kg/day of zinc. Therefore, the estimated total endogenous excretion of zinc is 64 μg/kg/ day for older infants and 48 μg/kg/day for children aged 1 through 3 years.

Requirements for Growth. These requirements have been estimated from chemical analyses of infants and adults, which give an average concentration of 20 μg/g wet weight of zinc (Widdowson and Dickerson, 1964). It is assumed that each gram of new lean and adipose tissue requires this amount of zinc. The average amount of new tissue accreted for older infants and young children is 13 and 6 g/ day, respectively (Kuczmarski et al., 2000).

With the estimates above, the total amount of absorbed zinc required for infants ages 7 through 12 months is 836 μg/day (Table 12-2). The corresponding value for children ages 1 through 3 years is 744 μg/day (Table 12-3).

Fractional Absorption of Dietary Zinc. Fractional absorption probably has the greatest variation of any of the above physiological factors, depending as it does on numerous factors including quantity of ingested zinc, nutritional status, and bioavailability. Although a "critical" average fractional absorption of 0.4 has been derived from the data sets used for adult men (see "Adults Ages 19 Years and Older"), a more conservative value of 0.3 is used for preadolescent children. This value is based on studies of infants and young children reported by Fairweather-Tait and coworkers (1995) and Davidsson and coworkers (1996). To calculate the dietary zinc requirement based on

TABLE 12-2 Requirement for Absorbed Zinc for Infants Aged 7 through 12 Months

Intestinal losses	50 µg/kg/day × 9 kg	= 450 µg/day
Urinary and integumental losses	14 µg/kg/day × 9 kg	= 126 µg/day
Requirement for growth	13 g/day × 20 µg/g	= 260 µg/day
Required absorbed zinc		= 836 µg/day

TABLE 12-3 Requirement for Absorbed Zinc for Children Aged 1 through 3 Years

Intestinal losses	34 µg/kg/day × 13 kg	= 442 µg/day
Urinary and integumental losses	14 µg/kg/day × 13 kg	= 182 µg/day
Requirement for growth	6 g/day × 20 µg/g	= 120 µg/day
Required absorbed zinc		= 744 µg/day

the fractional zinc absorption, it is assumed that the older infant continues to be fed human milk between 7 and 12 months of age along with complementary foods. The fractional absorption of zinc from human milk continues to approximate 0.5 (Abrams et al., 1997). Based on an average intake of 500 µg/day from human milk and a fractional absorption of 0.5, the amount of zinc ingested from milk is approximately 250 µg/day. Therefore the estimated absorbed zinc required from complementary foods is 586 µg/day (836 – 250). Applying a fractional absorption of 0.3, zinc intake required from complementary foods is 1.95 mg/day (586 ÷ 0.3). Therefore, the EAR for infants ages 7 through 12 months is 2.5 mg/day (0.5 + 1.95). For children ages 1 through 3 years, a fractional absorption of 0.3 is used to estimate the required dietary zinc resulting in an EAR of 2.5 mg/day (744 ÷ 0.3), after rounding.

Extrapolation from Adults. An average requirement of 2.3 and 3.0 mg/day for older infants and young children, respectively, is calculated with use of the method described in Chapter 2 that extrapolates from the adult EAR based on body size.

Growth. Limited dietary zinc data are available for children in this age group. In a 6-month, placebo-controlled, randomized zinc supplementation study (Walravens et al., 1989), a major criterion for inclusion was a weight-for-age less than the tenth percentile in apparently healthy young children with no organic disease and no detectable family dynamic issues that might explain failure to thrive. Compared with placebo-treated control subjects, the zinc-supplemented children had a significantly greater increase in mean weight-for-age Z-scores. Inspection of the individual data points indicated that 87.5 percent of zinc-supplemented subjects had an increase in weight-for-age Z-scores compared with 52 percent of control subjects. These results indicate that 35.5 percent of 10 percent, or 3.6 percent of the overall population in this age group, had growth-limiting zinc deficiency. The calculated mean dietary intake at baseline for the placebo-treated children was 4.1 ± 0.8 mg/day (standard deviation [SD]) of zinc. Subtraction of two SDs from this population mean gives an EAR of 2.5 mg/day. It is likely that this calculation errs on the low side because of the variability associated with 24-hour recall dietary information and because some children with weight-for-age greater than the tenth percentile are also likely to have mild growth-limiting zinc deficiency. Hence this value corresponds reasonably well with the EAR determined from the factorial approach.

Zinc EAR and RDA Summary, Ages 7 Months through 3 Years

EAR for Infants
  7–12 months   **2.5 mg/day of zinc**

EAR for Children
  1–3 years   **2.5 mg/day of zinc**

The Recommended Dietary Allowance (RDA) for zinc is set by using a coefficient of variation (CV) of 10 percent (see Chapter 1) because information is not available on the standard deviation of the requirement. The RDA is defined as equal to the EAR plus twice the CV to cover the needs of 97 to 98 percent of the individuals in the group (therefore, the zinc RDA is 120 percent of the EAR). The calculated RDA is rounded to the nearest 1 mg.

RDA for Infants
  7–12 months   **3 mg/day of zinc**

RDA for Children
  1–3 years   **3 mg/day of zinc**

Children Ages 4 through 8 Years

Evidence Considered in Estimating the Average Requirement

Factorial Analysis. Factorial analysis is used to determine the EAR for children ages 4 through 8 years. The nonintestinal endogenous losses and requirement for growth are based on data previously discussed (see "Infants and Children Ages 7 Months through 3 Years"). For this age group, the average intestinal losses are 34 µg/kg/day of zinc and the amount of new tissue accreted is 7 g/day (Kuczmarski et al., 2000). Based on the summation of zinc losses and requirements for growth, the required amount of absorbed zinc for this age group is approximately 1.2 mg/day (Table 12-4). With a fractional absorption of 0.3 based on studies in infants and young children (Davidsson et al., 1996; Fairweather-Tait et al., 1995), the EAR is 4.0 mg/day of zinc.

Extrapolation from Adults. The average requirement for zinc is 4 mg/day as determined by the method described in Chapter 2, which extrapolates from the adult EAR.

Growth. Some dietary data are available from children aged 4 through 8 years whose growth percentiles were at the lower end of the normal range and who were subjects in placebo-controlled, randomized trials of dietary zinc supplementation. In each of two studies, one in Canada (Gibson et al., 1989) and the other in the United States (Walravens et al., 1983), zinc supplementation was associated with greater linear growth gain. Mean dietary intakes of the placebo-treated controls in the Canadian and U.S. studies were 6.4 and 4.6 mg/day of zinc, respectively. No growth response was observed with zinc supplementation of healthy children of either gender, unselected for growth, whose average calculated zinc intake was 6.3 mg/day (Hambidge et al., 1979a). The SDs were too

TABLE 12-4 Requirement for Absorbed Zinc for Children Aged 4 through 8 Years

Intestinal losses	34 µg/kg/day × 22 kg	=	748 µg/day
Urinary and integumental losses	14 µg/kg/day × 22 kg	=	308 µg/day
Requirement for growth	7 g/day × 20 µg/g	=	140 µg/day
Required absorbed zinc		=	1,196 µg/day

large (likely attributable to methodological limitations) to use these data with any confidence in setting an EAR. However, these data are consistent with the EAR derived from a factorial approach.

Zinc EAR and RDA Summary, Ages 4 through 8 Years

EAR for Children

    4–8 years   **4 mg/day of zinc**

The RDA for zinc is set by using a CV of 10 percent (see Chapter 1) because information is not available on the standard deviation of the requirement. The RDA is defined as equal to the EAR plus twice the CV to cover the needs of 97 to 98 percent of the individuals in the group (therefore, the zinc RDA is 120 percent of the EAR). The calculated RDA was rounded to the nearest 1 mg.

RDA for Children

    4–8 years   **5 mg/day of zinc**

Children Ages 9 through 13 Years

Evidence Considered in Estimating the Average Requirement

Factorial Analysis. Estimates used for factorial analysis are similar for boys and girls, and therefore calculations are used to estimate a single average requirement for both genders. With use of the same values as for younger children, an average accretion of 10 g/day of new tissue (Kuczmarski et al., 2000), and a reference weight of 40 kg, the required amount of absorbed zinc is 2.1 mg/day (Table 12-5). Based on a fractional absorption of 0.3 observed in infants and young children (Davidsson et al., 1996; Fairweather-Tait et al., 1995), the EAR is 7 mg/day.

TABLE 12-5 Requirement for Absorbed Zinc for Children Aged 9 through 13 Years

Intestinal losses	34 µg/kg/day × 40 kg	= 1,360 µg/day
Urinary and integumental losses	14 µg/kg/day × 40 kg	= 560 µg/day
Requirement for growth	10 g/day × 20 µg/g	= 200 µg/day
Required absorbed zinc		= 2,120 µg/day

Extrapolation from Adults. As determined by the extrapolation method described in Chapter 2, the average requirement for boys and girls is 6.7 and 5.6 mg/day of zinc, respectively.

Zinc EAR and RDA Summary, Ages 9 through 13 Years

EAR for Boys
9–13 years   7 mg/day of zinc

EAR for Girls
9–13 years   7 mg/day of zinc

The RDA for zinc is set by using a CV of 10 percent (see Chapter 1) because information is not available on the standard deviation of the requirement. The RDA is defined as equal to the EAR plus twice the CV to cover the needs of 97 to 98 percent of the individuals in the group (therefore, the zinc RDA is 120 percent of the EAR). The calculated RDA is rounded to the nearest 1 mg.

RDA for Boys
9–13 years   8 mg/day of zinc

RDA for Girls
9–13 years   8 mg/day of zinc

Adolescents Ages 14 through 18 Years

Evidence Considered in Estimating the Average Requirement

Factorial Analysis. Endogenous losses are calculated as for younger age groups by using the reference weights (see Chapter 2) with the addition of 100 µg/day of zinc to allow for calculated average semen or menstrual losses (see "Adults Ages 19 Years and Older", which follows). For this age group, a fractional absorption of 0.4 is used; it corresponds to the average "critical" value for adult men from the data sets used in estimating adult requirements (see below). Gender differences are sufficient at this age for boys and girls requirements to be calculated separately. As determined by the summation of average zinc losses and the zinc requirement for growth (Kuczmarski et al., 2000; Widdowson and Dickerson, 1964), the amount of absorbed zinc that is required for boys and girls is approximately 3.4 and 3.0 mg/day, respectively (Table 12-6). On the basis of a fractional zinc absorption of 0.4 that was derived for men

TABLE 12-6 Requirement for Absorbed Zinc for Adolescent Boys and Girls Aged 14 through 18 Years

	Boys	Girls
Intestinal losses	34 µg/kg × 64 kg = 2,176 µg/day	34 µg/kg × 57 kg = 1,938 µg/day
Urinary and integumental losses	14 µg/kg × 64 kg = 896 µg/day	14 µg/kg × 57 kg = 798 µg/day
Semen or menstrual losses	100 µg/day	100 µg/day
Requirement for growth	10 g/day × 20µg/g = 200 µg	5 g/day × 20 µg/g = 100 µg/day
Required absorbed zinc	3,372 µg/day	2,936 µg/day

(see below), the EARs for adolescent boys and girls are calculated to be 8.5 and 7.3 mg/day of zinc, respectively.

Extrapolation from Adults. Based on the extrapolation method described in Chapter 2, the average requirement for adolescent boys and girls is 9.5 and 6.4 mg/day, respectively.

Zinc EAR and RDA Summary, Ages 14 through 18 Years

EAR for Boys
   14–18 years   **8.5 mg/day of zinc**

EAR for Girls
   14–18 years   **7.3 mg/day of zinc**

The RDA for zinc is set by using a CV of 10 percent (see Chapter 1) because information is not available on the standard deviation of the requirement. The RDA is defined as equal to the EAR plus twice the CV to cover the needs of 97 to 98 percent of the individuals in the group (therefore, the zinc RDA is 120 percent of the EAR). The calculated RDA is rounded up to the nearest 1 mg.

RDA for Boys
   14–18 years   **11 mg/day of zinc**

RDA for Girls
   14–18 years   **9 mg/day of zinc**

Adults Ages 19 Years and Older

Evidence Considered in Estimating the Average Requirement

As discussed earlier, there are no adequately documented functional or simple laboratory indexes of zinc nutriture that can provide a principal indicator of zinc requirements in adults. However, sufficient data are now available to apply a factorial approach to determine the EAR for adults. With this approach, the principal indicator selected is the minimal quantity of absorbed zinc that is adequate to replace endogenous zinc losses. The EAR is the average zinc intake that provides this quantity of absorbed zinc. An outline of these calculations follows.

Step 1: Calculation of Endogenous Losses of Zinc via Routes Other than the Intestine. Urinary zinc excretion declines only with extreme dietary zinc restriction and is not correlated with zinc ingested by young adult men over a range of 4 to 25 mg zinc/day (Baer and King, 1984; Behall et al., 1987; Coudray et al., 1997; Hallfrisch et al., 1987; Holbrook et al., 1989; Hunt JR et al., 1992; Jackson et al., 1984; Johnson et al., 1982, 1993; Lee et al., 1993; Mahalko et al., 1983; Milne et al., 1983; Snedeker et al., 1982; Spencer et al., 1979; Turnlund et al., 1984, 1986; Wada et al., 1985). In men, therefore, zinc excretion via the kidney should be regarded as a constant in calculating zinc requirements, the average excretion being 0.63 mg/ day. Though fewer data are available, the same constancy appears to be true for combined integumental and sweat losses (Johnson et al., 1993) and losses in semen (Hunt CD et al., 1992; Johnson et al., 1993) for which the zinc losses average 0.54 and 0.1 mg/day, respectively. Therefore, losses of endogenous zinc via routes other than the intestine can be regarded as a constant over the range of dietary zinc intake that encompasses zinc requirements. This average constant for men has been calculated to be 1.27 mg/day (0.63 + 0.54 + 0.1) of zinc. An equal quantity of zinc must be absorbed to match this loss.

In 10 studies, the mean urinary loss of zinc from women was 0.44 mg/day (Colin et al., 1983; Greger et al., 1978; Hallfrisch et al., 1987; Hunt JR et al., 1992, 1998; Miller et al., 1998; Swanson and King, 1982; Taper et al., 1980; Turnlund et al., 1991; Wisker et al., 1991). Reported integumental losses for men are multiplied by 0.86 to adjust for the different average surface area of women, and accordingly the average total zinc endogenous losses are 0.46 mg/ day for women. Menstrual zinc losses are assumed to average 0.1

mg/day (Hess et al., 1977). Therefore, the calculated total loss of endogenous zinc for women via routes other than the intestine is 1.0 mg/day (0.44 + 0.46 + 0.10).

Step 2: Relationship Between Excretion of Endogenous Zinc via the Intestine and Quantity of Zinc Absorbed. In contrast to other endogenous zinc losses, the quantity of endogenous zinc excreted via the intestine is positively correlated with the quantity of zinc absorbed over a wide range. This correlation is shown in Figure 12-1. This figure is based on 10 sets of balance data from seven studies (Hunt JR et al., 1992; Jackson et al., 1984; Lee et al., 1993; Taylor et al., 1991; Turnlund et al., 1984, 1986; Wada et al., 1985) of healthy young men, which also included isotopic tracer measurements of fractional zinc absorption. This correlation, in turn, allows for the quantification of daily zinc absorption and intestinal excretion of endogenous zinc. Importantly, this linear relationship, which indicates that for each milligram of zinc absorbed the intestine excretes approximately 0.6 mg/day of endogenous zinc, has been demonstrated only for zinc absorption ranging from 0.8 to 5.5 mg/day. It is also noted that most of these data were relatively short-term, and these variables were not examined while the participants were consuming habitual diets. However, the studies did extend as long as 6 months, a duration that suggests the observed relationship between absorption and endogenous losses via the intestine is a long-term phenomenon. Therefore, in contrast to other endogenous losses of zinc, losses from the intestine cannot be treated as a constant.

To achieve balance, absorption must match the sum of nonintestinal and intestinal endogenous zinc losses. The minimum amount of zinc that must be absorbed before absorption matches the losses is determined in step 3 below.

Corresponding data for women are both limited and divergent (Hunt JR et al., 1992, 1998; Sian et al., 1996; Turnlund et al., 1991). It has therefore been assumed that there are no significant gender differences for this relationship between absorbed zinc and intestinal excretion of endogenous zinc.

Step 3: Determination of Minimal Zinc Absorption Required to Replace Total Endogenous Zinc Excretion. The sum of nonintestinal endogenous zinc losses (1.27 mg/day for men and 1.0 mg/day for women) is added to the linear regression line for excretion of endogenous zinc in the feces versus absorbed zinc (Figure 12-1). These "adjusted" lines depict the quantitative relationship between absorbed zinc and total endogenous zinc losses for men and women.

The intercept between the dashed line (line of equality for absorbed zinc) and the gender-specific lines is then used to determine the minimal quantity of absorbed zinc required to replace endogenous zinc losses.

With this approach, the calculated average total minimal quantity of absorbed zinc required for the men in these studies is 3.84 mg/day (1.27 mg to match endogenous zinc losses from nonintestinal sources and, therefore, 2.57 mg/day to match intestinal endogenous zinc losses). The corresponding value for women is 3.3 mg/day (1.0 mg/day to match endogenous zinc losses from nonintestinal sources and, therefore, 2.3 mg/day to match intestinal endogenous zinc losses).

These calculated average minimal values for absorbed zinc are then used as the principal indicator for establishing an EAR in step 4.

Step 4: Determination of the Average Zinc Intake Required to Achieve Absorption of the Quantity of Zinc Necessary to Match Total Endogenous Losses. The EAR is determined from the asymptotic regression of absorbed zinc on zinc intake (Figure 12-2) that was derived from the same data sets used for Figure 12-1. Thus, if 3.84 mg/day of absorbed zinc is required for men, the amount of ingested zinc, and therefore the EAR, is 9.4 mg/day. When this approach is used for women, the EAR is 6.8 mg/day. This value corresponds to average fractional absorptions of 0.41 and 0.48 for men and women, respectively. A similar fractional absorption of 0.4 was observed for adult men fed experimental diets from which zinc bioavailability is likely to be favorable (August et al., 1989).

Other Criteria for Men. Zinc deficiency has not been documented in healthy adult men in North America with the assessment methods currently in use. Some supportive data have been derived from one of the studies included in the factorial approach outlined above (Wada et al., 1985). This study included six men who received a diet containing 5.5 mg/day of zinc for an 8-week period. At the end of this period, several zinc-responsive biochemical changes had occurred, including declines in serum retinol binding protein, albumin, prealbumin, and thyroxin concentrations (Wada and King, 1986).

Other data from experimental zinc depletion studies are also consistent but at lower levels of intake (zinc intakes of 3 to 5 mg/day). These data include decreased erythrocyte metallothionein (Grider et al., 1990; Thomas et al., 1992) and zinc concentrations, decreased

5′-nucleotidase activity (Beck et al., 1997a), and various abnormalities of laboratory indexes of immune status (Beck et al., 1997b).

Other Criteria for Women. Twenty-six percent of a group of apparently healthy Canadian omnivore women had prebreakfast serum zinc concentrations below the cut-off of 70 µg/dL (Gibson et al., 2000). The zinc intake of these subjects averaged 7.3 mg/day, which by this criterion is slightly above the EAR. These data are consistent with an EAR of 6.8 mg/day.

Elderly. Reported values on the fractional absorption of zinc in the elderly have been quite variable (Couzy et al., 1993; Hunt et al., 1995; Turnlund et al., 1982, 1986), and no consistent evidence indicates that aging affects absorption adversely. Results of balance studies are again, predictably, variable (Bunker et al., 1982; Hallfrisch et al., 1987; Wood and Zheng, 1997). No evidence suggests that the zinc requirements of the elderly are higher than those of younger adults, but possible differences in zinc metabolism (Wastney et al., 1986) merit further investigation.

Other Criteria for the Elderly. Zinc supplementation of 53 elderly men and women whose diet contained an average of 9.2 mg/day of zinc was not associated with any detectable benefits (Swanson et al., 1988). Specifically, there were no changes in circulating protein or immunoglobulin concentrations. In contrast, dietary zinc was positively correlated with serum albumin in a group of 82 elderly Canadians whose zinc intakes averaged 5 mg/day for women and 6.5 mg/day for men (Payette and Gray-Donald, 1991). Several studies in which improvements in laboratory indexes of zinc status with zinc supplementation were reported did not, unfortunately, include information on habitual zinc intake (Boukaiba et al., 1993; Cakman et al., 1997; Duchateau et al., 1981; Fortes et al., 1998). Fifteen older men and women whose habitual dietary zinc averaged 8.8 mg/day had a significant decline in the activity of 5′-nucleotidase activity after a 2-week period during which zinc intake was restricted to 4 mg/day (Bales et al., 1994). Subsequently, a 6-day supplementation period in which total zinc intake averaged 28 mg/day was associated with a significant increase in 5′-nucleotidase activity, but not beyond baseline levels. In 119 elderly women, serum IGF-1 concentration was weakly correlated with dietary zinc over a range of 5 to 17 mg/day (Devine et al., 1998). A nonplacebo controlled study of zinc supplementation in 13 elderly subjects, part of a larger group of 180 subjects whose average calculated zinc intake was 9 mg/day, was reported to result in normalization of zinc in granulocytes and lymphocytes and improvement in various immune parameters (Prasad et al., 1993). Ethanol tolerance tests indicated a change in ethanol metabolism when dietary zinc intake of postmenopausal women was restricted to 2.6 mg/day (Milne et al., 1987).

Zinc EAR and RDA Summary, Ages 19 Years and Older

EAR for Men
19–30 years	9.4 mg/day of zinc
31–50 years	9.4 mg/day of zinc
51–70 years	9.4 mg/day of zinc
> 70 years	9.4 mg/day of zinc

EAR for Women
19–30 years	6.8 mg/day of zinc
31–50 years	6.8 mg/day of zinc
51–70 years	6.8 mg/day of zinc
> 70 years	6.8 mg/day of zinc

The RDA for zinc is set by using a CV of 10 percent (see Chapter 1) because information is not available on the standard deviation of the requirement. The RDA is defined as equal to the EAR plus twice the CV to cover the needs of 97 to 98 percent of the individuals in the group (therefore, for zinc the RDA is 120 percent of the EAR). The calculated RDA was rounded to the nearest 1 mg.

RDA for Men
19–30 years	11 mg/day of zinc
31–50 years	11 mg/day of zinc
51–70 years	11 mg/day of zinc
> 70 years	11 mg/day of zinc

RDA for Women
19–30 years	8 mg/day of zinc
31–50 years	8 mg/day of zinc
51–70 years	8 mg/day of zinc
> 70 years	8 mg/day of zinc

Pregnancy

Evidence Considered in Estimating the Average Requirement

Factorial Approach. The average daily rates of zinc accumulation by maternal and embryonic/fetal tissues during the four quarters of pregnancy are 0.08, 0.24, 0.53, and 0.73 mg (Swanson and King, 1987). On the assumption of no compensatory change in intestinal excretion of endogenous zinc, it is concluded that increasing daily zinc absorption by these amounts is desirable.

The average fractional absorption of zinc was 27 percent for non-pregnant women from eight studies in which dietary zinc averaged 10 mg/day (Fung et al., 1997; Hunt JR et al., 1992, 1998; Miller et al., 1998; Sian et al., 1996; Turnlund et al., 1991). Increases in fractional absorption during pregnancy have been reported to be non-significant (Fung et al., 1997), but this outcome may reflect inadequate power of the study design. Therefore, increases in dietary zinc requirements during pregnancy are calculated to be the following:

First quarter	$0.08 \div 0.27 = 0.3$ mg/day of zinc
Second quarter	$0.24 \div 0.27 = 0.9$ mg/day of zinc
Third quarter	$0.53 \div 0.27 = 2.0$ mg/day of zinc
Fourth quarter	$0.73 \div 0.27 = 2.7$ mg/day of zinc

To set a single EAR for pregnant women, the EAR is based on the additional requirement during the fourth quarter (2.7 mg/day) of pregnancy plus the EAR for nonpregnant adolescent girls and women. It should be noted, however, that the zinc requirement during the first quarter of pregnancy is only minimally greater than the preconceptional requirement.

Other Criteria. Dietary supplementation reduced the decline in plasma/serum zinc concentration across pregnancy in a large cohort of Peruvian women whose dietary zinc intake was estimated to be 7 mg/day (Caulfield et al., 1999a), but not in North American women whose dietary zinc intake averaged 11 mg/day (Hambidge et al., 1983). Correlations observed between maternal biochemical indexes of zinc status and complications of pregnancy, delivery, and fetal development have been inconsistent.

Gravid women with a zinc intake of 6 mg/day or less were found to have a high incidence of premature deliveries (Scholl et al., 1993). Increased gestational age at delivery and increased birth size have been reported to result from zinc supplementation of pregnant African-American women whose baseline dietary zinc intake was calculated to be 13 mg/day (Goldenberg et al., 1995). This calculated dietary zinc intake is notably high in comparison with other data for African-American women (Mares-Perlman et al., 1995). Without additional supporting documentation, it is difficult to reconcile the implications of the results of this study (with respect to dietary zinc requirements during pregnancy) with the EARs derived from a factorial approach. Nor is it easy to reconcile these findings with the results of other intervention studies. For example, no effect of zinc supplements on birth size was observed in a recent large-scale study of Peruvian women whose dietary zinc intake was estimated to be 7 mg/day (Caulfield et al., 1999b). There was, however, evidence of improved fetal neurobehavioral development (Merialdi et al., 1998).

A report that zinc intakes of less than 7.5 mg/day during the third trimester are associated with lower zinc concentrations in human milk is consistent with the EAR (Ortega et al., 1997).

Zinc EAR and RDA Summary, Pregnancy

EAR for Pregnancy
14–18 years	10.0 mg/day of zinc
19–30 years	9.5 mg/day of zinc
31–50 years	9.5 mg/day of zinc

The RDA for zinc is set by using a CV of 10 percent (see Chapter 1) because information is not available on the standard deviation of the requirement. The RDA is defined as equal to the EAR plus twice the CV to cover the needs of 97 to 98 percent of the individuals in the group (therefore, for zinc the RDA is 120 percent of the EAR). The calculated RDA is rounded to the nearest 1 mg.

RDA for Pregnancy
14–18 years	12 mg/day of zinc
19–30 years	11 mg/day of zinc
31–50 years	11 mg/day of zinc

Lactation

Evidence Considered in Estimating the Average Requirement

Losses in Human Milk. Average concentrations of zinc in human milk decline physiologically from approximately 4 mg/L at 2 weeks postpartum to 3 mg/L at 4 weeks, 2 mg/L at 8 weeks, 1.5 mg/L at 12 weeks, and 1.2 mg/L at 24 weeks (Krebs et al., 1995; Moser-Veillon and Reynolds, 1990). With use of a standard volume of 0.78 L/day of human milk secreted per day (Chapter 2), calculated zinc losses via the mammary gland are 2.15 mg/day at 4 weeks, 1.56 mg/day at 8 weeks, 1.17 mg/day at 12 weeks, and 0.94 mg/day at 24 weeks.

Postpartum involution of the uterus and decreased maternal blood volume should release approximately 30 mg of zinc that has been accumulated during pregnancy (King and Turnlund, 1989); that is, an average of approximately 1 mg/day for the first month. It is reasonable to assume that this endogenous zinc is available for reutilization. Thus, 1 mg/day is subtracted from the amount of zinc lost during the first 4 weeks of lactation. The loss of zinc for weeks 8, 12 and 24 are averaged:

Week 4: $(2.15 - 1.0) = 1.15$ mg/day of zinc
Week 8: $(2.15 + 1.56) \div 2 = 1.85$ mg/day of zinc
Week 12: $(1.56 + 1.17) \div 2 = 1.36$ mg/day of zinc
Weeks 12–24: $(1.17 + 0.94) \div 2 = 1.05$ mg/day of zinc

The average calculated increased requirement for absorbed zinc during lactation is 1.35 mg/day.

Reported values for fractional absorption of zinc for adult women outside the reproductive cycle averages 27 percent (Fung et al., 1997; Hunt JR et al., 1992, 1998; Sian et al., 1996; Turnlund et al., 1991). If this value were applied to the calculation of increased dietary zinc required during lactation ($1.35 \div 0.27$), the average dietary requirement would increase by 5 mg/day. However, the fractional absorption of zinc increases during lactation by 0.107 (Fung et al., 1997). Therefore, the fractional absorption would be increased to 0.716 ($0.27 \div 0.377$) to give an additional requirement of 3.6 mg/day (5×0.716). This value is added to the EAR for adolescent girls and women to set the EAR during lactation.

Other Criteria. Typically, human milk zinc concentrations are not increased by the administration of a daily zinc supplement across lactation (Kirksey et al., 1979; Krebs et al., 1995; Moser-Veillon and Reynolds, 1990). In one study, however, a modest but statistically significant reduced rate of decline in zinc concentrations in milk across lactation was observed with a zinc supplement (Krebs et al., 1985). The dietary zinc in the placebo group averaged 10.7 mg/day. In a subsequent study, in which the average dietary zinc was higher at 13.0 mg/day, there was no evidence of an effect of zinc supplementation on zinc concentration in milk.

Zinc EAR and RDA Summary, Lactation

EAR for Lactation
14–18 years	10.9 mg/day of zinc
19–30 years	10.4 mg/day of zinc
31–50 years	10.4 mg/day of zinc

The RDA for zinc is set by using a CV of 10 percent (see Chapter 1) because information is not available on the standard deviation of the requirement. The RDA is defined as equal to the EAR plus twice the CV to cover the needs of 97 to 98 percent of the individuals in the group (therefore, for zinc the RDA is 120 percent of the EAR). The calculated RDA is rounded to the nearest 1 mg.

RDA for Lactation
14–18 years	13 mg/day of zinc
19–30 years	12 mg/day of zinc
31–50 years	12 mg/day of zinc

Special Considerations

Vegetarianism

Cereals are the primary source of dietary zinc for vegetarians (Gibson, 1994). The bioavailability of zinc in vegetarian diets is reduced if the phytate content in the diet is high (Gibson, 1994), and this may result in low zinc status (Freeland-Graves et al., 1980b). Absorption of zinc from vegetarian diets is lower than from nonvegetarian diets (Hunt et al., 1998; Kies, 1988); however, relatively minor changes to the diet can improve zinc absorption (Gibson et al., 1997; Harland et al., 1988). Vegetarian diets rich in calcium may negatively affect zinc bioavailability (Ellis et al., 1987).

Zinc intake from vegetarian diets has been found to be both similar to intake from nonvegetarian diets (Alexander et al., 1994; Berglund et al., 1994; Donovan and Gibson, 1996; Johansson and Widerstrom, 1994; Kelsay et al., 1988; Levin et al., 1986; Srikumar et al., 1992) and lower than intake from nonvegetarian diets (Faber et al., 1986; Freeland-Graves et al., 1980a; Harland and Peterson, 1978; Hunt et al., 1998; Janelle and Barr, 1995). In most older adult and elderly populations, vegetarians have lower zinc intakes than nonvegetarians (Brants et al., 1990; Hunt et al., 1988; Lowik et al., 1990). Among vegetarians, zinc concentrations in serum, plasma, hair, urine, and saliva are either the same as or lower than those of nonvegetarians (Anderson et al., 1981; Freeland-Graves et al., 1980a, 1980b; Hunt et al., 1998; Kadrabova et al., 1995; King et al., 1981; Krajcovicova-Kudlackova et al., 1995; Levin et al., 1986; Srikumar et al., 1992). The variations in these status indicators are most likely due to the amount of phytate, fiber, calcium, or other inhibitors of zinc absorption in the vegetarian diets. Individuals consuming vegetarian diets were found to be in positive zinc balance (Ganapathy et al., 1981; Hunt et al., 1998).

The requirement for dietary zinc may be as much as 50 percent greater for vegetarians and particularly for strict vegetarians whose major food staples are grains and legumes and whose dietary phytate:zinc molar ratio exceeds 15:1. At this time there are not sufficient data to set algorithms for establishing dietary requirements for zinc on the basis of the presence and concentration of other nutrients and food components.

Alcohol

Long-term alcohol consumption is associated with impaired zinc absorption and increased urinary zinc excretion. Low zinc status is observed in approximately 30 to 50 percent of alcoholics. Thus, with long-term alcohol consumption, the daily requirement for zinc will be greater than that estimated via the factorial approach.

INTAKE OF ZINC

Food Sources

The dietary sources of zinc vary widely. Zinc is abundant in red meats, certain seafood, and whole grains. Because zinc is mainly located in the germ and bran portions of grains, as much as 80 percent of the total zinc is lost during milling. Many breakfast cereals are fortified with zinc. Studies measuring zinc content in human milk are summarized in Table 12-1.

Dietary Intake

Data from nationally representative U.S. surveys are available to estimate zinc intakes (Appendix Tables C-25, C-26, D-4, E-9). Median intakes of zinc for adult men aged 19 to 50 years, based on the

Third National Health and Nutrition Examination Survey and the Continuing Survey of Food Intakes by Individuals, were approximately 14 mg/day (Appendix Tables C-25 and D-4). The median intakes for women in the same age range were approximately 9 mg/day. These values are similar to those found for zinc intakes of Canadian adults (Appendix Table F-3).

Intake from Supplements

In 1986, approximately 16 percent of Americans took supplements that contained zinc (Moss et al., 1989; see Table 2-2). The median total (food plus supplements) zinc intakes by adults taking supplements were similar to those of adults who did not take zinc supplements (Appendix Table C-26). Intake of zinc supplements, however, greatly increased the intakes in the upper quartile compared to those who did not take zinc supplements.

TOLERABLE UPPER INTAKE LEVELS

The Tolerable Upper Intake Level (UL) is the highest level of daily nutrient intake that is likely to pose no risk of adverse health effects for almost all individuals. Although members of the general population should be advised not to routinely exceed the UL, intake above the UL may be appropriate for investigation within well-controlled clinical trials. Clinical trials of doses above the UL should not be discouraged, as long as subjects participating in these trials have signed informed consent documents regarding possible toxicity and as long as these trials employ appropriate safety monitoring of trial subjects. In addition, the UL is not meant to apply to individuals who are receiving zinc under medical supervision.

Hazard Identification

Although no evidence of adverse effects from intake of naturally occurring zinc in food was found, the UL derived here applies to total zinc intake from food, water, and supplements (including fortified food). Adverse effects associated with chronic intake of supplemental zinc include suppression of immune response, decrease in high-density lipoprotein (HDL) cholesterol, and reduced copper status.

Adverse Effects

Acute Effects. Acute adverse effects of excess zinc have been reported. These include epigastric pain, nausea, vomiting, loss of appetite, abdominal cramps, diarrhea, and headaches (Prasad, 1976; Samman and Roberts, 1987). Fosmire (1990) estimated that an emetic dose of zinc sulfate was approximately 1 to 2 g of the salt (225 to 450 mg of zinc). Gastrointestinal distress has been reported at doses of 50 to 150 mg/day of supplemental zinc (Freeland-Graves et al., 1982).

Immunological Response. Intake of 300 mg/day of supplemental zinc as the sulfate for 6 weeks has been shown to cause some functional impairment in immunological response as well as significantly decreased concentrations of HDL cholesterol (Chandra, 1984).

Lipoprotein and Cholesterol. Two studies (Black et al., 1988; Hooper et al., 1980) have found that zinc at doses between 50 and 160 mg/day decreased serum lipoprotein and cholesterol concentrations in men. Samman and Roberts (1988), however, reported no depression of HDL concentrations in men at 150 mg/day of zinc and found some indication of a depression of low-density lipoproteins (LDL) in women. The different response to excess zinc in women was supported by an earlier study by Freeland-Graves and coworkers (1982). The reduction in HDL cholesterol concentration was shown to be transient and not dose related.

Reduced Copper Status. Reduced copper status has been associated with increased zinc intake (Boukaiba et al., 1993; Burke et al., 1981; Festa et al., 1985; Fischer et al., 1984; Prasad et al., 1978; Samman and Roberts, 1988; Yadrick et al., 1989) (Table 12-7). In all studies in which the interaction of excess zinc and copper was measured, there was a consistent decrease in erythrocyte copper-zinc superoxide dismutase (ESOD) activity, an erythrocyte enzyme indicative of copper status. Yadrick and coworkers (1989) reported this effect after total zinc intakes of about 60 mg/day (50-mg supplement plus 10 mg of dietary zinc) for up to 10 weeks. Although the clinical significance of the depressed ESOD activity is unknown, this marker enzyme is known to be a sensitive indicator of the effect of high zinc levels on copper homeostasis.

Zinc-Iron Interactions. Zinc and iron are known to interact, and Whittaker (1998) has reviewed the available studies (also see "Factors Affecting the Zinc Requirement"). The primary effect appears to be a decreased absorption of zinc at an iron:zinc ratio of 3:1 when the iron was administered in water. However, when iron was administered during a meal, no such effect was found. Similarly, when iron was present as heme iron, no effect was noted. One study found a 56 percent decline in iron absorption when the zinc:iron ratio was 5:1 and was administered in water (Rossander-Hulten et al., 1991). However, when this ratio of zinc and iron was administered in a hamburger meal, no effect on iron absorption was noted.

Other Endpoints. No evidence was found of reproductive effects in humans from zinc intake. There is one case report of three premature deliveries and one stillborn infant after excess zinc intake during pregnancy (Kumar, 1976). Because details on other contributing factors were not provided, interpretation of these results is limited. There is insufficient evidence of carcinogenicity from human or animal studies.

Summary

Although there are no data indicating adverse interactions between zinc and other nutrients when zinc is found in food, adverse nutrient interactions are present after feeding zinc in the form of dietary supplements. The adverse effect of excess zinc on copper metabolism (i.e., reduced copper status) was chosen as the critical effect on which to base a UL for total daily intake of zinc from food, water, and supplements in humans. This selection is based on (1) the consistency of findings from studies measuring the interaction of zinc and copper (Fischer et al., 1984; Samman and Roberts, 1988; Yadrick et al., 1989), (2) the sensitivity of ESOD activity as a marker for this effect, and (3) the quality and completeness of the database for this endpoint. The data on the effects of zinc on HDL cholesterol concentration were not consistent from study to study and therefore were not used to derive a UL.

Dose-Response Assessment

Adults

Data Selection. Data on reduced copper status in humans were used to derive a UL for zinc (Table 12-7). Studies measuring ESOD activity (which is a sensitive indicator of copper status) or other indicators

TABLE 12-7 Effect of Increasing Doses of Zinc (Zn) Intake on Copper (Cu) Status

Study	Subjects	Zinc Intake (mg/d)
Prasad et al., 1978	1 black man, 26 y w/sickle cell anemia	150–200
Greger et al., 1978	14 girls, 12–14 y	7.4 (food) 13.4 (food)
Burke et al., 1981	5 men, 6 women, 56–83 y	7.8 (fortified food) 23.26 (fortified food)
Fischer et al., 1984	26 healthy adult men	Placebo 50 (as gluconate)
Festa et al., 1985	9 healthy men, 21–27 y	1.8 (food) 4.0 (food) 6.0 (food) 8.0 (food) 18.5 (food)
Samman and Roberts, 1988	Healthy men and women	150 (as sulfate)
Yadrick et al., 1989	18 healthy women, 25–40 y	50 (as gluconate)
Boukaiba et al., 1993[c]	44 older adults, 73–106 y	Placebo 20

[a] The authors note it was not possible to separate the effects of sickle cell disease and copper depletion.

[b] Copper status was assessed by the activities of the copper-metalloenzymes, plasma ferroxidase (ceruloplasmin), and erythrocyte Cu,Zn-superoxide dismutase. No significant differences in the plasma copper levels or the ferroxidase activities between the supplemented and control groups could be detected at 2, 4, or 6 weeks. ESOD = erythrocyte copper-zinc superoxide dismutase.

of copper status (such as ceruloplasmin or serum copper concentration) were considered optimal for the dose-response assessment.

Identification of a No-Observed-Adverse-Effect Level (NOAEL) and Lowest-Observed-Adverse-Effect Level (LOAEL). A LOAEL of 60 mg/day is based on the study of Yadrick and coworkers (1989) who evaluated copper status after supplemental intake of 50 mg/day as zinc glu-

Duration	Cu Intake (mg/d)	Adverse Effects
2 y	Not provided	Cu deficiency anemia[a] Decreased serum Cu and ceruloplasmin
30 d	2.8 (food)	No significant change
30 d	2.8 (food)	No significant change
30 d	2.33 (fortified food)	Significant decrease in Cu retention
30 d	2.33 (fortified food)	
6 wk	Not provided	No effect
6 wk		Significant decrease in ESOD activity[b]
1 wk	2.6 (food)	No effect
1 wk	2.6 (food)	No effect
1 wk	2.6 (food)	No effect
1 wk	2.6 (food)	No effect
2 wk	2.6 (food)	Increase in Cu excretion/ decrease in retention
12 wk	Not provided	Decrease in ESOD (women only)
10 wk	Not provided	Significant decrease in ESOD activity
8 wk	Not provided	No effect
8 wk		Significant decrease in serum Cu

[c] Boukaiba et al. (1993) is a crossover study designed to determine the effects of low-dose zinc supplementation on food intake, nutritional status, immune and lipid indexes. The 16-week study period was divided into two experimental treatment periods, each lasting 8 weeks. Serum Zn concentrations were depressed.

conate in 18 healthy women (aged 25 to 40 years) for 10 weeks. ESOD activity was significantly lower than pretreatment values. Although no dietary zinc or copper intakes were reported, a level of dietary zinc can be estimated at approximately 10 mg/day for women (aged 19 to 50 years) from the 1988–1994 Third National Health and Nutrition Examination Survey (Appendix Table C-26). A LOAEL of 60 mg/day was calculated by adding the supplemental intake of 50 mg/day with the rounded estimate of dietary intake, 10 mg/day. Support for a LOAEL of 60 mg/day is provided by other studies showing altered copper balance after zinc supplementation (Fischer et al., 1984) (Table 12-7).

Uncertainty Assessment. An uncertainty factor (UF) of 1.5 was selected to account for interindividual variability in sensitivity and for extrapolation from a LOAEL to a NOAEL. Because reduced copper status is rare in humans, a higher UF was not justified.

Derivation of a UL. A LOAEL of 60 mg/day was divided by a UF of 1.5 to derive a UL of 40 mg/day for total intake of zinc from food, water, and supplements.

$$UL = \frac{LOAEL}{UF} = \frac{60 \text{ mg/day}}{1.5} = 40 \text{ mg/day}$$

Zinc UL Summary, Ages 19 Years and Older

UL for Adults
  ≥ 19 years   **40 mg/day of zinc**

Infants, Children, and Adolescents

Data Selection. There is only one case report of zinc-induced copper deficiency anemia in a young child (Botash et al., 1992): a 13-month-old girl was given 16 mg/day of zinc for 6 months followed by 24 mg/day for 1 month. There are no reports on the adverse effects of zinc on copper status in children or adolescents. The UL values for infants are based on a study by Walravens and Hambidge (1976).

Identification of a NOAEL. Walravens and Hambidge (1976) fed 68 healthy, full-term infants either formula containing 1.8 mg/L of zinc (control) or the same formula supplemented with an additional 4 mg/L (total of 5.8 mg/L) of zinc for 6 months. No effects of zinc on serum copper or cholesterol concentrations or other adverse effects were found. Thus, 5.8 mg/L is the NOAEL selected. Multiplying the NOAEL for infants 0 through 6 months of age by the estimated average intake of human milk of 0.78 L/day (Allen et al., 1991; Butte et al., 1984; Heinig et al., 1993) results in a NOAEL of 4.5 mg/day.

Uncertainty Assessment. The length of the study by Walravens and

Hambidge (1976) and the high number of infants justifies a UF of 1.0, given that there is no evidence that intakes from formula of 5.8 mg/L of zinc result in infant toxicity.

Derivation of a UL. The NOAEL of 4.5 mg/day was divided by a UF of 1.0 to obtain a UL of 4 mg/day (rounded down) for infants ages 0 through 6 months. No adverse effects of zinc in children and adolescents could be found. Due to a dearth of information, the UL for young infants was adjusted for older infants, children, and adolescents on the basis of relative body weight as described in Chapter 2 and using reference weights from Chapter 1 (Table 1-1). Values have been rounded down.

Zinc UL Summary, Ages 0 through 18 Years

UL for Infants
0–6 months	**4 mg/day of zinc**
7–12 months	**5 mg/day of zinc**

UL for Children
1–3 years	**7 mg/day of zinc**
4–8 years	**12 mg/day of zinc**
9–13 years	**23 mg/day of zinc**

UL for Adolescents
14–18 years	**34 mg/day of zinc**

Pregnancy and Lactation

Because the UL is based on reduced copper status and because there are inadequate data to justify a different UL for pregnant and lactating women, the UL for pregnant and lactating women is the same as that for nonpregnant and nonlactating women.

Zinc UL Summary, Pregnancy and Lactation

UL for Pregnancy
14–18 years	**34 mg/day of zinc**
19–50 years	**40 mg/day of zinc**

UL for Lactation
14–18 years	**34 mg/day of zinc**
19–50 years	**40 mg/day of zinc**

Special Considerations

Individuals with Menke's disease may be distinctly susceptible to the adverse effects of excess zinc intake. Since Menke's disease is a defect in the ATPase involved in copper efflux from enterocytes, supplying extra zinc will likely further limit copper absorption (Yuzbasiyan-Gurkan et al., 1992). Brewer and coworkers (1993) demonstrated the effectiveness of zinc therapy in reducing copper accumulation in individuals with Wilson's disease. The UL is not meant to apply to individuals who are being treated with zinc under close medical supervision.

Intake Assessment

Utilizing the Third National Health and Nutrition Examination Survey data, the highest reported intake of dietary zinc at the ninety-fifth percentile for all adults was 24 mg/day in men aged 19 to 30 years (Appendix Table C-25), which is lower than the UL of 40 mg/day. In 1986, approximately 17 percent of women and 15 percent of men consumed supplements that contained zinc (Moss et al., 1989; see Table 2-2). The ninety-fifth percentile intake of zinc coming from food and supplements for adult men and nonpregnant women was approximately 25 to 32 mg/day (Appendix Table C-26). For pregnant and lactating women, the zinc intake from food and supplements was approximately 40 and 47 mg/day, respectively, at the ninety-fifth percentile.

Risk Characterization

The risk of adverse effects resulting from excess zinc intake from food and supplements appears to be low at the highest intakes noted above. High intakes of zinc are due to the use of supplements, especially during lactation and pregnancy. Doses approaching or equal to the UL are currently being tested in the treatment of diarrhea, pneumonia, and acute respiratory infections, especially in developing countries. The UL is not meant apply to individuals who are receiving zinc for treatment purposes.

RESEARCH RECOMMENDATIONS FOR ZINC

• Biomarkers of zinc status based on functional outcomes; these may be gene products derived from zinc-influenced systems and may include transporter proteins that provide homeostatic regulation of zinc intake and cellular processing.

• Information on the relationship of oxidative stress to zinc status; zinc is used therapeutically for treatment of some medical problems, but how this relates to daily dietary zinc intake is not clear.

• Effectiveness and potential toxicity of zinc as a dietary supplement; on which systems should zinc's potential effectiveness be based, and which systems become dysfunctional with excessive zinc intake.

• The role of zinc and the immune system, particularly those related to T-cell function at marginal status.

• Quantitative data on human zinc homeostasis under a wide range of dietary conditions and at all ages using recent advances in zinc stable isotope methodology; quantification of what happens to zinc homeostasis as zinc intakes and absorption are increased and decreased beyond the range typically seen until recently; these metabolic studies need to be long-term.

REFERENCES

Abrams SA, Wen J, Stuff JE. 1997. Absorption of calcium, zinc, and iron from breast milk by five- to seven-month-old infants. *Pediatr Res* 41:384–390.

Aggett PJ. 1989. Severe zinc deficiency. In: Mills CF, ed. *Zinc in Human Biology*. New York: Springer-Verlag. Pp. 259–279.

Alexander D, Ball MJ, Mann J. 1994. Nutrient intake and haematological status of vegetarians and age-sex matched omnivores. *Eur J Clin Nutr* 48:538–546.

Alexander FW, Clayton BE, Delves HT. 1974. Mineral and trace-metal balances in children receiving normal and synthetic diets. *Quart J Med* 169:89–111.

Allen JC, Keller RP, Archer P, Neville MC. 1991. Studies in human lactation: Milk composition and daily secretion rates of macronutrients in the first year of lactation. *Am J Clin Nutr* 54:69–80.

Anderson BM, Gibson RS, Sabry JH. 1981. The iron and zinc status of long-term vegetarian women. *Am J Clin Nutr* 34:1042–1048.

Anderson RR. 1993. Longitudinal changes of trace elements in human milk during the first 5 months of lactation. *Nutr Res* 13:499–510.

Aquilio E, Spagnoli R, Seri S, Bottone G, Spennati G. 1996. Trace element content in human milk during lactation of preterm newborns. *Biol Trace Elem Res* 51:63–70.

Artacho R, Ruiz-Lopez MD, Gamez C, Puerta A, Lopez MC. 1997. Serum concentration and dietary intake of Zn in healthy institutionalized elderly subjects. *Sci Total Environment* 205:159–165.

August D, Janghorbani M, Young VR. 1989. Determination of zinc and copper absorption at three dietary Zn-Cu ratios by using stable isotope methods in young adult and elderly subjects. *Am J Clin Nutr* 50:1457–1463.

Baer MT, King JC. 1984. Tissue zinc levels and zinc excretion during experimental zinc depletion in young men. *Am J Clin Nutr* 39:556–570.

Bales CW, DiSilvestro RA, Currie KL, Plaisted CS, Joung H, Galanos AN, Lin PH. 1994. Marginal zinc deficiency in older adults: Responsiveness of zinc status indicators. *J Am Coll Nutr* 13:455–462.

Beck FW, Kaplan J, Fine N, Handschu W, Prasad AS. 1997a. Decreased expression of CD73 (ecto-5'-nucleotidase) in the CD8+ subset is associated with zinc deficiency in human patients. *J Lab Clin Med* 130:147–156.

Beck FW, Prasad AS, Kaplan J, Fitzgerald JT, Brewer GJ. 1997b. Changes in cytokine production and T cell subpopulations in experimentally induced zinc-deficient humans. *Am J Physiol* 272:E1002–E1007.

Behall KM, Scholfield DJ, Lee K, Powell AS, Moser PB. 1987. Mineral balance in adult men: Effect of four refined fibers. *Am J Clin Nutr* 46:307–314.

Berg JM, Shi Y. 1996. The galvanization of biology: A growing appreciation for the roles of zinc. *Science* 271:1081–1085.

Berglund M, Akesson A, Nermell B, Vahter M. 1994. Intestinal absorption of dietary cadmium in women depends on body iron stores and fiber intake. *Environ Health Perspect* 102:1058–1066.

Bhutta ZA, Nizami SQ, Isani Z. 1999. Zinc supplementation in malnourished children with persistent diarrhea in Pakistan. *Pediatrics* 103:e42. [Online]. Available: http://www.pediatrics.org/cgi/content/full/103/4/e42 [accessed June 5, 2000].

Biego GH, Joyeux M, Hartemann P, Debry G. 1998. Determination of mineral contents in different kinds of milk and estimation of dietary intake in infants. *Food Addit Contam* 15:775–781.

Black MR, Medeiros DM, Brunett E, Welke R. 1988. Zinc supplements and serum lipids in young adult white males. *Am J Clin Nutr* 47:970–975.

Bogden JD, Oleske JM, Munves EM, Lavenhar MA, Bruening KS, Kemp FW, Holding KJ, Denny TN, Louria DB. 1987. Zinc and immunocompetence in the elderly: Baseline data on zinc nutriture and immunity in supplemented subjects. *Am J Clin Nutr* 46:101–109.

Botash AS, Nasca J, Dubowy R, Weinberger HL, Oliphant M. 1992. Zinc-induced copper deficiency in an infant. *Am J Dis Child* 146:709–711.

Boukaiba N, Flament C, Acher S, Chappuis P, Piau A, Fusselier M, Dardenne M, Lemonnier D. 1993. A physiological amount of zinc supplementation: Effects on nutritional, lipid, and thymic status in an elderly population. *Am J Clin Nutr* 57:566–572.

Brants HA, Lowik MR, Westenbrink S, Hulshof KF, Kistemaker C. 1990. Adequacy of a vegetarian diet at old age (Dutch Nutrition Surveillance System). *J Am Coll Nutr* 9:292–302.

Brewer GJ, Yuzbasiyan-Gurkan V, Johnson V, Dick RD, Wang Y. 1993. Treatment of Wilson's Disease with zinc XII: Dose regimen requirements. *Am J Med Sci* 305:199–202.

Brown KH, Peerson JM, Allen LH. 1998. Effect of zinc supplementation on children's growth: A meta-analysis of intervention trials. *Bibl Nutr Dieta* 54:76–83.

Bunker VW, Lawson MS, Delves HT, Clayton BE. 1982. Metabolic balance studies for zinc and nitrogen in healthy elderly subjects. *Hum Nutr Clin Nutr* 36:213–221.

Burke DM, DeMicco FJ, Taper LJ, Ritchey SJ. 1981. Copper and zinc utilization in elderly adults. *J Gerontol* 36:558–563.

Butte NF, Garza C, Smith EO, Nichols BL. 1984. Human milk intake and growth in exclusively breast-fed infants. *J Pediatr* 104:187–195.

Cakman I, Kirchner H, Rink L. 1997. Zinc supplementation reconstitutes the production of interferon-α by leukocytes from elderly persons. *J Interferon Cytokine Res* 17:469–472.

Casey CE, Hambidge KM, Neville MC. 1985. Studies in human lactation: Zinc, copper, manganese and chromium in human milk in the first month of lactation. *Am J Clin Nutr* 41:1193–1200.

Casey CE, Neville MC, Hambidge KM. 1989. Studies in human lactation: Secretion of zinc, copper, and manganese in human milk. *Am J Clin Nutr* 49:773–785.

Caulfield LE, Zavaleta N, Figueroa A. 1999a. Adding zinc to prenatal iron and folate supplements improves maternal and neonatal zinc status in a Peruvian population. *Am J Clin Nutr* 69:1257–1263.

Caulfield LE, Zavaleta N, Figueroa A, Leon Z. 1999b. Maternal zinc supplementation does not affect size at birth or pregnancy duration in Peru. *J Nutr* 129:1563–1568.

Chandra RK. 1984. Excessive intake of zinc impairs immune responses. *J Am Med Assoc* 252:1443–1446.

Cheek DB, Reba RC, Woodward K. 1968. Cell growth and the possible role of trace minerals. In: Cheek DB, ed. *Human Growth; Body Composition, Cell Growth, Energy, and Intelligence*. Philadelphia: Lea and Febiger. Pp. 424–439.

Chen W, Chiang TP, Chen TC. 1991. Serum zinc and copper during long-term total parenteral nutrition. *J Formos Med Assoc* 90:1075–1080.

Chesters JK. 1997. Zinc. In: O'Dell BL, Sunde RA, eds. *Handbook of Nutritionally Essential Mineral Elements*. New York: Marcel Dekker. Pp. 185–230.

Cole TB, Wenzel HJ, Kafer KE, Schwartzkroin PA, Palmiter RD. 1999. Elimination of zinc from synaptic vesicles in the intact mouse brain by disruption of the ZnT3 gene. *Proc Natl Acad Sci USA* 96:1716–1721.

Colin MA, Taper LJ, Ritchey SJ. 1983. Effect of dietary zinc and protein levels on the utilization of zinc and copper by adult females. *J Nutr* 113:1480–1488.

Coudray C, Bellanger J, Castiglia-Delavaud C, Remesy C, Vermorel M, Rayssignuier Y. 1997. Effect of soluble or partly soluble dietary fibres supplementation on absorption and balance of calcium, magnesium, iron and zinc in healthy young men. *Eur J Clin Nutr* 51:375–380.

Cousins RJ. 1985. Absorption, transport, and hepatic metabolism of copper and zinc: Special reference to metallothionein and ceruloplasmin. *Physiol Rev* 65:238–309.

Cousins RJ. 1989a. Systemic transport of zinc. In: Mills CF, ed. *Zinc in Human Biology*. New York: Springer-Verlag. Pp. 79–93.

Cousins RJ. 1989b. Theoretical and practical aspects of zinc uptake and absorption. *Adv Exp Med Biol* 249:3–12.

Cousins RJ. 1994. Metal elements and gene expression. *Ann Rev Nutr* 14:449–469.

Cousins RJ. 1996. Zinc. In: Filer LJ, Ziegler EE, eds. *Present Knowledge in Nutrition*, 7th ed. Washington, DC: International Life Science Institute-Nutrition Foundation. Pp. 293–306.

Couzy F, Kastenmayer P, Mansourian R, Guinchard S, Munoz-Box R, Dirren H. 1993. Zinc absorption in healthy elderly humans and the effect of diet. *Am J Clin Nutr* 58:690–694.

Dalton TP, Bittel D, Andrews GK. 1997. Reversible activation of mouse metal response element-binding transcription factor 1 DNA binding involves zinc interaction with the zinc finger domain. *Molec Cell Biol* 17:2781–2789.

Davidsson L, Mackenzie J, Kastenmayer P, Aggett PJ, Hurrell RF. 1996. Zinc and calcium apparent absorption from an infant cereal: A stable isotope study in healthy infants. *Br J Nutr* 75:291–300.

Davis CD, Milne DB, Nielsen FH. 2000. Changes in dietary zinc and copper affect zinc-status indicators of postmenopausal women, notably extracellular superoxide dismutase and amyloid precursor proteins. *Am J Clin Nutr* 71:781–788.

Devine A, Rosen C, Mohan S, Baylink D, Prince RL. 1998. Effects of zinc and other nutritional factors on insulin-like growth factor I and insulin-like growth factor binding proteins in postmenopausal women. *Am J Clin Nutr* 68:200–206.

Dewey KG, Cohen RJ, Brown KH, Rivera LL. 1999. Age of introduction of complementary foods and growth of term, low-birth-weight, breast-fed infants: A randomized intervention study in Honduras. *Am J Clin Nutr* 69:679–686.

Donovan UM, Gibson RS. 1995. Iron and zinc status of young women aged 14 to 19 years consuming vegetarian and omnivorous diets. *J Am Coll Nutr* 14:463–472.

Donovan UM, Gibson RS. 1996. Dietary intakes of adolescent females consuming vegetarian, semi-vegetarian, and omnivorous diets. *J Adolesc Health* 18:292–300.

Duchateau J, Delepesse G, Vrijens R, Collet H. 1981. Beneficial effects of oral zinc supplementation on the immune response of old people. *Am J Med* 70:1001–1004.

Ellis R, Kelsay JL, Reynolds RD, Morris ER, Moser PB, Frazier CW. 1987. Phytate:zinc and phytate x calcium:zinc millimolar ratios in self-selected diets of Americans, Asian Indians, and Nepalese. *J Am Diet Assoc* 87:1043–1047.

Faber M, Gouws E, Spinnler Benade AJ, Labadarios D. 1986. Anthropometric measurements, dietary intake and biochemical data of South African lacto-ovovegetarians. *S Afr Med J* 69:733–738.

Failla ML. 1999. Considerations for determining "optimal nutrition" for copper, zinc, manganese and molybdenum. *Proc Nutr Soc* 58:497–505.

Fairweather-Tait SJ, Wharf SG, Fox TE. 1995. Zinc absorption in infants fed iron-fortified weaning food. *Am J Clin Nutr* 62:785–789.

Ferguson EL, Gibson RS, Opare-Obisaw C, Ounpuu S, Thompson LU, Lehrfeld J. 1993. The zinc nutriture of preschool children living in two African countries. *J Nutr* 123:1487–1496.

Festa MD, Anderson HL, Dowdy RP, Ellersieck MR. 1985. Effect of zinc intake on copper excretion and retention in men. *Am J Clin Nutr* 41:285–292.

Fischer PWF, Giroux A, L'Abbe MR. 1984. Effect of zinc supplementation on copper status in adult man. *Am J Clin Nutr* 40:743–746.

Fortes C, Forastiere F, Agabiti N, Fano V, Pacifici R, Virgili F, Piras G, Guidi L, Bartoloni C, Tricerri A, Zuccaro P, Ebrahim S, Perucci CA. 1998. The effect of zinc and vitamin A supplementation on immune response in an older population. *J Am Geriatr Soc* 46:19–26.

Fosmire GJ. 1990. Zinc toxicity. *Am J Clin Nutr* 51:225–227.

Fransson GB, Lonnerdal B. 1982. Zinc, copper, calcium, and magnesium in human milk. *J Pediatr* 101:504–508.

Freeland-Graves JH, Bodzy PW, Eppright MA. 1980a. Zinc status of vegetarians. *J Am Diet Assoc* 77:655–661.

Freeland-Graves JH, Ebangit ML, Hendrikson PJ. 1980b. Alterations in zinc absorption and salivary sediment zinc after a lacto-ovo-vegetarian diet. *Am J Clin Nutr* 33:1757–1766.

Freeland-Graves JH, Friedman BJ, Han WH, Shorey RL, Young R. 1982. Effect of zinc supplementation on plasma high-density lipoprotein cholesterol and zinc. *Am J Clin Nutr* 35:988–992.

Fung EB, Ritchie LD, Woodhouse LR, Roehl R, King JC. 1997. Zinc absorption in women during pregnancy and lactation: A longitudinal study. *Am J Clin Nutr* 66:80–88.

Ganapathy SN, Booker LK, Craven R, Edwards CH. 1981. Trace minerals, amino acids, and plasma proteins in adult men fed wheat diets. *J Am Diet Assoc* 78:490–497.

Gibson RS. 1994. Content and bioavailability of trace elements in vegetarian diets. *Am J Clin Nutr* 59:1223S–1232S.

Gibson RS, Vanderkooy PD, MacDonald AC, Goldman A, Ryan BA, Berry M. 1989. A growth-limiting, mild zinc-deficiency syndrome in some southern Ontario boys with low height percentiles. *Am J Clin Nutr* 49:1266–1273.

Gibson RS, Donovan UM, Heath AL. 1997. Dietary strategies to improve the iron and zinc nutriture of young women following a vegetarian diet. *Plant Foods Hum Nutr* 51:1–16.

Gibson RS, Heath AL, Prosser N, Parnell W, Donovan UM, Green T, McLaughlin KE, O'Connor DL, Bettger W, Skeaff CM. 2000. Are young women with low iron stores at risk of zinc as well as iron deficiency? In: Roussel AM, Anderson RA, Favrier A, eds. *Trace Elements in Man and Animals 10*. New York: Kluwer Academic. Pp. 323–328.

Goldenberg RL, Tamura T, Neggers Y, Copper RL, Johnston KE, DuBard MB, Hauth JC. 1995. The effect of zinc supplementation on preganancy outcome. *J Am Med Assoc* 274:463–468.

Greger JL, Snedeker SM. 1980. Effect of dietary protein and phosphorus levels on the utilization of zinc, copper and manganese by adult males. *J Nutr* 110:2243–2253.

Greger JL, Baligar P, Abernathy RP, Bennett OA, Peterson T. 1978. Calcium, magnesium, phosphorus, copper, and manganese balance in adolescent females. *Am J Clin Nutr* 31:117–121.

Grider A, Bailey LB, Cousins RJ. 1990. Erythrocyte metallothionein as an index of zinc status in humans. *Proc Natl Acad Sci USA* 87:1259–1262.

Günes C, Heuchel R, Georgiev O, Müller K-H, Lichtlen P, Blüthmann H, Marino S, Aguzzi A, Schaffner W. 1998. Embryonic lethality and liver degeneration in mice lacking the metal-responsive transcriptional activator MTF-1. *Embo J* 17:2846–2854.

Gunshin H, Mackenzie B, Berger UV, Gunshin Y, Romero MF, Boron WF, Nussberger S, Gollan JL, Hediger MA. 1997. Cloning and characterization of a mammalian proton-coupled metal-ion transporter. *Nature* 388:482–488.

Hallfrisch J, Powell A, Carafelli C, Reiser S, Prather ES. 1987. Mineral balances of men and women consuming high fiber diets with complex or simple carbohydrate. *J Nutr* 117:48–55.

Hambidge KM. 1989. Mild zinc deficiency in human subjects. In: Mills CF, ed. *Zinc in Human Biology*. New York: Springer-Verlag. Pp. 281–296.

Hambidge KM, Hambidge C, Jacobs M, Baum JD. 1972. Low levels of zinc in hair, anorexia, poor growth, and hypogeusia in children. *Pediatr Res* 6:868–874.

Hambidge KM, Chavez MN, Brown RM, Walravens PA. 1979a. Zinc nutritional status of young middle-income children and effects of consuming zinc-fortified breakfast cereals. *Am J Clin Nutr* 32:2532–2539.

Hambidge KM, Walravens PA, Casey CE, Brown RM, Bender C. 1979b. Plasma zinc concentrations of breast-fed infants. *J Pediatr* 94:607–608.

Hambidge KM, Krebs NF, Jacobs MA, Favier A, Guyette L, Ikle DN. 1983. Zinc nutritional status during pregnancy: A longitudinal study. *Am J Clin Nutr* 37:429–442.

Han O, Failla ML, Hill AD, Morris ER, Smith JC Jr. 1994. Inositol phosphates inhibit uptake and transport of iron and zinc by a human intestinal cell line. *J Nutr* 124:580–587.

Harland BF, Peterson M. 1978. Nutritional status of lacto-ovo vegetarian Trappist monks. *J Am Diet Assoc* 72:259–264.

Harland BF, Smith SA, Howard MP, Ellis R, Smith JC Jr. 1988. Nutritional status and phytate:zinc and phytate x calcium:zinc dietary molar ratios of lacto-ovo vegetarian Trappist monks: 10 years later. *J Am Diet Assoc* 88:1562–1566.

Heinig MJ, Nommsen LA, Peerson JM, Lonnerdal B, Dewey KG. 1993. Energy and protein intakes of breast-fed and formula-fed infants during the first year of life and their association with growth velocity: The DARLING Study. *Am J Clin Nutr* 58:152–161.

Hess FM, King JC, Margen S. 1977. Zinc excretion in young women on low zinc intakes and oral contraceptive agents. *J Nutr* 107:1610–1620.

Holbrook JT, Smith JC Jr, Reiser S. 1989. Dietary fructose or starch: Effects on copper, zinc, iron, manganese, calcium, and magnesium balances in humans. *Am J Clin Nutr* 49:1290–1294.

Hooper PL, Visconti L, Garry PJ, Johnson GE. 1980. Zinc lowers high-density lipoprotein-cholesterol levels. *J Am Med Assoc* 244:1960–1961.

Hunt CD, Johnson PE, Herbel J, Mullen LK. 1992. Effects of dietary zinc depletion on seminal volume and zinc loss, serum testosterone concentrations, and sperm morphology in young men. *Am J Clin Nutr* 56:148–157.

Hunt IF, Murphy NJ, Henderson C. 1988. Food and nutrient intake of Seventh-day Adventist women. *Am J Clin Nutr* 48:850–851.

Hunt JR. 1996. Bioavailability algorithms in setting recommended dietary allowances: Lessons from iron, applications to zinc. *J Nutr* 126:2345S–2353S.

Hunt JR, Mullen LK, Lykken GI. 1992. Zinc retention from an experimental diet based on the US FDA Total Diet Study. *Nutr Res* 12:1335–1344.

Hunt JR, Gallagher SK, Johnson LK, Lykken GI. 1995. High- versus low-meat diets: Effects on zinc absorption, iron status, and calcium, copper, iron, magnesium, manganese, nitrogen, phosphorus, and zinc balance in postmenopausal women. *Am J Clin Nutr* 62:621–632.

Hunt JR, Matthys LA, Johnson LK. 1998. Zinc absorption, mineral balance, and blood lipids in women consuming controlled lactoovovegetarian and omnivorous diets for 8 weeks. *Am J Clin Nutr* 67:421–430.

Huse M, Eck MJ, Harrison SC. 1998. A Zn^{2+} ion links the cytoplasmic tail of CD4 and the N-terminal region of Lck. *J Biol Chem* 273:18729–18733.

Jackson JL, Lesho E, Peterson C. 2000. Zinc and the common cold: A meta-analysis revisited. *J Nutr* 130:1512S-1515S.

Jackson MJ, Jones DA, Edwards RH, Swainbank IG, Coleman ML. 1984. Zinc homeostasis in man: Studies using a new stable isotope-dilution technique. *Br J Nutr* 51:199–208.

Jacob C, Maret W, Vallee BL. 1998. Control of zinc transfer between thionein, metallothionein, and zinc proteins. *Proc Natl Acad Sci USA* 95:3489–3494.

Janelle KC, Barr SI. 1995. Nutrient intakes and eating behavior scores of vegetarian and nonvegetarian women. *J Am Diet Assoc* 95:180–186, 189.

Johansson G, Widerstrom L. 1994. Change from mixed diet to lactovegetarian diet: Influence on IgA levels in blood and saliva. *Scand J Dent Res* 102:350–354.

Johnson MA, Baier MJ, Greger JL. 1982. Effects of dietary tin on zinc, copper, iron, manganese, and magnesium metabolism of adult males. *Am J Clin Nutr* 35:1332–1338.

Johnson PE, Evans GW. 1978. Relative zinc availability in human breast milk, infant formulas, and cow's milk. *Am J Clin Nutr* 31:416–421.

Johnson PE, Hunt CD, Milne DB, Mullen LK. 1993. Homeostatic control of zinc metabolism in men: Zinc excretion and balance in men fed diets low in zinc. *Am J Clin Nutr* 57:557–565.

Kadrabova J, Madaric A, Kovacikova Z, Ginter E. 1995. Selenium status, plasma zinc, copper, and magnesium in vegetarians. *Biol Trace Elem Res* 50:13–24.

Kaji M, Gotoh M, Takagi Y, Masuda H, Kimura Y, Uenoyama Y. 1998. Studies to determine the usefulness of the zinc clearance test to diagnose marginal zinc deficiency and the effects of oral zinc supplementation for short children. *J Am Coll Nutr* 17:388–391.

Kant AK, Moser-Veillon PB, Reynolds RD. 1989. Dietary intakes and plasma concentrations of zinc, copper, iron, magnesium, and selenium of young, middle aged, and older men. *Nutr Res* 9:717–724.

Kauwell GP, Bailey LB, Gregory JF 3rd, Bowling DW, Cousins RJ. 1995. Zinc status is not adversely affected by folic acid supplementation and zinc intake does not impair folate utilization in human subjects. *J Nutr* 125:66–72.

Kelsay JL, Frazier CW, Prather ES, Canary JJ, Clark WM, Powell AS. 1988. Impact of variation in carbohydrate intake on mineral utilization by vegetarians. *Am J Clin Nutr* 48:875–879.

Kies CV. 1988. Mineral utilization of vegetarians: Impact of variation in fat intake. *Am J Clin Nutr* 48: 884–887.

King JC. 1990. Assessment of zinc status. *J Nutr* 120:1474–1479.

King JC, Keen CL. 1999. Zinc. In: Shils ME, Olson JA, Shike M, Ross AC, eds. *Modern Nutrition in Health and Disease,* 9th ed. Baltimore: Williams & Wilkins. Pp. 223–239.

King JC, Turnlund JR. 1989. Human zinc requirements. In: Mills CF, ed. *Zinc in Human Biology.* London: Springer-Verlag. Pp. 335–350.

King JC, Stein T, Doyle M. 1981. Effect of vegetarianism on the zinc status of pregnant women. *Am J Clin Nutr* 34:1049–1055.

King JC, Hambidge KM, Westcott JL, Kern DL, Marshall G. 1994. Daily variation in plasma zinc concentrations in women fed meals at six-hour intervals. *J Nutr* 124:508–516.

Kirksey A, Ernst JA, Roepke JL, Tsai TL. 1979. Influence of mineral intake and use of oral contraceptives before pregnancy on the mineral content of human colostrum and of more mature milk. *Am J Clin Nutr* 32:30–39.

Klug A, Schwabe JWR. 1995. Zinc fingers. *FASEB J* 9:597–604.

Krajcovicova-Kudlackova M, Simoncic R, Babinska K, Bederova A, Brtkova A, Magalova T, Grancicova E. 1995. Selected vitamins and trace elements in blood of vegetarians. *Ann Nutr Metab* 39:334–339.

Krebs NF, Hambidge KM. 1986. Zinc requirements and zinc intakes of breast-fed infants. *Am J Clin Nutr* 43:288–292.

Krebs NF, Hambidge KM, Jacobs MA, Rasbach JO. 1985. The effects of a dietary zinc supplement during lactation on longitudinal changes in maternal zinc status and milk zinc concentrations. *Am J Clin Nutr* 41:560–570.

Krebs NF, Reidinger CJ, Robertson AD, Hambidge KM. 1994. Growth and intakes of energy and zinc in infants fed human milk. *J Pediatr* 124:32–39.

Krebs NF, Reidinger CJ, Hartley S, Robertson AD, Hambidge KM. 1995. Zinc supplementation during lactation: Effects on maternal status and milk zinc concentrations. *Am J Clin Nutr* 61:1030–1036.

Krebs NF, Reidinger CJ, Miller LV, Hambidge KM. 1996. Zinc homeostasis in breast-fed infants. *Pediatr Res* 39:661–665.

Kuczmarski RJ, Ogden CL, Grummer-Strawn LM, Flegal KM, Guo SS, Wei R, Mei Z, Curtin LR, Roche AF, Johnson CL. 2000. *CDC Growth Charts: United States.* Advance data from vital health statistics. No. 314. Hyattesville, MD: National Center for Health Statistics.

Kumar S. 1976. Effect of zinc supplementation on rats during pregnancy. *Nutr Rpts Intl* 13:33–36.

Lee DY, Prasad AS, Hydrick-Adair C, Brewer G, Johnson PE. 1993. Homeostasis of zinc in marginal human zinc deficiency: Role of absorption and endogenous excretion of zinc. *J Lab Clin Med* 122:549–556.

Lee HH, Prasad AS, Brewer GJ, Owyang C. 1989. Zinc absorption in human small intestine. *Am J Physiol* 256:G87–G91.

Levin N, Rattan J, Gilat T. 1986. Mineral intake and blood levels in vegetarians. *Isr J Med Sci* 22:105–108.

Lin RS, Rodriguez C, Veillette A, Lodish HF. 1998. Zinc is essential for binding of p56[lck] to CD4 and CD8α. *J Biol Chem* 273:32878–32882.

Lonnerdal B. 1989. Intestinal absorption of zinc. In: Mills CF, ed. *Zinc in Human Biology.* New York: Springer-Verlag. Pp. 33–55.

Lonnerdal B, Keen CL, Hurley LS. 1981. Iron, copper, zinc and manganese in milk. *Ann Rev Nutr* 1:149–174.

Lonnerdal B, Bell JG, Hendrickx AG, Burns RA, Keen CL. 1988. Effect of phytate removal on zinc absorption from soy formula. *Am J Clin Nutr* 48:1301–1306.

Lowik MR, Schrijver J, Odink J, van den Berg H, Wedel M. 1990. Long-term effects of a vegetarian diet on the nutritional status of elderly people (Dutch Nutrition Surveillance System). *J Am Coll Nutr* 9:600–609.

Mahalko JR, Sandstead HH, Johnson LK, Milne DB. 1983. Effect of a moderate increase in dietary protein on the retention and excretion of Ca, Cu, Fe, Mg, P, and Zn by adult males. *Am J Clin Nutr* 37:8–14.

Mares-Perlman JA, Subar AF, Block G, Greger JL, Luby MH. 1995. Zinc intake and sources in the US adult population: 1976–1980. *J Am Coll Nutr* 14:349–357.

McCabe MJ Jr, Jiang SA, Orrenius S. 1993. Chelation of intracellular zinc triggers apoptosis in mature thymocytes. *Lab Invest* 69:101–110.

McKenna AA, Ilich JZ, Andon MB, Wang C, Matkovic V. 1997. Zinc balance in adolescent females consuming a low- or high-calcium diet. *Am J Clin Nutr* 65:1460–1464.

McMahon RJ, Cousins RJ. 1998. Mammalian zinc transporters. *J Nutr* 128:667–670.

Merialdi M, Caulfield LE, Zavaleta N, Figueroa A, DiPietro JA. 1998. Adding zinc to prenatal iron and folate tablets improves fetal neurobehavioral development. *Am J Obstet Gynecol* 180:483–490.

Miller LV, Hambidge KM, Naake VL, Hong Z, Westcott JL, Fennessey PV. 1994. Size of the zinc pools that exchange rapidly with plasma zinc in humans: Alternative techniques for measuring and relation to dietary zinc intake. *J Nutr* 124:268–276.

Miller LV, Krebs NF, Hambidge KM. 1998. Human zinc metabolism: Advances in the modeling of stable isotope data. *Adv Exp Med Biol* 445:253–269.

Milne DB, Canfield WK, Mahalko JR, Sandstead HH. 1983. Effect of dietary zinc on whole body surface loss of zinc: Impact on estimation of zinc retention by balance method. *Am J Clin Nutr* 38:181–186.

Milne DB, Canfield WK, Mahalko JR, Sandstead HH. 1984. Effect of oral folic acid supplements on zinc, copper, and iron absorption and excretion. *Am J Clin Nutr* 39:535–539.

Milne DB, Canfield WK, Gallagher SK, Hunt JR, Klevay LM. 1987. Ethanol metabolism in postmenopausal women fed a diet marginal in zinc. *Am J Clin Nutr* 46:688–693.

Moser PB, Reynolds RD. 1983. Dietary zinc intake and zinc concentrations of plasma, erythrocytes, and breast milk in antepartum and postpartum lactating and nonlactating women: A longitudinal study. *Am J Clin Nutr* 38:101–108.

Moser-Veillon PB, Reynolds RD. 1990. A longitudinal study of pyridoxine and zinc supplementation of lactating women. *Am J Clin Nutr* 52:135–141.

Moss AJ, Levy AS, Kim I, Park YK. 1989. *Use of Vitamin and Mineral Supplements in the United States: Current Users, Types of Products, and Nutrients*. Advance Data, Vital and Health Statistics of the National Center for Health Statistics, Number 174. Hyattsville, MD: National Center for Health Statistics.

Nakamura T, Nishiyama S, Futagoishi-Suginohara Y, Matsuda I, Higashi A. 1993. Mild to moderate zinc deficiency in short children: Effect of zinc supplementation on linear growth velocity. *J Pediatr* 123:65–69.

Neggers YH, Goldenberg RL, Tamura T, Johnston KE, Copper RL, DuBard M. 1997. Plasma and erythrocyte zinc concentrations and their relationship to dietary zinc intake and zinc supplementation during pregnancy in low-income African-American women. *J Am Diet Assoc* 97:1269–1274.

Ninh NX, Thissen JP, Collette L, Gerard G, Khoi HH, Ketelslegers JM. 1996. Zinc supplementation increases growth and circulating insulin-like growth factor I (IGF-I) in growth-retarded Vietnamese children. *Am J Clin Nutr* 63:514–519.

Oberleas D, Muhrer ME, O'Dell BL. 1966. Dietary metal-complexing agents and zinc availability in the rat. *J Nutr* 90:56–62.

O'Brien KO, Zavaleta N, Caulfield LE, Wen J, Abrams SA. 2000. Prenatal iron supplements impair zinc absorption in pregnant Peruvian women. *J Nutr* 130:2251–2255.

Ortega RM, Andres P, Martinez RM, Lopez-Sobaler AM, Quintas ME. 1997. Zinc levels in maternal milk: The influence of nutritional status with respect to zinc during the third trimester of pregnancy. *Eur J Clin Nutr* 51:253–258.

Paik HY, Joung H, Lee JY, Lee HK, King JC, Keen CL. 1999. Serum extracellular superoxide dismutase activity as an indicator of zinc status in humans. *Biol Trace Elem Res* 69:45–57.

Payette H, Gray-Donald K. 1991. Dietary intake and biochemical indices of nutritional status in an elderly population, with estimates of the precision of the 7-d food record. *Am J Clin Nutr* 54:478–488.

Picciano MF, Guthrie HA. 1976. Copper, iron, and zinc contents of mature human milk. *Am J Clin Nutr* 29:242–254.

Pironi L, Miglioli M, Cornia GL, Ursitti MA, Tolomelli M, Piazzi S, Barbara L. 1987. Urinary zinc excretion in Crohn's disease. *Dig Dis Sci* 32:358–362.

Prasad AS. 1976. Deficiency of zinc in man and its toxicity. In: Prasad AS, Oberleas D, eds. *Trace Elements in Human Health and Disease, Volume 1. Zinc and Copper*. New York: Academic Press. Pp. 1–20.

Prasad AS. 1991. Discovery of human zinc deficiency and studies in an experimental human model. *Am J Clin Nutr* 53:403–412.

Prasad AS, Brewer GJ, Schoomaker EB, Rabbani P. 1978. Hypocupremia induced by zinc therapy in adults. *J Am Med Assoc* 240:2166–2168.

Prasad AS, Fitzgerald JT, Hess JW, Kaplan J, Pelen F, Dardenne M. 1993. Zinc deficiency in elderly patients. *Nutrition* 9:218–224.

Prasad AS, Mantzoros CS, Beck FW, Hess JW, Brewer GJ. 1996. Zinc status and serum testosterone levels of healthy adults. *Nutrition* 12:344–348.

Roesijadi G, Bogumil R, Vasak M, Kagi JH. 1998. Modulation of DNA binding of a tramtrack zinc finger peptide by the metallothionein-thionein conjugate pair. *J Biol Chem* 273:17425–17432.

Rossander-Hulten L, Brune M, Sandstrom B, Lonnerdal B, Hallberg L. 1991. Competitive inhibition of iron absorption by manganese and zinc in humans. *Am J Clin Nutr* 54:152–156.

Roth HP, Kirchgessner M. 1985. Utilization of zinc from picolinic or citric acid complexes in relation to dietary protein source in rats. *J Nutr* 115:1641–1649.

Ruz M, Cavan KR, Bettger WJ, Gibson RS. 1992. Erythrocytes, erythrocyte membranes, neutrophils and platelets as biopsy materials for the assessment of zinc status in humans. *Br J Nutr* 68:515–527.

Samman S, Roberts DCK. 1987. The effect of zinc supplements on plasma zinc and copper levels and the reported symptoms in healthy volunteers. *Med J Aust* 146:246–249.

Samman S, Roberts DCK. 1988. The effect of zinc supplements on lipoproteins and copper status. *Atherosclerosis* 70:247–252.

Samman S, Soto S, Cooke L, Ahmad Z, Farmakalidis E. 1996. Is erythrocyte alkaline phosphatase activity a marker of zinc status in humans? *Biol Trace Elem Res* 51:285–291.

Sandstead HH, Penland JG, Alcock NW, Dayal HH, Chen XC, Li JS, Zhao F, Yang JJ. 1998. Effects of repletion with zinc and other micronutrients on neuropsychologic performance and growth of Chinese children. *Am J Clin Nutr* 68:470S–475S.

Sandstrom B, Lonnerdal B. 1989. Promoters and antagonists of zinc absorption. In: Mills CF, ed. *Zinc in Human Biology*. New York: Springer-Verlag. Pp. 57–78.

Sandstrom B, Cederblad A, Lonnerdal B. 1983. Zinc absorption from human milk, cow's milk, and infant formulas. *Am J Dis Child* 137:726–729.

Scholl TO, Hediger ML, Schall JI, Fischer RL, Khoo CS. 1993. Low zinc intake during pregnancy: Its association with preterm and very preterm delivery. *Am J Epidemiol* 137:1115–1124.

Seal CJ, Heaton FW. 1985. Effect of dietary picolinic acid on the metabolism of exogenous and endogenous zinc in the rat. *J Nutr* 115:986–993.

Shankar AH, Prasad AS. 1998. Zinc and immune function: The biological basis of altered resistance to infection. *Am J Clin Nutr* 68:447S–463S.

Sian L, Mingyan X, Miller LV, Tong L, Krebs NF, Hambidge KM. 1996. Zinc absorption and intestinal losses of endogenous zinc in young Chinese women with marginal zinc intakes. *Am J Clin Nutr* 63:348–353.

Sievers E, Oldigs HD, Dorner K, Schaub J. 1992. Longitudinal zinc balances in breast-fed and formula-fed infants. *Acta Paediatr* 81:1–6.

Singh H, Flynn A, Fox PF. 1989. Zinc binding in bovine milk. *J Dairy Res* 56:249–263.

Smit-Vanderkooy PD, Gibson RS. 1987. Food consumption patterns of Canadian preschool children in relation to zinc and growth status. *Am J Clin Nutr* 45:609–616.

Snedeker SM, Smith SA, Greger JL. 1982. Effect of dietary calcium and phosphorus levels on the utilization of iron, copper, and zinc by adult males. *J Nutr* 112:136–143.

Solomons NW, Jacob RA. 1981. Studies on the bioavailability of zinc in humans: Effects of heme and nonheme iron on the absorption of zinc. *Am J Clin Nutr* 34:475–482.

Spencer H, Asmussen CR, Holtzman RB, Kramer L. 1979. Metabolic balances of cadmium, copper, manganese, and zinc in man. *Am J Clin Nutr* 32:1867–1875.

Spencer H, Kramer L, Norris C, Osis D. 1984. Effect of calcium and phosphorus on zinc metabolism in man. *Am J Clin Nutr* 40:1213–1218.

Srikumar TS, Johansson GK, Ockerman PA, Gustafsson JA, Akesson B. 1992. Trace element status in healthy subjects switching from a mixed to a lactovegetarian diet for 12 months. *Am J Clin Nutr* 55:885–890.

Sullivan VK, Burnett FR, Cousins RJ. 1998. Metallothionein expression is increased in monocytes and erythrocytes of young men during zinc supplementation. *J Nutr* 128:707–713.

Swanson CA, King JC. 1982. Zinc utilization in pregnant and nonpregnant women fed controlled diets providing the zinc RDA. *J Nutr* 112:697–707.

Swanson CA, King JC. 1987. Zinc and pregnancy outcome. *Am J Clin Nutr* 46:763–771.

Swanson CA, Mansourian R, Dirren H, Rapin CH. 1988. Zinc status of healthy elderly adults: Response to supplementation. *Am J Clin Nutr* 48:343–349.

Taper LJ, Hinners ML, Ritchey SJ. 1980. Effects of zinc intake on copper balance in adult females. *Am J Clin Nutr* 33:1077–1082.

Taylor CM, Bacon JR, Aggett PJ, Bremner I. 1991. Homeostatic regulation of zinc absorption and endogenous losses in zinc-deprived men. *Am J Clin Nutr* 53:755–763.

Telford WG, Fraker PJ. 1995. Preferential induction of apoptosis in mouse CD4$^+$CD8$^+$αβTCR^{lo}CD3ε^{lo} thymocytes by zinc. *J Cell Physiol* 164:259–270.

Thomas AJ, Bunker VW, Hinks LJ, Sodha N, Mullee MA, Clayton BE. 1988. Energy, protein, zinc and copper status of twenty-one elderly inpatients: Analysed dietary intake and biochemical indices. *Br J Nutr* 59:181–191.

Thomas EA, Bailey LB, Kauwell GA, Lee D-Y, Cousins RJ. 1992. Erythrocyte metallothionein response to dietary zinc in humans. *J Nutr* 122:2408–2414.

Turnlund JR, Michel MC, Keyes WR, King JC, Margen S. 1982. Use of enriched stable isotopes to determine zinc and iron absorption in elderly men. *Am J Clin Nutr* 35:1033–1040.

Turnlund JR, King JC, Keyes WR, Gong B, Michel MC. 1984. A stable isotope study of zinc absorption in young men: Effects of phytate and alpha-cellulose. *Am J Clin Nutr* 40:1071–1077.

Turnlund JR, Durkin N, Costa F, Margen S. 1986. Stable isotope studies of zinc absorption and retention in young and elderly men. *J Nutr* 116:1239–1247.

Turnlund JR, Keyes WR, Hudson CA, Betschart AA, Kretsch MJ, Sauberlich HE. 1991. A stable-isotope study of zinc, copper, and iron absorption and retention by young women fed vitamin B-6-deficient diets. *Am J Clin Nutr* 54:1059–1064.

Udomkesmalee E, Dhanamitta S, Yhoung-Aree J, Rojroongwasinkul N, Smith JC Jr. 1990. Biochemical evidence suggestive of suboptimal zinc and vitamin A status in schoolchildren in northeast Thailand. *Am J Clin Nutr* 52:564–567.

Umeta M, West CE, Haidar J, Deurenberg P, Hautvast JGAJ. 2000. Zinc supplementation and stunted infants in Ethiopia: A randomised controlled trial. *Lancet* 355:2021–2026.

Valberg LS, Flanagan PR, Chamberlain MJ. 1984. Effects of iron, tin, and copper on zinc absorption in humans. *Am J Clin Nutr* 40:536–541.

Valberg LS, Flanagan PR, Kertesz A, Bondy DC. 1986. Zinc absorption in inflammatory bowel disease. *Dig Dis Sci* 31:724–731.

Vallee BL, Galdes A. 1984. The metallobiochemistry of zinc enzymes. *Adv Enzymol* 56:283–429.

Vuori E, Makinen SM, Kara R, Kuitunen P. 1980. The effects of the dietary intakes of copper, iron, manganese, and zinc on the trace element content of human milk. *Am J Clin Nutr* 33:227–231.

Wada L, King JC. 1986. Effect of low zinc intakes on basal metabolic rate, thyroid hormones and protein utilization in adult men. *J Nutr* 116:1045–1053.

Wada L, Turnlund JR, King JC. 1985. Zinc utilization in young men fed adequate and low zinc intakes. *J Nutr* 115:1345–1354.

Walling A, Householder M, Walling A. 1989. Acrodermatitis enteropathica. *Am Fam Physician* 39:151–154.

Walravens PA, Hambidge KM. 1976. Growth of infants fed a zinc supplemented formula. *Am J Clin Nutr* 29:1114–1121.

Walravens PA, Krebs NF, Hambidge KM. 1983. Linear growth of low income preschool children receiving a zinc supplement. *Am J Clin Nutr* 38:195–201.

Walravens PA, Hambidge KM, Koepfer DM. 1989. Zinc supplementation in infants with a nutritional pattern of failure to thrive: A double-blind, controlled study. *Pediatrics* 83:532–538.

Walravens PA, Chakar A, Mokni R, Denise J, Lemonnier D. 1992. Zinc supplements in breastfed infants. *Lancet* 340:683–685.

Wastney ME, Aamodt RL, Rumble WF, Henkin RI. 1986. Kinetic analysis of zinc metabolism and its regulation in normal humans. *Am J Physiol* 251:R398–R408.

Whittaker P. 1998. Iron and zinc interactions in humans. *Am J Clin Nutr* 68:442S–446S.

WHO (World Health Organization). 1996. *Trace Elements in Human Nutrition and Health*. Geneva: WHO. Pp. 72–104.

Widdowson EM, Dickerson JWT. 1964. Chemical composition of the body. In: Comar CL, Bronner F, eds. *Mineral Metabolism. An Advanced Treatise, Vol. II. The Elements, Part A*. New York: Academic Press. Pp. 1–247.

Williams AW, Erdman JW Jr. 1999. Food processing: Nutrition, safety, and quality balances. In: Shils ME, Olson JA, Shike M, Ross AC, eds. *Modern Nutrition in Health and Disease*, 9th ed. Baltimore: Williams & Wilkins. Pp. 1813–1821.

Wisker E, Nagel R, Tanudjaja TK, Feldheim W. 1991. Calcium, magnesium, zinc, and iron balances in young women: Effects of a low-phytate barley-fiber concentrate. *Am J Clin Nutr* 54:553–559.

Wood RJ, Zheng JJ. 1997. High dietary calcium intakes reduce zinc absorption and balance in humans. *Am J Clin Nutr* 65:1803–1809.

Yadrick MK, Kenney MA, Winterfeldt EA. 1989. Iron, copper, and zinc status: Response to supplementation with zinc or zinc and iron in adult females. *Am J Clin Nutr* 49:145–150.

Yokoi K, Alcock NW, Sandstead HH. 1994. Iron and zinc nutriture of premenopausal women: Associations of diet with serum ferritin and plasma zinc disappearance and of serum ferritin with plasma zinc and plasma zinc disappearance. *J Lab Clin Med* 124:852–861.

Yuzbasiyan-Gurkan V, Grider A, Nostrant T, Cousins RJ, Brewer GJ. 1992. Treatment of Wilson's disease with zinc: X. Intestinal metallothionein induction. *J Lab Clin Med* 120:380–386.

Zalewski PD, Forbes IJ, Seamark RF, Borlinghaus R, Betts WH, Lincoln SF, Ward AD. 1994. Flux of intracellular labile zinc during apoptosis (gene-directed cell death) revealed by a specific chemical probe, Zinquin. *Chem Biol* 1:153–161.

Ziegler EE, Edwards BB, Jensen RL, Filer LJ, Fomon SJ. 1978. Zinc balance studies in normal infants. In: Kirchgessner M, ed. *Trace Element Metabolism in Man and Animals—3*. Freising-Weihenstephan: Arbeitskreis fier Tierernahrungs-forschung. Pp. 292–295.

Zlotkin SH, Cherian MG. 1988. Hepatic metallothionein as a source of zinc and cystcine during the first year of life. *Pediatr Res* 24:326–329.

13

Arsenic, Boron, Nickel, Silicon, and Vanadium

SUMMARY

An Estimated Average Requirement (EAR) or Adequate Intake (AI) was not set for arsenic, boron, nickel, silicon, or vanadium. In the case of the vitamins and other minerals reviewed in this report, there are well-established studies typically based on observations from several laboratories. The data currently available for these vitamins and other minerals provide an understanding of the metabolic role of each and describe the consequences of their restriction in the diets of both laboratory animals and humans. There are also clearly defined, readily reproducible indicators in humans for these vitamins and other minerals that can be used to determine an EAR and calculate a Recommended Dietary Allowance, or to establish an AI. At present, such data do not exist for arsenic, boron, nickel, silicon, and vanadium.

In the case of arsenic, boron, nickel, silicon, and vanadium, there is evidence that they have a beneficial role in some physiological processes in some species. For boron, silicon, and vanadium, measurable responses of human subjects to variations in dietary intake have also been demonstrated. However, the available data are not as extensive (e.g., dose-response data are absent) and the responses are not as consistently observed as they are for the vitamins and other minerals. Thus, data are insufficient to determine an EAR for any of these minerals.

Estimates of dietary intakes of arsenic, boron, nickel, silicon, and vanadium by the North American adult population are available and could have been used to establish an AI. However, establishing an AI also requires a clearly defined, reproducible indicator in humans sensitive to a range of intakes. Indicators that meet this criterion for establishing an AI are not currently available for any of these minerals, and therefore no AI was set.

Notwithstanding, observations of deficiency effects (e.g., on growth and development) in multiple animal species and data from limited human studies suggest beneficial roles for arsenic, boron, nickel, silicon, and vanadium in human health. These data clearly indicate a need for continued study of these elements to determine their metabolic role, identify sensitive indicators, and more fully characterize specific functions in human health.

Estimates of Tolerable Upper Intake Levels (UL) were set for boron, nickel, and vanadium. The ULs for boron and vanadium are based on animal data and have been set for adults at 20 mg/day and 1.8 mg/day, respectively. The UL for nickel is 1 mg/day. There were insufficient data using the model described in Chapter 3 to set a UL for arsenic and silicon.

ARSENIC

BACKGROUND INFORMATION

Function

There have been no studies to determine the nutritional importance of arsenic for humans. Although the metabolic function of arsenic is not well understood, one study in rats suggests that arsenic may have a role in the metabolism of methionine (Uthus and Poellot, 1992). Arsenic deprivation was associated with an increase in hepatic S-adenosyl-homocystine concentrations and a decrease in hepatic S-adenosyl-methionine concentrations. Arsenic deprivation has also been associated with impaired growth and abnormal reproduction in rats, hamsters, chicks, goats, and miniature pigs (Anke, 1986; Uthus, 1994). Arsenic has also been suggested to be involved with the regulation of gene expression (Meng and Meng, 1994). Arsenite is associated with changes in the methylation of core histones and therefore is active at the transcriptional level (Desrosiers and Tanguay, 1986).

Physiology of Absorption, Metabolism, and Excretion

The absorption of inorganic arsenic is related to the solubility of the compound ingested (Vahter, 1983). In humans, more than 90 percent of inorganic arsenite and arsenate from water is absorbed (Vahter, 1983), and approximately 60 to 70 percent of dietary arsenic is absorbed (Hopenhayn-Rich et al., 1993). Once absorbed, inorganic arsenic is transported to the liver where it is reduced to arsenite and then methylated. The majority of ingested arsenic is rapidly excreted in the urine. The proportion of the various forms of arsenic in urine can vary; however, the common forms present are inorganic arsenic, monomethylarsonic acid, dimethylarsinic acid, and trimethylated arsenic (Yamato, 1988).

FINDINGS BY LIFE STAGE AND GENDER GROUP

Because of the lack of human data to identify a biological role of arsenic in humans, neither an Estimated Average Requirement, Recommended Dietary Allowance, nor Adequate Intake were established.

INTAKE OF ARSENIC

Food Sources

Dairy products can contribute as much as 31 percent of arsenic in the diet; meat, poultry, fish, grains and cereal products collectively contribute approximately 56 percent (Mahaffey et al., 1975). Based on a national survey conducted in six Canadian cities from 1985 to 1988, it was reported that foods containing the highest concentrations of arsenic were fish (1,662 ng/g), meat and poultry (24.3 ng/g), bakery goods and cereals (24.5 ng/g), and fats and oils (19 ng/g) (Dabeka et al., 1993). The substantial portion of arsenic present in fish is in the organic form. The major contributors of inorganic arsenic are raw rice (74 ng/g), flour (11 ng/g), grape juice (9 ng/g), and cooked spinach (6 ng/g) (Schoof et al., 1999).

Dietary Intake

Results of the analysis of 265 core foods conducted by the Food and Drug Administration (1991–1997), and analysis of foods and intake data from the U.S. Department of Agriculture Continuing Survey of Food Intakes by Individuals (1994–1996), indicate that the intakes of arsenic for all age groups ranged from 0.5 to 0.81 µg/ kg/day (Gunderson, 1995) and that the median intake of arsenic by adult men and by women was approximately 2.0 to 2.9 µg/day and 1.7 to 2.1 µg/day, respectively (Appendix Table E-2). Adams and coworkers (1994) reported lower intakes for adults (23 to 58 µg/day) from 1982 to 1991. There was not a marked difference in the arsenic consumption between various age groups. Gartrell and coworkers (1985) reported a similar mean U.S. intake of arsenic of 62 µg/day, and Tao and Bolger (1999) reported intakes ranging from 28 to 72 µg/day for adults from 1987 to 1988.

Data on the concentration of arsenic in human milk are limited; however, studies have reported mean concentrations ranging from 0.2 to 6 µg/kg wet weight (Byrne et al., 1983; Dang et al., 1983; Grimanis et al., 1979).

TOLERABLE UPPER INTAKE LEVELS

The Tolerable Upper Intake Level (UL) is the highest level of daily nutrient intake that is likely to pose no risk of adverse health effects for almost all individuals. Although members of the general population should be advised not to routinely exceed the UL, intake above the UL may be appropriate for investigation within well-controlled clinical trials. Clinical trials of doses above the UL should not be discouraged, as long as subjects participating in these trials have signed informed consent documents regarding possible toxicity and as long as these trials employ appropriate safety monitoring of trial subjects. Arsenic is currently under investigation for the treatment of leukemia (Look, 1998).

Arsenic occurs in both inorganic and organic forms, with the inorganic forms that contain trivalent arsenite (III) or pentavalent arsenate (V) being of the greatest toxicological significance (Chan and Huff, 1997). No data on the possible adverse effects of organic arsenic compounds in food were found. Because the organic forms are usually less toxic than the inorganic (ATSDR, 1998), adverse effects of inorganic forms are described. It is unclear whether risk assessments should be developed for specific groups of inorganic arsenic compounds.

Adverse Effects

The adverse effects of arsenic in humans have been identified with exposure to inorganic arsenic, although in animals higher exposures to organic arsenic produces some of the same effects as lower exposures to inorganic arsenic (ATSDR, 1998). There is some evidence that arsenic III may be more toxic than arsenic V (Byron et al., 1967; Maitani et al., 1987). Animals do not appear to be good quantitative models for inorganic arsenic toxicity in humans (ATSDR, 1998), perhaps because of the species diversity of erythrocyte-binding of arsenic and inorganic arsenic methyltransferase activity, a detoxification mechanism (Aposhian, 1997; Goering et al., 1999).

Acute Effects

Inorganic arsenic is an established human poison. Ingestion of doses greater than 10 mg/kg/day leads to encephalopathy and gastrointestinal symptoms (Civantos et al., 1995; Levin-Scherz et al., 1987; Quatrehomme et al., 1992). Poisoning also occurs with arsenic doses of 1 mg/kg/day or greater and can be accompanied by anemia and hepatotoxicity (Armstrong et al., 1984; Fincher and Koerker, 1987).

Arsenicism

Chronic intake of 10 µg/kg/day or greater of inorganic arsenic produces arsenicism, a condition characterized by alteration of skin pigmentation and keratosis (NRC, 1999). In some regions, an occlusive peripheral vascular disease also occurs resulting in gangrene of the extremities, especially of the feet, thus termed blackfoot disease (Engel and Receveur, 1993; Tseng, 1977). It has been hypothesized that zinc deficiency may exacerbate the toxicity of arsenic (Engel and Receveur, 1993). Malnutrition has been associated with an increased risk of blackfoot disease (Yang and Blackwell, 1961). Because arsenicism may be associated with arsenic intakes higher than those causing other adverse effects (see "Carcinogenicity"), it was not selected as a critical adverse effect to set a UL.

Peripheral Neuropathy

Intermediate and chronic exposures of arsenic up to levels of 11 mg/L of water are associated with symmetrical peripheral neuropathy (Franzblau and Lilis, 1989; Huang et al., 1985; Wagner et al., 1979). However, in some populations exposures of 5 mg/L of water did not result in clinical or subclinical neuropathy (Kreiss et al., 1983).

Developmental Toxicity

Developmental effects in humans have not been demonstrated (ATSDR, 1998; NRC, 1999). In the hamster, single intragastric doses of 1.4 mg of arsenic/kg to pregnant females led to fetal mortality (Hood and Harrison, 1982). In the mouse, fetal mortality and teratogenicity were produced by single intragastric doses of 6 to 7 mg/kg (Hood, 1972) and 11 mg/kg (Hood and Bishop, 1972); oral doses of 23 mg/kg (Baxley et al., 1981) had the same effects. In the rat, an intraperitoneal dose of 5 to 10 mg/kg produced a high percentage of malformed fetuses (Beaudoin, 1974).

Genotoxicity

Sodium arsenite induced point mutations in two strains of *Escherichia coli* WP2; negative results were obtained in a *recA* strain. Arsenic trichloride and sodium arsenite gave positive results in a *rec* assay in *Bacillus subtilis* (Nishioka, 1975). Positive results were also obtained in this assay with arsenic trioxide and arsenic pentoxide (Kanematsu et al., 1980). Sodium methanearsonates were negative in this assay (Shirasu et al., 1976).

Potassium and sodium arsenite caused mitotic arrest and chromosomal aberrations, including chromatid gaps, breaks, translocations, dicentrics, and rings in cultured human peripheral leukocytes and human diploid fibroblast WI.38 and MRC5 lines (Oppenheim and Fishbein, 1965; Paton and Allison, 1972).

Some of the mutagenic effects of arsenic may be a consequence of the formation of reactive oxygen species (Hei et al., 1998).

Carcinogenicity

Ingestion of inorganic arsenic is associated with risk of cancers of the skin, bladder, and lung (IARC, 1980, 1987; NRC, 1999). Increased risks of other cancers such as kidney and liver have also been reported, but the strength of the association is not great (NRC, 1999). There are no studies of cancer in humans after exposure to organic arsenicals (ATSDR, 1998).

Most studies of a positive association with cancer involve intake of inorganic arsenic in drinking water. A large-scale survey of 40,421 inhabitants (19,269 men and 21,152 women) of an area on the southwest coast of Taiwan, where artesian well water with a high concentration of arsenic was consumed for more than 45 years, found that the overall prevalence rates for skin cancer, hyperpigmentation, and keratosis were 10.6, 183.5, and 71.0/1,000, respectively (Tseng et al., 1968). They also found that the male-to-female ratio for skin cancer was 2.9:1 and 1.1:1 for hyperpigmentation and keratosis. The prevalence appeared to increase progressively with age for all three conditions, although there was a decline in cancer and hyperpigmentation in women older than 69 years of age. The prevalence rates for skin cancer, hyperpigmentation, and keratosis showed an ascending gradient which correlated with the arsenic content of the well water. Blackfoot disease had an overall prevalence rate of 8.9/1,000 and, similar to skin cancer, displayed a dose-response relationship with the amount of arsenic in the well water. There was a significantly high association of blackfoot disease with hyperpigmentation, keratosis, and skin cancer.

The risk of bladder cancer in Taiwan was increased with intake of arsenic from water of 10 µg/kg/day (Chen et al., 1992). This increased risk has been confirmed in studies from Japan (Tsuda et al., 1995), Argentina (Hopenhayn-Rich et al., 1996), and Chile (Smith et al., 1998). Studies in U.S. populations exposed to arsenic in drinking water have not identified cancer increases (Morton et al., 1976; Southwick et al., 1981; Valentine et al., 1992).

These epidemiological associations have to some extent been replicated in animal experiments (Simeonova et al., 2000; Yamamoto et al., 1995). However, the mechanisms of arsenic carcinogenesis are not established, but may involve genetic effects (Goering et al., 1999) or perturbation of cellular signaling pathways (Simeonova et al., 2000).

Summary

Clearly, high intakes of inorganic arsenic are associated with various toxicities, including increased risks of several cancers with chronic exposure to high levels in drinking water. There is no evidence linking organic arsenic in food to any adverse effect, including cancer. Since there is no evidence available to define the mechanisms of arsenic carcinogenesis and no data to support a threshold, it is not possible to establish a health-based level of inorganic arsenic in drinking water and food. It should be noted that a recent report of the National Research Council recommended a downward revision from the current maximum contaminant level for arsenic in drinking water of 50 µg/L (NRC, 1999). Because organic forms of arsenic are less toxic than inorganic forms, any increased health risk from intake of organic arsenic from food products such as fish is unlikely.

Intake Assessment

The highest concentrations of arsenic in food are found in marine products, but these are in the organic form, usually arsenobetaine, which is not toxic. Various sources of exposure to inorganic arsenic, as arsenates or arsenites, exist. Occupational exposure to inorganic forms of arsenic occurs primarily by inhalation. Arsenic in drinking water is predominantly the trivalent and pentavalent forms as salts (EPA, 1988). Arsenic is also being used in the treatment of leukemias (Konig et al., 1997; Look, 1998).

The median intake of arsenic by men and by women was approximately 2.0 to 2.9 µg/day and 1.7 to 2.1 µg/day, respectively (Appendix Table E-2). Adams and coworkers (1994) reported lower intakes for adults (23 to 58 µg/day) from 1982 to 1991. The level of inorganic arsenic in water was about 2 µg/L (ATSDR, 1998). The drinking water for about 98 percent of the U.S. population was below 10 µg/L (Chappell et al., 1997). The U.S. Environmental Protection Agency (EPA) has a maximum contaminant level (MCL) of 50 µg/L for water supplies in the United States (EPA, 1975). However, the agency recently proposed a much lower MCL of 5 µg/L for arsenic in drinking water and is seeking comments on MCLs ranging from 3 to 20 µg/L (EPA, 2000). The EPA expects to promulgate a new, lower MCL in the near future. The average arsenic content of mineral drinking water in European countries is 21 µg/L (Zielhuis and Wibomo, 1984).

Risk Characterization

Although no UL was set for arsenic, there is no justification for adding arsenic to food and there may be a risk of adverse effects with consumption of organic arsenic in food or with intake of inorganic arsenic in water supplies at the current MCL of 50 µg/L in the United States. Substantial numbers of individuals in North America, however, are exposed to arsenic levels exceeding the MCL (Chappell et al., 1997; Grantham and Jones, 1977; Kreiss et al., 1983). Inhalation exposure occurs in occupational settings such as smelters and chemical plants, where the predominant form of airborne arsenic is arsenic trioxide dust (ATSDR, 1998).

RESEARCH RECOMMENDATIONS FOR ARSENIC

• A better understanding of species differences in biotransformation of arsenic and toxicity.

• The role of arsenic in methyl metabolism and genetic expression; identification of a reliable indicator of arsenic status in humans.

• Because relatively low serum arsenic concentrations have been associated with vascular diseases and central nervous system injury, more systematic investigation of the possible role of arsenic in these disorders.

BORON

BACKGROUND INFORMATION

Function

Of the five minerals discussed in this chapter, boron has received the most extensive study of its possible nutritional importance for animals and humans. Still, the collective body of evidence has yet to establish a clear biological function for boron in humans. There is evidence that boron is required by vascular plants and some microorganisms. The only known boron-containing compounds in nature are organoboron complexes from plants, some of which may have antibiotic properties (Hunt, 1998; Nielsen, 1997). Principles of bioinorganic chemistry predict that boron, which is primarily in the form of boric acid, $B(OH)_3$, at physiological pH, binds to cis-diols, perhaps with some specifically, and forms condensation products that are moderately labile in aqueous solutions (da Silva and Williams, 1991). The latter could theoretically provide stability to diol-rich molecules such as polysaccharides or steroids. Boron can act as an inhibitor of activity for a wide variety of enzymes in vitro (Hunt, 1998). However, no boron-containing enzyme has been identified.

In higher animals, boron has not been shown to have a sufficiently definitive pattern of effects to establish a function. Embryonic defects related to boron depletion have been reported for zebra fish (Rowe and Eckhert, 1999), frogs (Fort et al., 1998, 1999), and trout (Eckhert, 1998), and they suggest a function for boron in reproduction and development. However, boron-related developmental defects have not been found consistently in rodent models (Lanoue et al., 1998, 1999). Physiological effects, including changes in blood glucose and triglyceride concentrations and abnormal calcitriol ($1,25,OH_2D_3$) metabolism or function have been reported in boron-deficient chicks that have a concomitant vitamin D deficiency (Hunt, 1996). Higher insulin secretion from the pancreas of boron-deprived chicks has also been reported (Bakken, 1995). However, many of these studies found effects of boron only in the presence of secondary nutritional stressors, such as vitamin D deficiency.

Metabolism of vitamin D and estrogen, as measured by plasma metabolites, macromineral (especially calcium) metabolism, and immune function have been proposed as related to a function for boron in humans (Nielsen, 1998; Nielsen and Penland, 1999; Samman et al., 1998). Findings supporting these possible functions also have come from studies where another nutritional stressor was present or effects have not been consistently demonstrated. In one laboratory, several dietary boron deprivation studies in both rats and humans have consistently found an effect of boron intake on brain electrophysiology and, in humans, on performance of tasks measuring eye-hand coordination, attention, and short-term memory (Penland, 1998). However, these possible functions of boron have yet to be studied and confirmed by other laboratories.

Physiology of Absorption, Metabolism, and Excretion

Studies with animals and humans indicate that about 90 percent of boron is absorbed in the normal intake range (Hunt and Stoecker, 1996; Sutherland et al., 1998). Most dietary boron is hydrolyzed within the gut to yield $B(OH)_3$ which, as a neutral compound, is easily absorbed. The mechanism of boron absorption has not been studied, but a passive, nonmediated diffusion process involving $B(OH)_3$ is likely (da Silva and Williams, 1991). Some evidence for boron homeostasis exists. In a 42-day study in men with a boron intake average of 3.73 mg/day, urinary loss was 3.20 mg/day (86 percent of intake), whereas urinary boron loss was less when the boron intake was less than 3.20 mg/day and loss was more when the intake was more than that amount (Sutherland et al., 1998). In a study with postmenopausal women, 89 percent of boron from a low-boron diet (0.36 mg/day from food and 2.87 µg/day from a supplement) was excreted in the urine and 3 percent in the feces (Hunt and Stoecker, 1996). Other metabolic studies do not support homeostatic control. For example, urinary excretion was 86 and 84 percent when boron intake was 2.2 and 10 mg/day, respectively (Samman et al., 1998).

Boron chemistry suggests it is transported in the blood as $B(OH)_3$. Specifically, because boron forms labile complexes in aqueous solution, transport is probably as free boric acid rather than a complex (da Silva and Williams, 1991). The blood boron concentration is dependent on dietary intake as primarily shown by animal studies (Price et al., 1998; Samman et al., 1998). This reflects the relatively small boron pool that blood represents as well as efficient absorption and excretion. The excretory form of boron has not been studied. As a neutral molecule, blood borate should have high fractional renal clearance and easily enter the glomerular filtrate.

FINDINGS BY LIFE STAGE AND GENDER GROUP

There is evidence supporting a biological role of boron in some microroganisms. In higher animals, boron has been shown to have a role in reproduction and development. The collective body of evidence, however, has yet to establish a clear biological function for boron in humans. Therefore, neither an Estimated Average Requirement, Recommended Dietary Allowance, nor Adequate Intake was established for boron.

INTAKE OF BORON

Food Sources

Hunt and coworkers (1991) reported that the highest concentrations of boron were found in fruit-based beverages and products, tubers, and legumes. Depending on the geographic location, water could contribute a major portion of the dietary boron. Negligible or minimal amounts (less than 0.100 µg/g) were found in animal products, certain grain products, condiments, and confections. Similar findings were reported by Anderson and coworkers (1994). Meacham and Hunt (1998) reported that the ten foods with the highest concentration of boron were avocado, peanut butter, peanuts, prune and grape juice, chocolate powder, wine, pecans, and granola raisin and raisin bran cereals. Rainey and coworkers (1999), however, examined both the content and total food consumption (amount and frequency), reporting that the five major contributors of boron were coffee, milk, apples, dried beans, and potatoes, which collectively accounted for 27 percent of the dietary boron consumption. Although coffee and milk are low in boron, they were the top contributors due to the volumes consumed.

Dietary Intake

U.S. boron consumption was assessed by use of the Boron Nutrient Data Base linked to 2-day food records from respondents to the Third National Health and Nutrition Examination Survey (NHANES III) (Appendix Table C-12) and the Continuing Survey of Food Intakes by Individuals (CFSII) (Appendix Table D-1). In NHANES III, the median consumption of boron ranged from 0.75 to 0.96 mg/day for school-aged children and from 0.87 to 1.35 mg/day for adults. Median consumption of boron by pregnant women was 1.05 mg/day in NHANES III and 1.08 mg/day in CFSII. The median consumption of boron by lactating women was 1.27 mg/day in CFSII.

Anderson (1992) reported that the mean boron concentration of human milk from lactating women up to 5 months postpartum was 0.27 µg/L. Based on a mean secretion of 0.78 L/day of milk (Chapter 2), the amount of boron secreted is 0.21 mg/day.

Intake from Supplements

Information from NHANES III on supplement intake of boron is given in Appendix Table C-13. The adult median boron intake from supplements was approximately 0.14 mg/day. Based on dietary intake data provided in Appendix Table C-12, the median intake of dietary and supplemental boron was approximately 1.0 to 1.5 mg/day for adults.

TOLERABLE UPPER INTAKE LEVELS

The Tolerable Upper Intake Level (UL) is the highest level of daily nutrient intake that is likely to pose no risk of adverse health effects for almost all individuals. Although members of the general population should be advised not to routinely exceed the UL, intake above the UL may be appropriate for investigation within well-controlled clinical trials. Clinical trials of doses above the UL should not be discouraged, as long as subjects participating in these trials have signed informed consent documents regarding possible toxicity and as long as these trials employ appropriate safety monitoring of trial subjects.

Hazard Identification

It should be noted that because some studies report doses of boron while others report doses of boric acid or borax, comparison of experiments is facilitated by expressing all doses as boron equivalents (e.g., boric acid dose × 0.175; borax dose × 0.113).

Adverse Effects

No data are available on adverse health effects from ingestion of large amounts of boron from food and water. According to case reports of poisoning incidents and accidental ingestions of boric acid and borax, these compounds exhibit low toxicity. Stokinger (1981) reported that the minimal lethal dose of boric acid from ingestion is 640 mg/kg/day. The potential lethal dose has been reported to be 15 to 20 g/day for adults and 3 to 6 g/day for infants; however, in an examination of 784 cases of boric acid ingestion, Litovitz and coworkers (1988) found minimal or no toxicity at these or higher intake levels. Initial symptoms include nausea, gastric discomfort, vomiting, and diarrhea. At higher doses, skin flushing, excitation, convulsions, depression, and vascular collapse have been reported.

Human Data. Most of the toxicity data on repeated administration of boron (as boric acid or borax) comes from studies in laboratory animals. However, from reports on the use of borates to treat epilepsy where doses between 1,000 mg/day of boric acid (2.5 mg/kg/day) to 25 g/day of boric tartrate (24.8 mg/kg/day) were administered chronically, toxicity was expressed as dermatitis, alopecia, anorexia, and indigestion (Culver and Hubbard, 1996). On the basis of their review of the human data in adults, Culver and Hubbard (1996) reported no adverse effects at chronic intakes of 2.5 mg/kg/day (about 1 g of boric acid). On the basis of nine cases involving infants (Gordon et al., 1973; O'Sullivan and Taylor, 1983), there does not appear to be an increased sensitivity of response to chronic exposure of boron compounds.

Genotoxicity. On the basis of existing data, genotoxicity is not an area of concern after exposure of humans to boron compounds (ATSDR, 1992; Dieter, 1994).

Reproductive and Developmental Effects in Animals. Although not observed in humans, animal studies have shown that high doses of borax or boric acid produce adverse effects in the testis and affect male fertility (IPCS, 1998). Also, adverse effects have been found in the developing fetus (Heindel et al., 1992; IPCS, 1998; Price et al., 1996a). Effects on the testis have been observed in three species— rats, mice, and dogs—after supplementation with boric acid or borates in feed or drinking water (Fail et al., 1990, 1991; Green et al., 1973; Ku et al., 1993; Lee et al., 1978; Weir and Fisher, 1972). The effects tend to be similar in all three species and include inhibition of spermiation (release of spermatozoa into seminiferous tubule), loss of germ cells, changes in epididymal sperm morphology and caput sperm reserves, testicular atrophy, and decreased serum testosterone levels. Doses of 29 mg/kg/day in dogs and 58.5 mg/kg/day in rats have resulted in adverse reproductive effects. A comparison of the lowest-observed-adverse-effect levels (LOAELs) and no-observed-adverse-effect levels (NOAELs) for the key studies on reproduction is given in Table 13-1.

Pharmacokinetics. The pharmacokinetics of boron are very similar in animals and humans. There are several recent reviews of the available studies (Dourson et al., 1998; IPCS, 1998; Moore, 1997; Murray, 1998), and a summary of the key findings is presented here.

There is no evidence of boron accumulation in soft tissues of humans (Murray, 1998). In rats, boron increased more in bone than in plasma (Ku et al., 1991). Although methodological differences between studies preclude a clear-cut, cross-species comparison of blood boron concentrations in animals and humans at similar doses, IPCS (1998) reported a preliminary comparison between humans and rats after oral intakes of boron from diet or drinking water. Between 0.01 and 100 mg/kg/day, very similar blood levels were achieved at comparable intakes, further evidence that the kinetics of boron in humans and rats are alike.

Boron is rapidly excreted unchanged in the urine of humans and rodents regardless of the route of administration. In humans, the half-life for elimination was approximately 21 hours for both intravenously (Jansen et al., 1984a) and orally (Jansen et al., 1984b) administered boric acid. By using the data from Ku and coworkers (1991) and assuming first-order kinetics, the half-life in rats has been calculated in the range of 14 to 19 hours. As noted by Murray (1998) and Dourson and coworkers (1998), rats have mean glomerular filtration rates for boric acid three to four times that of humans, which could account for the small differences in blood (and, therefore, soft tissue) concentrations of boron noted by IPCS (1998).

Other Effects. Increased mortality was observed in mice fed dietary boric acid for periods of 13 weeks at boron levels of 563 mg/kg/day in females and 776 mg/kg/day in males (Dieter, 1994). Minimal to mild extramedullary hematopoiesis was noted at all doses for both sexes, and hyperkeratosis and hyperplasia of the forestomach also occurred at the highest doses for both sexes. Testicular atrophy or

TABLE 13-1 Ranking of Reproductive and Developmental Effects of Boron[a] by Increasing Dose

Reference	Species/ Duration[b]	Dose (mg boron/ kg body weight/d)[c]	Effect[d]
Price et al., 1996b	SD rat/gd 0–20	9.6	NOAEL for developmental effects immediately preterm
Price et al., 1996b	SD rat/gd 0–20	12.9	NOAEL for developmental effects measured at weaning
Heindel et al., 1992	SD rat/gd 0–20	13.3 13.6	LOAEL for reduced fetal weight, increased rib malformations/variations
Weir and Fisher, 1972	Male SD rat/ multigeneration	17.5	NOAEL for male sterility, testicular atrophy
Fail et al., 1991	CD-1 mouse/ multigeneration	19.2	LOAEL for reduced sperm motility, reduced F_2 pup weight
Price et al., 1996b	SD rat/gd 0–20	25.4	LOAEL for increased short rib XIII at weaning
Ku et al., 1993	Male SD rat/ 63 days	26	LOAEL for mild inhibited sperm release
Weir and Fisher, 1972	Male beagle dogs/ 2 years	29	Altered testis weight and histopathology LOAEL (reported NOAEL 8.8)
Price et al., 1996a	NZ white rabbits/ gd 6–19	21.9/43.7	NOAEL/LOAEL for decreased fetal body weight, increased fetal cardiovascular malformations and maternal toxicity
Heindel et al., 1992	CD-1 mouse/ gd 0–17	43 79	NOAEL for mouse developmental toxicity LOAEL for decreased fetal body weight
Ku et al., 1993	Male SD rat/ 63 days	52	LOAEL for testicular atrophy

[a] Administered as boric acid.
[b] SD = Sprague-Dawley rats, gd = gestational days, NZ = New Zealand.
[c] Boric acid was converted to boron.
[d] NOAEL = no-observed-adverse-effect level, LOAEL = lowest-observed-adverse-effect level.
SOURCE: IPCS (1998). Published here with permission of the World Health Organization.

degeneration was observed at doses of 141 mg/kg/day. These findings confirmed the earlier studies by Weir and Fisher (1972) in which rats fed 88 mg/kg/day of boron as borax or boric acid for 90 days developed testicular atrophy.

Summary

Based on the considerations of causality, relevance, and the quality and completeness of the database in animals, reproductive and developmental effects were selected as the critical endpoint on which to base a UL for adults. Because no data are available on adverse reproductive effects in humans from the consumption of large amounts of boron from food and water, animal data were utilized to estimate the UL. The following factors support the use of the laboratory animal studies listed in Table 13-1 to assess the developmental and reproductive risks from boron exposure in humans: (1) boric acid has been shown to cause developmental effects in four species of animals, (2) the toxicity of boric acid and borax correlates with their elemental boron content under physiological conditions, (3) the organs that are sensitive to the acute systemic effects of boron in humans and animals are similar, (4) the pattern of tissue distribution and excretion of boron is similar in animals and humans, and (5) the chronic effects of boron observed in mice, rats, and dogs and the effective doses are similar.

Dose-Response Assessment

Adults

Data Selection. In the absence of human data pertaining to a dose-response relationship, the animal data sets reporting developmental abnormalities are shown in Table 13-1. The studies showing developmental abnormalities at the lowest levels of intake are in dogs (Weir and Fisher, 1972) and rats (Price et al., 1996b). However, the study in dogs was not used directly in this risk assessment of boron due to problems in the design (few animals per treatment group and lack of information on food intake). The study of Price and coworkers (1996b) is considered the critical study to assess the risks to humans from exposure to boron.

Identification of a NOAEL and LOAEL. In the study by Price and coworkers (1996b), boric acid was fed to time-mated rats (60 per treatment group) from gestational days 0 to 20 at dosages of 3.3,

6.3, 9.6, 13.3, or 25 mg/kg/day. Maternal body weight did not differ among groups during gestation or lactation, and weight gain was not affected by the amount of boron in the diet. The most sensitive parameter of developmental toxicity was decreased fetal weights at gestational day 20, with significantly decreased fetal weights found only in the 13.3 and 25 mg/kg/day groups. Thus, a NOAEL of 9.6 mg/kg/day and a LOAEL of 13.3 mg/kg/day were reported.

In an earlier study in rats using a very similar experimental design, Heindel and coworkers (1992) reported an increase in fetal malformations with boric acid at dosages of 13.6, 28.5, and 57.7 mg/kg/day from gestational days 0 to 20. The most common malformations were enlargement of lateral ventricles in the brain, shortening of rib XIII, and wavy ribs. Although a LOAEL was found at the lowest dose tested (13.6 mg/kg/day), it is similar to the LOAEL of 13.3 mg/kg/day reported by Price and coworkers (1996b), a finding that provides additional support for the dose-response relationship for developmental toxicity as the critical effect.

Uncertainty Assessment. Five expert groups have assessed the risk to humans from boron using the NOAEL from Price and coworkers (1996b), and uncertainty factors (UFs) vary between 25 and 60 (Becking and Chen, 1998). There do not appear to be sufficient data to justify lowering the degree of uncertainty for extrapolating from experimental animals to humans from the 10 that is often used for nonessential chemicals. Thus, the usual value of 10 was selected. In view of the expected similarity in pharmokinetics among humans, however, a UF of 3 was chosen for intraspecies variability. These two UFs are multiplied to yield a UF of 30.

Derivation of a UL. The NOAEL for developmental effects in rats is 9.6 mg/kg/day. The UL for boron is calculated by dividing the NOAEL of 9.6 mg/kg/day by the UF of 30, resulting in an UL of 0.3 mg/kg/day. This value was multiplied by the average of the reference body weights for adult women, 61 kg, from Chapter 1 (Table 1-1). The resulting UL for adults is rounded to 20 mg/day.

$$UL = \frac{NOAEL}{UF} = \frac{9.6 \text{ mg/kg/day}}{30} = 0.32 \text{ mg/kg/day} \times 61 \text{ kg} \cong 20 \text{ mg/day}$$

Boron UL Summary, Ages 19 Years and Older

UL for Adults
  ≥ 19 years   **20 mg/day of boron**

Other Life Stage Groups

Infants. For infants, the UL was judged not determinable because of insufficient data on adverse effects in this age group and concern about the infant's ability to handle excess amounts. To prevent high levels of intake, the only source of intake for infants should be from food and formula.

Children and Adolescents. There are no reports of boron toxicity in children and adolescents. Given the dearth of information, the UL values for children and adolescents are extrapolated from those established for adults. Thus, the adult UL of 20 mg/day of boron was adjusted for children and adolescents on the basis of relative body weight as described in Chapter 2 using reference weights from Chapter 1 (Table 1-1). Values have been rounded.

Pregnancy and Lactation. Because the UL is based on adverse reproductive effects in animals and because there are no reports of boron toxicity in lactating females, the UL for pregnant and lactating females is the same as that for the nonpregnant and nonlactating female.

Boron UL Summary, Ages 0 through 18 Years, Pregnancy, Lactation

UL for Infants
    0–12 months   **Not possible to establish; source of intake should be from food and formula only**

UL for Children
    1–3 years   **3 mg/day of boron**
    4–8 years   **6 mg/day of boron**
    9–13 years   **11 mg/day of boron**

UL for Adolescents
    14–18 years   **17 mg/day of boron**

UL for Pregnancy
    14–18 years   **17 mg/day of boron**
    19–50 years   **20 mg/day of boron**

UL for Lactation
    14–18 years   **17 mg/day of boron**
    19–50 years   **20 mg/day of boron**

Intake Assessment

Humans can be exposed to boron from consumption of food, dietary supplements, and drinking water from natural, municipal, or bottled sources. Airborne boron contributes very little to the daily exposure of the general population. For humans not taking supplements, diet is the major source of boron followed by the intake from drinking water.

The ninety-fifth percentile dietary intake of boron in the United States is approximately 2.3 mg/day for men, 1.6 to 2.0 mg/day for women, 2.0 mg/day for pregnant women (Appendix Table C-12), 2.7 mg/day for vegetarian males, and 4.2 mg/day for vegetarian females (Rainey et al., 1999). These dietary intakes are slightly higher than those estimated by Meacham and Hunt (1998). The average intake of supplemental boron at the ninety-fifth percentile is approximately 0.4 mg/day for adults (Appendix Table C-13). A consumption of 1 L/day of municipal drinking water in the United States contributes 0.005 to 2 mg/day (mean of 0.2 mg/day) of boron (EPA, 1987), and bottled water can contribute an average of 0.75 mg/day (Allen et al., 1989). Percutaneous absorption of boron from consumer products through intact skin has been shown to contribute very little to the total daily intake (Wester et al., 1998).

At the ninety-fifth percentile, intake of boron from the diet and supplements is approximately 2.8 mg/day. Adding to that a maximum intake from water of 2 mg/day gives a total intake of less than 5 mg/day boron at this percentile.

Risk Characterization

At the ninety-fifth percentile intake, no segment of the U.S. population has a total (dietary, water, and supplemental) intake of boron greater than 5 mg/day (Appendix Tables C-13 and D-1). Those taking body-building supplements could consume an additional 1.5 to 20 mg/day (Moore, 1997). Therefore this supplemental intake may exceed the UL of 20 mg/day.

RESEARCH RECOMMENDATIONS FOR BORON

• The relationship between dietary boron and vitamin D metabolism; specifically, does boron influence the half-life of functional vitamin D metabolites and calcium metabolism as it relates to bone mineralization?

• The possible influence of boron on estrogen metabolism and function, particularly biological half-life, receptor-ligand inter-actions, and estrogen-inducible gene expression as related to bone mineral density.

• Studies of the possible role of boron in human neurophysio-logical and cognitive function that include delineation of a bio-chemical or other physiological basis for this function, in young as well as older populations.

NICKEL

BACKGROUND INFORMATION

Function

There have been no studies to determine the nutritional impor-tance of nickel in humans, nor has a biochemical function been clearly demonstrated for nickel in higher animals or humans (Uthus and Seaborn, 1996). Nickel may serve as a cofactor or structural component of specific metalloenzymes of various functions, includ-ing hydrolysis and redox reactions and gene expression (Andrews et al., 1988; Kim et al., 1991; Lancaster, 1988; Przybyla et al., 1992). Nickel may also serve as a cofactor facilitating ferric iron absorption or metabolism (Nielsen, 1985). Nickel is an essential trace element in animals, as demonstrated by deficiency signs reported in several species. Rats deprived of nickel exhibit retarded growth, low hemo-globin concentrations (Schnegg and Kirchgessner, 1975), and im-paired glucose metabolism (Nielsen, 1996). Nickel may interact with the vitamin B_{12}- and folic-acid dependent pathway of methionine synthesis from homocysteine (Uthus and Poellot, 1996).

Physiology of Absorption, Metabolism, and Excretion

The absorption of nickel is affected by the presence of certain foods and substances including milk, coffee, tea, orange juice, and ascorbic acid. Plasma ^{62}Ni was shown to peak between 1.5 and 2.5 hours after the ingestion of the stable isotope by four fasted, healthy men and women (Patriarca et al., 1997). The investigators reported no evidence that absorbed nickel was excreted via the gut. The percentage of nickel absorbed ranged from 29 to 40 percent. Uri-nary excretion of the ^{62}Ni dose ranged from 51 to 82 percent of the absorbed dose. Solomons and coworkers (1982) investigated absorp-tion of nickel ingested with food and found that the presence of food significantly decreased absorption. The absorption of dietary nickel is typically less than 10 percent.

Nickel is transported in blood bound primarily to albumin (Tabata and Sarkar, 1992). Although most tissues and organs do not significantly accumulate nickel, in humans the thyroid and adrenal glands have relatively high nickel concentrations (132 to 141 μg/kg dry weight) (Rezuke et al., 1987). Most organs contain less than 50 μg of nickel/kg dry weight.

Because of the poor absorption of nickel, the majority of ingested nickel is excreted in the feces. The majority of absorbed nickel is excreted in the urine with minor amounts excreted in sweat and bile.

FINDINGS BY LIFE STAGE AND GENDER GROUP

Nickel may serve as a cofactor or structural component of certain metalloenzymes and facilitate iron absorption or metabolism in microorganisms. No studies to determine the biological role of nickel in higher animals or humans have been reported. Therefore, neither an Estimated Average Requirement, Recommended Dietary Allowance, nor Adequate Intake was established for nickel.

INTAKE OF NICKEL

Food Sources

Major contributors to nickel intake are mixed dishes and soups (19 to 30 percent), grains and grain products (12 to 30 percent), vegetables (10 to 24 percent), legumes (3 to 16 percent), and desserts (4 to 18 percent) (Pennington and Jones, 1987). In food commodity groups, nickel concentrations are highest in nuts and legumes (128 and 55 μg/100 g, respectively), followed by sweeteners, including chocolate milk powder and chocolate candy. Of 234 foods analyzed, 66 percent had nickel concentrations less than 10 μg/100 g and 91 percent had concentrations less than 40 μg/100 g. Seven of these foods contained greater than 100 μg/100 g including nuts, legumes, and items with chocolate (Pennington and Jones, 1987). Major contributors of nickel to the Canadian diet include meat and poultry (37 percent), bakery goods and cereals (19 percent), soups (15 percent), and vegetables (11 percent) (Dabeka and McKenzie, 1995). Nielsen and Flyvholm (1983) suggested that nickel intakes in Denmark could reach over 900 μg/day by the consumption of certain foods based on the nickel composition and level of consumption of oatmeal, legumes (including soybeans), nuts, cocoa, and chocolate. Cooking foods in stainless steel utensils can increase the nickel content if the foods are acidic (Christensen and Moller, 1978).

Dietary Intake

Based on the Food and Drug Administration Total Diet Study of 1984, the mean nickel consumption of infants and young children was 69 to 90 µg/day (Pennington and Jones, 1987). For adolescents, the median consumption was approximately 71 to 97 µg/day, and the median consumption for adults and the elderly was approximately 74 to 100 µg/day and 80 to 97 µg/day, respectively (Appendix Table E-7). On the basis of a national survey conducted in five Canadian cities from 1986 to 1988, Dabeka and McKenzie (1995) reported that average nickel consumption for children was 190 to 251 µg/day; for adolescents, 248 to 378 µg/day; and for all adults, 207 to 406 µg/day.

At 38 days postpartum, the mean nickel concentration in human milk was reported to be 1.2 ng/mL (Casey and Neville, 1987). Based on an average secretion of 0.78 L/day (see Chapter 2), the mean secretion of nickel in human milk is approximately 1 µg/day. According to a report by Dabeka (1989), the average intake of nickel by 0- to 12-month-old Canadian infants was 38 µg/day, taking into account human milk as well as formula consumption.

Intake from Supplements

Information from the Third National Health and Nutrition Examination Survey on supplemental use of nickel is given in Appendix Table C-22. The median supplemental intake for adult men and women was approximately 5 µg/day. Therefore, adults consume approximately 79 to 105 µg/day of nickel from diet and supplements.

TOLERABLE UPPER INTAKE LEVELS

The Tolerable Upper Intake Level (UL) is the highest level of daily nutrient intake that is likely to pose no risk of adverse health effects for almost all individuals. Although members of the general population should be advised not to routinely exceed the UL, intake above the UL may be appropriate for investigation within well-controlled clinical trials. Clinical trials of doses above the UL should not be discouraged, as long as subjects participating in these trials have signed informed consent documents regarding possible toxicity and as long as these trials employ appropriate safety monitoring of trial subjects. In addition, the UL is not meant to apply to individuals who are receiving nickel under medical supervision.

Hazard Identification

Adverse Effects

There is no evidence in humans of adverse effects associated with exposure to nickel through consumption of a normal diet. The UL derived here applies to excess nickel intake as soluble nickel salts.

Human Data. A few case reports have documented the acute effects of the ingestion of high doses of soluble nickel salts. Twenty workers who accidentally ingested 0.5 to 2.5 g of nickel as nickel sulfate and chloride hexahydrate in contaminated water developed nausea, abdominal pain, diarrhea, vomiting, and shortness of breath among other symptoms (Sunderman et al., 1988). Ten of these subjects were found to have altered hematological parameters. In one other case report, one subject who ingested approximately 50 µg/kg of nickel as nickel sulfate in water was reported to have developed transient hemianopsia at the time of peak serum concentrations (Sunderman et al., 1989). In persons with hypersensitivity to nickel, oral exposure has been reported to result in contact dermatitis-like symptoms (Gawkrodger et al., 1986).

Animal Data. In oral subchronic (ABC, 1988) and chronic (Ambrose et al., 1976) studies with rats, exposure to soluble nickel compounds has been associated with increased mortality, clinical signs of general systemic toxicity (e.g., lethargy, ataxia, irregular breathing, hypothermia, and salivation), decreased body weight gains, and changes in absolute and relative organ weights (kidney, liver, spleen, and heart). Fetotoxicity associated with oral exposure to nickel chloride and nickel sulfate has been reported in two separate two-generation studies (RTI, 1988; Smith et al., 1993) and in one three-generation study (Schroeder and Mitchner, 1971). Nickel salts also have been shown to interfere with the reproductive capacity of male rats (Hoey, 1966; Laskey and Phelps, 1991; Waltschewa et al., 1972).

Summary

On the basis of considerations of data quality, sensitivity of the toxicological endpoint, and relevance to human dietary exposure, general systemic toxicity—in the form of decreased body weight gain reported in the subchronic and chronic rat studies (ABC, 1988; Ambrose et al., 1976)—was selected as the critical endpoint on which to base the derivation of the UL. Other data (e.g., hypersensitivity in humans and carcinogenic effects associated with inhalation exposure) were not considered relevant to human dietary exposure.

Dose-Response Assessment

Adults

Data Selection. A subchronic rat gavage study (ABC, 1988) and a chronic rat dietary study (Ambrose et al., 1976) were considered most suitable for establishing an UL for human dietary exposure to soluble nickel salts.

Identification of a No-Observed-Adverse-Effect Level (NOAEL) and a Lowest-Observed-Adverse Effect Level (LOAEL). A NOAEL of 5 mg/kg/day was identified for both the 90-day subchronic gavage study (ABC, 1988) and the 2-year chronic dietary study (Ambrose et al., 1976) in rats. In both cases, the NOAEL was established on the basis of decreased body weight gains and signs of systemic toxicity at higher dose levels.

In the ABC (1988) study, groups of male and female CD rats were administered nickel chloride by water gavage at doses of 0, 5, 35, and 100 mg/kg/day for 3 months. On the basis of findings of decreased body weights, mortality, and clinical signs at higher doses, 5 mg/kg/day was concluded to be the NOAEL.

In the chronic study rats were administered nickel sulfate in the diet at doses of 0, 100, 1,000, or 2,500 ppm nickel (about 0, 5, 50, and 125 mg/kg/day) for a period of 2 years (Ambrose et al., 1976). Effects of treatment included reduced body weight gain in high-dose animals (125 mg/kg/day). Sporadic significant decreases in body weight gains were also recorded in the mid-dose group (50 mg/kg/day). Rats fed high- and mid-dose levels of nickel were reported to have significantly higher relative heart weights and lower relative liver weights. Although the study was suitable in design and conduct for use in establishing a UL for human dietary exposure to soluble nickel salts, poor survivorship in controls does raise some concern about its interpretability.

The results of three reproductive studies, one three-generation study (Schroeder and Mitchener, 1971) and two two-generation studies (RTI, 1988; Smith et al., 1993), suggest potential for feto-toxicity after oral exposure to soluble nickel salts. The lowest LOAEL identified by Smith and coworkers (1993) was 1.3 mg/kg/day of nickel based on the total number of dead pups and the percentage of dead pups per litter. The Schroeder and Mitchener (1971) study concluded that exposure to nickel at a concentration of 5 mg/L, or about 0.4 mg/kg body weight/day (assuming 8 ml/100 g body weight), was associated with increased neonatal death; however, these conclusions were based on the results of only five non-randomized matings and therefore were not considered valid for use in determining a LOAEL for human dietary exposure to soluble nickel salts. In fact, all of the reproduction studies either were flawed or their interpretation was hampered by their statistical design and methodological and data-reporting limitations, as well as by incon-sistencies in the reported dose-response relationships. As a result, these studies were not suitable for use in the establishment of a UL.

In summary, taken together, the oral subchronic and chronic rat studies support a NOAEL of 5 mg/kg body weight/day for soluble nickel salts. The selection of this NOAEL is in agreement with the NOAEL selected in the toxicological assessment of oral nickel expo-sure performed by the U.S. Environmental Protection Agency (EPA, 2000).

Uncertainty Assessment. When determining an uncertainty factor (UF) for nickel, several sources of uncertainty were selected to extrapolate from the NOAEL from the long-term rat study to the general population. The first UF of 10, which was used to extrapo-late from the rat study to humans, incorporated uncertainties about the nature of the dose-response curve for nickel toxicity and uncer-tainties about the sensitivity of rats as compared with humans in respect to nickel toxicity. The second UF of 10 was to account for potential variation within the human population, especially in re-gard to the potential for nickel to induce hypersensitivity reactions in sensitive individuals. The third UF of 3 was introduced because of concerns raised by studies on reproductive effects, namely, that nickel may be a reproductive toxin at levels lower than the NOAEL observed for the chronic rat study. These three UFs were multiplied to yield the ultimate UF of 300 that would accommodate the gener-al population including women who are pregnant or lactating.

Derivation of a UL. The NOAEL of 5 mg/kg body weight/day was divided by the UF of 300 to obtain a UL of 0.017 mg/kg body weight/day for adult humans. This figure was multiplied by the average of the reference body weights for adult women, 61 kg, from Chapter 1 (Table 1-1). The resulting UL for adults is rounded down to 1.0 mg/day.

$$UL = \frac{NOAEL}{UF} = \frac{5\ mg/kg/day}{300} = 0.017\ mg/kg/day \times 61\ kg \cong 1.0\ mg/day$$

Nickel UL Summary, Ages 19 years and Older

UL for Adults
   ≥ 19 years   **1.0 mg/day of soluble nickel salts**

Other Life Stage Groups

Infants. For infants, the UL was judged not determinable because of the lack of data on adverse effects in this age group and concern about the infant's ability to handle excess amounts. To prevent high levels of intake, the only source of intake for infants should be from food and formula.

Children and Adolescents. There are no reports of nickel toxicity in children and adolescents. The UL values for children and adolescents were extrapolated from those established for adults. Thus, the adult UL of 1.0 mg/day of soluble nickel salts was adjusted for children and adolescents on the basis of relative body weight as described in Chapter 2 using reference weights from Chapter 1 (Table 1-1).

Pregnancy and Lactation. No data were found that could be used to identify a NOAEL or LOAEL and derive a UL for pregnant and lactating women. Therefore, the ULs for pregnant and lactating women are the same as for the nonpregnant and nonlactating women.

Nickel UL Summary, Ages 0 through 18 Years, Pregnancy, Lactation

UL for Infants
   0–12 months   **Not possible to establish; source of intake should be from food and formula only**

UL for Children
    1–3 years   0.2 mg/day of soluble nickel salts
    4–8 years   0.3 mg/day of soluble nickel salts
    9–13 years   0.6 mg/day of soluble nickel salts

UL for Adolescents
    14–18 years   1.0 mg/day of soluble nickel salts

UL for Pregnancy
    14–18 years   1.0 mg/day of soluble nickel salts
    19–50 years   1.0 mg/day of soluble nickel salts

UL for Lactation
    14–18 years   1.0 mg/day of soluble nickel salts
    19–50 years   1.0 mg/day of soluble nickel salts

Special Considerations

Individuals with preexisting nickel hypersensitivity (from previous dermal exposure) and kidney dysfunction are distinctly susceptible to the adverse effects of excess nickel intake (Gawkrodger et al., 1986). These individuals may not be protected by the UL for nickel intake for the general population.

Intake Assessment

Based on the Food and Drug Administration Total Diet Study (Appendix Table E-7), 0.5 mg/day was the highest intake at the ninety-ninth percentile of nickel from food reported for any life stage and gender group; this was the reported intake for pregnant females. Nickel intake from supplements provided only 9.6 to 15 µg/day at the ninety-ninth percentile for all age and gender groups (Appendix Table C-22).

Risk Characterization

The risk of adverse effects resulting from excess intakes of nickel from food and supplements appears to be very low at the highest intakes noted above. Increased risks are likely to occur from environmental exposures or from the consumption of contaminated water.

RESEARCH RECOMMENDATIONS FOR NICKEL

• Identification and clear characterization of a biochemical function for nickel in humans; identification of a reliable indicator of nickel status for use in future studies of nickel deficiency.

• Further exploration of the possible role of nickel in vitamin B_{12} and folate metabolism, including whether nickel nutrition should be a concern for pregnant women or people at risk for cardiovascular disease.

SILICON

BACKGROUND INFORMATION

Function

A functional role for silicon in humans has not yet been identified. In view of the distribution of silicon in the body, as well as the biochemical changes that occur in bone with a silicon deficiency, silicon appears to be involved with the formation of bone in chickens and rats (Carlisle, 1980a, 1980b, 1981; Schwarz and Milne, 1972). Silicon contributes to prolylhydrolase activity, which is important for collagen formation (Carlisle, 1984). Chicks fed a silicon-deficient diet exhibited structural abnormalities of the skull and long-bone (Carlisle, 1984). Rats deprived of silicon showed decreased bone hydroxyproline and alkaline and acid phosphatases (Seaborn and Nielsen, 1993, 1994). Silicon has been suggested to have a preventive role in atherogenesis (Mancinella, 1991).

Physiology of Absorption, Metabolism, and Excretion

Findings that as much as 50 percent of ingested silicon is excreted in the urine (Kelsay et al., 1979) suggest that some dietary forms of silicon are well absorbed. Silicon in blood exists almost entirely as silicic acid and is not bound to proteins. Various connective tissues including the aorta, trachea, bone, tendons, and skin contain most of the silicon present in the body (Carlisle, 1984). Significantly higher serum silicon concentrations were seen in patients with chronic renal failure (46 µmol/L) compared to controls (21 µmol/L) (Dobbie and Smith, 1986).

In a study by Popplewell et al. (1998), 48 hours after ingestion of [32]Si, 36 percent of the dose was excreted in the urine and elimination appeared to be complete. This study, however, did not eliminate the possibility of longer-term retention of additional [32]Si. Goldwater (1936) reported daily silicon excretion levels for five subjects averaging 10 mg/day and ranging from 5 to 17 mg/day. Kelsay and coworkers (1979) studied 11 men fed low- and high-fiber diets and found their urinary silicon excretion to be 12 and 16 mg/day, respectively, amounts which were not significantly different.

FINDINGS BY LIFE STAGE AND GENDER GROUP

Silicon appears to be involved in the formation of collagen and bone in animals. A biological role of silicon in humans has not yet been identified. Therefore, neither an Estimated Average Requirement, Recommended Dietary Allowance, nor Adequate Intake was established for silicon.

INTAKE OF SILICON

Food Sources

Concentrations of silicon are higher in plant-based foods than in animal-derived food products. Based on the Food and Drug Administration Total Diet Study, beverages, including beer, coffee, and water, are the major contributors of silicon (55 percent), followed by grains and grain products (14 percent), and vegetables (8 percent) (Pennington, 1991). Refining reduces the silicon content in foods. Silicate additives that have been increasingly used as antifoaming and anticaking agents can raise the silicon content in foods; however, the bioavailability of these additives is low.

Dietary Intake

Based on the Total Diet Study, the mean intakes of silicon in adult men and women were 40 and 19 mg/day, respectively (Pennington, 1991). Appendix Table E-8 indicates that the daily median intakes of silicon for adult men and women ranged from approximately 14 to 21 mg/day. Kelsay and coworkers (1979) found intakes of 46 mg/day from a high-fiber diet and 21 mg/day from a low-fiber diet.

The mean concentration of silicon in human milk was reported to be 0.47 mg/L in women up to 5 months postpartum (Anderson, 1992). Based on the mean secretion of 0.78 L of human milk per day (Chapter 2), the mean intake of silicon by infants receiving human milk is approximately 0.37 mg/day.

Intake from Supplements

Information from the Third National Health and Nutrition Examination Survey on supplement use of silicon is provided in Appendix Table C-23. The median intake of supplemental silicon by adults was approximately 2 mg/day.

TOLERABLE UPPER INTAKE LEVELS

The Tolerable Upper Intake Level (UL) is the highest level of daily nutrient intake that is likely to pose no risk of adverse health effects for almost all individuals. Although members of the general population should be advised not to routinely exceed the UL, intake above the UL may be appropriate for investigation within well-controlled clinical trials. Clinical trials of doses above the UL should not be discouraged, as long as subjects participating in these trials have signed informed consent documents regarding possible toxicity and as long as these trials employ appropriate safety monitoring of trial subjects.

Hazard Identification

There is no evidence that silicon that occurs naturally in food and water produces adverse health effects. Limited reports indicate that magnesium trisilicate (6.5 mg of elemental silicon per tablet) when used as an antacid in large amounts for long periods (i.e., several years) may be associated with the development of urolithiasis due to the formation, in vivo, of silicon-containing stones (Haddad and Kouyoumdjian, 1986). Less than 30 cases of urolithiasis reported to be associated with intake of silicates (in the form of antacids) could be found even though antacids containing silicon have been sold since the 1930s.

Takizawa and coworkers (1988) examined the carcinogenicity of amorphous silica (SiO_2) given by the oral route to rats and mice for approximately 2 years. There was no evidence that orally administered silica induced tumors.

Dose-Response Assessment

There are no adequate data demonstrating a no-observed-adverse-effect level (NOAEL) for silicon. Apart from scattered reports of silicate-induced urolithiasis, said to be associated with antacids, the limited toxicity data on silicon suggest that typical levels of intake have no risk of inducing adverse effects for the general population. Due to lack of data indicating adverse effects of silicon, it is not possible to establish a UL.

RESEARCH RECOMMENDATIONS FOR SILICON

• The physiological role of silicon and how this role relates to human health.

• The possible role of silicon in atherosclerosis and hypertension, several bone disorders, Alzheimer's disease, and other conditions common to the elderly because of the prevalence and cost of these disorders.

• The determination of a reliable indicator of silicon status.

VANADIUM

BACKGROUND INFORMATION

Function

A functional role for vanadium in higher animals and humans has not yet been identified. Vanadium mimics insulin and stimulates cell proliferation and differentiation (Heyliger et al., 1985; Nielsen and Uthus, 1990). Vanadium inhibits various ATPases, phosphatases, and phosphoryl-transfer enzymes (Nielsen, 1985). The response of thyroid peroxidase to changing dietary iodine concentrations has been shown to be altered in vanadium-deprived rats (Uthus and Nielsen, 1990). Vanadium-deprived goats show elevated abortion rates and decreased milk production (Anke et al., 1989). In vitro, vanadium in the form of vanadate regulates hormone, glucose, and lipid metabolism; however, vanadium most probably exists in the vanadyl form in vivo (Rehder, 1991).

Vanadium in the forms of vanadyl sulfate (100 mg/day) and sodium metavanadate (125 mg/day) has been used as a supplement for diabetic patients (Boden et al., 1996; Cohen et al., 1995; Goldfine et al., 1995). Although insulin requirements were decreased in patients with Type I diabetes, the doses of vanadium used in the supplements were about 100 times the usual intakes (Pennington and Jones, 1987), and they greatly exceed the Tolerable Upper Intake Level (UL) for vanadium.

Physiology of Absorption, Metabolism, and Excretion

The absorption of ingested vanadium is less than 5 percent, and therefore most ingested vanadium is found in the feces. Absorbed vanadate is converted to the vanadyl cation, which can complex with ferritin and transferrin in plasma and body fluids (Harris et al., 1984; Sabbioni et al., 1978). Highest concentrations of vanadium are found in the liver, kidney, and bone. However, very little of the absorbed vanadium is retained in the body. Patterson and coworkers (1986) investigated vanadium metabolism in sheep and suggested a compartmental model with certain tissues constituting a "slow turnover" pool where the turnover times for vanadium might exceed 400 days. Other tissues were suggested to constitute a "fast turnover" pool with vanadium residency of about 100 hours.

FINDINGS BY LIFE STAGE AND GENDER GROUP

In laboratory animals, vanadium mimics insulin (diminishes hyperglycemia and improves insulin secretion) and inhibits the activity of various enzymes. A deficiency of vanadium results in increased abortion rates. A biological role of vanadium in humans has not yet been identified. Therefore, neither an Estimated Average Requirement, Recommended Dietary Allowance, nor Adequate Intake was determined for vanadium.

INTAKE OF VANADIUM

Food Sources

Foods rich in vanadium include mushrooms, shellfish, black pepper, parsley, dill seed, and certain prepared foods. Myron and coworkers (1977) reported that processed foods contained more vanadium than nonprocessed foods. Byrne and Kosta (1978) also suggested that beer and wine may contribute an appreciable amount of vanadium to the diet. Commodity groups highest in vanadium are grains and grain products, sweeteners, and infant cereals. Analysis of data from the 1984 Food and Drug Administration Total Diet Study (Pennington and Jones, 1987) showed grains and grain products contributed 13 to 30 percent of the vanadium in adult diets. Beverages were also an important source for adults and elderly men (26 to 57 percent). This study also reported that 88 percent of the foods consumed had concentrations less than 2 µg/100 g. Canned apple juice and cereals were the major contributors of vanadium to the diets of infants and toddlers.

Dietary Intake

Pennington and Jones (1987) reported that vanadium intake ranged from 6.5 to 11 µg/day for infants, children, and adolescents. The intake of vanadium for adults and the elderly ranged from 6 to 18 µg/day.

Intake from Supplements

Information from the Third National Health and Nutrition Examination Survey on supplement use of vanadium is provided in Appendix Table C-24. The median intake of supplement vanadium by adults was approximately 9 µg/day. Vanadium in the forms of vanadyl sulfate (100 mg/day) and sodium metavanadate (125 mg/day) has been used as a supplement for diabetic patients (Boden et al., 1996; Cohen et al., 1995; Goldfine et al., 1995). Although insulin requirements were decreased in patients with Type I diabetes, the doses of vanadium used in the supplements were about 100 times the usual intakes (Pennington and Jones, 1987), and they greatly exceed the Tolerable Upper Intake Level (UL) for vanadium.

TOLERABLE UPPER INTAKE LEVELS

The Tolerable Upper Intake Level (UL) is the highest level of daily nutrient intake that is likely to pose no risk of adverse health effects for almost all individuals. Although members of the general population should be advised not to routinely exceed the UL, intake above the UL may be appropriate for investigation within well-controlled clinical trials. Clinical trials of doses above the UL should not be discouraged, as long as subjects participating in these trials have signed informed consent documents regarding possible toxicity and as long as these trials employ appropriate safety monitoring of trial subjects. In addition, the UL is not meant to apply to individuals who are receiving vanadium under medical supervision.

Hazard Identification

There is no evidence of adverse effects associated with vanadium intake from food, which is the major source of exposure to vanadium for the general population (Barceloux, 1999). There are data on adverse effects associated with vanadium intake from supplements and drinking water. Because the forms found in food and supplements are the same (i.e., tetravalent or vanadyl [VO_2+] and pentavalent or vanadate [VO_3-] forms), the UL value will apply to total vanadium intake from food, water, and supplements.

Most vanadium toxicity reports involve industrial exposure to high levels of airborne vanadium. The most toxic vanadium compound is vanadium pentoxide, but because vanadium pentoxide is not a normal constituent of food, supplements, or drinking water, it will not be considered in this review.

Weight training athletes use up to 60 mg/day of vanadyl sulfate supplements (or 18.6 mg of elemental vanadium) to improve performance (Barceloux, 1999). Furthermore, because vanadium may become useful in future treatment of diabetes, there is increased concern about its long-term toxicity.

Adverse Effects

Acute Toxicity. Acute vanadium poisoning has not been observed in humans. Acute poisoning from sodium vanadate in rats causes desquamative enteritis, mild liver congestion with fatty changes, and slight parenchymal degeneration of the renal convoluted tubules (Daniel and Lillie, 1938). In mice, a subcutaneous dose of 20 mg/kg of ammonium metavanadate produced acute tubular necrosis by 6 to 7 hours postinjection (Wei et al., 1982).

Renal Toxicity. Evidence of renal toxicity associated with high vanadium intake in humans was not found. There is evidence of kidney effects in animals (Table 13-2). Domingo and coworkers (1985) found histopathological lesions of the kidney and increased plasma urea and uric acid concentrations in rats exposed to 50 µg/mL in drinking water for 3 months. This finding suggests possible alterations in renal function. In a second study, Domingo and coworkers (1991) evaluated the toxicity of sodium metavanadate (0.15 mg/mL), sodium orthovanadate (0.23 mg/mL), and vanadyl sulfate pentahydrate (0.31 mg/mL) solutions given to diabetic rats for 28 days. In the vanadium-treated animals, they observed decreased weight gain and increased serum concentrations of urea and creatinine, as well as some deaths. A histopathological investigation was not performed.

Boscolo and coworkers (1994) reported that the lumen of the proximal tubules was narrowed and contained amorphous material in rats fed 40 µg/mL of sodium metavanadate in drinking water for

TABLE 13-2 Animal Data on Vanadium-Induced Renal Toxicity, by Increasing Dose

Study	Species	Form	Dose (µg/mL)	Dose (mg/kg/d)
Wei et al., 1982	Mouse	Vanadate	ND[a]	20
Boscolo et al., 1994	Rat	Vanadate	1	ND
		Vanadate	10	ND
		Vanadate	40	ND
Domingo et al., 1985	Rat	Vanadate	5	0.8
		Vanadate	10	1.5
		Vanadate	50	7.7[b]
Domingo et al., 1991	Rat	Vanadate	ND	6.1
		Vanadate	ND	15.6
		Vanadyl	ND	22.7

[a] ND = not determined.
[b] 7.7 mg/kg/d was calculated by using average weight of growing rats of 271 g and

6 or 7 months. Hydropic degeneration was also seen in some proximal and distal tubules and the loop of Henle. Because water intakes were not provided, this study could not be used to derive a dose. Acute tubular necrosis was observed in mice fed 20 mg/kg/day of ammonium metavanadate (Wei et al., 1982). The effect of supplemental vanadium intake on renal function needs further careful study.

Gastrointestinal Effects. There is human evidence of mild gastrointestinal effects (abdominal cramps, loose stool) primarily in patients with diabetes and animal evidence of more severe gastrointestinal effects (diarrhea, death) after ingestion of vanadium compounds (Boden et al., 1996; Dimond et al., 1963; Franke and Moxon, 1937; Goldfine et al., 1995). The human data are summarized in Table 13-3.

Hematological Effects. Vanadium compounds may cause anemia and changes in the leukocyte system. Animal studies of hemolytic activity of vanadium salts have conflicting results (Dai and McNeill, 1994; Dai et al., 1995; Hogan, 1990; Zaporowska and Wasilewski, 1992;

Duration	Results
6–7 hr	Acute tubular necrosis
≈ 7 mo	No effects
≈ 7 mo	Effects on kidney morphology (less evident)
≈ 6 mo	Effects on kidney morphology
3 mo	No effects
3 mo	Vanadium detected in kidneys
3 mo	Increased uric acid and urea; vanadium detected in kidneys
1 mo	Increased serum urea and creatinine
1 mo	Increased serum urea, but not creatinine
1 mo	Increased serum urea and creatinine

average drinking water consumption of 42 mL/day. 50 µg/mL × 42 mL/d × 1/0.27/kg body weight × 1 mg/1,000 µg = 7.7 mg/kg/day.

Zaporowska et al., 1993). Fawcett and coworkers (1997) showed no effects of oral vanadyl sulfate (0.5 mg/kg body weight/day) on hematological indexes, blood viscosity, and biochemistry in a 12-week, double-blind, placebo-controlled trial in 31 athletes.

Cardiovascular Effects. Exposure to vanadate induced an increase in blood pressure and heart rate in rats (Carmignani et al., 1991; Steffen et al., 1981). Boscolo and coworkers (1994) showed an increase in arterial blood pressure following chronic exposure of rats to 1, 10, and 40 µg/mL of vanadium for 6 or 7 months. These changes were not dose-dependent.

Reproductive Effects. No evidence of reproductive abnormalities after ingestion in humans was found. Two animal studies evaluating the reproductive toxicity of vanadium have been reported: in one, Llobet and coworkers (1993) observed that at 60 and 80 mg/kg body weight/day, a significant decrease in pregnancy rate occurred; in the other, Domingo and coworkers (1986) found no effects on fertility or reproduction in rats gavaged up to 20 mg/kg body weight/day with sodium metavanadate.

TABLE 13-3 Human Data on Vanadium-Induced Gastrointestinal Effect, by Increasing Dose

Study[a]	Subjects	Form	Dose[b] (mg V/d)	Dose[c] (mg/kg/d)
Dimond et al., 1963	6 adults	Vanadyl	5	0.07
			10	0.15
			15	0.2
			20	0.3
Cohen et al., 1995	6 adults	Vanadyl	31	0.5
Boden et al., 1996	8 adults	Vanadyl	31	0.5
Goldfine et al., 1995	10 adults	Vanadate	52	0.8

[a] Dimond was uncontrolled; Cohen, Boden, and Goldfine were noninsulin-dependent diabetics.

[b] mg vanadium (V)/d was calculated as follows: For Dimond, mg V/d = 51 (molecular weight of V) ÷ 250 (molecular weight of ammonium vanadyl tartrate [i.e., 150 for tartaric acid minus 1 for H = 149 for tartrate + 101 for ammonium vanadyl, i.e., 117 for ammonium vanadate minus 16 for oxygen = 250]) = 0.20 × 25 mg/d (amount of

Other Adverse Effects. Other adverse effects associated with vanadium intake in humans include green tongue, fatigue, lethargy, and focal neurological lesions (Barceloux, 1999). These effects, however, have not been consistently observed or dose-related. No studies were found evaluating the genotoxicity in humans or animals after ingestion of vanadium, and no evidence was found showing carcinogenicity of vanadium compounds in animals or humans. The U.S. Environmental Protection Agency recently set an oral reference dose of 0.009 mg/kg/day for vanadium pentoxide based on decreased hair cystine content. This finding is from a chronic oral rat study described by Stokinger (1981). Because it is not clear that reduced hair cystine is an adverse effect, data on reduced hair cystine were judged not relevant to the derivation of a UL for elemental vanadium.

Summary

On the basis of the quality and completeness of the database and the strength of the causal association, renal toxicity was selected as the critical adverse effect on which to base a UL. The data on other

Duration	Result
6–10 wk	Cramping, diarrhea, black loose stools ≥ 20 mg/d
3 wk	Mild gastrointestinal effects
4 wk	Mild gastrointestinal effects
2 wk	Mild gastrointestinal effects

compound given by Dimond) = 5 mg/d. For Cohen and Boden, mg V/d = 51 ÷ 163 (molecular weight of vanadyl sulfate) = 0.31 × 100 mg/d (amount of compound given by Cohen and Boden) = 31 mg/d. For Goldfine, mg V/day = 51 ÷ 122 (molecular weight for NaVO$_3$) = 0.42 × 125 (amount of compound given by Goldfine) = 52 mg/d.
c Body weight used was the average of the reference weights for adult men and women (76 and 61 kg, respectively).

effects such as hematological, cardiovascular, or reproductive effects are not consistent. While gastrointestinal effects appear to occur at lower doses in humans, the specificity of the observed effects and the dose-response relationship are not as clearly defined as the histopathological lesions and adverse kidney effects demonstrated in animals. While kidney effects have not been demonstrated in humans, excess vanadium has been shown in rats to accumulate in kidneys (Oster et al., 1993), and the evidence in different species (i.e., mice and rats) further supports a possible risk in humans. Because of the widespread use of high-dose (60 mg/day) supplemental vanadium by athletes and other subgroups (e.g., borderline diabetics) that are considered part of the apparently healthy general population (Barceloux, 1999), further research on vanadium toxicity is needed.

Dose-Response Assessment

Adults

Data Selection. The data in laboratory rats involving subchronic to chronic durations of intake were used to derive a UL. Studies that provided doses in units of concentration but provided no information on the body weights of the rats or the amount of water consumed were not used.

Identification of a No-Observed-Adverse-Effects Level (NOAEL) or Lowest-Observed-Adverse-Effects Level (LOAEL). A NOAEL of 0.8 mg/kg body weight/day and a LOAEL of 7.7 mg/kg body weight/day were determined on the basis of the results of Domingo and coworkers (1985). Vanadium could not be detected in the kidneys of animals receiving 5 µg/mL (or 0.8 mg/kg/day) (Table 13-2). Also, plasma urea, uric acid, and creatinine concentrations were within the normal range in this treatment group (Domingo et al., 1985). However, the study does not indicate whether there were kidney lesions at this level; therefore, whether this is a true NOAEL value for this study is uncertain. The same can be said for the treatment group given 10 µg/mL (or 1.5 mg/kg/day). The study does not provide enough detail about the findings at this dose level to ascertain whether it is a NOAEL or LOAEL.

The value of 7.7 mg/kg/day is the best estimate of a LOAEL from this data set. At this dose, there were evident lesions of the kidney and small, but significant, increases in plasma urea and uric acid. Furthermore, this LOAEL appears to be consistent with other studies (Boscolo et al., 1994; Domingo et al., 1991). Boscolo and coworkers (1994) failed to provide information on intakes (mg/kg/day), and therefore the study was judged not useful for deriving a UL. Nevertheless, both Domingo and coworkers (1991) and Boscolo and coworkers (1994) showed a similar dose-response relationship. The study by Domingo and coworkers (1991) in diabetic rats provides results that are fairly consistent with their earlier study (Domingo et al., 1985). Although Domingo and coworkers (1991) tested different compounds of vanadium and used a shorter duration, they observed increased serum urea and creatinine concentrations at similar doses (6.1 and 22.7 mg/kg/day).

Uncertainty Assessment. In determining an uncertainty factor (UF) for vanadium, several sources of uncertainty were considered and combined into the final UF. The severity of kidney lesions justifies a UF higher than 1, and so a UF of 3 was selected to extrapolate from the LOAEL to the NOAEL. A UF of 10 was selected to extrapolate from laboratory animals to humans because no human and little animal data were available to use in the dose-response assessment. Another UF of 10 was selected for intraspecies variability. The three

UFs are multiplied to yield an overall UF of 300 to extrapolate from the LOAEL in animals to derive a UL in humans.

Derivation of a UL. The LOAEL of 7.7 mg/kg/day was divided by a UF of 300 to obtain a UL of 0.026 mg/kg/day or 26 µg/kg/day for adult humans. This value was rounded and multiplied by the average of the reference body weights for adult men and women, 68.5 kg, from Chapter 1 (Table 1-1). The resulting UL for adults is 1.78 mg/day (which was rounded to 1.8 mg/day).

$$UL = \frac{LOAEL}{UF} = \frac{7.7 \text{ mg/kg/day}}{300} = 26 \text{ µg/kg/day} \times 68.5 \text{ kg} \cong 1.8 \text{ mg/day}$$

Vanadium UL Summary, Ages 19 Years and Older

UL for Adults
  ≥ 19 years   **1.8 mg/day of elemental vanadium**

Other Life Stage Groups

Given the severity of the critical effect for vanadium in adults, the lack of data on vanadium toxicity in other more sensitive life stage groups is of particular concern. Due to this lack of data, it was not possible to determine ULs for pregnant and lactating women, children, and infants. These individuals should be particularly cautious about consuming vanadium supplements. As indicated above, more research is needed on the renal effects of vanadium intake, particularly in these sensitive subgroups.

Vanadium UL Summary, Ages 0 through 18 Years, Pregnancy, Lactation

UL for Infants
  0–12 months   **Not possible to establish; source of intake should be from food and formula only**

UL for Children
  1–3 years   **Not possible to establish; source of intake should be from food only**
  4–8 years   **Not possible to establish; source of intake should be from food only**
  9–13 years   **Not possible to establish; source of intake should be from food only**

UL for Adolescents
    14–18 years   Not possible to establish; source of intake
                           should be from food only

UL for Pregnancy
    14–18 years   Not possible to establish; source of intake
                           should be from food only
    19–50 years   Not possible to establish; source of intake
                           should be from food only

UL for Lactation
    14–18 years   Not possible to establish; source of intake
                           should be from food only
    19–50 years   Not possible to establish; source of intake
                           should be from food only

Special Considerations

A review of the literature revealed no special subpopulations that are distinctly susceptible to the adverse effects of high vanadium intake.

Intake Assessment

Although percentile data are not available for dietary vanadium intakes from U.S. surveys, the highest mean intake of vanadium reported for the U.S. population was 18 µg/day (Pennington and Jones, 1987). The average intake of supplemental vanadium at the ninety-ninth percentile by adults was 20 µg/day, which is significantly lower than the adult UL for vanadium.

Risk Characterization

The risk of adverse effects resulting from excess intake of vanadium from food is very unlikely. Because of the high doses of vanadium present in some supplements, increased risks are likely to result from the chronic consumption of supplements containing large doses of vanadium. Currently, doses of vanadium greater than the UL are being tested for their benefits in treating diabetics. The UL is not meant to apply to individuals who are being treated with vanadium under close medical supervision.

RESEARCH RECOMMENDATIONS FOR VANADIUM

• Determination of the biochemical role of vanadium in both higher animals and humans and a reliable status indicator of vanadium for further work in humans.

• The efficacy and safety of the use of vanadium as a nutritional supplement.

REFERENCES

ABC (American Biogenics Corporation). 1988. *Ninety Day Gavage Study in Albino Rats Using Nickel.* Study 410-2520. Final report submitted to the U.S. Environmental Protection Agency, Office of Solid Waste, by Research Triangle Institute and American Biogenics Corporation under contract 68-01-7075.

Adams MA, Bolger PM, Gunderson EL. 1994. Dietary intake and hazards of arsenic. In: Chappell WR, Abernathy CO, Cothern CR, eds. *Arsenic: Exposure and Health.* Northwood, UK: Science and Technology Letters. Pp. 41–49.

Allen HE, Halley-Henderson MA, Hass CN. 1989. Chemical composition of bottled mineral water. *Arch Environ Health* 44:102–116.

Ambrose AM, Larson PS, Borzelleca JF, Hennigar GR. 1976. Long term toxicologic assessment of nickel in rats and dogs. *J Food Sci Technol* 13:181–187.

Anderson DL, Cunningham WC, Lindstrom TR. 1994. Concentrations and intakes of H, B, S, K, Na, Cl, and NaCl in foods. *J Food Comp Anal* 7:59–82.

Anderson RR. 1992. Comparison of trace elements in milk of four species. *J Dairy Sci* 75:3050–3055.

Andrews RK, Blakeley RL, Zerner B. 1988. Nickel in proteins and enzymes. In: Sigel H, Sigel A, eds. *Metal Ions in Biological Systems,* Vol. 23. New York: Marcel Dekker. Pp. 165–284.

Anke M. 1986. Arsenic. In: Mertz W, ed. *Trace Elements in Human and Animal Nutrition,* Vol. 2, 5th ed. Orlando, FL: Academic Press. Pp. 347–372.

Anke M, Groppel B, Gruhn K, Langer M, Arnhold W. 1989. The essentiality of vanadium for animals. In: Anke M, Bauman W, Braunlich H, eds. *6th International Trace Element Symposium,* Vol. 1. Jena, Germany: Friedrich-Schiller-Universitat. Pp. 17–27.

Aposhian HV. 1997. Enzymatic methylation of arsenic species and other new approaches to arsenic toxicity. *Annu Rev Pharmacol Toxicol* 37:397–419.

Armstrong CW, Stroube RB, Rubio T, Siudyla EA, Miller GB Jr. 1984. Outbreak of fatal arsenic poisoning caused by contaminated drinking water. *Arch Environ Health* 39:276–279.

ATSDR (Agency for Toxic Substances and Disease Registry). 1992. *Toxicological Profile for Boron.* Atlanta: U.S. Public Health Service, ATSDR.

ATSDR. 1998. *Toxicological Profile for Arsenic.* Atlanta: U.S. Public Health Service, ATSDR.

Bakken N. 1995. *Dietary Boron Modifies the Effects of Vitamin D Nutriture on Energy Metabolism and Bone Morphology in the Chick.* Masters of Science thesis, University of North Dakota, Grand Forks.

Barceloux DG. 1999. Vanadium. *J Toxicol Clin Toxicol* 37:265–278.

Baxley MN, Hood RD, Vedel GC, Harrison WP, Szczech GM. 1981. Prenatal toxicity of orally administered sodium arsenite in mice. *Bull Environ Contam Toxicol* 26:749–756.

Beaudoin AR. 1974. Teratogenicity of sodium arsenate in rats. *Teratology* 10:153–157.

Becking GC, Chen BH. 1998. International Programme on Chemical Safety (IPCS) environmental health criteria on boron human health risk assessment. *Biol Trace Elem Res* 66:439–452.

Boden G, Chen X, Ruiz J, van Rossum GD, Turco S. 1996. Effects of vanadyl sulfate on carbohydrate and lipid metabolism in patients with non-insulin-dependent diabetes mellitus. *Metabolism* 45:1130–1135.

Boscolo P, Carmignani M, Volpe AR, Felaco M, Del Rosso G, Porcelli G, Giuliano G. 1994. Renal toxicity and arterial hypertension in rats chronically exposed to vanadate. *Occup Environ Med* 51:500–503.

Byrne AR, Kosta L. 1978. Vanadium in foods and in human body fluids and tissues. *Sci Total Environ* 10:17–30.

Byrne AR, Kosta L, Dermelj M, Tusek-Znidaric M. 1983. Aspects of some trace elements in human milk. In: Bratter P, Schramel P, eds. *Trace Element Analytical Chemistry in Medicine and Biology*, Vol. 2. Berlin: Walter de Gruyter. Pp. 21–35.

Byron WR, Bierbower GW, Brouwer JB, Hansen WH. 1967. Pathologic changes in rats and dogs from two-year feeding of sodium arsenite or sodium arsenate. *Toxicol Appl Pharmacol* 10:132–147.

Carlisle EM. 1980a. A silicon requirement for normal skull formation in chicks. *J Nutr* 110:352–359.

Carlisle EM. 1980b. Biochemical and morphological changes associated with long bone abnormalities in silicon deficiency. *J Nutr* 110:1046–1055.

Carlisle EM. 1981. Silicon: A requirement in bone formation independent of vitamin D1. *Calcif Tissue Int* 33:27–34.

Carlisle EM. 1984. Silicon. In: Frieden E, ed, *Biochemistry of the Essential Ultratrace Elements*. New York: Plenum Press. Pp. 257–291.

Carmignani M, Boscolo P, Volpe AR, Togna G, Masciocco L, Preziosi P. 1991. Cardiovascular system and kidney as specific targets of chronic exposure to vanadate in the rat: Functional and morphological findings. *Arch Toxicol Suppl* 14:124–127.

Casey CE, Neville MC. 1987. Studies in human lactation 3: Molybdenum and nickel in human milk during the first month of lactation. *Am J Clin Nutr* 45:921–926.

Chan PC, Huff J. 1997. Arsenic carcinogenesis in animals and in humans: Mechanistic, experimental, and epidemiological evidence. *J Environ Sci Health* C15:83–122.

Chappell WR, Beck BD, Brown KG, Chaney R, Cothern CR, Irgolic KJ, North DW, Thornton I, Tsongas TA. 1997. Inorganic arsenic: A need and an opportunity to improve risk assessment. *Environ Health Perspect* 105:1060–1067.

Chen CJ, Chen CW, Wu MM, Kuo TL. 1992. Cancer potential in liver, lung, bladder and kidney due to ingested inorganic arsenic in drinking water. *Br J Cancer* 66:888–892.

Christensen OB, Moller H. 1978. Release of nickel from cooking utensils. *Contact Dermatitis* 4:343–346.

Civantos DP, Lopez Rodriguez A, Aguado-Borruey JM, Narvaez JA. 1995. Fulminant malignant arrythmia and multiorgan failure in acute arsenic poisoning. *Chest* 108:1774–1775.

Cohen N, Halberstam M, Shlimovich P, Chang CJ, Shamoon H, Rossetti L. 1995. Oral vanadyl sulfate improves hepatic and peripheral insulin sensitivity in patients with non-insulin-dependent diabetes mellitus. *J Clin Invest* 95:2501–2509.

Culver BD, Hubbard SA. 1996. Inorganic boron health effects in humans: An aid to risk assessment and clinical judgment. *J Trace Elem Exp Med* 9:175–184.

Dabeka RW. 1989. Survey of lead, cadmium, cobalt and nickel in infant formulas and evaporated milks and estimation of dietary intakes of the elements by infants 0–12 months old. *Sci Total Environ* 89:279–289.

Dabeka RW, McKenzie AD. 1995. Survey of lead, cadmium, fluoride, nickel, and cobalt in food composites and estimation of dietary intakes of these elements by Canadians in 1986–1988. *J AOAC Int* 78:897–909.

Dabeka RW, McKenzie AD, Lacroix GM, Cleroux C, Bowe S, Graham RA, Conacher HB, Verdier P. 1993. Survey of arsenic in total diet food composites and estimation of the dietary intake of arsenic by Canadian adults and children. *J AOAC Int* 76:14–25.

Dai S, McNeill JH. 1994. One-year treatment of non-diabetic and streptozotocin-diabetic rats with vanadyl sulphate did not alter blood pressure or haematological indices. *Pharmacol Toxicol* 74:110–115.

Dai S, Vera E, McNeill JH. 1995. Lack of haematological effect of oral vanadium treatment in rats. *Pharmacol Toxicol* 76:263–268.

Daniel EP, Lillie RD. 1938. Experimental vanadium poisoning in the white rat. *Public Health Rep* 53:765–777.

Dang HS, Jaiswal DD, Somasundaram S. 1983. Distribution of arsenic in human tissues and milk. *Sci Total Environ* 29:171–175.

da Silva FJ, Williams RJ. 1991. *The Biological Chemistry of the Elements: The Inorganic Chemistry of Life*. Oxford: Clarendon Press. Pp. 58–63.

Desrosiers R, Tanguay RM. 1986. Further characterization of the posttranslational modifications of core histones in response to heat and arsenite stress in *Drosophila*. *Biochem Cell Biol* 64:750–757.

Dieter MP. 1994. Toxicity and carcinogenicity studies of boric acid in male and female B6C3F$_1$ mice. *Environ Health Perspect Suppl* 102:93–97.

Dimond EG, Caravaca J, Benchimol A. 1963. Vanadium: Excretion, toxicity, lipid effect in man. *Am J Clin Nutr* 12:49–53.

Dobbie JW, Smith MB. 1986. Urinary and serum silicon in normal and uraemic individuals. *Ciba Found Symp* 121:194–213.

Domingo JL, Llobet JM, Tomas JM, Corbella J. 1985. Short-term toxicity studies of vanadium in rats. *J Appl Toxicol* 5:418–421.

Domingo JL, Paternain JL, Llobet JM, Corbella J. 1986. Effects of vanadium on reproduction, gestation, parturition and lactation in rats upon oral administration. *Life Sci* 39:819–824.

Domingo JL, Gomez M, Llobet JM, Corbella J, Keen CL. 1991. Oral vanadium administration to streptozotocin-diabetic rats has marked negative side-effects which are independent of the form of vanadium used. *Toxicology* 66:279–287.

Dourson M, Maier A, Meek B, Renwick A, Ohanian E, Poirier K. 1998. Boron tolerable intake: Re-evaluation of toxicokinetics for data-derived uncertainty factors. *Biol Trace Elem Res* 66:453–463.

Eckhert CD. 1998. Boron stimulates embryonic trout growth. *J Nutr* 128:2488–2493.

Engel RR, Receveur O. 1993. Re: "Arsenic ingestion and internal cancers: A review". *Am J Epidemiol* 138:896–897.

EPA (Environmental Protection Agency). 1975. Water programs: National interim primary drinking water regulations. *Fed Register* 40:59566.

EPA. 1987. *Health Effects Assessment for Boron and Compounds*. EPA/600/8-88/021. Cincinnati, OH: EPA.

EPA. 1988. *Special Report on Ingested Inorganic Arsenic: Skin Cancer; Nutritional Essentiality.* EPA 625/3-87/013. Washington, DC: EPA.

EPA. 2000. *Integrated Risk Information System Database.* United States Environmental Protection Agency. [Online.] Available: http://www.epa.gov/iris/subst/0271.htm [accessed November 10, 2000].

EPA. 2000. National primary drinking water regulations; Arsenic and clarifications to compliance and new source contaminants monitoring; Proposed rule. *Fed Register* 65:38887–38983.

Fail PA, George JD, Grizzle TB, Heindel JJ, Chapin RE. 1990. *Final Report on the Reproductive Toxicity of Boric Acid (CAS No. 10043-35-3) in CD-1 Swiss Mice.* Research Triangle Park, NC: Department of Health and Human Services, National Toxicology Program.

Fail PA, George JD, Seely JC, Grizzle TB, Heindel JJ. 1991. Reproductive toxicity of boric acid in Swiss (CD-1) mice: Assessment using the continuous breeding protocol. *Fundam Appl Toxicol* 17:225–239.

Fawcett JP, Farquhar SJ, Thou T, Shand BI. 1997. Oral vanadyl sulphate does not affect blood cells, viscosity or biochemistry in humans. *Pharmacol Toxicol* 80:202–206.

Fincher RM, Koerker RM. 1987. Long-term survival in acute arsenic encephalopathy. Follow-up using newer measures of electrophysiologic parameters. *Am J Med* 82:549–552.

Fort DJ, Propst TL, Stover EL, Strong PL, Murray FJ. 1998. Adverse reproductive and developmental effects in Xenopus from insufficient boron. *Biol Trace Elem Res* 66:237–259.

Fort DJ, Stover EL, Strong PL, Murray FJ, Keen CL. 1999. Chronic feeding of a low boron diet adversely affects reproduction and development in Xenopus laevis. *J Nutr* 129:2055–2060.

Franke KW, Moxon AL. 1937. The toxicity of orally ingested arsenic, selenium, tellurium, vanadium and molybdenum. *J Pharmacol Exp Ther* 61:89–102.

Franzblau A, Lilis R. 1989. Acute arsenic intoxication from environmental arsenic exposure. *Arch Environ Health* 44:385–390.

Gartrell MJ, Craun JC, Podrebarac DS, Gunderson EL. 1985. Pesticides, selected elements, and other chemicals in adult total diet samples, October 1978–September 1979. *J Assoc Off Anal Chem* 68:862–875.

Gawkrodger DJ, Cook SW, Fell GS, Hunter JAA. 1986. Nickel dermatitis: The reaction to oral nickel challenge. *Br J Dermatol* 115:33–38.

Goering PL, Aposhian HV, Mass MJ, Cebrian M, Beck BD, Waalkes MP. 1999. The enigma of arsenic carcinogenesis: Role of metabolism. *Toxicol Sci* 49:5–14.

Goldfine AB, Simonson DC, Folli F, Patti ME, Kahn CR. 1995. In vivo and in vitro studies of vanadate in human and rodent diabetes mellitus. *Molec Cell Biochem* 153:217–231.

Goldwater LJ. 1936. The urinary excretion of silica in non-silicotic humans. *J Ind Hyg Toxicol* 18:163–166.

Gordon AS, Prichard JS, Freedman MH. 1973. Seizure disorders and anemia associated with chronic borax intoxication. *Can Med Assoc J* 108:719–721.

Grantham DA, Jones JF. 1977. Arsenic contamination of water wells in Nova Scotia. *J Am Water Works Assoc* 69:653–657.

Green GH, Lott MD, Weeth HJ. 1973. Effects of boron water on rats. *Proc West Sect Am Soc Anim Sci* 24:254–258.

Grimanis AP, Vassilaki-Grimani M, Alexiou D, Papadatos C. 1979. Determination of seven trace elements in human milk, powdered cow's milk and infant foods by neutron activation analysis. In: Byrne AR, Kosta L, Ravnik V, Stupar J, Hudnik V, eds. *Nuclear Activation Techniques in the Life Sciences 1978.* Vienna: International Atomic Energy Agency. Pp. 241–253.

Gunderson EL. 1995. FDA Total Diet Study, July 1986–April 1991, dietary intakes of pesticides, selected elements, and other chemicals. *J AOAC Int* 78:1353–1363.

Haddad FS, Kouyoumdjian A. 1986. Silica stones in humans. *Urol Int* 41:70–76.

Harris WR, Friedman SB, Silberman D. 1984. Behavior of vanadate and vanadyl ion in canine blood. *J Inorg Biochem* 20:157–169.

Hei TK, Liu SX, Waldren C. 1998. Mutagenicity of arsenic in mammalian cells: Role of reactive oxygen species. *Proc Natl Acad Sci USA* 95:8103–8107.

Heindel JJ, Price CJ, Field EA, Marr MC, Myers CB, Morrissey RE, Schwetz BA. 1992. Developmental toxicity of boric acid in mice and rats. *Fundam Appl Toxicol* 18:266–277.

Heyliger CE, Tahiliani AG, McNeill JH. 1985. Effect of vanadate on elevated blood glucose and depressed cardiac performance of diabetic rats. *Science* 227:1474–1477.

Hoey MJ. 1966. The effects of metallic salts on the histology and functioning of the rat testis. *J Reprod Fertil* 12:461–471.

Hogan GR. 1990. Peripheral erythrocyte levels, hemolysis and three vanadium compounds. *Experientia* 46:444–446.

Hood RD. 1972. Effects of sodium arsenite on fetal development. *Bull Environ Contam Toxicol* 7:216–222.

Hood RD, Bishop SL. 1972. Teratogenic effects of sodium arsenate in mice. *Arch Environ Health* 24:62–65.

Hood RD, Harrison WP. 1982. Effects of prenatal arsenite exposure in the hamster. *Bull Environ Contam Toxicol* 29:671–678.

Hopenhayn-Rich C, Smith AH, Goeden HM. 1993. Human studies do not support the methylation threshold hypothesis for the toxicity of inorganic arsenic. *Environ Res* 60:161–177.

Hopenhayn-Rich C, Biggs ML, Fuchs A, Bergoglio R, Tello EE, Nicolli H, Smith AH. 1996. Bladder cancer mortality associated with arsenic in drinking water in Argentina. *Epidemiology* 7:117–124.

Huang YZ, Qian XC, Wang GQ, Xiao BY, Ren DD, Feng ZY, Wu JY, Xu RJ, Zhang FE. 1985. Endemic chronic arsenism in Xinjiang. *Chin Med J* 98:219–222.

Hunt CD. 1996. Biochemical effects of physiological amounts of dietary boron. *J Trace Elem Exp Med* 9:185–213.

Hunt CD. 1998. Regulation of enzymatic activity. One possible role of dietary boron in higher animals and humans. *Biol Trace Elem Res* 66:205–225.

Hunt CD, Stoecker BJ. 1996. Deliberations and evaluations of the approaches, endpoints and paradigms for boron, chromium and fluoride dietary recommendations. *J Nutr* 126:2441S–2451S.

Hunt CD, Shuler TR, Mullen LM. 1991. Concentration of boron and other elements in human foods and personal-care products. *J Am Diet Assoc* 91:558–568.

IARC (International Agency for Research on Cancer). 1980. *Some Metals and Metallic Compounds.* IARC Monographs on the Evaluation of Carcinogenic Risks to Humans, Vol. 23. Lyon, France: IARC.

IARC. 1987. *Overall Evaluations of Carcinogenicity: An Updating of IARC Monographs Volumes 1 to 42.* IARC Monographs on the Evaluation of Carcinogenic Risks to Humans, Supplement 7. Lyon, France: IARC.

IPCS (International Programme on Chemical Safety). 1998. *Environmental Health Criteria: 204: Boron.* Geneva: World Health Organization.

Jansen JA, Andersen J, Schou JS. 1984a. Boric acid single dose pharmacokinetics after intravenous administration to man. *Arch Toxicol* 55:64–67.

Jansen JA, Schou JS, Aggerbeck A. 1984b. Gastro-intestinal absorption and in vitro release of boric acid from water-emulsifying ointments. *Food Chem Toxicol* 22:49–53.

Kanematsu N, Hara M, Kada T. 1980. Rec assay and mutagenicity studies on metal compounds. *Mutat Res* 77:109–116.

Kelsay JL, Behall KM, Prather ES. 1979. Effect of fiber from fruits and vegetables on metabolic responses of human subjects. II. Calcium, magnesium, iron and silicon balances. *Am J Clin Nutr* 32:1876–1880.

Kim H, Yu C, Maier RJ. 1991. Common cis-acting region responsible for transcriptional regulation of Bradyrhizobium japonicum hydrogenase by nickel, oxygen, and hydrogen. *J Bacteriol* 173:3993–3999.

Konig A, Wrazel L, Warrell RP Jr, Rivi R, Pandolfi PP, Jakubowski A, Gabrilove JL. 1997. Comparative activity of melarsoprol and arsenic trioxide in chronic B-cell leukemia lines. *Blood* 90:562–570.

Kreiss K, Zack MM, Landrigan PJ, Feldman RG, Niles CA, Chirico-Post J, Sax DS, Boyd MH, Cox DH. 1983. Neurologic evaluation of a population exposed to arsenic in Alaskan well water. *Arch Environ Health* 38:116–121.

Ku WW, Chapin RE, Moseman RF, Brink RE, Pierce KD, Adams KY. 1991. Tissue disposition of boron in male Fischer rats. *Toxicol Appl Pharmacol* 111:145–151.

Ku WW, Shih LM, Chapin RE. 1993. The effects of boric acid (BA) on testicular cells in culture. *Reprod Toxicol* 7:321–331.

Lancaster JR. 1988. *The Bioinorganic Chemistry of Nickel.* New York: VCH Publishers.

Lanoue L, Taubeneck MW, Muniz J, Hanna LA, Strong PL, Murray FJ, Nielsen FH, Hunt CD, Keen CL. 1998. Assessing the effects of low boron diets on embryonic and fetal development in rodents using in vitro and in vivo model systems. *Biol Trace Elem Res* 66:271–298.

Lanoue L, Strong PL, Keen CL. 1999. Adverse effects of a low boron environment on the preimplanation development of mouse embryos in vitro. *J Trace Elem Exp Med* 12:235–250.

Laskey JW, Phelps PV. 1991. Effect of cadmium and other metal cations on in vitro Leydig cell testosterone production. *Toxicol Appl Pharmacol* 108:296–306.

Lee IP, Sherrins RJ, Dixon RL. 1978. Evidence for induction of germinal aplasia in male rats by environmental exposure to boron. *Toxicol Appl Pharmacol* 45:577–590.

Levin-Scherz JK, Patrick JD, Weber FH, Garabedian C Jr. 1987. Acute arsenic ingestion. *Ann Emerg Med* 16:702–704.

Litovitz TL, Klein-Schwartz W, Oderda GM, Schmitz BF. 1988. Clinical manifestations of toxicity in a series of 784 boric acid ingestions. *Am J Emerg Med* 6:209–213.

Llobet JM, Colomina MT, Sirvent JJ, Domingo JL, Corbella J. 1993. Reproductive toxicity evaluation of vanadium in male mice. *Toxicology* 80:199–206.

Look AT. 1998. Arsenic and apoptosis in the treatment of acute promyelocytic leukemia. *J Natl Cancer Inst* 90:86–88.

Mahaffey KR, Corneliussen PE, Jelinek CF, Fiorino JA. 1975. Heavy metal exposure from foods. *Environ Health Perspect* 12:63–69.

Maitani T, Saito N, Abe M, Uchiyama S, Saito Y. 1987. Chemical form-dependent induction of hepatic zinc-thionein by arsenic administration and effect of co-administered selenium in mice. *Toxicol Lett* 39:63–70.

Mancinella A. 1991. Silicon, a trace element essential for living organisms. Recent knowledge on its preventive role in atherosclerotic process, aging and neo-plasms. *Clin Ter* 137:343–350.

Meacham SL, Hunt CD. 1998. Dietary boron intakes of selected populations in the United States. *Biol Trace Elem Res* 66:65–78.

Meng Z, Meng N. 1994. Effects of inorganic arsenicals on DNA synthesis in unsensitized human blood lymphocytes in vitro. *Biol Trace Elem Res* 42:201–208.

Moore JA. 1997. An assessment of boric acid and borax using the IEHR Evaluative Process for Assessing Human Developmental and Reproductive Toxicity of Agents. *Reprod Toxicol* 11:123–160.

Morton W, Starr G, Pohl D, Stoner J, Wagner S, Weswig D. 1976. Skin cancer and water arsenic in Lane County, Oregon. *Cancer* 37:2523–2532.

Murray FJ. 1998. A comparative review of the pharmacokinetcis of boric acid in rodents and humans. *Biol Trace Elem Res* 66:331–341.

Myron DR, Givand SH, Nielsen FH. 1977. Vanadium content of selected foods as determined by flameless atomic absorption spectroscopy. *J Agric Food Chem* 25:297–300.

Nielsen FH. 1985. The importance of diet composition in ultratrace element research. *J Nutr* 115.1239–1247.

Nielsen FH. 1996. How should dietary guidance be given for mineral elements with beneficial actions or suspected of being essential? *J Nutr* 126:2377S–2385S.

Nielsen FH. 1997. Boron. In: O'Dell BL, Sunde RA, eds. *Handbook of Nutritionally Essential Mineral Elements*. New York: Marcel Dekker. Pp. 453–464.

Nielsen FH. 1998. The justification for providing dietary guidance for the nutritional intake of boron. *Biol Trace Elem Res* 66:319–330.

Nielsen FH, Flyvholm M. 1983. Risks of high nickel intake with diet. In: Sunderman FW Jr, ed. *Nickel in the Human Environment*. IARC Scientific Publications No. 53. Lyon, France: International Agency for Research on Cancer. Pp. 333–338.

Nielsen FH, Penland JG. 1999. Boron supplementation of peri-menopausal women affects boron metabolism and indicies associated with macromineral metabolism, hormonal status and immune function. *J Trace Elem Exp Med* 12:251–261.

Nielsen FH, Uthus EO. 1990. The essentiality and metabolism of vanadium. In: Chasteen ND, ed. *Vanadium in Biological Systems*. Dordrecht, The Netherlands: Kluwer Academic. Pp. 51–62.

Nishioka H. 1975. Mutagenic activities of metal compounds in bacteria. *Mutat Res* 31:185–189.

NRC (National Research Council). 1999. *Arsenic in Drinking Water*. Washington, DC: National Academy Press.

Oppenheim JJ, Fishbein WN. 1965. Induction of chromosome breaks in cultured normal human leukocytes by potassium arsenite, hydroxyurea and related compounds. *Cancer Res* 25:980–985.

Oster MH, Llobet JM, Domingo JL, German JB, Keen CL. 1993. Vanadium treatment of diabetic Sprague-Dawley rats results in tissue vanadium accumulation and pro-oxidant effects. *Toxicology* 83:115–130.

O'Sullivan K, Taylor M. 1983. Chronic boric acid poisoning in infants. *Arch Dis Child* 58:737–749.

Paton GR, Allison AC. 1972. Chromosome damage in human cell cultures induced by metal salts. *Mutat Res* 16:332–336.

Patriarca M, Lyon TD, Fell GS. 1997. Nickel metabolism in humans investigated with an oral stable isotope. *Am J Clin Nutr* 66:616–621.

Patterson BW, Hansard SL, Ammerman CB, Henry PR, Zech LA, Fisher WR. 1986. Kinetic model of whole-body vanadium metabolism: Studies in sheep. *Am J Physiol* 251:R325–R332.

Penland JG. 1998. The importance of boron nutrition for brain and psychological function. *Biol Trace Elem Res* 66:299–317.

Pennington JA. 1991. Silicon in foods and diets. *Food Addit Contam* 8:97–118.

Pennington JA, Jones JW. 1987. Molybdenum, nickel, cobalt, vanadium, and strontium in total diets. *J Am Diet Assoc* 87:1644–1650.

Popplewell JF, King SJ, Day JP, Ackrill P, Fifield LK, Cresswell RG, di Tada ML, Liu K. 1998. Kinetics of uptake and elimination of silicic acid by a human subject: A novel application of ^{32}Si and accelerator mass spectrometry. *J Inorg Biochem* 69:177–180.

Price CJ, Marr MC, Myers CB, Seely JC, Heindel JJ, Schwetz BA. 1996a. The developmental toxicity of boric acid in rabbits. *Fundam Appl Toxicol* 34:176–187.

Price CJ, Strong PL, Marr MC, Myers CB, Murray FJ. 1996b. Developmental toxicity NOAEL and postnatal recovery in rats fed boric acid during gestation. *Fundam Appl Toxicol* 32:179–193.

Price CJ, Strong PL, Murray FJ, Goldberg MM. 1998. Developmental effects of boric acid in rats related to maternal blood boron concentrations. *Biol Trace Elem Res* 66:359–372.

Przybyla AE, Robbins J, Menon N, Peck HD. 1992. Structure-function relationships among the nickel-containing hydrogenases. *FEMS Microbiol Rev* 8:109–135.

Quatrehomme G, Ricq O, Lapalus P, Jacomet Y, Ollier A. 1992. Acute arsenic intoxication: Forensic and toxicologic aspects (an observation). *J Forensic Sci* 37:1163–1171.

Rainey CJ, Nyquist LA, Christensen RE, Strong PL, Culver BD, Coughlin JR. 1999. Daily boron intake from the American diet. *J Am Diet Assoc* 99:335–340.

Rehder D. 1991. The bioinorganic chemistry of vanadium. *Angew Chem Int Ed Engl* 30:148–167.

Rezuke WN, Knight JA, Sunderman FW. 1987. Reference values for nickel concentrations in human tissues and bile. *Am J Ind Med* 11:419–426.

Rowe RI, Eckhert CD. 1999. Boron is required for zebrafish embryogenesis. *J Exp Biol* 202:1649–1654.

RTI (Research Triangle Institute). 1988. *Two Generation Reproduction and Fertility Study of Nickel Chloride Administered to CD Rats in the Drinking Water: Fertility and Reproductive Performance of the P_0 Generation. Final Study Report.* Report to Office of Solid Waste Management, US Environmental Protection Agency by Research Triangle Institute. RTI Project No. 472U-3228-07. Research Triangle Park, NC: RTI.

Sabbioni E, Marafante E, Amantini L, Ubertalli L, Birattari C. 1978. Similarity in metabolic patterns of different chemical species of vanadium in the rat. *Bioinorg Chem* 8:503–515.

Samman S, Naghii MR, Lyons Wall PM, Verus AP. 1998. The nutritional and metabolic effects of boron in humans and animals. *Biol Trace Elem Res* 66:227–235.

Schnegg A, Kirchgessner M. 1975. Changes in hemoglobin content, erythrocyte count and hematocrit in nickel deficiency. *Nutr Metab* 19:268–278.

Schoof RA, Yost LJ, Eickhoff J, Crecelius EA, Cragin DW, Meacher DM, Menzel DB. 1999. A market basket survey of inorganic arsenic in food. *Food Chem Toxicol* 37:839–846.

Schroeder HA, Mitchener M. 1971. Toxic effects of trace elements on the reproduction of mice and rats. *Arch Environ Health* 23:102–106.

Schwarz K, Milne DB. 1972. Growth-promoting effects of silicon in rats. *Nature* 239:333–334.

Seaborn CD, Nielsen FH. 1993. Silicon: A nutritional beneficence for bones, brains and blood vessels? *Nutr Today* 28:13–18.

Seaborn CD, Nielsen FH. 1994. Dietary silicon affects acid and alkaline phosphatase and [45]calcium uptake in bone of rats. *J Trace Elem Exp Med* 7:11–18.

Shirasu Y, Moriya M, Kato K, Furuhashi A, Kada T. 1976. Mutagenicity screening of pesticides in the microbial system. *Mutat Res* 40:19–30.

Simeonova PP, Wang S, Toriuma W, Kommineni V, Matheson J, Unimye N, Kayama F, Harki D, Ding M, Vallyathan V, Luster MI. 2000. Arsenic mediates cell proliferation and gene expression in the bladder epithelium: Association with activating protein-1 transactivation. *Cancer Res* 60:3445–3453.

Smith AH, Goycolea M, Haque R, Biggs ML. 1998. Marked increase in bladder and lung cancer mortality in a region of Northern Chile due to arsenic in drinking water. *Am J Epidemiol* 147:660–669.

Smith MK, George EL, Stober JA, Feng HA, Kimmel GL. 1993. Perinatal toxicity associated with nickel chloride exposure. *Environ Res* 61:200–211.

Solomons NW, Viteri F, Shuler TR, Nielsen FH. 1982. Bioavailability of nickel in man: Effects of foods and chemically-defined dietary constituents on the absorption of inorganic nickel. *J Nutr* 112:39–50.

Southwick JW, Western AE, Beck MM, Whitley T, Isaacs R. 1981. *Community Health Associated with Arsenic in Drinking Water in Millard County, Utah.* EPA-600/1-81-064. Cincinnati, OH: US Environmental Protection Agency, Health Effects Research Laboratory.

Steffen RP, Pamnani MB, Clough DL, Huot SJ, Muldoon SM, Haddy FJ. 1981. Effect of prolonged dietary administration of vanadate on blood pressure in the rat. *Hypertension* 3:I173–I178.

Stokinger HE. 1981. The halogens and nonmetals boron and silicon. In: Clayton GD, Clayton FE, eds. *Patty's Industrial Hygiene and Toxicology,* Vol. 2B. New York: John Wiley and Sons. Pp. 2978–3005.

Sunderman FW Jr, Dingle B, Hopfer SM, Swift T. 1988. Acute nickel toxicity in electroplating workers who accidently ingested a solution of nickel sulfate and nickel chloride. *Am J Ind Med* 14:257–266.

Sunderman FW Jr, Hopfer SM, Sweeney KR, Marcus AH, Most BM, Creason J. 1989. Nickel absorption and kinetics in human volunteers. *Proc Soc Exp Biol Med* 191:5–11.

Sutherland B, Strong P, King JC. 1998. Determining human dietary requirements for boron. *Biol Trace Elem Res* 66:193–204.

Tabata M, Sarkar B. 1992. Specific nickel(II)-transfer process between the native sequence peptide representing the nickel(II)-transport site of human serum albumin and L-histidine. *J Inorg Biochem* 45:93–104.

Takizawa Y, Hirasawa F, Noritomi E, Aida M, Tsunoda H, Uesugi S. 1988. Oral ingestion of SYLOID to mice and rats and its chronic toxicity and carcinogenicity. *Acta Med Biol* 36:27–56.

Tao SS, Bolger PM. 1999. Dietary arsenic intakes in the United States: FDA Total Diet Study, September 1991–December 1996. *Food Addit Contam* 16:465–472.

Tseng WP. 1977. Effects and dose-response relationships of skin cancer and black-foot disease with arsenic. *Environ Health Perspect* 19:109–119.

Tseng WP, Chu HM, How SW, Fong JM, Lin CS, Yeh S. 1968. Prevalence of skin cancer in an endemic area of chronic arsenicism in Taiwan. *J Natl Cancer Inst* 40:453–463.

Tsuda T, Babazono A, Yamanoto E, Kurumatani N, Mino Y, Ogawa T, Kishi Y, Aoyama H. 1995. Ingested arsenic and internal cancer: A historical cohort study followed for 33 years. *Am J Epidemiol* 141:198–209.

Uthus EO. 1994. Diethyl maleate, an in vivo chemical depletor of glutathione, affects the response of male and female rats to arsenic deprivation. *Biol Trace Elem Res* 46:247–259.

Uthus EO, Nielsen FH. 1990. Effect of vanadium, iodine and their interaction on growth, blood variables, liver trace elements and thyroid status indices in rats. *Magnes Trace Elem* 9:219–226.

Uthus EO, Poellot R. 1992. Effect of dietary pyridoxine on arsenic deprivation in rats. *Magnes Trace Elem* 10:339–347.

Uthus EO, Poellot RA. 1996. Dietary folate affects the response of rats to nickel deprivation. *Biol Trace Elem Res* 52:23–35.

Uthus EO, Seaborn CD. 1996. Deliberations and evaluations of the approaches, endpoints and paradigms for dietary recommendations of the other trace elements. *J Nutr* 126:2452S–2459S.

Vahter M. 1983. Metabolism of arsenic. In: Fowler BA, ed. *Biological and Environmental Effects of Arsenic.* Amsterdam: Elsevier. Pp. 171–198.

Valentine JL, He SY, Reisbord LS, Lachenbruch PA. 1992. Health response by questionnaire in arsenic-exposed populations. *J Clin Epidemiol* 45:487–494.

Wagner SL, Maliner JS, Morton WE, Braman RS. 1979. Skin cancer and arsenical intoxication from well water. *Arch Dermatol* 115:1205–1207.

Waltschewa W, Slatewa M, Michailow I. 1972. Testicular changes due to long-term administration of nickel sulfate in rats. *Exp Pathol* 6:116–121.

Wei CI, Al Bayati MA, Culbertson MR, Rosenblatt LS, Hansen LD. 1982. Acute toxicity of ammonium metavanadate in mice. *J Toxicol Environ Health* 10:673–687.

Weir RJ, Fisher RS. 1972. Toxicologic studies on borax and boric acid. *Toxicol Appl Pharmacol* 23:351–364.

Wester RC, Hui X, Maibach HI, Bell K, Schell MJ, Northington DJ, Strong P, Culver BD. 1998. In vivo percutaneous absorption of boron as boric acid, borax, and disodium octaborate tetrahydrate in humans: A summary. *Biol Trace Elem Res* 66:101–109.

Yamamoto S, Konishi Y, Matsuda T, Murai T, Shibata MA, Matsui-Yuasa I, Otani S, Kuroda K, Endo G, Fukushina S. 1995. Cancer induction by an organic arsenic compound, dimethylarsinic acid (cacodylic acid), in F344/DuCrj rats after pretreatment with five carcinogens. *Cancer Res* 55:1271–1276.

Yamato N. 1988. Concentrations and chemical species of arsenic in human urine and hair. *Bull Environ Contam Toxicol* 40:633–640.

Yang TH, Blackwell RQ. 1961. Nutritional and environmental conditions in the endemic Blackfoot area. *Formosan Sci* 15:101–129.

Zaporowska H, Wasilewski W. 1992. Haematological results of vanadium intoxication in Wistar rats. *Comp Biochem Physiol C* 101:57–61.

Zaporowska H, Wasilewski W, Slotwinska M. 1993. Effect of chronic vanadium administration in drinking water to rats. *Biometals* 6:3–10.

Zielhuis RL, Wibomo AA. 1984. Standard setting and metal speciation: Arsenic. In: Nriagu JO, ed. *Changing Metal Cycles and Human Health.* New York: Springer-Verlag. Pp. 323–344.

14

Uses of
Dietary Reference Intakes

OVERVIEW

The Dietary Reference Intakes (DRIs) may be used for many purposes, most of which fall into two broad categories: assessing existing nutrient intakes and planning for future nutrient intakes. Each category may be further subdivided into uses for individual diets and uses for diets of groups (Figure 14-1).

For example, the Recommended Dietary Allowance (RDA), Estimated Average Requirement (EAR), and Tolerable Upper Intake Level (UL) may be used as one aspect in the assessment of the diet of an individual. The RDA and Adequate Intake (AI) may be used as a basis for planning an improved diet for the same individual. Likewise, the EARs and ULs may be used to assess the nutrient intakes of a group of individuals, such as those participating in a dietary survey regularly conducted as part of the National Nutrition Monitoring System. The EAR and UL can also be used to plan nutritionally adequate diets for groups of people receiving meals in nursing homes, schools, and other group-feeding settings.

In the past, RDAs in the United States and Recommended Nutrient Intakes (RNIs) in Canada were the primary values available to health professionals for assessing and planning the diets of individuals and groups, and for making judgments about inadequate and excessive intake. However, the RDAs and RNIs alone were not ideally suited for many of these purposes (IOM, 1994). The DRIs provide a more complete set of reference values. The transition from using RDAs

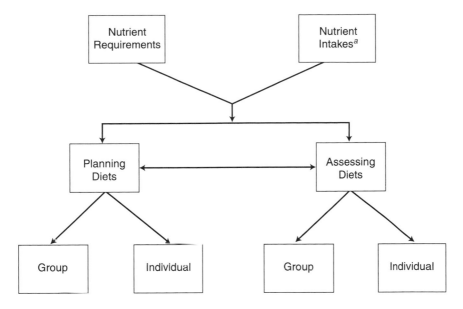

FIGURE 14-1 Conceptual framework—uses of Dietary Reference Intakes.
^a Food plus supplements.

and RNIs alone to appropriately using all of the DRIs will require time and effort by health professionals and others.

Appropriate uses of each of the new DRIs are described briefly in this chapter and in more detail in two reports on the applications of the DRIs in assessment (IOM, 2000) and planning. Also included in this chapter are specific applications to the nutrients discussed in this report. Details on how the DRIs are set with reference to specific life stage and gender groups and the primary criterion that defines adequacy for each of these nutrients are given in Chapters 4 through 13.

ASSESSING NUTRIENT INTAKES OF INDIVIDUALS

Using the Recommended Dietary Allowance and the Estimated Average Requirement for Individuals

The Dietary Reference Intakes (DRIs) were not designed to be used alone in assessing the adequacy of the diet of a specific individual because there is variability in the requirement estimate. The

Estimated Average Requirement (EAR) estimates the median of a distribution of requirements for a life stage and gender group, but it is not possible to know where an individual falls on this distribution without further physiological or biochemical measures. Thus, from dietary data alone, it is only possible to estimate the *likelihood* of nutrient adequacy or inadequacy. Furthermore, the rarity of having precise and representative data on the usual intake of an individual adds further uncertainty to the evaluation of an individual's dietary adequacy.

Dietary assessment methods have several inherent inaccuracies. One is that individuals underreport their intakes (Mertz et al., 1991; Schoeller, 1999), and it appears that obese individuals often do so to a greater extent than do normal-weight individuals (Heitmann and Lissner, 1995). Currently, a method for adjusting intakes based on underreporting by individuals is not available and much work is needed to develop an acceptable method.

Furthermore, large day-to-day variations in intake, which occur for almost all individuals, mean that it often takes a prohibitively large number of days of intake measurement to approximate usual intake (Basiotis et al., 1987). As a result, substantial caution must be used when interpreting nutrient assessments based on self-reported dietary data covering relatively few days of intake. Data on nutrient intakes should almost always be interpreted in combination with typical food usage patterns.

An approach for using data from dietary records or recalls to estimate the likelihood that an individual's nutrient intake is adequate is presented in the report *Dietary Reference Intakes: Applications in Dietary Assessment* (IOM, 2000). This approach, which is appropriate for nutrients with symmetrical requirement distributions, requires the following data:

- the individual's mean nutrient intakes during a given number of days;
- the day-to-day standard deviation of intakes for each nutrient of interest, as estimated from larger data sets for the appropriate life stage and gender group;
- the EAR; and
- the standard deviation of the nutrient requirement in the individual's life stage and gender group.

From this information, a ratio is computed that compares the magnitude of difference between the individual's intake and the EAR to an estimate of variability of intake and requirements. The bigger the difference between intake and EAR and the lower the variability of intakes and requirements, the greater the degree of certainty one has in assessing whether the individual's nutrient intake is adequate or inadequate. This approach is preferred because of its relative accuracy and should be used when the data indicated above are available.

However, when the estimate of usual intake is not based on specific recalls or records, a more qualitative interpretation of intakes could be used. For example, many practitioners use the diet history method to construct a usual day's intake, but the error structure associated with this method is unknown. Thus, a practitioner should be cautious when using this method to approximate usual intakes.

For practical purposes, many users of the DRIs may find it useful to consider that observed intakes below the EAR very likely need to be improved (because the probability of adequacy is 50 percent or less), and those between the EAR and the Recommended Dietary Allowance (RDA) probably need to be improved (because the probability of adequacy is less than 97.5 percent). Only if intakes have been observed for a large number of days and are at or above the RDA, or observed intakes for fewer days are well above the RDA, should one have a high level of confidence that the intake is adequate.

For example, a 40-year-old man who usually consumes 8 mg/day of zinc from his food and who takes a multiple vitamin and mineral supplement containing 15 mg of zinc 3 days a week would average 14.4 mg/day (8 mg + [15 mg × 3 ÷ 7]). Thus, his diet alone (8 mg/day) would put him at a high risk of inadequacy since it is below the EAR of 9.4 mg/day. The addition of the supplement, however, provides an amount above the RDA of 11 mg/day, thus suggesting little likelihood that intake is inadequate if dietary assessment represents his true usual food and supplement intake. If this same man took his multiple vitamin and mineral supplement every day, his usual intake from supplements alone would exceed the RDA, and one could conclude that he has little likelihood of inadequate zinc intake even without knowledge of his intake of zinc from food.

Using the Adequate Intake for Individuals

Adequate Intakes (AIs) have been set for all nutrients for infants through 6 months of age. By definition and observation, infants born at term who are exclusively fed human milk by healthy mothers are consuming an adequate nutrient intake. Infants who are consuming formulas with a nutrient profile similar to human milk (after adjustment for differences in bioavailability) are also consuming adequate levels. When an infant formula contains lower nutrient levels than human milk, the likelihood of nutrient adequacy for infants consuming this formula cannot be determined because data on infants at lower concentrations of intake are not available for review.

AIs have also been established for older individuals for several nutrients. Of the nutrients considered in this report, AIs have been developed for vitamin K, chromium, and manganese. Usual individual intakes equal to or above the AI can be assumed adequate. However, the likelihood of inadequacy of usual intakes below the AI cannot be determined.

Using the Tolerable Upper Intake Level for Individuals

The Tolerable Upper Intake Level (UL) is used to examine the possibility of overconsumption of a nutrient. If an individual's usual nutrient intake remains below the UL, there is little or no risk of adverse effects from excessive intake. At intakes above the UL, the risk of adverse effects may increase. However, the intake at which a given individual will develop adverse effects as a result of taking large amounts of a nutrient is not known with certainty. For example, an adult with usual zinc intakes that exceed the UL (40 mg/day) may be at increased risk of the adverse effect of reduced copper status. There is no established benefit for healthy individuals in consuming amounts of nutrients that exceed the RDA or AI.

ASSESSING NUTRIENT INTAKES OF GROUPS

Using the Estimated Average Requirement for Groups

The prevalence of nutrient inadequacy for a group of individuals may be estimated by comparing the distribution of usual intakes with the distribution of requirements. The Estimated Average Requirement (EAR) is the appropriate Dietary Reference Intake (DRI) to use for this purpose. In most situations, a cut-point approach may be used to estimate the prevalence of inadequate intakes. This approach is a simplification of the full probability method of calculating the prevalence of inadequacy described by the National Research Council (NRC, 1986). The cut-point approach allows the prevalence of inadequate intakes in a population to be approximated by determining the percentage of individuals in the group whose usual intakes are less than the EAR for the nutrient of interest. This approach assumes that the intake and requirement distributions are independent, an assumption made for the nutrients addressed in this report. It further assumes that the variability of intakes among individuals within the group under study is at least as large as the variability of their requirements. This assumption is warranted in free-living populations. Finally, it assumes that the requirement distribution is symmetrical. This is thought to be true for all nutrients discussed in this report except iron, for which requirement distributions are skewed. Additional information on assessing the adequacy of group intakes of iron is provided in the section on "Nutrient-Specific Considerations".

Before determining the percentage of the group whose intake is below the EAR, the intake distribution should be adjusted to remove the effect of day-to-day variation in intake. This can be accomplished either by collecting dietary data for each individual over a large number of days or by statistical adjustments to the intake distribution that are based on assumptions about the day-to-day variation (derived from repeat measurements of a representative subset of the group under study) (Nusser et al., 1996). When this adjustment is performed and observed intakes are thus more representative of the usual diet, the intake distribution narrows, giving a more precise estimate of the proportion of the group with usual intakes below the EAR (Figure 14-2). An explanation of this adjustment procedure has been presented in two previous reports (IOM, 2000; NRC, 1986).

An example of using the EAR cut-point approach to assess the dietary zinc adequacy of women aged 51 to 70 years follows. Dietary intake data are available from the Third National Health and Nutrition Examination Survey (NHANES III), which includes intakes from both food and supplements. Although the NHANES food-intake data were based on a single 24-hour recall for all individuals, replicate 24-hour recalls were conducted on a subset of the participants, and these estimates of day-to-day variation have been used to adjust the intake distributions (see Appendix Tables C-25 and C-26). The EAR for zinc for women is 6.8 mg/day. In the U.S. population, about 25 percent of adult women aged 51 to 70 years did not consume adequate amounts of zinc from food sources alone (Appendix Table C-25), as this proportion had estimated intakes below the EAR. When dietary supplements were included, there was little difference in the proportion below the EAR, suggesting that few individuals with low zinc intakes use zinc supplements.

The assessment of nutrient adequacy for groups of people requires unbiased, quantitative information on the intake of the nu-

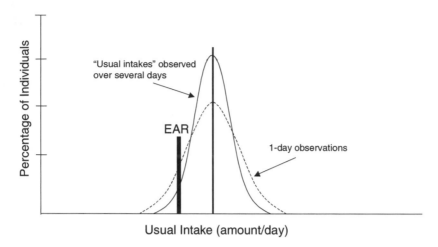

FIGURE 14-2 Comparison of 1-day and usual intakes for estimating the proportion of a group consuming intakes below the Estimated Average Requirement (EAR).

trient of interest by individuals in the group. Care must be taken to ensure the quality of the information upon which assessments are made so that they are not underestimates or overestimates of total nutrient intake. Estimates of total nutrient intake, including amounts from supplements, should be obtained. For some of the nutrients discussed in this report, drinking water may also be a significant nutrient source. It is also important to use appropriate food composition tables with accurate nutrient values for the foods as consumed. In the example for zinc, both a database of representative zinc values for all foods that contribute substantially to the intakes of this nutrient and a supplement database with the zinc composition of the specific supplements consumed by the population under study are required.

Overestimates of the prevalence of inadequate intakes could result if the data used are based on intakes that are systematically underreported or if foods rich in zinc are underreported. Such underreporting is common in national surveys (Briefel et al., 1997). Currently, a method for adjusting intakes based on underreporting by individuals is not available and much work is needed to develop an acceptable method. Conversely, underestimates of the prevalence of inadequacy would result if zinc-rich foods were overreported. A more extensive discussion of potential sources of error in self-reported dietary data can be found in the report *Dietary Reference Intakes: Applications in Dietary Assessment* (IOM, 2000).

Using the Recommended Dietary Allowance for Groups

The Recommended Dietary Allowances (RDAs) are not useful in estimating the prevalence of inadequate intakes for groups. As described above, the EAR should be used for this purpose.

Using the Adequate Intake for Groups

In this report, Adequate Intakes (AIs) are assigned for infants, and they reflect the average intake for infants receiving human milk through 6 or 12 months of age. Human milk and formulas with the same nutrient composition as human milk (after adjustment for bioavailability) provide the appropriate levels of nutrients for full-term infants of healthy, well-nourished mothers. Groups of infants consuming formulas with lower levels of nutrients than human milk may be at some risk of inadequacy, but the prevalence of inadequacy cannot be quantified.

AIs are assigned to all age groups in this report for vitamin K, chromium, and manganese. For vitamin K and manganese, AIs were based on median intakes of apparently healthy populations as assessed in large national surveys. By definition, this means that groups with median intakes equal to or above the AI can be assumed to have a low prevalence of inadequacy (provided that variability in intake does not exceed that of the healthy group used to establish the AI). However, it should be noted that group median intakes below the AI cannot be assumed to be inadequate. For chromium, the AI was established by using an estimated amount of chromium/ 1,000 kcal of nutritionally balanced meals and median energy intakes from NHANES III (Briefel et al., 1997). Thus, there is less certainty about concluding that the prevalence of nutrient inadequacy is low in groups with mean usual intakes equal to or above the AI for chromium.

Using the Tolerable Upper Intake Level for Groups

The proportion of the population with usual intakes below the Tolerable Upper Intake Level (UL) is likely to be at no risk of adverse effects due to overconsumption, but the proportion above the UL may be at some risk. In the case of zinc, for example, the UL for adults is 40 mg/day. The NHANES III data in Appendix Table

C-26, which include reported intakes from supplements, illustrate that the proportion of U.S. women aged 51 to 70 years who exceed this UL is just over 1 percent. In contrast, when data from food alone are examined, the proportion of the population with intakes above the UL is less than 1 percent (Appendix Table C-25).

In typical North American food-based diets, ULs for vitamin A, iodine, iron, manganese, molybdenum, and zinc can rarely be exceeded. The UL for copper pertains to food sources and copper supplements. Use of dietary supplements containing these nutrients would be the primary reason for exceeding the ULs.

The mean intake of a population cannot be used to evaluate the prevalence of intakes above the UL. A distribution of usual intakes, including intakes from supplements and drinking water, is required to assess the proportion of the population that might be at risk of overconsumption.

PLANNING NUTRIENT INTAKES OF INDIVIDUALS

Using the Recommended Dietary Allowance for Individuals

Individuals should use the Recommended Dietary Allowance (RDA) as the target for their daily nutrient intakes if an RDA has been established. For example, to increase their vitamin A consumption to meet the RDA (900 and 700 µg/day for men and women, respectively), adults can increase their intake of foods that provide preformed vitamin A (including dairy products, eggs, margarine, liver) and carotenoids like β-carotene (deep green and yellow fruits and vegetables). An 8-ounce glass of milk contains about 65 µg of preformed vitamin A, and a half-cup serving of carrots contains the equivalent of approximately 950 µg of vitamin A as β-carotene.

Using the Adequate Intake for Individuals

Adequate Intakes (AIs) are set for infants through 6 months of age for all nutrients, and for all nutrients except iron and zinc, for infants 7 through 12 months of age. Human milk will supply the AI for a nutrient for term infants through 6 months of age, and so it is not necessary to plan additional sources of intakes for infants exclusively fed human milk. Likewise, an infant formula with a nutrient profile similar to human milk (after adjustment for differences in bioavailability) should supply adequate nutrients for an infant.

In this report, AIs are also set for children, adolescents, and adults for vitamin K, chromium, and manganese. Accordingly, individuals should use the AI as their goal for intake of these nutrients.

PLANNING NUTRIENT INTAKES OF GROUPS

Using the Estimated Average Requirement and the Tolerable Upper Intake Level for Groups

For those nutrients with Estimated Average Requirements (EARs), the EAR may also be used as a basis for planning or making recommendations for the nutrient intakes of groups. The mean intake of a group should be high enough so that only a small percent of the group would have intakes below the EAR, thus indicating a low prevalence of dietary inadequacy. Traditionally, a prevalence of inadequacy below 2 to 3 percent has been used as a target. For nutrients with a statistically normal requirement distribution, this goal would be attained by planning for a group mean *intake* equal to the EAR plus 2 standard deviations (SD) of the intake distribution. Because the variability of intakes generally exceeds the variability of requirements, this target group mean intake will usually exceed the Recommended Dietary Allowance (RDA) (which equals the EAR plus 2 SDs of the *requirement* distribution). Prevalences of inadequacy more or less than 2 to 3 percent could also be considered, and mean intakes needed to attain these prevalences would be estimated by determining the number of SDs of intake that would result in the desired prevalence below the EAR. This is done by consulting tables that list areas of the standard normal distribution in relation to standard deviation scores (z scores).

When it is known that requirements for a nutrient are not normally distributed (for example, iron requirements) and one wants to ensure a low group prevalence of inadequacy, examination of the distributions of both intakes and requirements would be needed to determine a median intake at which the proportion of individuals below the EAR is low.

Using the EAR and Tolerable Upper Intake Level (UL) in planning intakes of groups involves a number of key decisions and the analysis of issues such as the following:

• determination of the current nutrient intake distribution of the group of interest;
• an evaluation of possible interventions to shift the current distribution, if necessary, so there is an acceptably low prevalence of intakes below the EAR, as well as an acceptably low prevalence of

intakes above the UL; some interventions may increase the intake of only those most at risk (usually by individual intervention), while others may increase the intake of the entire group (such as fortification of the food supply); and

• the selection of the degree of risk that can be tolerated when planning for the group (for example, a 2 to 3 percent prevalence versus a higher or lower prevalence).

Using the Adequate Intake for Groups

Adequate Intakes (AIs) have been established as mean or median intakes of healthy groups for some nutrients discussed in this report. This includes all nutrients for infants fed human milk through 6 months of age and the nutrients vitamin K and manganese for adults. Planning a group intake that meets the AI should, by definition, be associated with a low prevalence of inadequacy. This, of course, assumes that the group being planned for has similar characteristics to the group used to establish the AI. For chromium, the only nutrient in this report with an AI that is not based on the mean or median intake of healthy groups, there is less certainty that group mean intakes equal to or above the AI will be associated with a low prevalence of inadequacy.

NUTRIENT-SPECIFIC CONSIDERATIONS

Vitamin A

A major change in the extent to which provitamin A carotenoids can be used to form vitamin A is the replacement of retinol equivalents (µg RE) with retinol activity equivalents (µg RAE) for the provitamin A carotenoids. The RAEs for dietary β-carotene, α-carotene, and β-cryptoxanthin are 12, 24, and 24 µg, respectively, compared to corresponding REs of 6, 12, and 12 µg reported by the National Research Council (NRC, 1989). It is recommended that future food composition and intake tables use actual weights (µg) of provitamin A carotenoids rather than use converted data based on the equivalency to vitamin A. This prevents confusion as to whether the RE or RAE has been used for determining the total vitamin A content of a food or for estimating total vitamin A intakes. This change raises two issues: (1) how vitamin A intakes can be determined using the currently available U.S. Department of Agriculture's (USDA) Nutrient Database for Standard Reference, and (2) how to interpret published data on vitamin A intakes of various population groups.

Determining the Vitamin A Content of Foods with Current Nutrient Databases

Nutrient databases will need to be revised to give total vitamin A activity in µg RAE. In addition, developers of nutrient databases may choose to provide the amount (µg) of preformed vitamin A and of individual carotenoids. Thus, if the vitamin A activity for provitamin A carotenoids changes in the future, it will be possible to recalculate total vitamin A. In the meantime, it is possible to estimate total vitamin A activity in µg RAE from existing tables in µg RE. For foods, such as liver, containing only vitamin A activity from preformed vitamin A (retinol), no adjustment is necessary. Vitamin A values for foods (e.g., carrots) containing only plant sources (provitamin A carotenoids) of vitamin A can be adjusted by dividing the µg RE by two. For foods that are mixtures containing both plant and animal sources of vitamin A (e.g., a casserole containing meat and vegetables), the adjustment process is more complex. If the recipe for a mixture is known, the new vitamin A value may be calculated after adjusting the vitamin A content of each ingredient, as necessary. Alternatively, if the nutrient database contains values as µg RE for both total vitamin A and carotenoids, then it is possible to calculate a new value for both carotenoids and for total vitamin A. For example, USDA's Nutrient Database for Individual Surveys contains both these variables. To determine a revised total vitamin A value, the retinol value is calculated as the difference between the original total vitamin A value and the original carotenoid value. The revised total vitamin A content is then calculated as the sum of the retinol value and the adjusted carotenoid value, which is the original carotenoid value in µg RE divided by two. As discussed in the following section, this same procedure may be used to adjust intake data that have been analyzed using other databases.

As shown in Figure 4-2, supplemental β-carotene has a higher bioconversion to vitamin A than does dietary β-carotene. With low doses, the conversion is as high as 2:1, and developers of composition information for dietary supplements should use this higher conversion factor. Little is known about the bioconversion of the forms of β-carotene that are added to foods, so fortification forms of β-carotene should be assumed to have the same bioconversion as food forms, 12:1. Food and supplement labels usually state vitamin A levels in International Units (IU). One IU of retinol is equivalent to 0.3 µg of retinol, or 0.3 µg RAE. One IU of β-carotene in supplements is equivalent to 0.5 IU of retinol or 0.15 µg RAE (0.3×0.5). One IU of dietary β-carotene is equivalent to 0.165 IU retinol or

0.05 μg RAE (0.3 × 0.165). One IU of other dietary provitamin A carotenoids is equivalent to 0.025 μg RAE.

Interpreting Published Data on Vitamin A Intakes of Various Population Groups

Existing data on vitamin A intakes of individuals and groups will need to be reinterpreted because of the changes in the retinol molar equivalency ratios for carotenoids to μg RAE. Two scenarios are possible: (1) the existing data provide values for both total vitamin A and carotenoid intake, and (2) the existing data provide values only for total vitamin A intake.

Existing Data Provide Values for Both Total Vitamin A and Carotenoids. Data from some dietary surveys, such as the 1994–1996 Continuing Survey of Food Intakes of Individuals (CSFII) and the Third National Health and Nutrition Examination Survey (NHANES III), include REs for both total vitamin A and for carotenoids. The data manipulations required depend on the type of information that is sought (for example, mean intakes versus the proportion of a group with inadequate intakes). A way to approximate the mean intake of a group follows:

1a. Find the group mean intake for total vitamin A intake (e.g., for women aged 30 to 39 years in the CSFII, mean intake was 895 μg RE). Subtract the group mean intake of carotenoids (e.g., for women aged 30 to 39 years in the CSFII, mean carotene intake was 500 μg RE). Thus, preformed vitamin A intake would be estimated as 395 μg (895 – 500).
1b. Divide the group mean intake of carotenoids by 2 (in this example, 500 ÷ 2 = 250 μg RAE). This represents the corrected value for provitamin A intake.
1c. Add the corrected provitamin A intake determined in Step 1b to the preformed vitamin A intake determined in Step 1a. In this example, the mean vitamin A intake of women aged 30 to 39 years in the CSFII would be 645 μg RAE (250 + 395).

To determine the group prevalence of inadequate vitamin A intakes, one would need to have access to the individual intake data from which the group means were determined. For each person in the group, Steps 1a through 1c would be followed. Then the proportion of individuals with intakes below the Estimated Average

Requirement (EAR) can be determined. For vitamin A, the EAR for women is 500 µg, and thus the proportion of the group with intakes below this level would reflect the group prevalence of inadequate intakes.

Existing Data Provide Values for Only Total Vitamin A Intake. In this situation, there will be more uncertainty associated with estimates of both group mean intakes and the proportion of a group with inadequate intakes. This is because of the lack of information on the proportion of the total vitamin A intake that was derived from carotenoids. In this situation, a possible approach to approximating group mean intakes follows:

2a. Use other published data from a similar subject life stage and gender group that provide intakes of both total vitamin A and carotenoids to perform the calculations in Steps 1a through 1c above. For example, if the group of interest was 30- to 39-year-old women, data for this group from the CSFII could be used.

2b. Calculate the adjusted vitamin A intake for this group as a percentage of the unadjusted mean intake. For the example of 30- to 39-year-old women, the adjusted mean intake was 645 µg, and the unadjusted mean was 895 µg. Thus the adjusted vitamin A intake would be 0.72 (645 ÷ 895), or 72 percent.

2c. Apply the adjustment factor to the mean intake of the group of interest. For example, if the group's mean intake had been reported as 1,100 µg, the adjusted intake would be 792 µg (1,100 × 0.72).

This method could also be used to estimate the group prevalence of inadequacy, again with access to the individual intake data from which the group means were determined. In this case, the adjustment factor (in the example above, 72 percent) would be applied to data for each individual, and used in Steps 2a through 2c. The resulting distribution of intakes would then be examined to approximate the proportion of intakes below the EAR. In this situation, the approximate nature of this approach should be emphasized to an even greater extent. Given that the proportion of vitamin A derived from preformed vitamin A and from carotenoids will differ among individuals, use of an "average" adjustment factor has the potential to introduce errors that may not be random.

Implications Arising from the Development of Retinol Activity Equivalents (RAE)

The vitamin A activity of provitamin A carotenoids found in darkly colored fruits and green leafy vegetables is half that previously assumed. Consequently, individuals who rely on plant foods for the majority of their vitamin A needs should ensure that they consume foods that are rich in carotenoids (specifically, deep yellow and green vegetables and fruits) on a regular basis.

Another implication of the reduced contribution from the pro-vitamin A carotenoids is that vitamin A intakes of most population groups are lower than was previously believed. For example, in the CSFII survey, the reported mean proportion of vitamin A derived from carotenoids was 47 percent. Using the new conversion factors would thus reduce the population mean vitamin A intake by about 23 to 24 percent, or from 982 µg RE to 751 µg RAE.

Multiple EARs for Vitamin A

A second (lower) EAR has been set for vitamin A for each age group and gender, primarily for those populations with limited access to vitamin A-rich foods. The functional endpoint for this EAR is the correction of abnormal dark adaptation, rather than assuring adequate stores. Users may wish to utilize this lower EAR to assess the population prevalence of intakes that are inadequate to support normal dark adaptation, but this EAR is not intended to be used for planning intakes of groups in the United States and Canada.

Vitamin K

Because habitual vitamin K intake may modulate warfarin dosage in patients using this anticoagulant, these individuals should maintain their normal dietary and supplementation patterns once an effective dose has been established. Short-term, day-to-day variability in the intake of vitamin K from food sources does not appear to interfere with anticoagulant status and therefore does not need to be carefully monitored. However, changes in supplemental vitamin K intake should be avoided, as bioavailability of synthetic (supplemental) phylloquinone is considerably greater than bioavailability of phylloquinone from food sources.

Chromium

Because the chromium content of foods is not included in existing food composition databases, the intakes of individuals and groups cannot be assessed unless duplicate portions of ingested meals are directly analyzed. The lack of a readily available, accurate biochemical method of assessing chromium status further complicates the use of the Adequate Intake (AI) for assessment and planning purposes.

Iron

As described in Chapters 1 and 9, iron requirements were estimated through the use of factorial models involving the summation of estimates of component losses and deposition of iron. Since it is expected that the distribution of requirements would not fit the normal distribution, a process involving Monte Carlo simulation of a very large (100,000 individuals) data set was undertaken, with each "person" assigned a random value of the distribution of each component of iron need.

These needs were summed at the level of the individual to yield an estimated distribution of total requirements among individuals (see Appendix Tables I-3 and I-4). The EAR and Recommended Dietary Allowance (RDA) estimates were then derived from those distributions, as the fiftieth and ninety-seventh and one-half percentiles, respectively.

Very few data were available with which to estimate the *distribution* of basal iron losses. For this reason, variability in body size (weight in adults, surface area in children) was used as a proxy for direct measurement of variability in basal losses. The rationale for this approach stems from the fact that dermal, intestinal, and urinary losses (components of basal losses) are related to body size. However, even though body weight was used to obtain information on the distribution of losses, it is not appropriate to adjust the iron EAR or RDA for body size because variability of body weight was taken into account when these numbers were derived. Although populations with a body size distribution that differs substantially from those in the United States and Canada may have different iron requirements, a method for making such adjustments is not available.

Assessing the Adequacy of Intakes of Groups

Information on the distribution of iron requirements (rather than knowledge of the EAR) is needed to estimate the prevalence of inadequate intakes in a population. Because iron is one nutrient for which it is known with certainty that the requirement distributions are not symmetrical for all life stage and gender groups, the proportion of individuals with intakes below the EAR will not reflect the population prevalence of nutrient inadequacy. Instead, the full probability approach must be used.

The Probability Approach. Using the probability approach requires knowledge of both the distribution of requirements and the distribution of usual intakes for the population of interest. As described previously (IOM, 2000; NRC, 1986), the probability approach involves (1) determining the risk of inadequacy for each individual in the population, and then (2) averaging the individual probabilities across the group. For iron, Appendix Tables I-5, I-6, and I-7 give the probability of inadequacy at various intakes. These tables may be used to calculate the risk of inadequacy for each individual, and then the estimated prevalence of inadequacy for a population. In addition, Appendix C of *Dietary Reference Intakes: Applications in Dietary Assessment* (IOM, 2000) demonstrates how to carry out the necessary calculations to obtain a prevalence estimate for a group, and statistical programs (SAS or similar software) can be used to carry out these procedures.

A simplified estimate that could also be determined manually is illustrated in Table 14-1 for a hypothetical group of 1,000 menstruating women not taking oral contraceptives and consuming a typical omnivorous diet. The first and second columns of this table are based on information in Appendix Tables I-4 and I-7. Intakes below 4.42 mg/day are assumed to have a 100 percent probability of inadequacy (risk = 1.0). Those with intakes above 18.23 mg/day are assumed to have a zero risk of inadequacy. For intakes between these two extremes, the risk of inadequacy is calculated as 100 minus the midpoint of the percentile of requirement. For example, intakes between 4.42 and 4.88 fall between the 2.5 and 5th percentile of requirement. The midpoint is 3.75, and the probability of inadequacy is $100 - 3.75 \cong 96.3$ percent, or a risk of 0.96. The appropriate risk of inadequacy is then multiplied by the number of women with intakes in that range. In this example, only one woman had an intake between 4.42 and 4.88 mg/day, so the number of women with inadequate intake is 0.96 (1×0.96). In the next range (4.89

TABLE 14-1 Illustration of the Full Probability Approach to Estimate the Prevalence of Dietary Iron Inadequacy in a Group of 1,000 Menstruating Women (Not Using Oral Contraceptives and Following an Omnivorous Diet)

Percentiles of Requirement Distribution	Range of Usual Intake Associated with Requirement Percentiles (mg/d)	Risk of Inadequate Intake	Number of Women with Intake in Range	Number of Women with Inadequate Intake
< 2.5	< 4.42	1.0	1	1
2.5–5.0	4.42–4.88	0.96	1	0.96
5–10	4.89–5.45	0.93	3	2.79
10–20	5.46–6.22	0.85	10	8.5
20–30	6.23–6.87	0.75	15	11.25
30–40	6.88–7.46	0.65	20	13
40–50	7.47–8.07	0.55	23	12.65
50–60	8.08–8.76	0.45	27	12.15
60–70	8.77– 9.63	0.35	50	17.5
70–80	9.64–10.82	0.25	150	37.5
80–90	10.83–13.05	0.15	200	30.0
90–95	13.06–15.49	0.08	175	14
95–97.5	15.50–18.23	0.04	125	5
> 97.5	> 18.23	0.0	200	0
Total			1,000	165

mg/day to 5.45 mg/day, or between the fifth and tenth percentiles) there were three women, with an associated number of women with inadequate intake of 2.79 (3 × 0.93). If this is done for each intake range, the total number of women with inadequate intakes can be determined. In this example, 165 of the 1,000 women have inadequate intakes, for an estimated prevalence of inadequacy of 16.5 percent. It is important to remember that this approach does not identify the specific women with inadequate intakes, but is rather a statistical calculation of the prevalence of inadequate intakes. Thus, it cannot be used to screen individuals at risk of inadequacy.

Note that the prevalence of nutrient inadequacy that is estimated by the full probability approach differs considerably from that estimated by the cut-point method (the proportion with intakes below the EAR). In this example, the EAR (median requirement) is 8.07 mg/day, and only 73 women have intakes below this amount. Thus, the cut-point method would lead to an estimated prevalence of in-adequacy of 7.3 percent, which differs considerably from the estimate of 16.5 percent obtained by using the full probability approach. The reason for the discrepancy is that one of the conditions needed for the cut-point approach (a symmetrical requirement distribution) is not true for iron requirements of menstruating women.

Comparison of Assessments Using the Probability Approach to Biochemical Assessment. If requirement estimates are correct and both the dietary data and biochemical measures are reliable estimates of true usual intake and true blood concentrations in the same population, then the prevalence of apparently inadequate dietary intakes and bio-chemical deficiency should be similar, as discussed in Chapter 9. In the example above, one would expect to observe a prevalence of low serum ferritin concentrations (< 15 µg/L) that approximates the prevalence of inadequate intakes, or about 16.5 percent. The individuals with low serum ferritin concentrations are not necessarily the same as the individuals with low intake values, so the probability approach is not appropriate for identifying specific individuals with low serum ferritin values.

Special Situations in Which the EAR and RDA May Vary

Special situations in which iron requirements may vary are sum-marized in Table 14-2 along with suggestions on how to adjust esti-mates of requirements.

Zinc

Bioavailability of zinc is known to vary greatly, depending on the intakes of other dietary components, most notably phytate, that inhibit absorption. The World Health Organization (WHO, 1996) suggested that bioavailability of zinc might range from 15 percent in a diet with low bioavailability to a high of 50 percent in diets with high bioavailability. Characteristics associated with diets varying in bioavailability are summarized in Table 14-3. Gibson and Ferguson (1998) have reviewed the use of the phytate:zinc ratio for assessing dietary zinc intake. Table 14-3 indicates that diets of most North Americans would have "medium" bioavailability, approximating the fractional absorption rate of 38 percent that was used in estimating the EAR for adults. It also indicates that diets of some strict vegetar-ians may have low bioavailability, with the result that their dietary requirements for zinc would be increased. A quantitative estimate

TABLE 14-2 Situations in which the Iron Requirement May Vary

Special Consideration	Recommended Iron Intake
Infants who do not receive human milk, 0 through 6 months	The Adequate Intake (AI) of 0.27 mg/day does not apply. For infants who do not receive human milk, it is recommended that iron-containing formula (4–12 mg/L) be used from birth through 12 months.
Preterm infants	Even if they receive human milk, the AI is not adequate for preterm infants as their iron stores are low. Supplementation is recommended.
Menarche before (or after) age 14 in girls	The Estimated Average Requirement (EAR) and Recommended Dietary Allowance (RDA) for girls ages 9 to 13 years make no allowance for menstrual losses. Girls who reach menarche before age 14 years should consume an additional 2.5 mg/day. Conversely, the RDA for girls ages 14 to 18 years assumes that menstruation is occurring. It thus follows that girls 14 years and older who have not reached menarche would have a lower recommended intake of iron.
Teens/preteens in the growth spurt	Because the rate of growth during the adolescent growth spurt can be more than double the average rate for boys, and up to 50 percent higher for girls, it is recommended that boys' intakes during the growth spurt increase by 2.9 mg/day and girls' intakes by 1.1 mg/day.
Oral contraceptive users	Because blood losses are reduced by approximately 60 percent in women who habitually use oral contraceptive agents, the iron requirement and thus recommended intake for adolescent girls and women taking oral contraceptives would be lower.
Postmenopausal women using cyclic hormone replacement therapy (HRT)	Postmenopausal women who use HRT may be treated with use of either cyclic (a given number of days on active hormones followed by a week or so without hormones) or continuous protocols. Women using cyclic protocols frequently experience withdrawal bleeding in the week without hormones and thus would have higher iron requirements than women not using HRT or using continuous HRT. Few data are available on the magnitude and variability of HRT-associated blood loss, but it is probably between the losses experienced by premenopausal women who use oral contraceptives and those of postmenopausal women who do not bleed.

continued

TABLE 14-2 Continued

Special Consideration	Recommended Iron Intake
Vegetarians	Iron bioavailability is reduced in vegetarian diets, both because of the absence of easily absorbed heme iron and because of the presence of inhibitors of iron absorption. The percent bioavailability was estimated at 10 percent (versus 18 percent in omnivorous diets). Thus, the iron requirement for vegetarians would be approximately 1.8 times higher than the values established for omnivores, and recommended intakes could be adjusted using a similar factor.
Athletes	Basal losses of iron by athletes performing intense exercise on a daily basis are elevated, with estimates ranging from a 30 to 70 percent increase. Therefore, the iron requirement is increased for those who exercise intensely on a daily basis. It should be noted, however, that much of the research conducted with respect to iron needs of athletes has been done with runners. The postulated mechanisms of increased basal losses (hematuria and fecal blood loss) may not occur to as great an extent in athletes who participate in other sports.
Blood donors	The donation of 1 unit of blood/year is estimated to increase the need for absorbed iron by 0.6 to 0.7 mg/day, which, assuming 18 percent absorption, suggests that intake would need to be 3 to 4 mg/day higher. Thus, individuals who donate blood on a regular basis will have an increased iron requirement. Presumably, iron needs of frequent donors would increase in proportion to the amount of blood donated.

of the average requirement of individuals consuming diets with low zinc bioavailability cannot be made at this time. However, it seems reasonable to suggest that such individuals should be counseled to consume intakes that are at least equal to the RDA, and perhaps up to as much as twice the RDA.

The Tolerable Upper Intake Level (UL) for zinc for adults is 40 mg, which exceeds the RDA for men by somewhat less than four-fold and for women by five-fold. Although intakes of zinc above 40 mg/day from food alone are uncommon (the ninety-ninth percen-

TABLE 14-3 Qualitative Bioavailability of Zinc According to Diet Characteristics[a]

Bioavailability	Dietary Characteristics
High	Refined diets low in cereal fiber and phytic acid, with adequate protein primarily from meats and fish
	Phytate/zinc molar ratio < 5
Medium	Mixed diets containing animal or fish protein
	Vegetarian diets not based primarily on unrefined, unfermented cereal grains
	Phytate/zinc molar ratio 5–15
Low	Diets high in unrefined, unfermented, and ungerminated cereal grains, especially when animal protein intake is negligible
	High-phytate soy protein products are the primary protein source
	Diets in which ≥ 50 percent of energy is provided by high phytate foods (high extraction rate [90 percent] flours and grains, legumes)
	Phytate/zinc molar ratio > 15
	High intake of inorganic calcium (> 1 g/day) potentiates the inhibitory effects of these diets, especially when animal protein intake is low

[a] The phytate content of foods is provided by Hallberg and Hulthen (2000). The zinc content of foods is available from the U.S. Department of Agriculture at http://www.nal.usda.gov/fnic/foodcomp.
SOURCE: Modified from WHO (1996).

tiles for intake were less than 40 mg/day for all adults in both the NHANES III and CSFII surveys), when intake from supplements is added, higher proportions are above the UL. This is not unexpected, as many multiple vitamin-mineral supplements contain 15 mg of zinc. On the other hand, zinc intakes below the EAR are also fairly common. The dilemma, then, is how to ensure adequate zinc nutriture in the population while avoiding intakes in excess of the UL. Even in populations with low mean zinc intakes, care must be taken not to intervene in ways that would move a substantial proportion of the population above the UL. For example, widespread fortification of the food supply with zinc may not be appropriate, even if the prevalence of inadequacy in a population is high. More targeted approaches, such as increased consumption of zinc-rich foods by those at a high risk of inadequacy, should be considered.

Trace Elements

Previous editions of the RDAs in the United States (NRC, 1980, 1989) established a category of estimated safe and adequate daily dietary intakes (ESADDI) for essential nutrients with databases that were insufficient for developing an RDA, but where evidence of potentially toxic intakes was known. The values for ESADDI typically were ranges of intakes. The DRI process has taken a different approach. If the data required to establish intake recommendations (either an EAR and RDA, or an AI) were not available, as is the case for arsenic, boron, nickel, silicon, and vanadium in this report, no requirement is set. However, the database was adequate to establish ULs for boron, nickel, and vanadium. Therefore, for these nutrients an upper limit has been set, but not a lower limit. Accordingly, when intake data are available, users can estimate the proportion of the population that may be at risk from excessive intakes of these elements.

SUMMARY

The Dietary Reference Intakes (DRIs) may be used to assess nutrient intakes as well as for planning nutrient intakes. Box 14-1 summarizes the appropriate uses of the DRIs for individuals and groups.

For the nutrients presented in this report, only iron requires the use of the full probability approach to estimate the prevalence of inadequacy due to skewedness of the requirement distributions. Guidance is provided for adjustments to the iron requirement for several special situations, including onset of menarche before age 14 years in girls, onset of the growth spurt in adolescent males and females, use of oral contraceptives, athletes, vegetarians, and frequent blood donors.

Adjustments to zinc requirements are also recommended on the basis of the impact of the zinc:phytate ratio on bioavailability of zinc.

Examples are provided of ways to determine the appropriate adjustments to estimates of the usual intake of vitamin A considering the change in the vitamin A activity of provitamin A carotenoids.

BOX 14-1 Uses of Dietary Reference Intakes for Healthy Individuals and Groups

Type of Use	For an Individual[a]	For a Group[b]
Assessment	**EAR:** use to examine the probability that usual intake is inadequate.	**EAR:** use to estimate the prevalence of inadequate intakes within a group.
	RDA: usual intake at or above this level has a low probability of inadequacy.	**RDA:** do not use to assess intakes of groups.
	AI[c]: usual intake at or above this level has a low probability of inadequacy.	**AI**[c]: mean usual intake at or above this level implies a low prevalence of inadequate intakes.
	UL: usual intake above this level may place an individual at risk of adverse effects from excessive nutrient intake.	**UL:** use to estimate the percentage of the population at potential risk of adverse effects from excess nutrient intake.
Planning	**RDA:** aim for this intake.	**EAR:** use to plan an intake distribution with a low prevalence of inadequate intakes.
	AI[c]: aim for this intake.	**AI**[c]: use to plan mean intakes.
	UL: use as a guide to limit intake; chronic intake of higher amounts may increase the potential risk of adverse effects.	**UL:** use to plan intake distributions with a low prevalence of intakes potentially at risk of adverse effects.

RDA = Recommended Dietary Allowance
EAR = Estimated Average Requirement
AI = Adequate Intake
UL = Tolerable Upper Level

[a] Evaluation of true status requires clinical, biochemical, and anthropometric data.

continued

BOX 14-1 Continued

b Requires statistically valid approximation of distribution of usual intakes.
c For the nutrients in this report, AIs are set for infants for all nutrients, and for other age groups for vitamin K, chromium, and manganese. The AI may be used as a guide for infants as it reflects the average intake from human milk. Infants consuming formulas with the same nutrient composition as human milk are consuming an adequate amount after adjustments are made for differences in bioavailability. When the AI for a nutrient is not based on mean intakes of healthy populations, this assessment of adequacy is made with less confidence.

REFERENCES

Basiotis PP, Welsh SO, Cronin FJ, Kelsay JL, Mertz W. 1987. Number of days of food intake records required to estimate individual and group nutrient intakes with defined confidence. *J Nutr* 117:1638–1641.

Briefel RR, Sempos CT, McDowell MA, Chien S, Alaimo K. 1997. Dietary methods research in the Third National Health and Examination Survey: Underreporting of energy intake. *Am J Clin Nutr* 65:1203S–1209S.

Gibson RS, Ferguson EL. 1998. Assessment of dietary zinc in a population. *Am J Clin Nutr* 68:430S–434S.

Hallberg L, Hulthen L. 2000. Prediction of dietary iron absorption: An algorithm for calculating absorption and bioavailability of dietary iron. *Am J Clin Nutr* 71:1147–1160.

Heitmann BL, Lissner L. 1995. Dietary underreporting by obese individuals—Is it specific or non-specific? *Br Med J* 311:986–989.

IOM (Institute of Medicine). 1994. *How Should the Recommended Dietary Allowances be Revised?* Washington, DC: National Academy Press.

IOM. 2000. *Dietary Reference Intakes: Applications in Dietary Assessment.* Washington, DC: National Academy Press.

Mertz W, Tsui JC, Judd JT, Reiser S, Hallfrisch J, Morris ER, Steele PD, Lashley E. 1991. What are people really eating? The relation between energy intake derived from estimated diet records and intake determined to maintain body weight. *Am J Clin Nutr* 54:291–295.

NRC (National Research Council). 1980. *Recommended Dietary Allowances,* 9th ed. Washington, DC: National Academy Press.

NRC. 1986. *Nutrient Adequacy. Assessment Using Food Consumption Surveys.* Washington, DC: National Academy Press.

NRC. 1989. *Recommended Dietary Allowances,* 10th ed. Washington, DC: National Academy Press.

Nusser SM, Carriquiry AL, Dodd KW, Fuller WA. 1996. A semiparametric transformation approach to estimating usual daily intake distributions. *J Am Stat Assoc* 91:1440–1449.

Schoeller DA. 1999. Recent advances from application of doubly labeled water to measurement of human energy expenditure. *J Nutr* 129:1765–1768.

USDA (U.S. Department of Agriculture). 1999. *USDA Nutrient Database for Standard Reference,* Release 13. [Online.] Available: http://www.nal.usda.gov/fnic/foodcomp [accessed February 2000].

WHO (World Health Organization). 1996. Zinc. In: *Trace Elements in Human Nutrition and Health.* Geneva: WHO. Pp. 72–104.

15

A Research Agenda

The Panel on Micronutrients and the Standing Committee on the Scientific Evaluation of Dietary Reference Intakes were charged with developing a research agenda to provide a basis for public policy decisions related to recommended intakes of vitamin A, vitamin K, arsenic, boron, chromium, copper, iodine, iron, manganese, molybdenum, nickel, silicon, vanadium, and zinc, and ways to achieve the recommendations. This chapter describes the approach used to develop the research agenda, briefly summarizes gaps in knowledge, and presents a prioritized research agenda. A section at the end of each nutrient chapter (Chapters 4 through 13) presents a prioritized list of research topics for the nutrient.

APPROACH

The following approach resulted in the research agenda identified in this chapter:

1. Identify gaps in knowledge to understand the role of the nutrients in human health, functional and biochemical indicators to assess nutrient requirements, methodological problems related to the assessment of intake of these micronutrients and to the assessment of adequacy of intake, relationships of nutrient intake to chronic disease, and adverse effects of nutrients;

2. Examine data to identify major discrepancies between intake and the Estimated Average Requirements (EARs) and consider possible reasons for such discrepancies;

3. Consider the need to protect individuals with extreme or distinct vulnerabilities due to genetic predisposition or disease conditions; and

4. Weigh the alternatives and set priorities based on expert judgment.

MAJOR KNOWLEDGE GAPS

Requirements

To derive an Estimated Average Requirement (EAR), the criterion must be known for a particular status indicator or combination of indicators that is consistent with impaired status as defined by some clinical consequence. For the micronutrients considered in this report, there is a dearth of information on the biochemical values that reflect abnormal function. A priority should be the determination of the relationship of existing status indicators to clinical endpoints in the same subjects to determine if a correlation exists. For some micronutrients, either new clinical endpoints or intermediate endpoints of impaired function need to be identified and related to status indicators.

The depletion-repletion research paradigms and balance studies, although not ideal, are still probably the best approach to determining requirements for many of the trace minerals. However, these studies should be designed to meet three important criteria:

1. An indicator of nutrient status is needed for which a cutoff point has been identified, below which nutrient status is documented to be impaired. (In the case of manganese, serum manganese concentrations appear to be sensitive to large variations in manganese intake; however, there is a lack of information to indicate that this indicator reflects manganese status.)

2. The depletion and repletion periods and balance studies should be sufficiently long to allow a new steady state to be reached. For iodine and chromium, long-term balance studies are lacking. Study design should allow examination of the effects of initial status on response to maintenance or depletion-repletion.

3. Repletion regimen intakes should bracket the expected EAR intake to assess the EAR more accurately and to allow for a measure of variance. In addition, an accurate assessment of variance requires a sufficient number of subjects.

A relatively new and increasingly popular approach to determining requirements is kinetic modeling of body pools, using steady-state compartmental analyses. This approach is unlikely to supplant depletion-repletion studies because it suffers from a number of drawbacks. Several assumptions that cannot be tested experimentally are often needed, and the numbers obtained for body pool sizes are inherently imprecise. Even if accurate assessments of body pools were possible and were obtained, such information would be useful in setting a requirement only if one could establish the body pool size at which functional deficiency occurs. The amount needed for restoration of biochemical status indicators to baseline values is not necessarily equivalent to the requirement for the nutrient.

For many of the nutrients under review, useful data are seriously lacking for setting requirements for infants, children, adolescents, pregnant and lactating women, and the elderly. Studies should use graded levels of nutrient intake and a combination of response indexes, and they should consider other points raised above. For some of these nutrients, studies should examine whether the requirement varies substantially by trimester of pregnancy. Data are lacking about gender issues with respect to metabolism and requirements of these nutrients.

More information is needed on the vitamin A activity of carotenoids from plant foods and mixed meals, including meat. Field trials, studying the vitamin A efficacy of plant foods, are needed in which preformed vitamin A (positive control) is used at a supplementation level equivalent to plant food interventions. Assessment of the bioconversion and retinol molar equivalency ratio of carotenoids has mostly been conducted on single foods, rather than on a mixture of fruits and vegetables. Newer methods, such as stable isotopic methods, to evaluate the bioconversion of provitamin A carotenoids to vitamin A are encouraged. With such data, more information can be obtained about the relative contribution of dietary provitamin A carotenoids and dietary preformed vitamin A to vitamin A nutrition.

Further research is needed to evaluate the impact of non-nutritional factors on nutrient indicators. Evidence from national survey data provided in this report suggests that body mass index and plasma glucose concentration are positively correlated with indicators of iron status. Such non-nutritional factors may markedly affect the interpretation of the survey data for certain subpopulations where the prevalence of non-nutritional factors is high.

There is increasing evidence to suggest that the interaction between many of these nutrients and other food components affect nutrient absorption and metabolic utilization (bioavailability), but these interactions are not well understood in relation to the maintenance of normal nutritional status. These interactions may affect the dietary requirement for one or more of the nutrients.

Role of Nutrients in Human Health

There is evidence that arsenic, boron, nickel, silicon, and vanadium have a role in some physiological processes in some species, and for boron, silicon, and vanadium, measurable responses of human subjects to variation in dietary intake have been demonstrated. However, the available data are not as extensive and the responses are not as consistently observed as they are for the other micronutrients. Therefore, further research is needed to evaluate the metabolic role of these five trace minerals in human health.

Methodology

For some micronutrients, serious limitations exist in the methods available to analyze laboratory values indicative of micronutrient status or to determine the micronutrient content of foods, or both. Furthermore, the standardization of indicators in relation to functional outcome is needed. These methodological limitations have slowed progress in conducting or interpreting studies of nutrient requirements. Because of the difficulty in measuring chromium in food samples, data on chromium intake in North America are limited. There is a need for further standardization of thyroid volume and urinary iodine excretion to varying levels of iodine consumption. Further studies are needed for identifying the best indicator for assessing the effect of iron deficiency anemia on cognitive development.

Potential sources of error in self-reported intake data include underreporting of portion sizes and frequency of intake, omission of foods, and inaccuracies related to the use of food composition tables. At the current time, a method for adjusting intakes based on underreporting is not available and much work is needed to develop an acceptable method.

Relationships of Intake to Chronic Disease

There are major gaps in knowledge linking the intake of some micronutrients and the prevention and retardation of certain chronic diseases common in North America. Although a number of studies have been conducted to evaluate the role of vitamin K in maintenance of bone health, its role is still not well understood. A number of studies have demonstrated a beneficial effect of chromium on insulin action and circulating glucose levels; however, further information is needed to relate the intake of chromium to the prevention and reversal of diabetes. Although information on vitamin K and chromium is insufficient, even less information is available for the other nutrients, and therefore EARs are based on indicators other than functional ones.

Adverse Effects

Considering these micronutrients as a group, only a few studies have been conducted that were explicitly designed to address adverse effects of chronic high intake. For four nutrients—vitamin K, arsenic, chromium, and silicon—data were insufficient to set a Tolerable Upper Intake Level (UL). Because of insufficient human data, the UL for three nutrients—boron, molybdenum, and vanadium— were based on animal data. Thus, information on which to base a UL is extremely limited for some micronutrients.

THE RESEARCH AGENDA

Five major types of information gaps were noted: (1) a lack of data demonstrating a role of some of these nutrients in human health, (2) a dearth of studies designed specifically to estimate average requirements in presumably healthy humans, (3) a lack of data on the nutrient needs of infants, children, adolescents, the elderly, and pregnant women, (4) a lack of studies to determine the role of these nutrients in reducing the risk of certain chronic diseases, and (5) a lack of studies designed to detect adverse effects of chronic high intakes of these nutrients.

Highest priority is given to research that has the potential to prevent or retard human disease processes and to prevent deficiencies with functional consequences. The following four areas for research were assigned the highest priority (other research recommendations are found at the ends of Chapters 4 through 13):

• studies to identify and further understand the functional (e.g., cognitive function, regulation of insulin, bone health, and immune function) and biochemical endpoints that reflect sufficient and insufficient body stores of these micronutrients;
• studies to further identify and quantify the effect of interactions between nutrients and interactions between micronutrients and

other food components, the food matrix, food processing, and age on nutrient bioavailability and therefore dietary requirement;

• studies to further investigate the roles of arsenic, boron, nickel, silicon, and vanadium in human health; and

• studies to investigate the influence of non-nutritional factors (e.g., body mass index, glucose intolerance, infection) on the biochemical indicators for micronutrients such as iron and vitamin A that are currently measured by U.S. and Canadian nutritional surveys.

Because of a lack of sufficient data, a Tolerable Upper Intake Level (UL) could not be established for vitamin K, arsenic, chromium, and silicon. Furthermore, there was a lack of data from humans to establish a UL for boron, molybdenum, and vanadium, and therefore a UL was based on animal data. Thus, research is needed concerning the ULs for these micronutrients. However, it was concluded that higher priority should be given to the areas listed above because of low suspicion of toxicity at intakes consumed from food and supplements in the United States and Canada.

A

Origin and Framework of the Development of Dietary Reference Intakes

This report is one in a series of publications resulting from the comprehensive effort being undertaken by the Food and Nutrition Board's (FNB) Standing Committee on the Scientific Evaluation of Dietary Reference Intakes (DRI Committee) and its panels and sub-committees.

ORIGIN

This initiative began in June 1993, when the FNB organized a symposium and public hearing entitled "Should the Recommended Dietary Allowances Be Revised?" Shortly thereafter, to continue its collaboration with the larger nutrition community on the future of the Recommended Dietary Allowances (RDAs), the FNB took two major steps: (1) it prepared, published, and disseminated the concept paper "How Should the Recommended Dietary Allowances Be Revised?" (IOM, 1994), which invited comments regarding the proposed concept, and (2) it held several symposia at nutrition-focused professional meetings to discuss the FNB's tentative plans and to receive responses to this initial concept paper. Many aspects of the conceptual framework of the DRIs came from the United Kingdom's *Dietary Reference Values for Food Energy and Nutrients for the United Kingdom* report (COMA, 1991).

The five general conclusions presented in the FNB's 1994 concept paper are:

1. Sufficient new information has accumulated to support a reassessment of the RDAs.

2. Where sufficient data for efficacy and safety exist, reduction in the risk of chronic degenerative disease is a concept that should be included in the formulation of future recommendations.

3. Upper levels of intake should be established where data exist regarding risk of toxicity.

4. Components of food of possible benefit to health, although not meeting the traditional concept of a nutrient, should be reviewed, and if adequate data exist, reference intakes should be established.

5. Serious consideration must be given to developing a new format for presenting future recommendations.

Subsequent to the symposium and the release of the concept paper, the FNB held workshops at which invited experts discussed many issues related to the development of nutrient-based reference values, and FNB members have continued to provide updates and engage in discussions at professional meetings. In addition, the FNB gave attention to the international uses of the earlier RDAs and the expectation that the scientific review of nutrient requirements should be similar for comparable populations.

Concurrently, Health Canada and Canadian scientists were reviewing the need for revision of the *Recommended Nutrient Intakes* (RNIs) (Health Canada, 1990). Consensus following a symposium for Canadian scientists cosponsored by the Canadian National Institute of Nutrition and Health Canada in April 1995 was that the Canadian government should pursue the extent to which involvement with the developing FNB process would be of benefit to both Canada and the United States in terms of leading toward harmonization.

Based on extensive input and deliberations, the FNB initiated action to provide a framework for the development and possible international harmonization of nutrient-based recommendations that would serve, where warranted, for all of North America. To this end, in December 1995, the FNB began a close collaboration with the government of Canada and took action to establish the DRI Committee. It is hoped that representatives from Mexico will join in future deliberations.

THE CHARGE TO THE COMMITTEE

In 1995, the DRI Committee was appointed to oversee and conduct this project. The DRI Committee devised a plan involving the work of seven or more expert nutrient group panels and two over-arching subcommittees (Figure A-1). The process described below, used to develop this report, is expected to be used for subsequent reports.

The Panel on Micronutrients, composed of experts on those nutrients, was appointed in January 1999. It was responsible to (1) review the scientific literature concerning micronutrients and selected components of foods that may influence the bioavailability of these nutrients; (2) develop dietary reference levels of intake for the selected dietary micronutrients that are compatible with good nutrition throughout the lifespan and that may decrease risk of developmental abnormalities and chronic disease; (3) address the safety of high intakes of these dietary micronutrients and, when appropriate, determine tolerable upper intake limits; and (4) identify a research agenda to provide a basis for public policy decisions related to recommended intakes and ways to achieve those intakes.

The panel was charged with analyzing the literature, evaluating possible criteria or indicators of adequacy, and providing substantive rationales for their choices of each criterion. Using the criterion

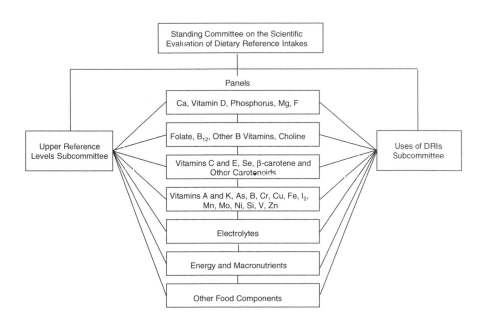

FIGURE A-1 Dietary Reference Intakes project structure.

chosen for each stage of the lifespan, the panel estimated the average requirement for each nutrient or food component reviewed, where adequate data were available. As the panel members reviewed data on Tolerable Upper Intake Levels (ULs), they also interacted with the Subcommittee on Upper Reference Levels, which assisted the panel in applying the risk assessment model (see Chapter 3) to each selected nutrient. The DRI values in this report are a product of the joint efforts of the DRI Committee, the Panel on Micronutrients, the Subcommittee on Upper Reference Levels of Nutrients, and the Subcommittee on Interpretation and Uses of Dietary Reference Intakes.

REFERENCES

COMA (Committee on Medical Aspects of Food Policy). 1991. *Dietary Reference Values for Food Energy and Nutrients for the United Kingdom.* Report on Health and Social Subjects, No. 41. London: HMSO.
Health Canada. 1990. *Nutrition Recommendations. The Report of the Scientific Review Committee 1990.* Ottawa: Canadian Government Publishing Centre.
IOM (Institute of Medicine). 1994. *How Should the Recommended Dietary Allowances be Revised?* Washington, DC: National Academy Press.

B

Acknowledgments

The Panel on Micronutrients, the Subcommittee on Upper Reference Levels of Nutrients, the Subcommittee on Interpretation and Uses of Dietary Reference Intakes, the Standing Committee on the Scientific Evaluation of Dietary Reference Intakes, and the Food and Nutrition Board (FNB) staff are grateful for the time and effort of the many contributors to the report and the workshops and meetings leading up to the report. Through openly sharing their considerable expertise and different outlooks, these individuals and organizations brought clarity and focus to the challenging task of setting Dietary Reference Intakes (DRIs) for vitamins A and K, boron, chromium, copper, iodine, iron, manganese, molybdenum, nickel, vanadium, and zinc. The list below mentions those individuals who worked closely with the members and staff, but many others also deserve heartfelt thanks. Those individuals made important contributions to the report by offering suggestions and opinions at the many professional meetings and workshops the members attended. The panel, subcommittee, and committee members, as well as the FNB staff thank the following named (as well as unnamed) individuals and organizations:

591

INDIVIDUALS

Carol Ballew
Neil Binkley
Sarah Booth
Barbara Bowman
Lewis Braverman
Gary Brittenham
James Cook
James Coughlin
Francoise Delange
Kay Dewey
Judy Douglas
Curtis Eckhert
Mark Failla
Jeanne Freeland-
    Graves
James Friel
Victor Gordeuk
Michael Green

John Hathcock
James Heimbach
Terresita Hernandez
Curtiss Hunt
Janet Hunt
Cliff Johnson
Bo Lonnerdal
Anne Looker
Henry Lukaski
John McNeill
David Milne
Phylis Moser-Veillon
Joe Mulinare
Mary Murphy
Richard Nelson
Forrest Nielsen
Donald Oberleas
Cynthia Ogden

James Olson
Charlene Rainey
Helen Rasmussen
Harold Sandstead
Leon Schurgers
Chris Sempos
Anuraj Shankar
Dianne Soprano
Anne Sowell
Charles Stephensen
Phillip Strong
Guangwen Tang
Eric Uthus
Karin van het Hof
Clive West
Ulf Wiegand
Jan Wolff

FEDERAL ADVISORY STEERING COMMITTEE

Barbara Bowman
Elizabeth Castro
Margaret Cheney
Carolyn Clifford
Paul Coates
Rebecca Costello
Kathleen Ellwood
Nancy Ernst

Peter Fischer
Elizabeth Frazao
Karl Friedl
Nancy Gaston
Jay Hirschman
Van Hubbard
Clifford Johnson
Christine Lewis
Jean Lloyd

Melvin Mathias
Linda Meyers
Esther Myers
Cynthia Ogden
Susan Pilch
Pamela Starke-Reed
Jacqueline Wright
Elizabeth Yetley

ORGANIZATIONS

American Dietetic Association
American Society for Nutritional Sciences
Council for Responsible Nutrition
Federation of American Scientists for Experimental Biology
Health Canada
Institute of Food Technologists
Nutrition Coordinating Center, University of Minnesota

C

Dietary Intake Data from the Third National Health and Nutrition Examination Survey (NHANES III), 1988–1994

TABLE C-1 Mean and Percentiles for One-Day Intake of α-Carotene (µg/day) from Food, NHANES III (1988–1994)

Sex/Age Category[a]	Number of Persons Examined	Mean	Percentile	
			5th	10th
Both sexes, 2 to 6 mo	793	359	0	0
Both sexes, 7 to 12 mo	827	589	0	1
Both sexes, 1 to 3 y	3,309	221	1	2
Both sexes, 4 to 8 y	3,448	207	1	3
M 9 to 13 y	1,219	343	1	3
M 14 to 18 y	909	239	0	<1
M 19 to 30 y	1,902	425	<1	2
M 31 to 50 y	2,533	457	<1	2
M 51 to 70 y	1,942	582	<1	2
M 71+ y	1,255	535	<1	3
F 9 to 13 y	1,216	307	1	1
F 14 to 18 y	949	203	0	1
F 19 to 30 y	1,901	246	<1	1
F 31 to 50 y	2,939	468	<1	2
F 51 to 70 y	2,065	592	1	3
F 71+ y	1,368	588	1	4
F Pregnant	346	376	1	3
F Lactating	99	417	1	2
All Individuals	28,575	407	<1	2
All Indiv (+P/L)	29,015	406	<1	2

594

25th	50th	75th	90th	95th	99th
0	3	210	1,107	2,066	3,894
6	91	638	1,596	3,194	5,417
6	17	56	655	1,376	3,443
9	22	58	366	1,190	3,443
8	25	68	291	1,202	5,846
8	29	76	257	1,638	4,476
9	39	128	1,386	2,355	7,207
10	51	191	1,457	2,464	6,620
13	58	308	2,028	3,174	6,053
13	51	262	1,681	3,135	5,758
7	19	60	400	1,719	5,171
4	21	58	295	1,348	2,927
7	29	97	567	1,327	3,718
10	44	208	1,460	2,712	6,960
15	59	354	1,823	3,240	7,427
14	58	488	2,250	3,266	4,966
9	41	166	1,175	1,836	6,735
10	43	111	483	2,132	6,735
9	36	144	1,184	2,416	5,689
9	36	144	1,184	2,389	5,689

continued

TABLE C-1 Continued

Sex/Age Category[a]	Number of Persons Examined	Mean	Percentile	
			1st	5th

NOTE: Data are limited to individuals who provided a complete and reliable 24-hour dietary recall on day 1. Estimates represent the unadjusted distribution of the intake reported per individual (the distribution of the data does not meet the assumptions of the Iowa State University method, i.e., the C-Side program). The mean and percentiles for all distributions were calculated using SAS PROC UNIVARIATE. All sample weights greater than 40,000 were truncated to 40,000 to reduce the influence of extreme intake patterns. Food composition data are from the NDS-R Food and Nutrient Database, Version 30, 1999, Nutrition Coordinating Center, University of Minnesota. Infants and children fed human milk and females who had "blank but applicable" pregnancy and

10th	25th	50th	75th	90th	95th	99th

lactating status data or who responded "I don't know" to questions on pregnancy and lactating status were excluded from all analyses. Females who were both pregnant and lactating were included in both the Pregnant and Lactating categories. The sample sizes for the Pregnant and Lactating categories were very small so their estimates of usual intake distributions are not reliable.

[a] M = male, F = female, P/L = pregnant and lactating.

SOURCE: ENVIRON International Corporation and Iowa State University Department of Statistics, 2000, Revised.

TABLE C-2 Mean and Percentiles for Usual Intake of β-Carotene (µg/day) from Food, NHANES III (1988–1994)

Sex/Age Category[a]	Number of Persons Examined	Mean	Percentile 5th	Percentile 10th
Both sexes, 2 to 6 mo	793	1,159	1	1
Both sexes, 7 to 12 mo	827	1,950	42	79
Both sexes, 1 to 3 y	3,309	1,020	75	110
Both sexes, 4 to 8 y	3,448	1,722	1,037	1,148
Standard error		353	174	202
M 9 to 13 y	1,219	1,694	461	575
Standard error		499	89	124
M 14 to 18 y	909	1,420	492	600
Standard error		190	51	67
M 19 to 30 y	1,902	2,146	726	885
Standard error		164	63	71
M 31 to 50 y	2,533	2,299	736	913
Standard error		139	48	54
M 51 to 70 y	1,942	2,622	826	1,026
Standard error		163	73	82
M 71+ y	1,255	2,733	800	1,009
Standard error		166	64	72
F 9 to 13 y	1,216	1,826	584	720
Standard error		667	141	186
F 14 to 18 y	949	1,183	411	502
Standard error		124	35	44
F 19 to 30 y	1,901	1,595	538	660
Standard error		169	38	50
F 31 to 50 y	2,939	2,144	763	929
Standard error		100	46	49
F 51 to 70 y	2,065	2,665	931	1,141
Standard error		336	64	71
F 71+ y	1,368	2,634	983	1,196
Standard error		133	65	72
Pregnant	346	1,531	654	778
Standard error		217	112	138
Lactating	99	1,568	789	900
Standard error		425	147	176
All Individuals	28,575	1,985	617	774
Standard error		45	23	25
All Indiv (+P/L)	29,015	1,978	615	771
Standard error		44	23	25

NOTE: Data are limited to individuals who provided a complete and reliable 24-hour dietary recall on day 1. The intake distributions for 2–6 months, 7–12 months, and 1–3 years of age are unadjusted. Means and percentiles for these groups were computed using SAS PROC UNIVARIATE. For all other groups, data were adjusted using the Iowa State University method. Mean, standard errors, and percentiles were obtained using C-Side. Standard errors were estimated via jackknife replication. Each standard error has 49 degrees of freedom. Food composition data are from the NDS-R Food and Nutrient Database, Version 30, 1999, Nutrition Coordinating Center, University of Minnesota. Infants and children fed human milk and females who had "blank but applicable"

25th	50th	75th	90th	95th	99th
6	77	1,274	4,240	6,658	10,365
236	711	2,166	5,684	7,974	13,208
198	411	931	2,279	3,920	8,583
1,362	1,649	2,001	2,386	2,653	3,247
256	332	426	531	606	777
839	1,300	2,069	3,218	4,230	7,173
206	353	612	1,030	1,420	2,630
833	1,201	1,749	2,484	3,082	4,670
101	153	236	358	466	778
1,231	1,793	2,663	3,831	4,759	7,101
88	124	199	321	429	728
1,306	1,942	2,886	4,110	5,068	7,479
69	103	170	288	409	848
1,470	2,199	3,302	4,741	5,861	8,603
100	134	198	297	381	596
1,479	2,261	3,457	5,029	6,262	9,334
91	134	213	335	448	794
1,023	1,519	2,269	3,278	4,099	6,278
296	495	834	1,350	1,810	3,190
700	1,014	1,472	2,062	2,523	3,692
64	96	154	260	370	737
929	1,359	1,989	2,805	3,447	5,083
78	128	214	338	444	739
1,289	1,857	2,678	3,713	4,502	6,414
57	78	129	205	266	428
1,598	2,317	3,339	4,612	5,580	7,943
100	186	400	811	1,230	2,560
1,653	2,351	3,304	4,431	5,250	7,138
91	123	168	224	266	379
1,031	1,388	1,866	2,456	2,902	3,972
178	204	258	368	468	760
1,121	1,435	1,862	2,391	2,798	3,812
239	348	530	800	1,040	1,700
1,110	1,665	2,491	3,580	4,444	6,641
29	40	55	78	100	167
1,106	1,659	2,483	3,567	4,428	6,614
29	39	54	76	97	161

pregnancy and lactating status data or who responded "I don't know" to questions on pregnancy and lactating status were excluded from all analyses. Females who were both pregnant and lactating were included in both the Pregnant and Lactating categories. The sample sizes for the Pregnant and Lactating categories were very small so their estimates of usual intake distributions are not reliable.

[a] M = male, F = female, P/L = pregnant and lactating.

SOURCE: ENVIRON International Corporation and Iowa State University Department of Statistics, 2000.

TABLE C-3 Mean and Percentiles for One-Day Intake of β-Cryptoxanthin (µg/day) from Food, NHANES III (1988–1994)

Sex/Age Category[a]	Number of Persons Examined	Mean	Percentile	
			5th	10th
Both sexes, 2 to 6 mo	793	18	0	0
Both sexes, 7 to 12 mo	827	43	0	1
Both sexes, 1 to 3 y	3,309	83	0	1
Both sexes, 4 to 8 y	3,448	84	0	1
M 9 to 13 y	1,219	101	0	0
M 14 to 18 y	909	121	0	1
M 19 to 30 y	1,902	136	0	1
M 31 to 50 y	2,533	117	0	1
M 51 to 70 y	1,942	122	0	1
M 71+ y	1,255	135	0	1
F 9 to 13 y	1,216	94	0	0
F 14 to 18 y	949	88	0	0
F 19 to 30 y	1,901	98	0	0
F 31 to 50 y	2,939	84	0	1
F 51–70 y	2,065	107	0	1
F 71+ y	1,368	105	0	1
F Pregnant	346	159	1	2
F Lactating	99	172	0	1
All Individuals	28,575	104	0	1
All Indiv (+P/L)	29,015	105	0	1

NOTE: Data are limited to individuals who provided a complete and reliable 24-hour dietary recall on day 1. Estimates represent the unadjusted distribution of the intake reported per individual (the distribution of the data does not meet the assumptions of the Iowa State University method, i.e., the C-Side program). The mean and percentiles for all distributions were calculated using SAS PROC UNIVARIATE. All sample weights greater than 40,000 were truncated to 40,000 to reduce the influence of extreme intake patterns. Food composition data are from the NDS-R Food and Nutrient Database, Version 30, 1999, Nutrition Coordinating Center, University of Minnesota. Infants and children fed human milk and females who had "blank but applicable" pregnancy and

25th	50th	75th	90th	95th	99th
0	7	23	45	65	177
8	23	51	103	143	258
4	39	113	213	326	544
3	27	120	239	337	596
3	20	139	263	373	662
3	14	167	334	463	1,376
4	19	177	392	556	1,262
5	27	152	326	476	982
4	34	160	312	442	892
4	39	154	278	384	1,336
3	23	147	266	344	787
3	13	92	266	422	836
3	13	118	260	421	1,009
3	18	100	245	357	738
4	41	157	266	383	715
5	52	153	273	345	635
6	46	184	367	813	1,357
16	91	179	474	1,003	1,003
4	24	134	277	410	830
4	24	135	279	413	850

lactating status data or who responded "I don't know" to questions on pregnancy and lactating status were excluded from all analyses. Females who were both pregnant and lactating were included in both the Pregnant and Lactating categories. The sample sizes for the Pregnant and Lactating categories were very small so their estimates of usual intake distributions are not reliable.

[a] M = male, F = female, P/L = pregnant and lactating.

SOURCE: ENVIRON International Corporation and Iowa State University Department of Statistics, 2000, Revised.

TABLE C-4 Mean and Percentiles for Usual Intake of Lutein and Zeaxanthin (µg/day) from Food, NHANES III (1988–1994)

Sex/Age Category[a]	Number of Persons Examined	Mean	Percentile	
			5th	10th
Both sexes, 2 to 6 mo	793	457	0	0
Both sexes, 7 to 12 mo	827	790	60	98
Both sexes, 1 to 3 y	3,309	927	159	217
Both sexes, 4 to 8 y	3,448	1,277	530	616
Standard error		93	24	32
M 9 to 13 y	1,219	1,330	674	770
Standard error		68	30	38
M 14 to 18 y	909	1,418	693	801
Standard error		84	39	45
M 19 to 30 y	1,902	2,032	881	1,040
Standard error		353	71	95
M 31 to 50 y	2,533	2,192	929	1,097
Standard error		151	57	70
M 51 to 70 y	1,942	2,264	880	1,046
Standard error		110	29	36
M 71+ y	1,255	2,088	788	937
Standard error		132	44	52
F 9 to 13 y	1,216	1,280	569	668
Standard error		306	72	70
F 14 to 18 y	949	1,162	448	526
Standard error		102	34	37
F 19 to 30 y	1,901	1,704	532	645
Standard error		243	19	30
F 31 to 50 y	2,939	2,013	690	848
Standard error		102	32	39
F 51 to 70 y	2,065	1,960	691	840
Standard error		96	24	29
F 71+ y	1,368	1,921	675	817
Standard error		108	26	33
Pregnant	346	1,455	649	754
Standard error		132	50	60
Lactating	99	1,850	958	1,098
Standard error		277	144	171
All Individuals	28,575	1,719	583	714
Standard error		49	13	16
All Indiv (+P/L)	29,015	1,712	581	712
Standard error		44	11	14

NOTE: Data are limited to individuals who provided a complete and reliable 24-hour dietary recall on day 1. The intake distributions for 2–6 months, 7–12 months, and 1–3 years of age are unadjusted. Means and percentiles for these groups were computed using SAS PROC UNIVARIATE. For all other groups, data were adjusted using the Iowa State University method. Mean, standard errors, and percentiles were obtained using C-Side. Standard errors were estimated via jackknife replication. Each standard error has 49 degrees of freedom. Food composition data are from the NDS-R Food and Nutrient Database, Version 30, 1999, Nutrition Coordinating Center, University of Minnesota. Infants and children fed human milk and females who had "blank but applicable"

25th	50th	75th	90th	95th	99th
1	94	353	1,083	2,407	5,703
214	398	832	1,512	2,788	5,673
365	624	1,068	1,823	2,572	7,542
801	1,099	1,537	2,135	2,625	3,965
48	74	119	190	261	471
960	1,228	1,583	2,009	2,328	3,099
52	65	84	113	138	217
1,016	1,317	1,707	2,159	2,487	3,247
57	76	104	144	179	284
1,366	1,839	2,469	3,240	3,834	5,342
126	234	554	880	1,090	1,700
1,443	1,957	2,669	3,560	4,251	5,986
94	130	186	269	339	539
1,405	1,966	2,776	3,825	4,656	6,800
51	83	140	228	308	543
1,261	1,778	2,552	3,590	4,430	6,649
72	107	168	260	342	582
866	1,152	1,544	2,038	2,426	3,408
135	298	130	547	669	1,210
699	993	1,421	1,989	2,452	3,700
57	79	128	210	292	608
906	1,353	2,071	3,111	4,026	6,743
65	142	296	558	819	1,730
1,185	1,712	2,486	3,514	4,346	6,541
55	82	127	199	266	473
1,167	1,684	2,437	3,404	4,161	6,077
43	65	111	226	363	857
1,130	1,634	2,381	3,359	4,133	6,124
50	82	137	228	320	626
973	1,306	1,767	2,335	2,764	3,811
80	113	166	243	311	502
1,373	1,750	2,217	2,730	3,087	3,874
220	278	340	406	457	593
1,004	1,466	2,144	3,021	3,711	5,470
23	36	61	99	133	231
1,001	1,461	2,135	3,007	3,694	5,442
20	32	55	91	123	218

pregnancy and lactating status data or who responded "I don't know" to questions on pregnancy and lactating status were excluded from all analyses. Females who were both pregnant and lactating were included in both the Pregnant and Lactating categories. The sample sizes for the Pregnant and Lactating categories were very small so their estimates of usual intake distributions are not reliable.

[a] M = male, F = female, P/L = pregnant and lactating.

SOURCE: ENVIRON International Corporation and Iowa State University Department of Statistics, 2000.

TABLE C-5 Mean and Percentiles for One-Day Intake of
Lycopene (μg/day) from Food, NHANES III (1988–1994)

Sex/Age Category[a]	Number of Persons Examined	Mean	Percentile	
			5th	10th
Both sexes, 2 to 6 mo	793	164	0	0
Both sexes, 7 to 12 mo	827	1,873	0	0
Both sexes, 1 to 3 y	3,309	5,278	0	0
Both sexes, 4 to 8 y	3,448	6,951	0	0
M 9 to 13 y	1,219	10,111	0	0
M 14 to 18 y	909	11,547	0	0
M 19 to 30 y	1,902	12,656	0	0
M 31 to 50 y	2,533	9,882	0	0
M 51 to 70 y	1,942	6,635	0	0
M 71+ y	1,255	6,666	0	0
F 9 to 13 y	1,216	8,262	0	0
F 14 to 18 y	949	7,980	0	0
F 19 to 30 y	1,901	7,438	0	0
F 31 to 50 y	2,939	5,972	0	0
F 51 to 70 y	2,065	5,388	0	0
F 71+ y	1,368	4,332	0	0
F Pregnant	346	8,713	0	0
F Lactating	99	9,513	0	0
All Individuals	28,575	7,753	0	0
All Indiv (+P/L)	29,015	7,774	0	0

NOTE: Data are limited to individuals who provided a complete and reliable 24-hour dietary recall on day 1. Estimates represent the unadjusted distribution of the intake reported per individual (the distribution of the data does not meet the assumptions of the Iowa State University method, i.e., the C-Side program). The mean and percentiles for all distributions were calculated using SAS PROC UNIVARIATE. All sample weights greater than 40,000 were truncated to 40,000 to reduce the influence of extreme intake patterns. Food composition data are from the NDS-R Food and Nutrient Database, Version 30, 1999, Nutrition Coordinating Center, University of Minnesota. Infants and children fed human milk and females who had "blank but applicable" pregnancy and

25th	50th	75th	90th	95th	99th
0	0	0	188	666	2,707
0	0	780	7,520	11,481	21,577
0	1,361	6,366	16,629	23,756	43,262
23	2,902	9,125	19,566	30,234	52,255
242	4,301	12,771	24,775	41,509	89,687
133	5,211	15,355	30,456	38,538	123,299
511	5,079	16,000	33,447	47,460	110,395
0	2,902	11,832	29,126	46,342	76,642
0	1,625	6,853	19,600	30,456	60,917
0	1,376	5,627	20,557	29,938	83,429
0	2,902	11,482	23,962	34,292	50,216
0	2,902	10,179	20,804	31,449	72,465
0	2,420	9,709	20,760	29,933	62,806
0	1,836	7,053	15,350	28,061	57,600
0	1,361	4,877	15,741	27,594	47,917
0	842	3,409	13,084	22,550	52,255
696	3,802	13,467	25,101	27,943	71,038
1,625	3,969	12,058	33,520	37,942	48,076
0	2,141	9,152	22,290	33,325	65,522
0	2,167	9,226	22,398	33,325	65,517

lactating status data or who responded "I don't know" to questions on pregnancy and lactating status were excluded from all analyses. Females who were both pregnant and lactating were included in both the Pregnant and Lactating categories. The sample sizes for the Pregnant and Lactating categories were very small so their estimates of usual intake distributions are not reliable.

[a] M = male, F = female, P/L = pregnant and lactating.

SOURCE: ENVIRON International Corporation and Iowa State University Department of Statistics, 2000, Revised.

TABLE C-6 Mean and Percentiles for Usual Intake of Retinol (μg/day) from Food, NHANES III (1988–1994)

Sex/Age Category[a]	Number of Persons Examined	Mean	Percentile	
			5th	10th
Both sexes, 2 to 6 mo	793	530	220	297
Both sexes, 7 to 12 mo	827	515	198	246
Both sexes, 1 to 3 y	3,309	496	83	139
Both sexes, 4 to 8 y	3,448	610	423	459
Standard error		15	10	11
M 9 to 13 y	1,219	673	291	348
Standard error		23	11	13
M 14 to 18 y	909	689	248	309
Standard error		36	16	19
M 19 to 30 y	1,902	598	199	241
Standard error		36	9	14
M 31 to 50 y	2,533	636	206	260
Standard error		31	9	11
M 51 to 70 y	1,942	682	216	277
Standard error		40	14	17
M 71+ y	1,255	658	229	281
Standard error		35	13	14
F 9 to 13 y	1,216	576	227	279
Standard error		34	18	22
F 14 to 18 y	949	440	147	186
Standard error		22	10	12
F 19 to 30 y	1,901	429	141	177
Standard error		19	7	9
F 31 to 50 y	2,939	441	146	179
Standard error		19	4	7
F 51 to 70 y	2,065	527	159	192
Standard error		40	7	10
F 71+ y	1,368	543	188	231
Standard error		41	9	9
Pregnant	346	600	233	282
Standard error		132	23	25
Lactating	99	931	480	577
Standard error		134	125	158
All Individuals	28,575	547	216	263
Standard error		8	4	4
All Indiv (+P/L)	29,015	550	217	264
Standard error		8	4	4

NOTE: Data are limited to individuals who provided a complete and reliable 24-hour dietary recall on day 1. The intake distributions for 2–6 months, 7–12 months, and 1–3 years of age are unadjusted. Means and percentiles for these groups were computed using SAS PROC UNIVARIATE. For all other groups, data were adjusted using the Iowa State University method. Mean, standard errors, and percentiles were obtained using C-Side. Standard errors were estimated via jackknife replication. Each standard error has 49 degrees of freedom. Food composition data are from the NDS-R Food and Nutrient Database, Version 30, 1999, Nutrition Coordinating Center, University of Minnesota. Infants and children fed human milk and females who had "blank but applicable"

25th	50th	75th	90th	95th	99th
417	523	641	744	881	1,175
345	481	632	785	906	1,424
245	404	602	836	1,058	2,069
523	602	687	771	823	929
13	15	17	20	22	27
462	619	823	1,063	1,238	1,645
15	20	30	44	57	92
437	624	869	1,150	1,351	1,802
24	32	45	65	82	128
346	534	763	1,039	1,231	1,707
16	35	53	85	91	166
376	557	807	1,109	1,333	1,863
15	24	39	63	83	138
410	607	862	1,160	1,395	2,040
24	37	58	184	223	270
395	571	818	1,130	1,378	2,031
17	26	44	75	108	219
373	526	711	946	1,089	1,502
25	29	53	118	99	286
269	393	559	752	892	1,212
16	21	28	38	49	81
255	378	545	742	888	1,245
11	19	25	38	48	83
254	383	551	779	935	1,366
8	15	23	55	64	148
274	428	655	969	1,243	1,951
17	25	49	102	140	316
324	468	673	937	1,149	1,716
19	29	61	99	139	317
387	540	746	990	1,169	1,591
32	49	118	321	581	1,620
733	895	1,079	1,314	1,503	1,974
176	140	133	184	228	387
361	502	684	889	1,034	1,358
5	7	10	14	17	26
362	505	688	895	1,041	1,368
6	8	10	14	18	26

pregnancy and lactating status data or who responded "I don't know" to questions on pregnancy and lactating status were excluded from all analyses. Females who were both pregnant and lactating were included in both the Pregnant and Lactating categories. The sample sizes for the Pregnant and Lactating categories were very small so their estimates of usual intake distributions are not reliable.

[a] M = male, F = female, P/L = pregnant and lactating.

SOURCE: ENVIRON International Corporation and Iowa State University Department of Statistics, 2000.

TABLE C-7 Mean and Percentiles for Usual Intake of Total Vitamin A (μg RE^a/day) from Food, NHANES III (1988–1994)

Sex/Age Category^b	Number of Persons Examined	Mean	Percentile 5th	10th
Both sexes, 2 to 6 mo	793	755	318	381
Both sexes, 7 to 12 mo	827	893	298	362
Both sexes, 1 to 3 y	3,309	691	149	213
Both sexes, 4 to 8 y	3,448	849	585	632
Standard error		32	20	22
M 9 to 13 y	1,219	965	404	477
Standard error		46	15	18
M 14 to 18 y	909	950	381	462
Standard error		49	24	28
M 19 to 30 y	1,902	1,005	377	463
Standard error		58	20	21
M 31 to 50 y	2,533	1,111	387	470
Standard error		62	12	16
M 51 to 70 y	1,942	1,146	415	512
Standard error		46	17	22
M 71+ y	1,255	1,182	451	549
Standard error		48	17	19
F 9 to 13 y	1,216	836	387	453
Standard error		58	18	21
F 14 to 18 y	949	660	282	337
Standard error		39	19	22
F 19 to 30 y	1,901	740	302	365
Standard error		35	13	16
F 31 to 50 y	2,939	838	355	424
Standard error		21	10	11
F 51 to 70 y	2,065	1,013	409	492
Standard error		68	22	22
F 71+ y	1,368	1,040	460	542
Standard error		41	17	20
Pregnant	346	947	423	497
Standard error		156	44	63
Lactating	99	1,253	717	811
Standard error		263	369	435
All Individuals	28,575	922	445	517
Standard error		12	6	7
All Indiv (+P/L)	29,015	924	446	518
Standard error		12	6	7

NOTE: Data are limited to individuals who provided a complete and reliable 24-hour dietary recall on day 1. The intake distributions for 2–6 months, 7–12 months, and 1–3 years of age are unadjusted. Means and percentiles for these groups were computed using SAS PROC UNIVARIATE. For all other groups, data were adjusted using the Iowa State University method. Mean, standard errors, and percentiles were obtained using C-Side. Standard errors were estimated via jackknife replication. Each standard error has 49 degrees of freedom. Food composition data are from the NDS-R Food and Nutrient Database, Version 30, 1999, Nutrition Coordinating Center, University of Minnesota. Infants and children fed human milk and females who had "blank but applicable" pregnancy and lactating status data or who responded "I don't know" to questions on

25th	50th	75th	90th	95th	99th
493	624	881	1,315	1,732	2,586
516	721	1,034	1,631	2,021	3,093
351	537	804	1,198	1,570	2,796
719	829	958	1,090	1,177	1,356
27	31	36	45	55	90
628	859	1,178	1,571	1,880	2,689
26	33	61	106	152	322
629	870	1,182	1,538	1,789	2,356
36	47	62	81	96	139
638	914	1,273	1,643	1,917	2,647
44	48	135	126	104	157
652	949	1,380	1,926	2,367	3,582
24	46	85	130	176	352
713	1,012	1,425	1,937	2,332	3,307
30	35	69	97	127	231
750	1,047	1,457	1,972	2,371	3,357
26	38	60	97	138	284
587	776	1,016	1,290	1,490	1,964
28	46	77	122	162	280
450	610	815	1,045	1,208	1,571
28	36	48	62	74	105
490	668	907	1,200	1,424	1,969
22	30	43	65	83	131
565	764	1,027	1,341	1,574	2,132
14	19	26	39	51	88
664	913	1,245	1,648	1,954	2,714
29	60	101	138	168	307
710	954	1,271	1,640	1,911	2,562
24	34	54	86	118	223
648	861	1,139	1,485	1,760	2,484
106	157	198	259	336	628
988	1,215	1,477	1,745	1,922	2,289
426	279	237	332	362	542
662	863	1,118	1,402	1,601	2,046
8	11	15	20	25	36
663	865	1,120	1,405	1,605	2,051
8	11	15	20	25	36

pregnancy and lactating status were excluded from all analyses. Females who were both pregnant and lactating were included in both the Pregnant and Lactating categories. The sample sizes for the Pregnant and Lactating categories were very small so their estimates of usual intake distributions are not reliable.

[a] RE = retinol equivalents. 1 μg RE = 6 μg β-carotene and 12 μg α-carotene or β-cryptoxanthin.

[b] M = male, F = female, P/L = pregnant and lactating.

SOURCE: ENVIRON International Corporation and Iowa State University Department of Statistics, 2000.

TABLE C-8 Mean and Percentiles for Usual Intake of Total Vitamin A (μg RAE^a/day) from Food, NHANES III (1988–1994)

Sex/Age Category^b	Number of Persons Examined	Mean	Percentile	
			5th	10th
Both sexes, 2 to 6 mo	793	643	305	362
Both sexes, 7 to 12 mo	827	704	260	331
Both sexes, 1 to 3 y	3,309	593	123	181
Both sexes, 4 to 8 y	3,448	728	588	615
Standard error		25	21	23
M 9 to 13 y	1,219	818	354	422
Standard error		29	13	15
M 14 to 18 y	909	819	322	392
Standard error		41	20	23
M 19 to 30 y	1,902	803	295	367
Standard error		59	13	19
M 31 to 50 y	2,533	898	309	368
Standard error		58	7	8
M 51 to 70 y	1,942	910	330	405
Standard error		36	13	15
M 71+ y	1,255	909	360	435
Standard error		33	13	14
F 9 to 13 y	1,216	706	323	381
Standard error		44	16	21
F 14 to 18 y	949	549	228	275
Standard error		30	15	18
F 19 to 30 y	1,901	583	236	287
Standard error		24	9	12
F 31 to 50 y	2,939	640	266	320
Standard error		23	12	9
F 51 to 70 y	2,065	771	299	361
Standard error		43	12	15
F 71+ y	1,368	793	354	408
Standard error		34	15	15
Pregnant	346	757	346	405
Standard error		147	37	46
Lactating	99	1,094	603	686
Standard error		217	270	333
All Individuals	28,575	733	343	402
Standard error		9	4	5
All Indiv (+P/L)	29,015	736	344	404
Standard error		9	4	5

NOTE: Data are limited to individuals who provided a complete and reliable 24-hour dietary recall on day 1. The intake distributions for 2–6 months, 7–12 months, and 1–3 years of age are unadjusted. Means and percentiles for these groups were computed using SAS PROC UNIVARIATE. For all other groups, data were adjusted using the Iowa State University method. Mean, standard errors, and percentiles were obtained using C-Side. Standard errors were estimated via jackknife replication. Each standard error has 49 degrees of freedom. Food composition data are from the NDS-R Food and Nutrient Database, Version 30, 1999, Nutrition Coordinating Center, University of Minnesota. Infants and children fed human milk and females who had "blank but applicable"

25th	50th	75th	90th	95th	99th
468	590	761	1,009	1,170	1,587
468	636	841	1,144	1,338	1,930
304	484	707	1,014	1,259	2,131
663	722	787	850	890	968
24	25	26	27	30	38
557	746	996	1,301	1,530	2,081
18	24	35	58	81	149
538	749	1,023	1,333	1,553	2,048
30	39	51	70	87	133
516	744	1,024	1,292	1,487	2,028
48	47	163	140	90	121
515	759	1,104	1,584	1,964	3,002
21	42	71	141	198	392
565	811	1,141	1,523	1,818	2,602
19	29	48	77	107	209
587	810	1,117	1,500	1,794	2,517
17	24	41	71	101	191
497	660	863	1,086	1,244	1,614
28	37	57	88	116	208
371	507	681	877	1,015	1,322
22	28	37	48	57	83
388	530	717	943	1,112	1,517
16	22	31	45	57	92
428	583	795	1,030	1,191	1,583
9	24	31	96	113	125
491	685	959	1,281	1,516	2,125
20	31	57	101	132	218
532	716	967	1,264	1,493	2,068
25	23	41	89	125	299
523	691	916	1,188	1,394	1,893
69	111	170	308	483	1,190
845	1,054	1,299	1,555	1,725	2,085
343	233	191	260	289	484
521	687	894	1,123	1,283	1,636
6	8	11	15	19	28
523	689	897	1,128	1,288	1,644
6	8	11	15	19	28

pregnancy and lactating status data or who responded "I don't know" to questions on pregnancy and lactating status were excluded from all analyses. Females who were both pregnant and lactating were included in both the Pregnant and Lactating categories. The sample sizes for the Pregnant and Lactating categories were very small so their estimates of usual intake distributions are not reliable.

[a] RAE = retinol activity equivalents. 1 µg RAE = 12 µg β-carotene and 24 µg α-carotene or β-cryptoxanthin.

[b] M = male, F = female, P/L = pregnant and lactating.

SOURCE: ENVIRON International Corporation and Iowa State University Department of Statistics, 2000.

TABLE C-9 Mean and Percentiles for Usual Intake of Total Vitamin A (µg RAE[a]/day) from Supplements NHANES III (1988–1994)

Sex/Age Category[b]	Number of Persons Examined	Mean	SEM[c]	Percentile 5th
Both sexes, 1 to 8 y	1,677	804	51	193
Both sexes, 9 to 18 y	437	906	58	75
M 19+ years	1,041	1,304	38	145
F 19+ years	1,463	1,338	63	171
F Pregnant/Lactating	148	1,106	36	567[d]
All Individuals	4,618	1,185	35	150
All Indiv (+P/L)	4,766	1,182	33	150

NOTE: Means, standard errors, and percentiles were calculated with WesVar Complex Samples 3.0. Children fed human milk and females who had "blank but applicable" pregnancy and lactating status data or who responded "I don't know" to questions on pregnancy and lactating status were excluded from all analyses.

[a] RAE = retinol activity equivalents. 1 µg RAE = 12 µg β-carotene and 24 µg α-carotene or β-cryptoxanthin.

[b] M = male, F = female, P/L = pregnant and lactating.

10th	25th	50th	75th	90th	95th	99th
323	438	721	745	1,439	1,482	2,511
191	431	751	1,437	1,492	1,676	3,713[d]
250	779	1,439	1,485	1,756	3,003	4,494[d]
298	818	1,422	1,501	1,531	2,543	4,120
854	866	1,027	1,146	1,420	1,492[d]	2,894[d]
293	647	1,172	1,501	1,501	2,390	4,449
294	651	1,174	1,501	1,501	2,383	4,367

[c] SEM = standard error of the mean.

[d] These values are potentially unreliable in a statistical sense based on an insufficient sample size as recommended in statistical reporting standards (Life Sciences Research Office/Federation of American Societies for Experimental Biology. 1995. *Third Report on Nutrition Monitoring in the United States*. Washington, DC: US Government Printing Office).

SOURCE, ENVIRON International Corporation, 2000.

TABLE C-10 Mean and Percentiles of Usual Intake of
Vitamin K (µg/day) from Food, NHANES III (1988–1994)

Sex/Age Category[a]	Number of Persons Examined	Mean	Percentile 5th	Percentile 10th
Both sexes, 2 to 6 mo	793	62.6	19.8	29.8
Both sexes, 7 to 12 mo	827	53.1	6.7	9.3
Both sexes, 1 to 3 y	3,309	38.7	5.3	8.3
Both sexes, 4 to 8 y	3,448	59.2	32.0	36.0
Standard error		6.2	2.3	2.9
M 9 to 13 y	1,219	65.1	35.0	40.0
Standard error		3.6	1.7	1.6
M 14 to 18 y	909	79.4	43.0	49.0
Standard error		4.4	2.3	2.6
M 19 to 30 y	1,902	105.8	54.0	62.0
Standard error		12.6	2.4	2.9
M 31 to 50 y	2,533	125.4	63.0	72.0
Standard error		11.4	5.6	6.8
M 51 to 70 y	1,942	120.0	55.0	64.0
Standard error		8.5	3.4	4.2
M 71+ y	1,255	97.8	44.0	52.0
Standard error		8.1	3.8	4.4
F 9 to 13 y	1,216	63.4	27.0	31.0
Standard error		6.3	1.5	2.1
F 14 to 18 y	949	66.6	29.0	35.0
Standard error		3.6	1.6	2.0
F 19 to 30 y	1,901	98.0	32.0	40.0
Standard error		14.6	2.5	3.7
F 31 to 50 y	2,939	99.6	38.0	46.0
Standard error		3.3	1.2	1.4
F 51 to 70 y	2,065	97.2	36.0	44.0
Standard error		4.4	1.3	1.6
F 71+ y	1,368	93.8	32.0	39.0
Standard error		4.3	1.5	1.9
Pregnant	346	87.8	38.0	45.0
Standard error		12.5	5.7	7.7
Lactating	99	78.6	38.0	44.0
Standard error		11.1	6.1	7.4
Pregnant/Lactating	440	87.0	37.0	44.0
Standard error		8.5	4.1	5.4
All Individuals	28,575	93.9	38.0	45.0
Standard error		3.1	1.0	1.3
All Individuals (+P/L)	29,015	93.7	38.0	45.0
Standard error		3.0	1.0	1.3

NOTE: Data are limited to individuals who provided a complete and reliable 24-hour dietary recall on day 1. The intake distributions for 2–6 months, 7–12 months, and 1–3 years of age are unadjusted. Means and percentiles for these groups were computed using SAS PROC UNIVARIATE. For all other groups, data were adjusted using the Iowa State University method. Mean, standard errors, and percentiles were obtained using C-Side. Standard errors were estimated via jackknife replication. Each standard error has 49 degrees of freedom. Food composition data are from the NDS-R Food and Nutrient Database, Version 30, 1999, Nutrition Coordinating Center, University of Minnesota. Infants and children fed human milk and females who had "blank but applicable"

25th	50th	75th	90th	95th	99th
41.4	54.2	71.9	99.1	119.8	274.2
20.9	45.1	67.0	95.5	119.2	246.2
14.3	25.8	44.1	77.1	111.9	308.7
44.0	55.0	70.0	87.0	101.0	132.0
4.1	5.6	7.7	10.5	12.9	18.5
49.0	61.0	77.0	95.0	108.0	139.0
1.8	2.7	4.4	7.6	10.8	22.1
60.0	75.0	94.0	116.0	131.0	166.0
3.2	4.1	5.3	7.0	8.3	11.7
77.0	98.0	126.0	158.0	183.0	241.0
5.1	10.2	17.5	26.0	32.5	51.3
91.0	117.0	150.0	189.0	217.0	282.0
8.6	10.6	13.1	16.9	20.9	34.8
82.0	109.0	145.0	189.0	223.0	303.0
5.7	7.7	10.5	14.2	17.2	25.1
67.0	89.0	119.0	155.0	181.0	243.0
5.7	7.6	10.1	13.0	15.3	22.3
41.0	56.0	77.0	104.0	125.0	181.0
3.2	4.9	7.7	12.2	16.3	28.4
45.0	60.0	81.0	106.0	125.0	174.0
2.7	3.4	4.5	6.4	8.4	14.5
56.0	82.0	121.0	173.0	217.0	340.0
6.2	10.9	19.7	31.2	41.6	77.5
63.0	88.0	123.0	167.0	201.0	288.0
2.0	2.8	4.1	6.2	8.2	14.3
60.0	85.0	121.0	165.0	200.0	284.0
2.3	3.5	5.6	8.9	11.9	20.3
55.0	79.0	116.0	165.0	204.0	308.0
2.7	3.8	5.4	8.8	13.4	31.7
59.0	80.0	107.0	140.0	166.0	229.0
10.3	11.7	13.3	17.8	24.7	52.9
57.0	74.0	95.0	119.0	136.0	172.0
9.8	12.5	14.4	14.7	14.5	18.7
59.0	79.0	106.0	139.0	164.0	225.0
6.9	7.8	9.2	12.7	17.6	37.5
60.0	83.0	115.0	155.0	186.0	264.0
1.8	2.6	3.8	5.9	8.0	14.7
60.0	83.0	115.0	155.0	186.0	263.0
1.7	2.5	3.7	5.8	7.8	14.5

pregnancy and lactating status data or who responded "I don't know" to questions on pregnancy and lactating status were excluded from all analyses. Females who were both pregnant and lactating were included in both the Pregnant and Lactating categories. The sample sizes for the Pregnant and Lactating categories were very small so their estimates of usual intake distributions are not reliable.

[a] M = male, F = female, P/L = pregnant and lactating.

SOURCE: ENVIRON International Corporation and Iowa State University Department of Statistics, 2000.

TABLE C-11 Mean and Percentiles of Usual Intake of Vitamin K (µg/day) from Food and Supplements, NHANES III (1988–1994)

Sex/Age Category[a]	Number of Persons Examined	Mean	Percentile	
			5th	10th
Both sexes, 2 to 6 mo	793	62.6	19.8	29.8
Both sexes, 7 to 12 mo	827	53.1	6.8	9.5
Both sexes, 1 to 3 y	3,309	38.9	6.2	8.9
Both sexes, 4 to 8 y	3,448	59.5	32.5	36.1
M 9 to 13 y	1,219	65.7	35.2	39.7
M 14 to 18 y	909	80.3	42.4	50.0
M 19 to 30 y	1,902	107.8	56.2	62.9
M 31 to 50 y	2,533	126.9	64.6	74.4
M 51 to 70 y	1,942	122.3	56.2	64.5
M 71+ y	1,255	99.8	43.6	52.6
F 9 to 13 y	1,216	63.7	26.9	32.4
F 14 to 18 y	949	67.2	29.8	34.1
F 19 to 30 y	1,901	99.6	32.6	39.1
F 31 to 50 y	2,939	101.9	39.1	47.3
F 51 to 70 y	2,065	100.3	36.9	45.0
F 71+ y	1,368	97.3	33.7	40.5
Pregnant	346	88.4	38.2	45.6
Lactating	99	79.1	37.9	43.6
Pregnant/Lactating	440	87.4	36.4	44.4
All Individuals	28,575	95.5	38.5	45.7
All Individuals (+P/L)	29,015	95.3	38.5	45.7

NOTE: Data are limited to individuals who provided a complete and reliable 24-hour dietary recall on day 1. The intake distributions for 2–6 months, 7–12 months, and 1–3 years of age are unadjusted. Means and percentiles for these groups were computed using SAS PROC UNIVARIATE. For all other groups, data were adjusted using the Iowa State University method. Mean, standard errors, and percentiles were obtained using C-Side. Standard errors were estimated via jackknife replication. Each standard error has 49 degrees of freedom. Food composition data are from the NDS-R Food and Nutrient Database, Version 30, 1999, Nutrition Coordinating Center, University of Minnesota. Infants and children fed human milk and females who had "blank but applicable"

25th	50th	75th	90th	95th	99th
41.2	53.7	71.9	98.3	115.8	227.4
23.4	46.2	66.5	96.5	121.3	278.5
14.7	25.9	43.9	77.7	107.9	241.2
44.1	55.0	70.2	88.4	97.9	137.7
48.9	62.1	77.8	94.3	112.4	138.3
60.3	76.5	96.5	116.3	131.0	162.3
78.4	101.1	129.1	160.4	181.3	233.8
92.1	118.6	151.1	189.3	217.2	296.3
85.0	110.7	146.7	191.1	229.9	316.5
68.3	92.7	119.0	153.8	182.8	249.1
41.4	56.7	77.8	102.3	126.3	173.8
45.1	60.4	82.1	105.9	122.4	176.1
56.6	82.3	128.0	173.1	211.5	367.0
64.3	90.2	126.3	167.1	201.4	290.4
62.3	87.4	125.9	168.0	195.7	286.0
57.0	82.5	121.7	168.9	202.5	328.5
59.9	79.5	110.6	137.1	169.7	249.4
62.0	72.3	94.8	114.1	123.7	206.9
60.2	79.2	107.8	139.6	165.1	239.5
61.5	85.0	116.9	158.2	186.6	264.2
61.4	84.9	116.8	157.7	185.6	262.8

pregnancy and lactating status data or who responded "I don't know" to questions on pregnancy and lactating status were excluded from all analyses. Females who were both pregnant and lactating were included in both the Pregnant and Lactating categories. The sample sizes for the Pregnant and Lactating categories were very small so their estimates of usual intake distributions are not reliable.

[a] M = male, F = female, P/L = pregnant and lactating.

SOURCE: ENVIRON International Corporation and Iowa State University Department of Statistics, 2000.

TABLE C-12 Mean and Percentiles for Usual Intake of Boron (mg/day) from Food, NHANES III (1988–1994)

Sex/Age Category[a]	Number of Persons Examined	Mean	Percentile	
			1st	5th
Both sexes, 6 to 8 y	1,512	0.85	0.33	0.43
Standard error		0.03	0.01	0.02
M 9 to 13 y	1,223	0.92	0.34	0.46
Standard error		0.03	0.02	0.02
M 14 to 18 y	913	1.06	0.34	0.47
Standard error		0.05	0.02	0.02
M 19 to 30 y	1,906	1.29	0.47	0.63
Standard error		0.04	0.03	0.02
M 31 to 50 y	2,536	1.42	0.57	0.76
Standard error		0.04	0.02	0.03
M 51 to 70 y	1,946	1.42	0.59	0.77
Standard error		0.04	0.02	0.02
M 71+ y	1,257	1.28	0.46	0.63
Standard error		0.04	0.02	0.02
F 9 to 13 y	1,241	0.84	0.33	0.43
Standard error		0.03	0.01	0.02
F 14 to 18 y	979	0.80	0.29	0.39
Standard error		0.03	0.01	0.02
F 19 to 30 y	1,975	0.92	0.33	0.44
Standard error		0.03	0.02	0.03
F 31 to 50 y	2,993	1.19	0.49	0.64
Standard error		0.06	0.04	0.03
F 51 to 70 y	2,080	1.16	0.49	0.64
Standard error		0.03	0.02	0.03
F 71+ y	1,370	1.03	0.42	0.55
Standard error		0.02	0.01	0.01
Pregnant	348	1.13	0.39	0.53
Standard error		0.10	0.03	0.04
All Individuals 6+	21,931	1.15	0.60	0.72
Standard error		0.01	0.03	0.02
All Indiv 6+ (+P)	22,279	1.15	0.60	0.73
Standard error		0.01	0.03	0.02

NOTE: Estimates were obtained using C-SIDE v1.02 (C-SIDE courtesy of Iowa State University Statistical Laboratory). Standard errors were estimated via jackknife replication. Each standard error has 43 degrees of freedom.

10th	25th	50th	75th	90th	95th	99th
0.50	0.63	0.80	1.02	1.27	1.45	1.89
0.03	0.04	0.03	0.03	0.05	0.07	0.18
0.53	0.68	0.86	1.09	1.38	1.59	2.10
0.02	0.02	0.02	0.03	0.05	0.07	0.14
0.56	0.73	0.98	1.30	1.67	1.93	2.54
0.03	0.04	0.05	0.06	0.09	0.12	0.22
0.72	0.91	1.20	1.58	1.97	2.25	2.97
0.03	0.04	0.05	0.06	0.07	0.08	0.15
0.87	1.08	1.35	1.67	2.05	2.34	3.01
0.03	0.03	0.03	0.04	0.06	0.08	0.14
0.87	1.08	1.34	1.68	2.05	2.32	2.95
0.02	0.02	0.03	0.05	0.07	0.09	0.14
0.73	0.94	1.20	1.53	1.91	2.20	2.88
0.03	0.03	0.04	0.05	0.07	0.09	0.16
0.50	0.63	0.79	0.99	1.23	1.40	1.80
0.02	0.02	0.03	0.03	0.04	0.06	0.09
0.45	0.56	0.75	1.00	1.21	1.36	1.77
0.02	0.02	0.03	0.04	0.06	0.07	0.12
0.51	0.66	0.87	1.11	1.40	1.61	2.14
0.03	0.02	0.04	0.05	0.06	0.07	0.14
0.73	0.90	1.13	1.40	1.72	1.95	2.47
0.02	0.05	0.09	0.08	0.07	0.08	0.12
0.73	0.89	1.10	1.36	1.64	1.85	2.32
0.03	0.03	0.03	0.03	0.05	0.06	0.09
0.63	0.78	0.98	1.22	1.48	1.66	2.04
0.02	0.02	0.02	0.03	0.04	0.05	0.07
0.62	0.80	1.05	1.38	1.74	2.00	2.59
0.05	0.07	0.08	0.12	0.18	0.23	0.39
0.80	0.94	1.12	1.33	1.55	1.70	2.03
0.02	0.02	0.01	0.02	0.03	0.04	0.07
0.80	0.94	1.12	1.33	1.55	1.70	2.02
0.02	0.02	0.01	0.02	0.03	0.04	0.07

[a] M = male, F = female, P = pregnant.

SOURCE: C. Rainey, Nutrition Research Group, and A. Carriquiry, Iowa State University, 1999.

TABLE C-13 Mean and Percentiles of Usual Intake of Boron (mg/day) from Supplements, NHANES III (1988–1994)

Sex/Age Category[a]	Number of Persons Examined	Mean	SEM[b]	Percentile 5th
Both sexes, 1 to 8 y	24	0.27[c]	0.08	0.01[c]
Both sexes, 9 to 18 y	78	0.16	0.03	0.00[c]
M 19+ y	521	0.17	0.01	0.02
F 19+ y	658	0.18	0.01	0.02
Pregnant/lactating	5	0.15[c]	0.00	0.13[c]
All individuals	1,281	0.18	0.01	0.02
All individuals (+P/L)	1,286	0.18	0.01	0.02

NOTE: Means, standard errors, and percentiles were calculated with WesVar Complex Samples 3.0. Children fed human milk and females who had "blank but applicable" pregnancy and lactating status data or who responded "I don't know" to questions on pregnancy and lactating status were excluded from all analyses.
[a] M = male, F = female, P/L = pregnant and lactating.
[b] SEM = standard error of the mean.

TABLE C-14 Mean and Percentiles of Usual Intake of Chromium (µg/day) from Supplements, NHANES III (1988–1994)

Sex/Age Category[a]	Number of Persons Examined	Mean	SEM[b]	Percentile 5th
Both sexes, 1 to 8 y	83	24.5	2.8	6.1[c]
Both sexes, 9 to 18 y	129	18.3	2.5	0.6[c]
M 19+ y	698	29.5	1.7	3.2
F 19+ y	915	30.0	1.6	4.4
F Pregnant/Lactating	33	23.7[c]	0.8	13.0[c]
All Individuals	1,825	28.9	1.1	3.3
All Individuals (+P/L)	1,858	28.8	1.1	3.3

NOTE: Means, standard errors, and percentiles were calculated with WesVar Complex Samples 3.0. Children fed human milk and females who had "blank but applicable" pregnancy and lactating status data or who responded "I don't know" to questions on pregnancy and lactating status were excluded from all analyses.
[a] M = male, F = female, P/L = pregnant and lactating.
[b] SEM = standard error of the mean.

10th	25th	50th	75th	90th	95th	99th
0.02[c]	0.08[c]	0.12[c]	0.28[c]	0.46[c]	0.65[c]	0.94[c]
0.01[c]	0.03	0.12	0.14	0.30[c]	0.47[c]	1.01[c]
0.04	0.12	0.14	0.14	0.15	0.41	1.08[c]
0.05	0.13	0.14	0.14	0.15	0.47	1.01[c]
0.13[c]	0.14[c]	0.14[c]	0.14[c]	0.15[c]	0.15[c]	0.15[c]
0.04	0.13	0.14	0.14	0.15	0.47	1.02[c]
0.04	0.13	0.14	0.15	0.15	0.47	1.02[c]

[c] These values are potentially unreliable in a statistical sense based on an insufficient sample size as recommended in statistical reporting standards (Life Sciences Research Office/Federation of American Societies for Experimental Biology. 1995. *Third Report on Nutrition Monitoring in the United States.* Washington, DC: US Government Printing Office).
SOURCE: ENVIRON International Corporation, 1999.

10th	25th	50th	75th	90th	95th	99th
10.1[c]	14.7	17.6	22.1	40.2[c]	57.9[c]	97.1[c]
1.2[c]	4.3	14.3	23.2	26.0[c]	45.9[c]	122.8[c]
6.3	13.8	22.7	24.7	48.5	100.0	204.1[c]
7.7	14.8	23.1	24.6	49.3	126.8	202.3[c]
14.3[c]	18.4[c]	20.7[c]	23.0[c]	24.4[c]	24.9[c]	29.4[c]
6.4	14.7	23.0	24.6	48.7	100.0	200.9
6.4	14.7	23.0	24.6	48.5	100.0	200.4

[c] These values are potentially unreliable in a statistical sense based on an insufficient sample size as recommended in statistical reporting standards (Life Sciences Research Office/Federation of American Societies for Experimental Biology. 1995. *Third Report on Nutrition Monitoring in the United States.* Washington, DC: US Government Printing Office).
SOURCE: ENVIRON International Corporation, 1999.

TABLE C-15 Mean and Percentiles for Usual Intake of Copper (mg/day) from Food, NHANES III (1988–1994)

Sex/Age Category[a]	Number of Persons Examined	Mean	Percentile	
			5th	10th
Both sexes, 2 to 6 mo	793	0.71	0.30	0.40
Both sexes, 7 to 12 mo	827	0.75	0.30	0.40
Both sexes, 1 to 3 y	3,309	0.74	0.30	0.40
Both sexes, 4 to 8 y	3,448	0.97	0.70	0.75
Standard error		0.02	0.03	0.03
M 9 to 13 y	1,219	1.24	0.86	0.93
Standard error		0.03	0.03	0.03
M 14 to 18 y	909	1.50	0.86	0.97
Standard error		0.05	0.04	0.04
M 19 to 30 y	1,902	1.70	0.96	1.08
Standard error		0.05	0.05	0.05
M 31 to 50 y	2,533	1.67	0.96	1.08
Standard error		0.03	0.02	0.02
M 51 to 70 y	1,942	1.54	0.86	0.97
Standard error		0.03	0.03	0.03
M 71+ y	1,255	1.33	0.75	0.85
Standard error		0.05	0.03	0.03
F 9 to 13 y	1,216	1.08	0.74	0.80
Standard error		0.03	0.03	0.03
F 14 to 18 y	949	1.10	0.61	0.69
Standard error		0.05	0.03	0.03
F 19 to 30 y	1,901	1.17	0.67	0.75
Standard error		0.10	0.14	0.13
F 31 to 50 y	2,939	1.18	0.68	0.76
Standard error		0.02	0.03	0.03
F 51 to 70 y	2,065	1.13	0.67	0.75
Standard error		0.02	0.02	0.02
F 71+ y	1,368	1.04	0.63	0.70
Standard error		0.02	0.03	0.02
Pregnant	346	1.28	0.76	0.85
Standard error		0.05	0.06	0.05
Lactating	99	1.62	0.97	1.09
Standard error		0.11	0.08	0.08
All Individuals	28,575	1.30	0.72	0.82
Standard error		0.04	0.03	0.03
All Indiv (+P/L)	29,015	1.30	0.72	0.82
Standard error		0.04	0.03	0.03

NOTE: Data are limited to individuals who provided a complete and reliable 24-hour dietary recall on day 1. The intake distributions for 2–6 months, 7–12 months, and 1–3 years of age are unadjusted. Means and percentiles for these groups were computed using SAS PROC UNIVARIATE. For all other groups, data were adjusted using the Iowa State University method. Mean, standard errors, and percentiles were obtained using C-Side. Standard errors were estimated via jackknife replication. Each standard error has 49 degrees of freedom. Infants and children fed human milk and females who had "blank but applicable" pregnancy and lactating status data or who responded "I don't

25th	50th	75th	90th	95th	99th
0.50	0.70	0.90	1.00	1.20	1.50
0.50	0.70	0.90	1.10	1.30	1.70
0.50	0.70	0.90	1.10	1.30	1.90
0.84	0.96	1.09	1.21	1.29	1.46
0.03	0.03	0.03	0.03	0.03	0.05
1.06	1.22	1.40	1.59	1.70	1.95
0.02	0.03	0.03	0.04	0.04	0.06
1.17	1.44	1.76	2.09	2.32	2.80
0.04	0.05	0.05	0.07	0.08	0.12
1.32	1.63	2.00	2.39	2.65	3.21
0.05	0.05	0.06	0.07	0.09	0.13
1.30	1.60	1.96	2.35	2.61	3.18
0.02	0.03	0.03	0.05	0.07	0.11
1.19	1.47	1.81	2.18	2.43	2.97
0.03	0.03	0.04	0.05	0.07	0.11
1.03	1.27	1.57	1.88	2.10	2.56
0.03	0.04	0.05	0.07	0.09	0.14
0.92	1.06	1.22	1.39	1.49	1.71
0.02	0.02	0.03	0.04	0.05	0.06
0.84	1.05	1.30	1.56	1.74	2.13
0.04	0.05	0.06	0.07	0.09	0.12
0.91	1.12	1.37	1.64	1.83	2.24
0.12	0.10	0.09	0.09	0.11	0.17
0.93	1.14	1.39	1.65	1.83	2.20
0.02	0.03	0.03	0.04	0.05	0.08
0.90	1.09	1.32	1.55	1.71	2.05
0.02	0.02	0.03	0.04	0.05	0.07
0.83	1.01	1.21	1.43	1.57	1.86
0.02	0.02	0.02	0.03	0.04	0.06
1.02	1.24	1.50	1.77	1.95	2.32
0.04	0.04	0.06	0.09	0.12	0.20
1.31	1.58	1.89	2.20	2.41	2.82
0.10	0.12	0.14	0.17	0.19	0.24
0.99	1.24	1.54	1.86	2.09	2.58
0.04	0.04	0.05	0.06	0.07	0.10
1.00	1.24	1.54	1.86	2.09	2.59
0.04	0.04	0.05	0.06	0.07	0.10

know" to questions on pregnancy and lactating status were excluded from all analyses. Females who were both pregnant and lactating were included in both the Pregnant and Lactating categories. The sample sizes for the Pregnant and Lactating categories were very small so their estimates of usual intake distributions are not reliable.

[a] M = male, F = female, P/L = pregnant and lactating.

SOURCE: ENVIRON International Corporation and Iowa State University Department of Statistics, 2000.

TABLE C-16 Mean and Percentiles for Usual Intake of Copper (mg/day) from Food and Supplements, NHANES III (1988–1994)

Sex/Age Category[a]	Number of Persons Examined	Mean	Percentile	
			5th	10th
Both sexes, 2 to 6 mo	793	0.71	0.30	0.40
Both sexes, 7 to 12 mo	827	0.75	0.30	0.40
Both sexes, 1 to 3 y	3,309	0.74	0.30	0.40
Both sexes, 4 to 8 y	3,448	1.05	0.69	0.75
M 9 to 13 y	1,219	1.28	0.87	0.94
M 14 to 18 y	909	1.58	0.90	0.99
M 19 to 30 y	1,900	1.85	0.97	1.13
M 31 to 50 y	2,533	1.85	1.03	1.11
M 51 to 70 y	1,942	1.79	0.91	1.00
M 71+ y	1,255	2.20	0.77	0.94
F 9 to 13 y	1,216	1.13	0.74	0.81
F 14 to 18 y	949	1.15	0.64	0.73
F 19 to 30 y	1,901	1.32	0.65	0.74
F 31 to 50 y	2,939	1.45	0.75	0.83
F 51 to 70 y	2,065	1.45	0.64	0.81
F 71+ y	1,368	1.52	0.63	0.71
Pregnant	346	1.86	0.86	1.01
Lactating	99	2.14	0.97	1.12
All Individuals	28,575	1.49	0.77	0.85
All Indiv (+P/L)	29,015	1.50	0.77	0.85

NOTE: Data are limited to individuals who provided a complete and reliable 24-hour dietary recall on day 1. The intake distributions for 2–6 months, 7–12 months, and 1–3 years of age are unadjusted; the total nutrient intake is the sum of the unadjusted food intake and the daily supplement intake. For all other groups, individual total nutrient intakes were obtained as the sum of the adjusted individual usual intake from food alone and the daily supplement intake. The mean and percentiles of the estimated usual intake distributions were computed using SAS PROC UNIVARIATE. Infants and children fed human milk and females who had "blank but applicable" pregnancy and

25th	50th	75th	90th	95th	99th
0.50	0.70	0.90	1.00	1.20	1.50
0.50	0.70	0.90	1.10	1.30	1.70
0.50	0.70	0.90	1.10	1.30	1.90
0.86	0.96	1.13	1.25	1.58	3.00
1.06	1.21	1.42	1.64	1.92	2.95
1.21	1.47	1.77	2.24	2.62	3.77
1.35	1.68	2.08	2.88	3.55	4.30
1.34	1.67	2.04	2.79	3.54	4.29
1.23	1.56	1.96	3.15	3.62	4.56
1.09	1.35	1.75	3.02	3.47	4.53
0.92	1.07	1.20	1.42	1.65	3.07
0.88	1.07	1.30	1.61	1.94	3.27
0.97	1.16	1.41	1.98	3.07	4.02
0.97	1.22	1.50	2.73	3.22	4.04
0.95	1.14	1.52	3.01	3.31	4.08
0.85	1.04	1.42	2.98	3.21	3.84
1.14	1.32	2.82	3.55	4.01	4.60
1.46	1.92	2.58	3.58	4.24	4.70
1.01	1.28	1.64	2.36	3.22	4.00
1.01	1.28	1.64	2.40	3.22	4.04

lactating status data or who responded "I don't know" to questions on pregnancy and lactating status were excluded from all analyses. Females who were both pregnant and lactating were included in both the Pregnant and Lactating categories. The sample sizes for the Pregnant and Lactating categories were very small so their estimates of usual intake distributions are not reliable.

[a] M = male, F = female, P/L = pregnant and lactating.

SOURCE: ENVIRON International Corporation and Iowa State University Department of Statistics, 2000.

TABLE C-17 Mean and Percentiles of Usual Intake of Iodine (µg/day) from Supplements, NHANES III (1988–1994)

Sex/Age Category[a]	Number of Persons Examined	Mean	SEM[b]	Percentile 5th
Both sexes, 1 to 8 y	289	117	8	19[c]
Both sexes, 9 to 18 y	154	94	8	5[c]
M 19+ y	749	126	4	18
F 19+ y	972	137	6	19
Pregnant/Lactating	63	158	4	76[c]
All Individuals	2,164	129	3	16
All Individuals (+P/L)	2,227	130	3	17

NOTE: Means, standard errors, and percentiles were calculated with WesVar Complex Samples 3.0. Children fed human milk and females who had "blank but applicable" pregnancy and lactating status data or who responded "I don't know" to questions on pregnancy and lactating status were excluded from all analyses.

[a] M = male, F = female, P/L = pregnant and lactating.
[b] SEM = standard error of the mean.

10th	25th	50th	75th	90th	95th	99th
27	67	106	130	143	148^c	563^c
9	25	74	129	144	150^c	288^c
36	75	135	143	148	150	306^c
44	103	142	146	149	152	304^c
82^c	99	128	155	169^c	173^c	260^c
34	74	141	146	149	150	304
35	74	141	146	149	152	304

^{c} These values are potentially unreliable in a statistical sense based on an insufficient sample size as recommended in statistical reporting standards (Life Sciences Research Office/Federation of American Societies for Experimental Biology. 1995. *Third Report on Nutrition Monitoring in the United States*. Washington, DC: US Government Printing Office).
SOURCE: ENVIRON International Corporation, 1999.

TABLE C-18 Mean and Percentiles for Usual Intake of Iron (mg/day) from Food, NHANES III (1988–1994)

Sex/Age Category[a]	Number of Persons Examined	Mean	Percentile	
			5th	10th
Both sexes, 2 to 6 mo	793	16.29	4.30	6.70
Both sexes, 7 to 12 mo	827	15.80	3.20	5.30
Both sexes, 1 to 3 y	3,309	10.36	3.60	4.60
Both sexes, 4 to 8 y	3,448	13.14	7.90	8.70
Standard error		0.18	0.14	0.15
M 9 to 13 y	1,219	16.51	9.70	10.90
Standard error		0.39	0.23	0.24
M 14 to 18 y	909	20.03	10.30	11.60
Standard error		1.35	0.34	0.40
M 19 to 30 y	1,902	19.06	10.60	11.90
Standard error		0.57	0.34	0.33
M 31 to 50 y	2,533	18.99	10.50	11.80
Standard error		0.34	0.17	0.18
M 51 to 70 y	1,942	18.19	9.60	10.90
Standard error		0.41	0.20	0.21
M 71+ y	1,255	16.85	8.80	10.00
Standard error		0.47	0.25	0.24
F 9 to 13 y	1,216	13.73	7.90	8.80
Standard error		0.55	0.33	0.33
F 14 to 18 y	949	12.22	6.60	7.50
Standard error		0.44	0.23	0.27
F 19 to 30 y	1,901	12.92	7.20	8.20
Standard error		0.30	0.18	0.23
F 31 to 50 y	2,939	12.77	7.40	8.30
Standard error		0.27	0.15	0.16
F 51 to 70 y	2,065	12.85	7.20	8.10
Standard error		0.29	0.16	0.14
F 71+ y	1,368	13.06	7.20	8.20
Standard error		0.32	0.38	0.37
Pregnant	346	15.34	9.00	10.20
Standard error		0.75	0.52	0.53
Lactating	99	20.87	10.10	11.70
Standard error		2.60	3.11	2.23
All Individuals	28,575	15.08	7.70	8.80
Standard error		0.12	0.12	0.11
All Indiv (+P/L)	29,015	15.13	7.70	8.90
Standard error		0.19	0.17	0.17

NOTE: Data are limited to individuals who provided a complete and reliable 24-hour dietary recall on day 1. The intake distributions for 2–6 months, 7–12 months, and 1–3 years of age are unadjusted. Means and percentiles for these groups were computed using SAS PROC UNIVARIATE. For all other groups, data were adjusted using the Iowa State University method. Mean, standard errors, and percentiles were obtained using C-Side. Standard errors were estimated via jackknife replication. Each standard error has 49 degrees of freedom. Infants and children fed human milk and females who had "blank but applicable" pregnancy and lactating status data or who responded "I don't

25th	50th	75th	90th	95th	99th
10.80	15.30	20.40	26.50	31.40	47.30
9.00	14.50	20.00	26.90	33.60	46.40
6.50	9.00	12.50	17.60	21.30	31.30
10.40	12.60	15.30	18.20	20.20	25.00
0.16	0.19	0.22	0.28	0.35	0.58
13.00	15.70	19.20	23.10	25.90	32.40
0.28	0.34	0.47	0.70	0.93	1.60
14.10	18.10	23.50	30.50	36.10	52.60
0.42	0.76	1.64	3.34	5.00	11.80
14.20	17.90	22.70	27.50	31.10	40.80
0.32	0.46	0.80	1.16	1.41	2.85
14.40	17.90	22.20	27.40	31.30	41.00
0.21	0.27	0.42	0.69	0.93	1.73
13.40	16.80	21.40	27.10	31.40	42.00
0.23	0.31	0.48	0.79	1.10	2.01
12.30	15.50	19.90	25.30	29.50	39.70
0.26	0.35	0.55	0.99	1.50	3.30
10.60	12.90	16.00	19.70	22.40	28.80
0.42	0.18	0.88	1.01	1.18	1.93
9.20	11.60	14.50	17.70	20.00	25.20
0.36	0.44	0.54	0.68	0.78	0.95
10.00	12.20	15.10	18.40	21.00	26.90
0.40	0.30	0.48	0.54	0.69	1.23
10.00	12.10	14.80	18.00	20.30	25.70
0.18	0.22	0.32	0.48	0.64	1.11
9.70	12.00	15.00	18.70	21.40	27.90
0.16	0.22	0.36	0.59	0.82	1.65
10.00	12.30	15.30	18.70	21.30	27.40
0.44	0.41	0.32	0.47	0.60	1.20
12.20	14.70	17.60	21.20	24.00	30.80
0.58	0.70	0.98	1.34	1.62	2.35
15.80	21.30	25.80	28.90	30.80	34.60
2.93	6.15	3.93	2.49	3.32	2.52
11.00	14.10	18.10	22.60	25.80	33.10
0.10	0.11	0.15	0.23	0.31	0.53
11.10	14.20	18.10	22.60	25.80	33.10
0.18	0.18	0.20	0.26	0.32	0.54

know" to questions on pregnancy and lactating status were excluded from all analyses. Females who were both pregnant and lactating were included in both the Pregnant and Lactating categories. The sample sizes for the Pregnant and Lactating categories were very small so their estimates of usual intake distributions are not reliable.

[a] M = male, F = female, P/L = pregnant and lactating.

SOURCE: ENVIRON International Corporation and Iowa State University Department of Statistics, 2000.

TABLE C-19 Mean and Percentiles for Usual Intake of Iron (mg/day) from Food and Supplements, NHANES III (1988–1994)

Sex/Age Category[a]	Number of Persons Examined	Mean	Percentile	
			5th	10th
Both sexes, 2 to 6 mo	793	16.29	4.30	6.70
Both sexes, 7 to 12 mo	827	15.80	3.20	5.30
Both sexes, 1 to 3 y	3,309	10.36	3.60	4.60
Both sexes, 4 to 8 y	3,448	14.68	7.97	8.81
M 9 to 13 y	1,219	18.05	10.03	11.01
M 14 to 18 y	909	20.88	10.58	11.77
M 19 to 30 y	1,902	20.87	10.64	12.23
M 31 to 50 y	2,533	21.09	11.00	12.12
M 51 to 70 y	1,942	20.64	9.95	11.30
M 71+ y	1,255	20.95	9.33	10.41
F 9 to 13 y	1,216	14.63	8.13	8.89
F 14 to 18 y	949	13.24	6.88	7.63
F 19 to 30 y	1,901	16.76	7.42	8.49
F 31 to 50 y	2,939	17.11	7.61	8.66
F 51 to 70 y	2,065	16.83	7.54	8.27
F 71+ y	1,368	19.01	7.38	8.41
Pregnant	346	48.97	9.90	10.59
Lactating	99	58.51	12.29	13.19
All Individuals	28,575	17.78	8.04	9.33
All Indiv (+P/L)	29,015	18.34	8.04	9.34

NOTE: Data are limited to individuals who provided a complete and reliable 24-hour dietary recall on day 1. The intake distributions for infants 2–6 months, 7–12 months, and 1–3 years of age are unadjusted; the total nutrient intake is the sum of the unadjusted food intake and the daily supplement intake. For all other groups, individual total nutrient intakes were obtained as the sum of the adjusted individual usual intake from food alone and the daily supplement intake. The mean and percentiles of the estimated usual intake distributions were computed using SAS PROC UNIVARIATE. Infants and children fed human milk and females who had "blank but applicable"

25th	50th	75th	90th	95th	99th
10.80	15.30	20.40	26.50	31.40	47.30
9.00	14.50	20.00	26.90	33.60	46.40
6.50	9.00	12.50	17.60	21.30	31.30
10.75	13.10	16.49	21.27	27.13	34.83
13.11	16.09	20.39	25.70	31.87	42.14
14.60	18.32	24.03	32.68	38.84	59.41
14.70	18.55	24.39	31.84	37.80	60.93
14.64	18.90	24.24	33.48	38.74	54.96
13.74	17.89	24.30	34.30	40.47	55.70
12.58	16.74	24.42	34.50	42.69	77.66
10.63	13.28	16.61	21.84	28.63	34.93
9.18	11.96	15.20	19.61	24.42	39.78
10.28	12.97	17.26	29.10	36.35	80.78
10.41	13.08	17.56	31.01	38.50	71.49
10.02	13.06	18.64	30.46	35.84	47.20
10.35	13.21	19.55	32.03	37.35	81.24
13.86	21.42	75.48	88.84	170.70	279.30
17.40	28.33	84.48	112.00	271.50	271.50
11.58	14.84	19.87	29.66	35.90	59.42
11.59	14.93	20.06	30.13	37.14	75.67

pregnancy and lactating status data or who responded "I don't know" to questions on pregnancy and lactating status were excluded from all analyses. Females who were both pregnant and lactating were included in both the Pregnant and Lactating categories. The sample sizes for the Pregnant and Lactating categories were very small so their estimates of usual intake distributions are not reliable.

[a] M = male, F = female, P/L = pregnant and lactating.

SOURCE: ENVIRON International Corporation and Iowa State University Department of Statistics, 2000.

TABLE C-20 Mean and Percentiles of Usual Intake of Manganese (mg/day) from Supplements, NHANES III (1988–1994)

Sex/Age Category[a]	Number of Persons Examined	Mean	SEM[b]	Percentile 5th
Both sexes, 1 to 8 y	97	1.16	0.15	0.06[c]
Both sexes, 9 to 18 y	137	1.64	0.16	0.07[c]
M 19+ y	736	2.63	0.11	0.34
F 19+ y	958	2.73	0.11	0.32
Pregnant/Lactating	33	4.72[c]	0.17	1.25[c]
All Individuals	1,928	2.57	0.07	0.24
All Individuals (+P/L)	1,961	2.61	0.07	0.24

NOTE: Means, standard errors, and percentiles were calculated with WesVar Complex Samples 3.0. Children fed human milk and females who had "blank but applicable" pregnancy and lactating status data or who responded "I don't know" to questions on pregnancy and lactating status were excluded from all analyses.
[a] M = male, F = female, P/L = pregnant and lactating.
[b] SEM = standard error of the mean.

TABLE C-21 Mean and Percentiles of Usual Intake of Molybdenum (µg/day) from Supplements, NHANES III (1988–1994)

Sex/Age Category[a]	Number of Persons Examined	Mean	SEM[b]	Percentile 5th
Both sexes, 1 to 8 y	79	26.0	3.7	6.1[c]
Both sexes, 9 to 18 y	128	19.5	3.1	0.5[c]
M 19+ y	667	28.8	1.9	3.4
F 19+ y	880	29.8	1.5	3.6
Pregnant/Lactating	33	23.8[c]	0.8	13.0[c]
All Individuals	1,754	28.6	1.2	3.2
All Individuals (+P/L)	1,787	28.5	1.2	3.2

NOTE: Means, standard errors, and percentiles were calculated with WesVar Complex Samples 3.0. Children fed human milk and females who had "blank but applicable" pregnancy and lactating status data or who responded "I don't know" to questions on pregnancy and lactating status were excluded from all analyses.
[a] M = male, F = female, P/L = pregnant and lactating.
[b] SEM = standard error of the mean.

10th	25th	50th	75th	90th	95th	99th
0.24[c]	0.64	0.86	1.34	2.36[c]	2.44[c]	2.94[c]
0.09[c]	0.33	1.16	2.37	3.32[c]	4.30[c]	5.88[c]
0.69	1.54	2.49	2.50	4.64	5.07	8.30[c]
0.70	1.82	2.37	2.50	4.80	5.07	7.88[c]
2.09[c]	3.70[c]	4.15[c]	4.59[c]	4.86[c]	4.94[c]	6.89[c]
0.57	1.39	2.49	2.50	4.73	5.00	8.09
0.58	1.42	2.49	2.50	4.78	5.00	8.08

[c] These values are potentially unreliable in a statistical sense based on an insufficient sample size as recommended in statistical reporting standards (Life Sciences Research Office/Federation of American Societies for Experimental Biology. 1995. *Third Report on Nutrition Monitoring in the United States.* Washington, DC: US Government Printing Office).
SOURCE: ENVIRON International Corporation, 1999.

10th	25th	50th	75th	90th	95th	99th
9.2[c]	14.5	17.4	21.1	44.9[c]	66.1[c]	120.9[c]
2.0[c]	3.9	14.4	22.9	31.7[c]	50.4[c]	145.9[c]
6.4	14.0	22.7	24.6	36.4	79.6	159.3[c]
7.4	14.7	23.9	24.7	37.7	83.7	161.0[c]
14.3[c]	21.9[c]	23.0[c]	24.1[c]	24.7[c]	24.9[c]	31.5[c]
6.5	14.5	23.9	24.7	38.3	79.1	160.3
6.5	14.7	23.9	24.7	33.7	78.9	160.2

[c] These values are potentially unreliable in a statistical sense based on an insufficient sample size as recommended in statistical reporting standards (Life Sciences Research Office/Federation of American Societies for Experimental Biology. 1995. *Third Report on Nutrition Monitoring in the United States.* Washington, DC: US Government Printing Office).
SOURCE: ENVIRON International Corporation, 1999.

TABLE C-22 Mean and Percentiles of Usual Intake of Nickel (µg/day) from Supplements, NHANES III (1988–1994)

Sex/Age Category[a]	Number of Persons Examined	Mean	SEM[b]	Percentile 5th
Both sexes, 1 to 8 y	26	5.65[c]	0.98	0.66[c]
Both sexes, 9 to 18 y	89	3.97	0.50	0.17[c]
M 19+ y	571	4.46	0.13	0.71
F 19+ y	737	4.80	0.13	0.82
Pregnant/Lactating	8	5.55[c]	0.65	2.09[c]
All Individuals	1,423	4.62	0.10	0.63
All Individuals (+P/L)	1,431	4.63	0.10	0.63

NOTE: Means, standard errors, and percentiles were calculated with WesVar Complex Samples 3.0. Children fed human milk and females who had "blank but applicable" pregnancy and lactating status data or who responded "I don't know" to questions on pregnancy and lactating status were excluded from all analyses.
[a] M = male, F = female, P/L = pregnant and lactating.
[b] SEM = standard error of the mean.

TABLE C-23 Mean and Percentiles of Usual Intake of Silicon (mg/day) from Supplements, NHANES III (1988–1994)

Sex/Age Category[a]	Number of Persons Examined	Mean	SEM[b]	Percentile 5th
Both sexes, 1 to 8 y	20	1.57[c]	0.21	0.10[c]
Both sexes, 9 to 18 y	85	2.69	0.89	0.07[c]
M 19+ y	560	4.32	0.82	0.29
F 19+ y	727	7.04	0.89	0.26
Pregnant/Lactating	8	68.59[c]	17.83	0.44[c]
All Individuals	1,392	5.66	0.71	0.24
All Individuals (+P/L)	1,400	5.85	0.72	0.24

NOTE: Means, standard errors, and percentiles were calculated with WesVar Complex Samples 3.0. Children fed human milk and females who had "blank but applicable" pregnancy and lactating status data or who responded "I don't know" to questions on pregnancy and lactating status were excluded from all analyses.
[a] M = male, F = female, P/L = pregnant and lactating.
[b] SEM = standard error of the mean.

10th	25th	50th	75th	90th	95th	99th
1.28[c]	3.44[c]	4.30[c]	5.55[c]	7.22[c]	11.62[c]	14.52[c]
0.36[c]	0.82	4.55	4.83	5.00[c]	9.33[c]	15.18[c]
1.32	3.63	4.68	4.86	4.97	6.56	10.14[c]
1.60	4.53	4.70	4.87	4.98	7.27	15.18[c]
2.26[c]	2.79[c]	3.68[c]	4.56[c]	6.02[c]	8.01[c]	9.60[c]
1.41	4.50	4.69	4.87	4.98	7.09	14.62[c]
1.41	4.50	4.69	4.87	4.98	7.10	14.61[c]

[c] These values are potentially unreliable in a statistical sense based on an insufficient sample size as recommended in statistical reporting standards (Life Sciences Research Office/Federation of American Societies for Experimental Biology. 1995. *Third Report on Nutrition Monitoring in the United States.* Washington, DC: US Government Printing Office).
SOURCE: ENVIRON International Corporation, 1999.

10th	25th	50th	75th	90th	95th	99th
0.71[c]	0.94[c]	1.24[c]	1.69[c]	1.96[c]	2.01[c]	2.03[c]
0.09[c]	0.29	1.26	1.75	1.96[c]	2.63[c]	44.36[c]
0.54	1.40	1.78	1.91	1.99	8.48	65.22[c]
0.66	1.75	1.85	1.95	4.35	73.08	78.69[c]
0.79[c]	1.83[c]	31.32[c]	63.83[c]	96.31[c]	128.15[c]	153.63[c]
0.58	1.58	1.84	1.94	2.03	32.10	78.19[c]
0.58	1.61	1.84	1.94	2.48	33.09	78.33[c]

[c] These values are potentially unreliable in a statistical sense based on an insufficient sample size as recommended in statistical reporting standards (Life Sciences Research Office/Federation of American Societies for Experimental Biology. 1995. *Third Report on Nutrition Monitoring in the United States.* Washington, DC: US Government Printing Office).
SOURCE: ENVIRON International Corporation, 1999.

TABLE C-24 Mean and Percentiles of Usual Intake of Vanadium (µg/day) from Supplements, NHANES III (1988–1994)

Sex/Age Category[a]	Number of Persons Examined	Mean	SEM[b]	Percentile 5th
Both sexes, 1 to 8 y	26	6.09[c]	1.51	0.10[c]
Both sexes, 9 to 18 y	89	6.50	0.94	0.12[c]
M 19+ y	571	8.37	0.26	0.89
F 19+ y	742	8.61	0.19	0.91
Pregnant/Lactating	8	11.01[c]	1.33	0.55[c]
All Individuals	1,428	8.37	0.18	0.80
All Individuals (+P/L)	1,436	8.38	0.18	0.80

NOTE: Means, standard errors, and percentiles were calculated with WesVar Complex Samples 3.0. Children fed human milk and females who had "blank but applicable" pregnancy and lactating status data or who responded "I don't know" to questions on pregnancy and lactating status were excluded from all analyses.

[a] M = male, F = female, P/L = pregnant and lactating.

[b] SEM = standard error of the mean.

10th	25th	50th	75th	90th	95th	99th
0.52[c]	0.90[c]	5.09[c]	7.57[c]	9.06[c]	9.55[c]	9.95[c]
0.25[c]	1.12	6.25	8.79	9.75[c]	13.36[c]	20.90[c]
2.08	6.14	8.85	9.45	9.81	9.93	19.29[c]
2.12	7.80	9.34	9.69	9.90	9.97	20.03[c]
1.12[c]	2.84[c]	5.71[c]	8.57[c]	12.04[c]	16.02[c]	19.20[c]
1.68	5.68	9.31	9.68	9.89	9.97	19.99[c]
1.69	5.72	9.31	9.68	9.89	9.97	19.98[c]

[c] These values are potentially unreliable in a statistical sense based on an insufficient sample size as recommended in statistical reporting standards (Life Sciences Research Office/Federation of American Societies for Experimental Biology. 1995. *Third Report on Nutrition Monitoring in the United States*. Washington, DC: US Government Printing Office).
SOURCE: ENVIRON International Corporation, 1999.

TABLE C-25 Mean and Percentiles for Usual Intake of Zinc (mg/day) from Food, NHANES III (1988–1994)

Sex/Age Category[a]	Number of Persons Examined	Mean	Percentile	
			5th	10th
Both sexes, 2 to 6 mo	793	5.51	2.60	3.20
Both sexes, 7 to 12 mo	827	6.11	2.90	3.50
Both sexes, 1 to 3 y	3,309	6.94	3.00	3.60
Both sexes, 4 to 8 y	3,448	8.95	6.40	6.90
Standard error		0.13	0.11	0.11
M 9 to 13 y	1,219	11.83	8.20	8.90
Standard error		0.25	0.19	0.19
M 14 to 18 y	909	15.12	8.30	9.30
Standard error		0.67	0.28	0.32
M 19 to 30 y	1,902	15.40	8.80	9.90
Standard error		0.36	0.25	0.25
M 31 to 50 y	2,533	14.83	8.60	9.60
Standard error		0.26	0.17	0.18
M 51 to 70 y	1,942	13.77	7.60	8.60
Standard error		0.27	0.16	0.17
M 71+ y	1,255	12.17	6.70	7.50
Standard error		0.53	0.20	0.22
F 9 to 13 y	1,216	9.64	6.50	7.10
Standard error		0.32	0.17	0.18
F 14 to 18 y	949	9.26	5.20	5.90
Standard error		0.32	0.19	0.20
F 19 to 30 y	1,901	9.52	5.40	6.10
Standard error		0.22	0.14	0.14
F 31 to 50 y	2,939	9.67	5.70	6.40
Standard error		0.17	0.10	0.10
F 51 to 70 y	2,065	9.19	5.30	5.90
Standard error		0.18	0.11	0.11
F 71+ y	1,368	8.62	5.00	5.50
Standard error		0.19	0.10	0.11
Pregnant	346	11.24	6.90	7.70
Standard error		0.50	0.47	0.47
Lactating	99	14.78	9.30	10.30
Standard error		0.93	0.60	0.61
All Individuals	28,575	11.27	6.10	6.90
Standard error		0.12	0.12	0.12
All Indiv (+P/L)	29,015	11.29	6.20	7.00
Standard error		0.13	0.14	0.14

NOTE: Data are limited to individuals who provided a complete and reliable 24-hour dietary recall on day 1. The intake distributions for 2–6 months, 7–12 months, and 1–3 years of age are unadjusted. Means and percentiles for these groups were computed using SAS PROC UNIVARIATE. For all other groups, data were adjusted using the Iowa State University method. Mean, standard errors, and percentiles were obtained using C-Side. Standard errors were estimated via jackknife replication. Each standard error has 49 degrees of freedom. Infants and children fed human milk and females who had "blank but applicable" pregnancy and lactating status data or who responded "I don't

25th	50th	75th	90th	95th	99th
4.20	5.30	6.60	8.10	8.90	11.60
4.50	5.90	7.30	8.90	10.10	12.90
4.80	6.40	8.40	10.60	12.90	17.80
7.70	8.80	10.00	11.20	12.00	13.60
0.11	0.13	0.14	0.16	0.18	0.23
10.10	11.60	13.30	15.10	16.20	18.50
0.20	0.23	0.30	0.40	0.48	0.68
11.40	14.30	17.90	22.00	24.90	31.40
0.39	0.54	0.86	1.39	1.85	3.13
12.00	14.80	18.10	21.60	23.90	28.90
0.28	0.33	0.44	0.61	0.75	1.12
11.50	14.20	17.40	20.90	23.30	28.60
0.21	0.25	0.31	0.41	0.51	0.78
10.50	13.10	16.30	19.80	22.30	27.80
0.18	0.23	0.35	0.55	0.73	1.21
9.10	11.40	14.40	17.90	20.40	26.30
0.27	0.40	0.66	1.05	1.39	2.30
8.10	9.40	10.90	12.50	13.50	15.50
0.21	0.28	0.39	0.54	0.66	0.95
7.20	8.90	10.90	13.10	14.50	17.50
0.23	0.29	0.40	0.57	0.72	1.08
7.40	9.20	11.20	13.40	14.90	18.10
0.16	0.20	0.26	0.36	0.44	0.67
7.60	9.30	11.30	13.40	14.80	17.90
0.12	0.15	0.21	0.31	0.40	0.62
7.10	8.80	10.80	13.00	14.50	17.80
0.12	0.15	0.23	0.37	0.48	0.80
6.70	8.20	10.10	12.20	13.60	16.70
0.13	0.17	0.24	0.33	0.41	0.63
9.10	10.90	13.00	15.20	16.60	19.60
0.47	0.49	0.55	0.68	0.82	1.19
12.20	14.50	17.10	19.60	21.30	24.60
0.68	0.88	1.19	1.59	1.88	2.56
8.50	10.70	13.40	16.30	18.40	23.00
0.12	0.12	0.13	0.17	0.21	0.33
8.50	10.70	13.40	16.30	18.40	23.00
0.14	0.13	0.14	0.17	0.20	0.33

know" to questions on pregnancy and lactating status were excluded from all analyses. Females who were both pregnant and lactating were included in both the Pregnant and Lactating categories. The sample sizes for the Pregnant and Lactating categories were very small so their estimates of usual intake distributions are not reliable.

[a] M = male, F = female, P/L = pregnant and lactating.

SOURCE: ENVIRON International Corporation and Iowa State University Department of Statistics, 2000.

TABLE C-26 Mean and Percentiles for Usual Intake of Zinc (mg/day) from Food and Supplements, NHANES III (1988–1994)

Sex/Age Category[a]	Number of Persons Examined	Mean	Percentile	
			5th	10th
Both sexes, 2 to 6 mo	793	5.51	2.60	3.20
Both sexes, 7 to 12 mo	827	6.11	2.90	3.50
Both sexes, 1 to 3 y	3,309	6.94	3.00	3.60
Both sexes, 4 to 8 y	3,448	9.56	6.56	6.94
M 9 to 13 y	1,219	12.34	8.18	8.85
M 14 to 18 y	909	15.83	8.55	9.56
M 19 to 30 y	1,902	16.94	8.81	10.21
M 31 to 50 y	2,533	16.44	8.74	10.02
M 51 to 70 y	1,942	16.29	7.94	9.07
M 71+ y	1,255	15.08	7.08	7.94
F 9 to 13 y	1,216	10.17	6.68	7.35
F 14 to 18 y	949	9.78	5.19	6.18
F 19 to 30 y	1,901	11.23	5.60	6.33
F 31 to 50 y	2,939	12.14	5.98	6.63
F 51 to 70 y	2,065	12.15	5.36	6.22
F 71+ y	1,368	12.08	5.05	5.66
Pregnant	346	19.97	7.09	8.31
Lactating	99	24.67	10.05	10.60
All Individuals	28,575	13.00	6.34	7.23
All Indiv (+P/L)	29,015	13.14	6.35	7.24

NOTE: Data are limited to individuals who provided a complete and reliable 24-hour dietary recall on day 1. The intake distributions for 2–6 months, 7–12 months, and 1–3 years of age are unadjusted; the total nutrient intake is the sum of the unadjusted food intake and the daily supplement intake. For all other groups, individual total nutrient intakes were obtained as the sum of the adjusted individual usual intake from food alone and the daily supplement intake. The mean and percentiles of the estimated usual intake distributions were computed using SAS PROC UNIVARIATE. Infants and children fed human milk and females who had "blank but applicable" pregnancy and

25th	50th	75th	90th	95th	99th
4.20	5.30	6.60	8.10	8.90	11.60
4.50	5.90	7.30	8.90	10.10	12.90
4.80	6.40	8.40	10.60	12.90	17.80
7.88	8.95	10.22	11.64	14.22	24.36
10.26	11.71	13.34	15.42	17.30	30.35
11.82	14.80	18.33	22.11	26.16	39.03
12.71	15.34	19.52	25.75	29.76	43.00
12.10	14.77	18.87	25.18	30.46	42.60
11.07	13.90	18.10	26.95	31.55	59.70
9.73	12.12	16.93	26.13	30.05	56.85
8.26	9.55	11.01	12.87	14.48	25.52
7.49	8.98	11.11	13.39	15.54	26.26
7.81	9.64	12.09	18.58	24.64	36.90
8.02	10.08	12.67	22.49	25.76	36.73
7.48	9.52	13.04	23.73	26.13	37.26
7.07	8.92	12.41	23.97	26.20	49.72
10.11	13.09	31.35	37.49	39.86	47.97
13.08	20.42	38.59	42.64	46.70	46.70
8.86	11.21	14.55	21.67	26.39	38.29
8.87	11.22	14.61	22.24	26.82	39.37

lactating status data or who responded "I don't know" to questions on pregnancy and lactating status were excluded from all analyses. Females who were both pregnant and lactating were included in both the Pregnant and Lactating categories. The sample sizes for the Pregnant and Lactating categories were very small so their estimates of usual intake distributions are not reliable.

[a] M = male, F = female, P/L = pregnant and lactating.

SOURCE: ENVIRON International Corporation and Iowa State University Department of Statistics, 2000.

TABLE C-27 Mean and Percentiles for Drinking Water Intake (mL/day), NHANES III (1988–1994)

Sex/Age Category[a]	Number of Persons Examined	Mean	SEM[b]	Percentile 5th
Both sexes, 2 to 6 mo	784	115	8	0
Both sexes, 7 to 12 mo	809	172	8	0
Both sexes, 1 to 3 y	3,172	382	10	0
Both sexes, 4 to 8 y	3,247	620	24	0
M 9 to 13 y	1,188	1,107	42	64
M 14 to 18 y	891	1,402	59	0
M 19 to 30 y	1,872	1,389	41	0
M 31 to 50 y	2,495	1,294	35	0
M 51 to 70 y	1,872	1,253	41	0
M 71+ y	1,186	1,198	39	0
F 9 to 13 y	1,181	1,008	45	56
F 14 to 18 y	937	1,117	43	0
F 19 to 30 y	1,885	1,163	33	0
F 31 to 50 y	2,906	1,219	30	0
F 51 to 70 y	2,002	1,278	32	0
F 71+ y	1,317	1,147	25	0
Pregnant	341	1,413	79	147
Lactating	98	1,628	147	225[c]
P/L	434	1,462	69	166
All Individuals	27,744	1,144	13	0
All Indiv (+P/L)	28,178	1,149	13	0

NOTE: Means, standard errors, and percentiles were calculated with WesVar Complex Samples 3.0. Children fed human milk and females who had "blank but applicable" pregnancy and lactating status data or who responded "I don't know" to questions on pregnancy and lactating status were excluded from all analyses.

[a] M = male, F = female, P/L = pregnant and lactating.
[b] SEM = standard error of the mean.

10th	25th	50th	75th	90th	95th	99th
0	0	54	131	230	457	876[c]
0	0	107	205	446	472	902[c]
0	104	228	467	903	1,135	1,789
98	206	453	848	1,265	1,686	2,638
204	453	877	1,383	2,347	2,726	4,105[c]
211	608	1,038	1,772	2,648	3,642	5,612[c]
208	435	939	1,824	2,803	3,729	7,195
101	435	921	1,835	2,760	3,623	6,206
172	454	941	1,703	2,623	3,533	5,440
215	602	942	1,657	2,258	2,819	3,730[c]
178	351	709	1,320	2,103	2,628	4,371[c]
62	337	857	1,519	2,537	2,946	4,972[c]
94	368	889	1,704	2,603	3,128	4,717
95	334	897	1,734	2,645	3,411	4,723
189	468	966	1,768	2,614	3,341	4,625
222	470	945	1,545	2,064	2,634	3,724[c]
315	661	1,136	1,900	2,621	2,831	5,057[c]
453[c]	951	1,301	1,914	3,121[c]	3,721[c]	4,717[c]
353	694	1,251	1,902	2,665	3,562	4,865[c]
99	343	878	1,610	2,530	3,240	5,261
100	347	884	1,614	2,538	3,244	5,258

[c] These values are potentially unreliable in a statistical sense based on an insufficient sample size as recommended in statistical reporting standards (Life Sciences Research Office/Federation of American Societies for Experimental Biology. 1995. *Third Report on Nutrition Monitoring in the United States.* Washington, DC: US Government Printing Office).
SOURCE: ENVIRON International Corporation, 2000.

D

Dietary Intake Data from the Continuing Survey of Food Intakes by Individuals (CSFII), 1994–1996

TABLE D-1 Mean and Percentiles for Usual Intake of Boron (mg/day) from Food, CSFII (1994–1996)

Sex/Age Category[a]	Number of Persons Examined	Mean	Percentile	
			1st	5th
Both sexes, 0 to 6 mo	195	0.75	0.03	0.06
Standard error		0.14	0.01	0.01
Both sexes, 7 to 12 mo	130	0.99	0.12	0.20
Standard error		0.12	0.02	0.02
Both sexes, 1 to 3 y	1,834	0.86	0.25	0.35
Standard error		0.02	0.01	0.01
Both sexes, 4 to 8 y	1,650	0.80	0.33	0.43
Standard error		0.01	0.01	0.01
M 9 to 13 y	552	0.90	0.38	0.49
Standard error		0.03	0.02	0.02
M 14 to 18 y	446	1.02	0.34	0.47
Standard error		0.04	0.03	0.02
M 19 to 30 y	853	1.15	0.37	0.51
Standard error		0.03	0.02	0.02
M 31 to 50 y	1,684	1.33	0.42	0.58
Standard error		0.03	0.02	0.02
M 51 to 70 y	1,606	1.34	0.39	0.56
Standard error		0.02	0.02	0.02
M 71+ y	674	1.25	0.31	0.46
Standard error		0.03	0.02	0.02

10th	25th	50th	75th	90th	95th	99th
0.09	0.15	0.29	0.76	1.89	2.95	6.40
0.01	0.01	0.05	0.15	0.44	0.63	1.99
0.27	0.42	0.71	1.21	2.00	2.70	4.77
0.03	0.05	0.09	0.15	0.27	0.41	0.91
0.42	0.57	0.78	1.07	1.41	1.66	2.24
0.01	0.01	0.01	0.02	0.04	0.05	0.08
0.49	0.61	0.76	0.95	1.15	1.29	1.58
0.01	0.01	0.01	0.01	0.02	0.03	0.04
0.56	0.69	0.86	1.07	1.28	1.43	1.74
0.02	0.02	0.02	0.03	0.05	0.06	0.09
0.55	0.72	0.96	1.25	1.57	1.79	2.28
0.02	0.03	0.03	0.05	0.07	0.09	0.14
0.61	0.80	1.06	1.40	1.79	2.05	2.66
0.02	0.02	0.03	0.04	0.06	0.08	0.12
0.69	0.91	1.22	1.63	2.09	2.42	3.18
0.02	0.02	0.02	0.04	0.06	0.09	0.15
0.67	0.89	1.22	1.66	2.16	2.52	3.34
0.02	0.02	0.02	0.03	0.06	0.08	0.13
0.56	0.78	1.11	1.56	2.12	2.53	3.51
0.02	0.02	0.02	0.03	0.07	0.10	0.20

continued

TABLE D-1 Continued

Sex/Age Category[a]	Number of Persons Examined	Mean	Percentile	
			1st	5th
F 9 to 13 y	560	0.83	0.34	0.44
Standard error		0.03	0.02	0.02
F 14 to 18 y	436	0.78	0.26	0.36
Standard error		0.04	0.02	0.02
F 19 to 30 y	760	0.87	0.30	0.40
Standard error		0.03	0.02	0.02
F 31 to 50 y	1,614	1.00	0.31	0.44
Standard error		0.02	0.01	0.01
F 51 to 70 y	1,539	1.11	0.32	0.46
Standard error		0.02	0.01	0.01
F 71+ y	623	0.98	0.27	0.39
Standard error		0.03	0.02	0.02
F Pregnant	70	1.16	0.37	0.52
Standard error		0.09	0.06	0.07
F Lactating	41	1.39	0.38	0.55
Standard error		0.16	0.10	0.12
All Individuals	15,156	1.06	0.28	0.41
Standard error		0.01	0.00	0.00
All Indiv (+P/L)	15,267	1.06	0.28	0.41
Standard error		0.01	0.00	0.00

NOTE: Estimates were obtained using C-SIDE v1.02 (C-SIDE courtesy of Iowa State University Statistical Laboratory, Iowa State University). Standard errors were estimated via jackknife replication. Each standard error has 43 degrees of freedom.
[a] M = male, F = female, P/L = pregnant and lactating.
SOURCE: C. Rainey, Nutrition Research Group, and A. Carriquiry, Iowa State University, 1999.

10th	25th	50th	75th	90th	95th	99th
0.50	0.62	0.79	0.99	1.21	1.35	1.68
0.02	0.02	0.02	0.03	0.05	0.06	0.09
0.42	0.55	0.73	0.96	1.22	1.40	1.80
0.02	0.02	0.03	0.05	0.07	0.08	0.13
0.48	0.62	0.81	1.06	1.34	1.54	1.97
0.02	0.02	0.03	0.04	0.06	0.08	0.13
0.52	0.69	0.93	1.23	1.58	1.83	2.39
0.01	0.01	0.02	0.02	0.03	0.04	0.07
0.55	0.73	1.01	1.38	1.81	2.13	2.87
0.01	0.01	0.02	0.03	0.05	0.07	0.12
0.47	0.64	0.89	1.21	1.59	1.86	2.47
0.02	0.02	0.03	0.04	0.06	0.09	0.15
0.62	0.81	1.08	1.42	1.79	2.06	2.64
0.07	0.08	0.09	0.11	0.16	0.20	0.33
0.67	0.92	1.27	1.73	2.26	2.64	3.49
0.13	0.14	0.15	0.20	0.31	0.43	0.75
0.50	0.68	0.96	1.32	1.75	2.07	2.79
0.00	0.00	0.01	0.01	0.02	0.03	0.05
0.50	0.68	0.95	1.32	1.75	2.06	2.79
0.00	0.00	0.01	0.01	0.02	0.03	0.05

TABLE D-2 Mean and Percentiles for Usual Intake of Copper (mg/day) from Food, CSFII (1994–1996)

Sex/Age Category[a]	Number of Persons Examined	Mean	Percentile 5th	Percentile 10th
Both sexes, 0 to 6 mo	157	0.61	0.40	0.44
Standard error		0.02	0.02	0.02
Both sexes, 7 to 12 mo	112	0.77	0.49	0.55
Standard error		0.05	0.04	0.04
Both sexes, 1 to 3 y	1,791	0.71	0.41	0.47
Standard error		0.01	0.01	0.01
Both sexes, 4 to 8 y	1,650	0.88	0.55	0.61
Standard error		0.01	0.01	0.01
M 9 to 13 y	552	1.17	0.69	0.78
Standard error		0.04	0.02	0.02
M 14 to 18 y	446	1.45	0.81	0.92
Standard error		0.05	0.03	0.03
M 19 to 30 y	854	1.52	0.81	0.92
Standard error		0.03	0.03	0.03
M 31 to 50 y	1,684	1.50	0.84	0.95
Standard error		0.02	0.01	0.02
M 51 to 70 y	1,606	1.44	0.78	0.89
Standard error		0.03	0.02	0.02
M 71+ y	674	1.25	0.67	0.77
Standard error		0.03	0.02	0.02
F 9 to 13 y	560	0.99	0.64	0.71
Standard error		0.02	0.02	0.02
F 14 to 18 y	436	1.07	0.62	0.69
Standard error		0.05	0.04	0.05
F 19 to 30 y	760	1.05	0.60	0.68
Standard error		0.02	0.02	0.02
F 31 to 50 y	1,614	1.06	0.62	0.70
Standard error		0.01	0.01	0.01
F 51 to 70 y	1,539	1.05	0.63	0.70
Standard error		0.02	0.01	0.01
F 71+ y	623	1.00	0.56	0.64
Standard error		0.04	0.02	0.02
F Pregnant	71	1.17	0.76	0.83
Standard error		0.06	0.04	0.04
F Lactating	42	1.35	0.84	0.92
Standard error		0.11	0.09	0.09
All Individuals	15,058	1.17	0.58	0.67
Standard error		0.01	0.01	0.01
All Indiv (+P/L)	15,170	1.17	0.58	0.67
Standard error		0.01	0.01	0.01

NOTE: Data are limited to individuals who provided two 24-hour dietary recalls and were adjusted using the Iowa State University method. Mean, standard errors, and percentiles were obtained using C-Side. Standard errors were estimated via jackknife replication. Each standard error has 43 degrees of freedom. Infants and children fed human milk were excluded from all analyses. One female was pregnant and lactating and was included in both the Pregnant and Lactating categories. The sample sizes for

25th	50th	75th	90th	95th	99th
0.51	0.60	0.70	0.80	0.88	1.05
0.02	0.02	0.03	0.03	0.04	0.05
0.65	0.75	0.86	0.99	1.10	1.38
0.05	0.04	0.06	0.07	0.11	0.27
0.56	0.68	0.83	0.98	1.09	1.33
0.01	0.01	0.01	0.02	0.02	0.04
0.73	0.86	1.01	1.18	1.29	1.56
0.01	0.02	0.02	0.02	0.03	0.05
0.94	1.13	1.35	1.60	1.79	2.24
0.04	0.03	0.07	0.07	0.07	0.13
1.12	1.38	1.69	2.05	2.32	2.95
0.03	0.04	0.06	0.09	0.12	0.19
1.14	1.44	1.81	2.19	2.47	3.14
0.06	0.03	0.08	0.05	0.06	0.12
1.16	1.43	1.77	2.13	2.40	3.05
0.02	0.02	0.03	0.04	0.05	0.08
1.08	1.35	1.69	2.08	2.40	3.10
0.02	0.03	0.04	0.06	0.11	0.17
0.95	1.18	1.48	1.80	2.03	2.63
0.04	0.03	0.05	0.07	0.10	0.27
0.82	0.96	1.13	1.31	1.43	1.72
0.02	0.02	0.02	0.03	0.04	0.06
0.82	1.02	1.27	1.49	1.65	2.09
0.03	0.05	0.06	0.15	0.16	0.18
0.82	1.01	1.24	1.47	1.63	2.00
0.02	0.02	0.03	0.05	0.05	0.09
0.84	1.02	1.24	1.46	1.60	1.91
0.01	0.01	0.02	0.03	0.03	0.05
0.83	1.01	1.21	1.44	1.61	1.98
0.01	0.02	0.02	0.03	0.05	0.08
0.75	0.95	1.17	1.42	1.62	2.04
0.02	0.03	0.04	0.09	0.09	0.19
0.96	1.13	1.33	1.54	1.68	1.97
0.05	0.05	0.07	0.08	0.10	0.13
1.08	1.30	1.55	1.83	2.01	2.42
0.09	0.10	0.13	0.17	0.20	0.29
0.85	1.10	1.41	1.76	2.01	2.54
0.01	0.01	0.01	0.02	0.03	0.04
0.85	1.10	1.41	1.76	2.00	2.54
0.01	0.01	0.01	0.02	0.03	0.04

the Pregnant and Lactating categories were very small so their estimates of usual intake distributions are not reliable.

[a] M = male, F = female, P/L = pregnant and lactating.

SOURCE: ENVIRON International Corporation and Iowa State University Department of Statistics, 2000.

TABLE D-3 Mean and Percentiles for Usual Intake of Iron (mg/day) from Food, CSFII (1994–1996)

Sex/Age Category[a]	Number of Persons Examined	Mean	Percentile	
			5th	10th
Both sexes, 0 to 6 mo	157	14.6	7.6	8.9
Standard error		0.6	0.8	0.8
Both sexes, 7 to 12 mo	112	17.3	9.2	10.6
Standard error		0.7	0.5	0.5
Both sexes, 1 to 3 y	1,791	10.9	5.6	6.5
Standard error		0.2	0.1	0.1
Both sexes, 4 to 8 y	1,650	13.5	7.6	8.6
Standard error		0.2	0.2	0.1
M,9 to 13 y	552	18.2	10.0	11.4
Standard error		0.5	0.4	0.4
M 14 to 18 y	446	20.7	10.6	12.2
Standard error		0.8	0.4	0.4
M 19 to 30 y	854	19.2	10.3	11.9
Standard error		0.6	0.4	0.4
M 31 to 50 y	1,684	19.1	10.2	11.5
Standard error		0.4	0.3	0.2
M 51 to 70 y	1,606	17.5	9.3	10.7
Standard error		0.4	0.2	0.2
M 71+ y	674	16.4	8.5	9.7
Standard error		0.4	0.2	0.2
F 9 to 13 y	560	14.3	8.2	9.2
Standard error		0.4	0.2	0.2
F 14 to 18 y	436	13.5	7.4	8.5
Standard error		0.6	0.4	0.4
F 19 to 30 y	760	13.1	6.9	7.9
Standard error		0.4	0.2	0.3
F 31 to 50 y	1,614	13.1	7.1	8.0
Standard error		0.2	0.1	0.2
F 51 to 70 y	1,539	12.5	7.1	8.0
Standard error		0.2	0.1	0.1
F 71+ y	623	12.4	6.8	7.7
Standard error		0.3	0.2	0.2
F Pregnant	71	14.3	8.0	9.1
Standard error		4.3	4.1	4.3
F Lactating	42	18.6	9.5	10.8
Standard error		2.5	1.0	1.2
All Individuals	15,058	15.3	7.4	8.6
Standard error		0.1	0.1	0.1
All Indiv (+P/L)	15,170	15.3	7.4	8.6
Standard error		0.1	0.1	0.1

NOTE: Data are limited to individuals who provided two 24-hour dietary recalls and were adjusted using the Iowa State University method. Mean, standard errors, and percentiles were obtained using C-Side. Standard errors were estimated via jackknife replication. Each standard error has 43 degrees of freedom. Infants and children fed human milk were excluded from all analyses. One female was pregnant and lactating and was included in both the Pregnant and Lactating categories. The sample sizes for

25th	50th	75th	90th	95th	99th
11.1	13.9	17.5	21.5	24.2	29.7
0.5	0.6	0.7	0.9	1.0	2.8
13.4	16.8	20.7	24.5	27.0	31.9
0.6	0.6	0.8	1.2	1.4	2.1
8.1	10.3	13.0	16.2	18.5	23.5
0.1	0.2	0.3	0.4	0.5	1.0
10.4	12.8	15.9	19.3	21.7	27.5
0.1	0.2	0.3	0.4	0.6	0.9
14.1	17.2	21.0	26.0	29.9	39.3
0.3	0.4	0.6	1.0	1.3	2.2
15.3	19.3	24.5	30.8	35.5	46.5
0.5	0.7	1.1	1.6	2.0	3.1
14.7	18.1	22.5	27.8	31.8	41.0
0.5	0.5	0.9	1.0	1.2	2.1
14.1	17.8	22.5	28.1	32.3	42.7
0.2	0.3	0.4	0.7	1.0	1.8
13.2	16.5	20.6	25.5	29.2	37.6
0.3	0.3	0.5	0.7	0.9	1.4
12.1	15.5	19.6	24.2	27.4	34.5
0.3	0.4	0.6	0.8	1.0	1.5
11.1	13.7	16.8	20.0	22.2	27.0
0.3	0.3	0.4	0.5	0.6	0.8
10.4	12.7	15.7	19.4	22.2	28.8
0.8	0.5	1.1	1.1	1.2	2.2
9.8	12.4	15.7	19.2	21.7	28.0
0.6	0.4	0.9	0.8	1.0	1.7
9.8	12.3	15.5	19.0	21.5	27.5
0.2	0.2	0.3	0.4	0.5	0.7
9.6	11.9	14.7	17.7	19.9	24.9
0.2	0.2	0.3	0.4	0.5	0.7
9.5	11.9	14.8	17.9	20.0	24.5
0.2	0.3	0.3	0.4	0.6	0.8
11.2	13.9	17.0	20.1	22.2	26.6
4.5	4.6	4.4	4.1	3.9	3.5
13.3	17.1	22.2	28.3	32.8	43.6
1.6	2.2	3.1	4.3	5.3	8.1
11.0	14.3	18.5	23.3	26.7	34.2
0.1	0.1	0.2	0.3	0.4	0.6
11.0	14.3	18.6	23.3	26.7	34.2
0.1	0.1	0.2	0.3	0.4	0.6

the Pregnant and Lactating categories were very small so their estimates of usual intake distributions are not reliable.

[a] M = male, F = female, P/L = pregnant and lactating.

SOURCE: ENVIRON International Corporation and Iowa State University Department of Statistics, 2000.

TABLE D-4 Mean and Percentiles for Usual Intake of Zinc (mg/day) from Food, CSFII (1994–1996)

Sex/Age Category[a]	Number of Persons Examined	Mean	Percentile 5th	10th
Both sexes, 0 to 6 mo	157	6.1	4.0	4.3
Standard error		0.2	0.2	0.2
Both sexes, 7 to 12 mo	112	6.8	4.5	5.0
Standard error		0.2	0.2	0.2
Both sexes, 1 to 3 y	1,791	7.5	4.4	4.9
Standard error		0.1	0.1	0.1
Both sexes, 4 to 8 y	1,650	9.3	5.5	6.1
Standard error		0.1	0.1	0.1
M 9 to 13 y	552	12.6	7.6	8.5
Standard error		0.2	0.2	0.2
M 14 to 18 y	446	15.0	8.4	9.6
Standard error		0.6	0.5	0.7
M 19 to 30 y	854	14.6	8.1	9.2
Standard error		0.3	0.3	0.3
M 31 to 50 y	1,684	14.5	8.1	9.1
Standard error		0.3	0.1	0.2
M 51 to 70 y	1,606	13.0	7.2	8.0
Standard error		0.3	0.1	0.2
M 71+ y	674	11.4	6.3	7.1
Standard error		0.4	0.2	0.2
F 9 to 13 y	560	10.1	6.2	6.9
Standard error		0.2	0.2	0.2
F 14 to 18 y	436	9.9	5.5	6.3
Standard error		0.4	0.3	0.3
F 19 to 30 y	760	9.3	5.2	5.8
Standard error		0.3	0.2	0.2
F 31 to 50 y	1,614	9.5	5.4	6.1
Standard error		0.2	0.1	0.1
F 51 to 70 y	1,539	8.7	5.2	5.8
Standard error		0.1	0.1	0.1
F 71+ y	623	8.2	4.9	5.4
Standard error		0.2	0.2	0.2
F Pregnant	71	10.4	6.1	6.9
Standard error		2.0	1.8	1.9
F Lactating	42	12.2	7.3	8.1
Standard error		1.3	0.7	0.8
All Individuals	15,058	11.0	5.5	6.3
Standard error		0.1	0.1	0.1
All Indiv (+P/L)	15,170	11.0	5.5	6.3
Standard error		0.1	0.1	0.1

NOTE: Data are limited to individuals who provided two 24-hour dietary recalls and were adjusted using the Iowa State University method. Mean, standard errors, and percentiles were obtained using C-Side. Standard errors were estimated via jackknife replication. Each standard error has 43 degrees of freedom. Infants and children fed human milk were excluded from all analyses. One female was pregnant and lactating and was included in both the Pregnant and Lactating categories. The sample sizes for

25th	50th	75th	90th	95th	99th
5.0	5.9	7.0	8.1	8.8	10.4
0.2	0.2	0.3	0.4	0.4	0.6
5.7	6.7	7.8	8.9	9.6	11.0
0.2	0.2	0.3	0.4	0.5	0.7
5.9	7.2	8.8	10.5	11.7	14.6
0.1	0.1	0.2	0.3	0.4	0.6
7.3	9.0	10.9	12.8	14.1	17.1
0.1	0.1	0.2	0.2	0.3	0.5
10.2	12.2	14.5	17.2	19.2	23.5
0.2	0.2	0.3	0.4	0.5	0.9
11.7	14.3	17.5	21.2	24.0	30.3
0.8	0.6	0.6	0.9	1.2	3.2
11.2	14.0	17.3	20.8	23.2	29.1
0.3	0.3	0.4	0.5	0.6	1.0
11.0	13.7	17.1	21.1	23.8	30.7
0.2	0.2	0.4	0.5	0.8	1.3
9.8	12.3	15.3	18.8	21.2	26.9
0.2	0.2	0.4	0.6	0.8	1.1
8.7	10.8	13.4	16.3	18.3	23.3
0.2	0.3	0.5	0.8	1.0	1.9
8.1	9.7	11.6	13.7	15.1	18.4
0.2	0.2	0.3	0.4	0.5	0.9
7.7	9.5	11.7	14.0	15.5	18.7
0.4	0.3	0.4	0.6	0.8	1.5
7.1	8.9	11.0	13.1	14.6	18.1
0.2	0.2	0.3	0.4	0.6	0.9
7.3	9.1	11.1	13.4	14.9	18.5
0.1	0.1	0.2	0.3	0.4	0.6
6.9	8.4	10.2	12.1	13.4	16.4
0.2	0.1	0.2	0.2	0.4	0.7
6.5	8.0	9.6	11.4	12.5	15.0
0.2	0.2	0.2	0.3	0.3	0.5
8.4	10.2	12.2	14.2	15.4	18.0
2.0	2.1	2.0	1.9	1.8	1.6
9.6	11.6	14.2	17.0	18.9	23.2
1.0	1.3	1.6	2.0	2.3	3.0
8.0	10.4	13.3	16.6	18.8	23.9
0.1	0.1	0.1	0.2	0.2	0.4
8.0	10.4	13.3	16.5	18.8	23.8
0.1	0.1	0.1	0.2	0.2	0.4

the Pregnant and Lactating categories were very small so their estimates of usual intake distributions are not reliable.

[a] M = male, F = female, P/L = pregnant and lactating.

SOURCE: ENVIRON International Corporation and Iowa State University Department of Statistics, 2000.

E

Dietary Intake Data from the U.S. Food and Drug Administration Total Diet Study, 1991–1997

TABLE E-1 Mean and Percentiles for Usual Intake of Vitamin K (µg/day) from Food, Total Diet Study (1991–1997)

Sex/Age Category[a]	Number of Persons Examined	Mean	Percentile	
			1st	5th
Both sexes, 0 to 6 mo	204	111.39	0.01	0.11
Standard error		4.73	0.05	0.14
Both sexes, 7 to 12 mo	139	95.12	0.40	4.57
Standard error		6.96	0.00	0.38
Both sexes, 1 to 3 y	1,908	32.11	2.89	5.97
Standard error		1.03	0.19	0.11
Both sexes, 4 to 8 y	1,711	36.64	4.54	8.71
Standard error		1.17	0.30	0.12
M 9 to 13 y	574	48.08	8.51	11.35
Standard error		2.06	0.44	0.18
M 14 to 18 y	474	65.58	5.46	12.39
Standard error		4.34	0.57	0.28
M 19 to 30 y	920	69.47	5.72	11.55
Standard error		2.59	0.47	0.22
M 31 to 50 y	1,805	81.15	4.31	11.81
Standard error		2.18	0.30	0.18
M 51 to 70 y	1,680	95.47	4.19	11.10
Standard error		3.35	0.35	0.19
M 71+ y	722	81.58	3.89	8.00
Standard error		3.87	0.51	0.21

654

10th	25th	50th	75th	90th	95th	99th
9.52	47.96	98.58	124.98	156.01	189.39	270.99
0.76	0.83	0.43	0.41	0.60	1.02	2.43
8.10	17.20	71.48	110.89	138.01	174.22	300.69
0.41	0.50	0.83	0.43	0.76	1.31	4.57
8.51	11.87	17.89	26.67	43.27	74.11	130.96
0.09	0.07	0.07	0.09	0.17	0.32	0.59
11.44	15.45	21.98	31.78	48.19	75.64	129.14
0.09	0.08	0.08	0.09	0.16	0.32	0.72
14.33	19.46	29.03	44.01	68.21	99.01	167.13
0.21	0.15	0.15	0.21	0.32	0.54	1.41
16.42	22.90	34.10	54.40	87.08	136.98	266.04
0.24	0.18	0.19	0.27	0.40	0.96	2.05
17.26	26.34	39.93	63.03	96.41	148.37	262.23
0.20	0.15	0.15	0.19	0.31	0.62	1.46
18.65	27.91	44.07	71.39	116.26	186.22	332.43
0.14	0.12	0.12	0.16	0.24	0.51	1.03
17.90	27.07	44.06	74.38	134.39	252.35	429.42
0.14	0.12	0.13	0.17	0.33	0.67	1.13
13.29	23.30	38.36	64.60	116.93	219.68	404.46
0.21	0.19	0.17	0.25	0.45	0.89	1.66

continued

TABLE E-1 Continued

Sex/Age Category[a]	Number of Persons Examined	Mean	Percentile	
			1st	5th
F 9 to 13 y	586	43.63	5.44	9.11
Standard error		2.30	0.57	0.22
F 14 to 18 y	455	50.96	3.17	7.05
Standard error		3.18	0.62	0.22
F 19 to 30 y	880	56.87	4.24	7.65
Standard error		2.78	0.38	0.17
F 31 to 50 y	1,733	73.43	4.30	10.01
Standard error		2.42	0.34	0.16
F 51 to 70 y	1,605	82.85	3.89	8.49
Standard error		2.90	0.29	0.17
F 71+ y	669	79.42	2.06	6.47
Standard error		4.20	0.40	0.22
F Pregnant	81	46.37	5.62	10.71
Standard error		4.69	0.00	0.86
F Lactating	44	85.43	0.00	12.65
Standard error		17.85	0.00	1.37
All Individuals	15,941	66.05	3.44	8.24
Standard error		0.74	0.10	0.05
All Indiv (+P/L)	16,065	66.01	3.46	8.26
Standard error		0.74	0.10	0.05

[a] M = male, F = female, P/L = pregnant and lactating.
SOURCE: Health Technomics, Inc., 2000.

10th	25th	50th	75th	90th	95th	99th
12.64	17.06	24.10	36.70	57.87	89.57	180.64
0.19	0.14	0.14	0.18	0.30	0.61	1.77
11.03	16.83	27.00	43.01	67.99	112.05	216.91
0.24	0.19	0.19	0.23	0.38	0.87	1.88
11.96	18.20	29.19	46.96	76.47	124.47	240.14
0.19	0.13	0.14	0.18	0.31	0.55	1.51
14.79	20.68	34.25	59.02	103.07	179.95	347.92
0.11	0.10	0.11	0.15	0.25	0.57	1.07
14.58	22.60	37.25	64.78	120.67	215.82	394.82
0.13	0.11	0.12	0.17	0.32	0.62	1.05
11.34	19.37	33.20	61.84	116.75	227.76	395.35
0.21	0.18	0.18	0.26	0.53	0.94	1.84
14.11	17.69	26.26	44.57	68.09	110.45	165.89
0.48	0.38	0.45	0.57	0.85	2.21	4.52
18.50	23.78	33.07	60.77	129.08	286.29	510.99
0.91	0.59	0.61	1.21	1.86	7.99	12.56
12.45	18.65	30.51	53.14	95.41	159.43	302.27
0.04	0.03	0.03	0.05	0.08	0.16	0.35
12.48	18.66	30.50	53.10	95.35	159.30	301.84
0.04	0.03	0.03	0.05	0.08	0.16	0.35

TABLE E-2 Mean and Percentiles for Usual Intake of Arsenic (μg/day) from Food, Total Diet Study (1991–1997)

Sex/Age Category[a]	Number of Persons Examined	Mean	Percentile	
			1st	5th
Both sexes, 0 to 6 mo	204	1.17	0.00	0.00
Standard error		0.14	0.00	0.00
Both sexes, 7 to 12 mo	139	5.87	0.00	0.13
Standard error		2.04	0.00	0.12
Both sexes, 1 to 3 y	1,908	13.80	0.09	0.28
Standard error		1.31	0.05	0.03
Both sexes, 4 to 8 y	1,711	17.25	0.15	0.32
Standard error		1.46	0.06	0.03
M 9 to 13 y	574	28.32	0.11	0.37
Standard error		4.90	0.12	0.06
M 14 to 18 y	474	29.77	0.13	0.36
Standard error		5.95	0.11	0.06
M 19 to 30 y	920	36.17	0.10	0.35
Standard error		3.77	0.09	0.04
M 31 to 50 y	1,805	56.30	0.13	0.38
Standard error		3.95	0.06	0.03
M 51 to 70 y	1,680	63.24	0.05	0.30
Standard error		4.27	0.05	0.04
M 71+ y	722	60.31	0.06	0.27
Standard error		6.41	0.08	0.05
F 9 to 13 y	586	19.67	0.13	0.31
Standard error		3.10	0.11	0.06
F 14 to 18 y	455	24.39	0.08	0.24
Standard error		3.79	0.12	0.05
F 19 to 30 y	880	32.99	0.10	0.26
Standard error		3.58	0.08	0.04
F 31 to 50 y	1,733	39.39	0.09	0.25
Standard error		2.85	0.05	0.03
F 51 to 70 y	1,605	53.96	0.06	0.26
Standard error		3.97	0.05	0.04
F 71+ y	669	44.45	0.06	0.22
Standard error		5.42	0.08	0.05
F Pregnant	81	27.61	0.33	0.38
Standard error		10.45	0.00	0.13
F Lactating	44	29.73	0.00	0.35
Standard error		11.01	0.00	0.45
All Individuals	15,941	37.93	0.03	0.25
Standard error		1.02	0.01	0.01
All Indiv (+P/L)	16,065	37.86	0.03	0.25
Standard error		1.01	0.01	0.01

[a] M = male, F = female, P/L = pregnant and lactating.
SOURCE: Health Technomics, Inc., 2000.

10th	25th	50th	75th	90th	95th	99th
0.00	0.00	0.16	0.77	2.07	4.95	7.20
0.00	0.00	0.05	0.06	0.16	0.23	0.43
0.34	0.68	1.38	2.49	4.72	8.62	41.55
0.08	0.09	0.09	0.10	0.21	0.57	2.60
0.48	0.83	1.75	3.79	11.23	32.82	103.28
0.02	0.02	0.03	0.05	0.13	0.28	0.89
0.53	0.90	1.70	3.87	14.67	44.88	158.83
0.03	0.03	0.03	0.05	0.17	0.31	1.01
0.61	1.07	1.89	5.22	22.87	65.50	234.10
0.05	0.05	0.05	0.12	0.35	0.71	2.65
0.61	1.01	1.95	5.28	20.12	69.43	245.28
0.05	0.05	0.06	0.12	0.37	1.01	2.90
0.59	1.06	2.55	7.99	38.45	112.06	323.83
0.04	0.04	0.05	0.12	0.37	0.74	1.83
0.68	1.26	2.89	9.91	54.42	209.97	554.39
0.03	0.03	0.04	0.10	0.30	0.91	1.32
0.63	1.18	2.03	11.70	74.55	251.96	586.92
0.03	0.03	0.04	0.13	0.36	0.95	1.50
0.51	0.95	2.01	8.91	66.80	237.84	596.56
0.05	0.04	0.05	0.19	0.50	1.45	2.01
0.48	0.75	1.48	3.82	15.63	53.95	166.30
0.04	0.04	0.05	0.10	0.29	0.72	1.80
0.41	0.76	1.73	4.82	18.66	73.48	246.51
0.05	0.05	0.06	0.13	0.36	0.93	2.16
0.46	0.85	1.91	5.66	30.21	93.76	355.42
0.04	0.04	0.05	0.11	0.35	0.68	2.00
0.47	0.93	2.11	7.48	40.65	122.39	403.66
0.03	0.03	0.04	0.09	0.25	0.65	1.34
0.50	0.92	2.02	7.89	54.91	219.60	521.01
0.03	0.03	0.04	0.11	0.33	0.92	1.35
0.45	0.83	1.73	5.04	41.26	158.11	451.34
0.05	0.04	0.05	0.12	0.45	1.50	1.72
0.54	1.03	2.17	8.74	32.55	69.02	193.49
0.14	0.13	0.17	0.53	0.94	1.64	8.18
0.89	1.53	2.95	6.63	47.36	129.29	299.80
0.26	0.22	0.33	0.42	1.98	4.46	11.43
0.49	0.92	1.98	5.81	32.47	113.75	388.39
0.01	0.01	0.01	0.03	0.08	0.21	0.46
0.49	0.92	1.98	5.82	32.50	113.34	387.04
0.01	0.01	0.01	0.03	0.08	0.21	0.46

TABLE E-3 Mean and Percentiles for Usual Intake of Copper (mg/day) from Food, Total Diet Study (1991–1997)

Sex/Age Category[a]	Number of Persons Examined	Mean	Percentile 1st	5th
Both sexes, 0 to 6 mo	204	0.63	0.00	0.02
Standard error		0.02	0.03	0.04
Both sexes, 7 to 12 mo	139	0.65	0.05	0.11
Standard error		0.04	0.00	0.07
Both sexes, 1 to 3 y	1,908	0.49	0.08	0.15
Standard error		0.01	0.04	0.02
Both sexes, 4 to 8 y	1,711	0.63	0.16	0.24
Standard error		0.01	0.04	0.02
M 9 to 13 y	574	0.85	0.23	0.34
Standard error		0.03	0.08	0.04
M 14 to 18 y	474	0.96	0.22	0.34
Standard error		0.02	0.10	0.04
M 19 to 30 y	920	1.10	0.18	0.32
Standard error		0.04	0.08	0.03
M 31 to 50 y	1,805	1.13	0.15	0.32
Standard error		0.05	0.06	0.03
M 51 to 70 y	1,680	1.11	0.14	0.28
Standard error		0.04	0.06	0.03
M 71+ y	722	0.91	0.11	0.22
Standard error		0.04	0.08	0.04
F 9 to 13 y	586	0.70	0.19	0.27
Standard error		0.02	0.10	0.04
F 14 to 18 y	455	0.71	0.12	0.22
Standard error		0.02	0.06	0.04
F 19 to 30 y	880	0.73	0.15	0.23
Standard error		0.02	0.06	0.03
F 31 to 50 y	1,733	0.79	0.13	0.22
Standard error		0.03	0.05	0.02
F 51 to 70 y	1,605	0.76	0.11	0.22
Standard error		0.03	0.05	0.02
F 71+ y	669	0.79	0.11	0.21
Standard error		0.05	0.07	0.03
F Pregnant	81	0.86	0.21	0.28
Standard error		0.05	0.00	0.09
F Lactating	44	0.96	0.00	0.31
Standard error		0.07	0.00	0.17
All Individuals	15,941	0.82	0.10	0.22
Standard error		0.01	0.02	0.01
All Indiv (+P/L)	16,065	0.82	0.11	0.22
Standard error		0.01	0.02	0.01

[a] M = male, F = female, P/L = pregnant and lactating.
SOURCE: Health Technomics, Inc., 2000.

10th	25th	50th	75th	90th	95th	99th
0.08	0.30	0.58	0.72	0.90	1.06	1.34
0.04	0.06	0.03	0.03	0.05	0.08	0.15
0.15	0.26	0.54	0.74	0.90	1.05	1.26
0.04	0.05	0.05	0.04	0.05	0.08	0.18
0.21	0.28	0.39	0.51	0.67	0.82	1.01
0.01	0.01	0.01	0.01	0.01	0.02	0.03
0.31	0.38	0.49	0.64	0.80	0.96	1.20
0.01	0.01	0.01	0.01	0.01	0.02	0.05
0.41	0.51	0.66	0.85	1.09	1.32	1.69
0.03	0.02	0.02	0.02	0.03	0.05	0.09
0.44	0.57	0.76	1.02	1.31	1.63	2.04
0.04	0.03	0.03	0.03	0.04	0.06	0.11
0.44	0.59	0.79	1.09	1.46	1.92	2.56
0.03	0.02	0.02	0.02	0.03	0.05	0.11
0.45	0.59	0.80	1.06	1.41	1.80	2.52
0.02	0.01	0.01	0.01	0.02	0.03	0.08
0.39	0.53	0.73	0.99	1.31	1.63	3.25
0.02	0.01	0.01	0.02	0.02	0.03	0.18
0.31	0.45	0.63	0.87	1.14	1.45	2.57
0.03	0.02	0.02	0.02	0.03	0.05	0.22
0.34	0.43	0.56	0.71	0.88	1.06	1.43
0.02	0.02	0.02	0.02	0.03	0.05	0.09
0.30	0.41	0.55	0.72	0.95	1.21	1.57
0.04	0.02	0.02	0.02	0.04	0.06	0.11
0.31	0.41	0.55	0.76	1.00	1.22	1.53
0.02	0.02	0.02	0.02	0.03	0.03	0.07
0.30	0.40	0.56	0.75	0.99	1.25	1.64
0.02	0.01	0.01	0.01	0.02	0.03	0.06
0.31	0.40	0.54	0.72	0.94	1.19	1.73
0.02	0.01	0.01	0.01	0.02	0.03	0.10
0.27	0.36	0.50	0.68	0.89	1.08	2.91
0.02	0.02	0.02	0.02	0.03	0.04	0.31
0.35	0.47	0.67	0.93	1.25	1.48	1.75
0.09	0.06	0.07	0.07	0.09	0.08	0.30
0.43	0.60	0.80	0.94	1.25	1.71	2.55
0.00	0.11	0.07	0.07	0.14	0.23	0.22
0.30	0.41	0.57	0.79	1.07	1.39	1.92
0.01	0.00	0.00	0.00	0.01	0.01	0.02
0.30	0.41	0.57	0.79	1.07	1.39	1.92
0.01	0.00	0.00	0.00	0.01	0.01	0.02

TABLE E-4 Mean and Percentiles for Usual Intake of Iodine (mg/day) from Food, Total Diet Study (1991–1997)

Sex/Age Category[a]	Number of Persons Examined	Mean	Percentile 1st	Percentile 5th
Both sexes, 0 to 6 mo	204	0.08	0.00	0.00
Standard error		0.00	0.02	0.01
Both sexes, 7 to 12 mo	139	0.14	0.00	0.02
Standard error		0.01	0.00	0.04
Both sexes, 1 to 3 y	1,908	0.30	0.05	0.10
Standard error		0.00	0.03	0.01
Both sexes, 4 to 8 y	1,711	0.38	0.09	0.13
Standard error		0.01	0.03	0.01
M 9 to 13 y	574	0.49	0.09	0.15
Standard error		0.01	0.04	0.03
M 14 to 18 y	474	0.53	0.09	0.15
Standard error		0.02	0.04	0.03
M 19 to 30 y	920	0.41	0.05	0.11
Standard error		0.01	0.04	0.02
M 31 to 50 y	1,805	0.37	0.06	0.12
Standard error		0.01	0.03	0.01
M 51 to 70 y	1,680	0.33	0.05	0.11
Standard error		0.00	0.04	0.01
M 71+ y	722	0.30	0.05	0.10
Standard error		0.01	0.04	0.02
F 9 to 13 y	586	0.38	0.08	0.13
Standard error		0.01	0.06	0.02
F 14 to 18 y	455	0.33	0.06	0.09
Standard error		0.01	0.05	0.02
F 19 to 30 y	880	0.29	0.04	0.08
Standard error		0.01	0.04	0.02
F 31 to 50 y	1,733	0.26	0.04	0.08
Standard error		0.00	0.03	0.01
F 51 to 70 y	1,605	0.24	0.05	0.08
Standard error		0.00	0.03	0.01
F 71+ y	669	0.23	0.05	0.08
Standard error		0.01	0.03	0.02
F Pregnant	81	0.37	0.05	0.12
Standard error		0.02	0.00	0.05
F Lactating	44	0.41	0.00	0.11
Standard error		0.04	0.00	0.07
All Individuals	15,941	0.32	0.04	0.09
Standard error		0.00	0.01	0.00
All Indiv (+P/L)	16,065	0.33	0.04	0.09
Standard error		0.00	0.01	0.00

[a] M = male, F = female, P/L = pregnant and lactating.
SOURCE: Health Technomics, Inc., 2000.

10th	25th	50th	75th	90th	95th	99th
0.01	0.04	0.07	0.09	0.12	0.15	0.18
0.02	0.02	0.01	0.01	0.02	0.03	0.04
0.05	0.08	0.11	0.14	0.20	0.24	0.33
0.03	0.02	0.02	0.02	0.03	0.05	0.11
0.13	0.16	0.22	0.30	0.42	0.54	0.75
0.01	0.01	0.01	0.01	0.01	0.02	0.04
0.16	0.20	0.27	0.38	0.56	0.73	0.96
0.01	0.01	0.01	0.01	0.02	0.02	0.04
0.20	0.25	0.33	0.46	0.73	1.03	1.30
0.02	0.02	0.01	0.02	0.03	0.05	0.09
0.20	0.26	0.34	0.49	0.73	1.14	1.60
0.02	0.02	0.02	0.02	0.04	0.07	0.11
0.16	0.22	0.30	0.41	0.57	0.77	1.15
0.02	0.01	0.01	0.01	0.02	0.04	0.08
0.16	0.21	0.29	0.39	0.51	0.65	0.87
0.01	0.01	0.01	0.01	0.01	0.02	0.04
0.15	0.20	0.26	0.35	0.45	0.54	0.66
0.01	0.01	0.01	0.01	0.01	0.02	0.03
0.13	0.18	0.24	0.31	0.40	0.48	0.70
0.01	0.01	0.01	0.01	0.01	0.03	0.07
0.16	0.21	0.27	0.38	0.54	0.72	0.95
0.02	0.01	0.01	0.02	0.03	0.04	0.07
0.11	0.16	0.22	0.32	0.49	0.70	0.97
0.02	0.01	0.01	0.02	0.03	0.06	0.09
0.11	0.15	0.21	0.29	0.40	0.56	0.79
0.01	0.01	0.01	0.01	0.02	0.03	0.06
0.11	0.15	0.20	0.27	0.35	0.46	0.61
0.01	0.01	0.01	0.01	0.01	0.02	0.03
0.11	0.14	0.19	0.25	0.32	0.40	0.54
0.01	0.01	0.01	0.01	0.01	0.02	0.04
0.10	0.14	0.19	0.24	0.31	0.38	0.51
0.01	0.01	0.01	0.01	0.01	0.03	0.06
0.14	0.20	0.29	0.38	0.51	0.65	0.86
0.05	0.05	0.04	0.04	0.06	0.11	0.17
0.14	0.21	0.29	0.41	0.58	0.76	1.35
0.12	0.08	0.05	0.07	0.11	0.23	0.42
0.12	0.17	0.23	0.33	0.46	0.62	0.86
0.00	0.00	0.00	0.00	0.00	0.01	0.01
0.12	0.17	0.23	0.33	0.46	0.62	0.86
0.00	0.00	0.00	0.00	0.00	0.01	0.01

TABLE E-5 Mean and Percentiles for Usual Intake of Iron (mg/day) from Food, Total Diet Study (1991–1997)

Sex/Age Category[a]	Number of Persons Examined	Mean	Percentile	
			1st	5th
Both sexes, 0 to 6 mo	204	13.71	0.02	0.42
Standard error		0.60	0.09	0.19
Both sexes, 7 to 12 mo	139	15.92	0.82	2.65
Standard error		0.83	0.00	0.34
Both sexes, 1 to 3 y	1,908	9.86	1.37	2.85
Standard error		0.12	0.14	0.09
Both sexes, 4 to 8 y	1,711	12.27	2.90	4.63
Standard error		0.14	0.25	0.08
M 9 to 13 y	574	16.54	4.04	6.39
Standard error		0.34	0.42	0.17
M 14 to 18 y	474	18.60	3.72	6.35
Standard error		0.50	0.48	0.18
M 19 to 30 y	920	17.00	2.70	5.47
Standard error		0.31	0.29	0.15
M 31 to 50 y	1,805	16.03	2.67	5.38
Standard error		0.19	0.24	0.10
M 51 to 70 y	1,680	14.89	2.16	5.03
Standard error		0.18	0.25	0.10
M 71+ y	722	13.77	2.34	4.34
Standard error		0.28	0.38	0.15
F 9 to 13 y	586	12.54	3.10	4.73
Standard error		0.24	0.40	0.14
F 14 to 18 y	455	12.30	2.36	3.68
Standard error		0.37	0.31	0.16
F 19 to 30 y	880	11.99	2.28	3.63
Standard error		0.22	0.23	0.12
F 31 to 50 y	1,733	11.00	1.82	3.53
Standard error		0.14	0.20	0.08
F 51 to 70 y	1,605	10.79	1.88	3.47
Standard error		0.14	0.19	0.09
F 71+ y	669	10.76	1.73	3.12
Standard error		0.22	0.23	0.14
F Pregnant	81	14.74	3.10	5.43
Standard error		0.95	0.00	0.62
F Lactating	44	17.33	0.00	5.89
Standard error		1.37	0.00	0.70
All Individuals	15,941	13.03	1.74	3.83
Standard error		0.06	0.07	0.03
All Indiv (+P/L)	16,065	13.05	1.75	3.84
Standard error		0.06	0.07	0.03

[a] M = male, F = female, P/L = pregnant and lactating.
SOURCE: Health Technomics, Inc., 2000.

10th	25th	50th	75th	90th	95th	99th
1.63	5.04	11.04	15.08	21.48	28.03	33.20
0.21	0.26	0.17	0.16	0.27	0.36	0.55
4.05	6.61	12.59	17.54	22.75	30.23	40.30
0.28	0.23	0.22	0.22	0.29	0.57	1.26
4.13	5.47	7.46	10.44	14.03	17.78	22.31
0.06	0.04	0.04	0.05	0.06	0.10	0.17
5.82	7.36	9.59	12.79	16.74	21.54	27.41
0.06	0.05	0.04	0.05	0.07	0.12	0.20
7.94	9.81	12.74	16.99	23.38	28.19	37.26
0.12	0.09	0.09	0.11	0.15	0.24	0.45
8.06	10.26	13.75	18.73	26.30	34.94	45.69
0.13	0.12	0.10	0.12	0.20	0.30	0.50
7.43	9.74	12.85	17.41	23.80	30.42	41.23
0.10	0.07	0.07	0.09	0.13	0.19	0.37
7.29	9.39	12.49	16.57	22.07	29.11	36.88
0.08	0.05	0.05	0.06	0.08	0.14	0.21
6.67	8.48	11.51	15.57	20.98	26.70	33.76
0.07	0.05	0.05	0.06	0.09	0.14	0.21
5.80	7.74	10.39	14.12	19.36	25.64	32.96
0.10	0.08	0.07	0.08	0.13	0.19	0.34
6.04	7.58	9.96	13.20	17.10	21.43	26.92
0.11	0.08	0.08	0.09	0.11	0.23	0.34
5.06	6.84	9.21	12.49	16.93	22.58	29.76
0.14	0.09	0.09	0.10	0.16	0.26	0.46
4.99	6.58	9.14	12.53	16.39	21.70	29.92
0.09	0.07	0.06	0.07	0.10	0.20	0.33
4.71	6.26	8.41	11.33	15.26	19.83	26.68
0.06	0.05	0.04	0.05	0.07	0.12	0.23
4.72	6.11	8.27	11.23	15.22	19.42	24.68
0.05	0.05	0.04	0.05	0.07	0.11	0.20
4.45	6.08	8.20	11.26	15.32	19.68	24.62
0.10	0.07	0.07	0.08	0.12	0.19	0.28
6.65	8.49	11.04	14.15	19.74	33.86	38.77
0.19	0.26	0.21	0.24	0.39	0.83	0.69
6.62	8.14	12.36	19.68	26.28	33.92	38.17
0.43	0.26	0.44	0.57	0.42	1.09	0.98
5.27	7.03	9.74	13.51	18.48	24.26	31.65
0.02	0.02	0.02	0.02	0.03	0.04	0.07
5.28	7.04	9.75	13.53	18.51	24.32	31.76
0.02	0.02	0.02	0.02	0.03	0.04	0.07

TABLE E-6 Mean and Percentiles for Usual Intake of
Manganese (mg/day) from Food, Total Diet Study (1991–1997)

Sex/Age Category[a]	Number of Persons Examined	Mean	Percentile 1st	Percentile 5th
Both sexes, 0 to 6 mo	204	0.22	0.00	0.00
Standard error		0.02	0.00	0.00
Both sexes, 7 to 12 mo	139	0.79	0.00	0.11
Standard error		0.04	0.00	0.11
Both sexes, 1 to 3 y	1,908	1.60	0.17	0.45
Standard error		0.02	0.07	0.03
Both sexes, 4 to 8 y	1,711	1.89	0.40	0.63
Standard error		0.02	0.08	0.03
M 9 to 13 y	574	2.48	0.53	0.82
Standard error		0.05	0.13	0.06
M 14 to 18 y	474	2.89	0.60	0.81
Standard error		0.08	0.14	0.06
M 19 to 30 y	920	3.07	0.31	0.71
Standard error		0.07	0.14	0.06
M 31 to 50 y	1,805	3.27	0.41	0.79
Standard error		0.05	0.09	0.04
M 51 to 70 y	1,680	3.07	0.29	0.73
Standard error		0.04	0.10	0.04
M 71+ y	722	2.82	0.36	0.63
Standard error		0.06	0.10	0.06
F 9 to 13 y	586	2.05	0.46	0.72
Standard error		0.04	0.16	0.06
F 14 to 18 y	455	2.13	0.34	0.57
Standard error		0.07	0.13	0.07
F 19 to 30 y	880	2.34	0.34	0.57
Standard error		0.05	0.09	0.05
F 31 to 50 y	1,733	2.43	0.34	0.64
Standard error		0.03	0.08	0.03
F 51 to 70 y	1,605	2.42	0.34	0.66
Standard error		0.03	0.08	0.04
F 71+ y	669	2.35	0.25	0.57
Standard error		0.05	0.12	0.06
F Pregnant	81	2.87	0.69	0.79
Standard error		0.18	0.00	0.15
F Lactating	44	3.30	0.00	0.80
Standard error		0.28	0.00	0.25
All Individuals	15,941	2.43	0.07	0.49
Standard error		0.01	0.02	0.01
All Indiv (+P/L)	16,065	2.43	0.07	0.49
Standard error		0.01	0.02	0.01

[a] M = male, F = female, P/L = pregnant and lactating.
SOURCE: Health Technomics, Inc., 2000.

10th	25th	50th	75th	90th	95th	99th
0.00	0.00	0.06	0.21	0.44	0.65	0.95
0.00	0.01	0.03	0.03	0.05	0.07	0.15
0.23	0.36	0.57	0.80	1.15	1.66	2.28
0.08	0.05	0.04	0.05	0.08	0.19	0.20
0.63	0.87	1.22	1.71	2.32	2.96	3.64
0.02	0.02	0.02	0.02	0.03	0.04	0.06
0.84	1.09	1.48	2.00	2.67	3.32	4.11
0.02	0.02	0.02	0.02	0.03	0.05	0.08
1.07	1.40	1.91	2.59	3.50	4.52	5.71
0.05	0.04	0.03	0.04	0.06	0.10	0.13
1.05	1.48	2.17	3.04	4.15	5.32	7.04
0.06	0.05	0.04	0.05	0.07	0.11	0.22
1.06	1.51	2.17	3.15	4.52	6.01	8.15
0.04	0.03	0.03	0.04	0.06	0.09	0.16
1.14	1.58	2.31	3.42	4.83	6.32	8.33
0.03	0.03	0.03	0.03	0.04	0.06	0.12
1.07	1.56	2.26	3.30	4.55	5.66	6.85
0.04	0.03	0.02	0.03	0.04	0.06	0.09
0.97	1.41	2.13	3.09	4.22	5.23	6.36
0.05	0.04	0.04	0.05	0.06	0.09	0.12
0.90	1.18	1.57	2.14	2.93	3.59	4.58
0.04	0.03	0.03	0.04	0.05	0.09	0.14
0.81	1.09	1.55	2.20	3.00	3.90	5.23
0.05	0.04	0.04	0.05	0.06	0.11	0.20
0.82	1.12	1.64	2.45	3.53	4.59	5.95
0.04	0.03	0.03	0.04	0.05	0.07	0.14
0.86	1.20	1.77	2.58	3.60	4.63	5.88
0.03	0.02	0.02	0.03	0.04	0.05	0.09
0.89	1.25	1.82	2.59	3.54	4.46	5.65
0.03	0.02	0.02	0.03	0.04	0.05	0.09
0.86	1.19	1.75	2.60	3.47	4.30	5.22
0.05	0.04	0.04	0.04	0.05	0.08	0.13
1.06	1.39	2.10	3.13	4.18	5.88	6.88
0.14	0.12	0.13	0.12	0.16	0.40	0.36
1.04	1.55	2.56	3.42	5.16	5.79	8.55
0.33	0.18	0.19	0.18	0.24	0.22	0.49
0.79	1.15	1.71	2.53	3.65	4.79	6.20
0.01	0.01	0.01	0.01	0.01	0.02	0.03
0.79	1.15	1.72	2.54	3.65	4.80	6.21
0.01	0.01	0.01	0.01	0.01	0.02	0.03

TABLE E-7 Mean and Percentiles for Usual Intake of Nickel (µg/day) from Food, Total Diet Study (1991–1997)

Sex/Age Category[a]	Number of Persons Examined	Mean	Percentile 1st	Percentile 5th
Both sexes, 0 to 6 mo	204	8.96	0.00	0.00
Standard error		1.03	0.00	0.00
Both sexes, 7 to 12 mo	139	39.33	0.00	4.92
Standard error		2.23	0.00	0.74
Both sexes, 1 to 3 y	1,908	81.75	6.57	18.89
Standard error		1.24	0.47	0.21
Both sexes, 4 to 8 y	1,711	99.29	17.03	30.52
Standard error		1.36	0.48	0.23
M 9 to 13 y	574	127.91	24.84	42.00
Standard error		2.92	1.15	0.44
M 14 to 18 y	474	136.87	16.03	32.21
Standard error		3.95	1.19	0.55
M 19 to 30 y	920	139.71	9.64	25.69
Standard error		3.33	0.74	0.33
M 31 to 50 y	1,805	147.23	13.35	31.05
Standard error		2.41	0.51	0.28
M 51 to 70 y	1,680	140.74	9.88	26.61
Standard error		2.15	0.55	0.26
M 71+ y	722	135.58	10.89	24.04
Standard error		3.13	0.69	0.43
F 9 to 13 y	586	108.69	19.74	31.28
Standard error		2.48	0.98	0.36
F 14 to 18 y	455	101.36	13.12	24.71
Standard error		3.29	0.73	0.51
F 19 to 30 y	880	107.25	13.12	24.84
Standard error		2.37	0.65	0.33
F 31 to 50 y	1,733	106.17	11.15	23.27
Standard error		1.60	0.53	0.21
F 51 to 70 y	1,605	109.36	12.75	27.76
Standard error		1.63	0.58	0.25
F 71+ y	669	108.97	10.19	27.23
Standard error		2.40	0.95	0.37
F Pregnant	81	120.76	19.41	26.36
Standard error		8.10	0.00	1.11
F Lactating	44	162.19	0.00	33.97
Standard error		16.90	0.00	2.94
All Individuals	15,941	114.16	1.03	20.15
Standard error		0.62	0.10	0.09
All Indiv (+P/L)	16,065	114.33	1.09	20.24
Standard error		0.62	0.10	0.09

[a] M = male, F = female, P/L = pregnant and lactating.
SOURCE: Health Technomics, Inc., 2000.

10th	25th	50th	75th	90th	95th	99th
0.00	0.00	0.23	5.16	20.35	37.15	51.83
0.00	0.00	0.07	0.26	0.42	0.74	0.70
12.39	17.76	27.22	41.79	58.05	79.72	113.17
0.52	0.30	0.33	0.36	0.57	1.07	1.66
27.38	39.77	59.69	85.82	120.99	155.12	198.55
0.14	0.13	0.12	0.14	0.20	0.27	0.52
38.85	51.77	73.78	104.25	144.15	183.76	231.61
0.15	0.14	0.13	0.16	0.22	0.32	0.64
53.35	69.75	97.34	134.79	179.94	228.54	293.55
0.33	0.28	0.26	0.29	0.41	0.67	1.23
49.11	67.89	97.55	140.45	200.81	281.32	352.81
0.43	0.31	0.31	0.37	0.52	0.97	1.25
40.53	61.37	93.53	143.95	208.64	287.08	398.16
0.33	0.23	0.23	0.28	0.38	0.71	1.26
46.83	66.49	100.12	151.98	223.17	299.03	392.21
0.20	0.17	0.17	0.20	0.30	0.44	0.88
41.33	63.94	100.51	149.37	215.60	276.92	353.50
0.21	0.18	0.17	0.20	0.29	0.41	0.74
39.56	62.58	97.52	142.65	211.21	268.70	331.36
0.35	0.28	0.25	0.32	0.44	0.60	0.95
45.46	58.96	80.26	112.36	158.03	210.82	254.62
0.36	0.23	0.24	0.28	0.44	0.62	1.05
34.30	47.49	71.35	105.61	149.98	197.88	254.14
0.28	0.27	0.29	0.33	0.47	0.80	0.99
33.49	48.42	74.77	112.69	161.32	212.00	275.40
0.23	0.21	0.21	0.25	0.35	0.51	0.90
33.71	49.46	74.37	110.73	162.93	215.07	267.32
0.19	0.15	0.14	0.18	0.25	0.35	0.62
38.36	52.83	78.89	116.14	161.62	210.29	272.22
0.17	0.15	0.15	0.17	0.25	0.37	0.66
37.77	53.91	80.73	116.99	160.46	206.57	261.05
0.28	0.25	0.23	0.27	0.35	0.60	0.86
37.19	55.66	86.57	131.37	183.69	227.98	311.58
1.09	0.81	0.76	0.86	1.25	2.72	4.42
48.80	62.71	106.45	171.89	249.36	362.28	500.11
0.78	1.28	1.24	1.65	1.76	5.22	3.37
33.70	51.18	78.68	118.66	172.94	231.80	304.12
0.06	0.05	0.05	0.06	0.09	0.13	0.22
33.77	51.25	78.77	118.83	173.23	232.16	304.61
0.06	0.05	0.05	0.06	0.09	0.13	0.22

TABLE E-8 Mean and Percentiles for Usual Intake of Silicon (mg/day) from Food, Total Diet Study (1991–1997)

Sex/Age Category[a]	Number of Persons Examined	Mean	Percentile	
			1st	5th
Both sexes, 0 to 6 mo	204	51.33	0.13	0.73
Standard error		3.43	0.23	0.27
Both sexes, 7 to 12 mo	139	43.42	2.25	4.15
Standard error		3.37	0.00	0.43
Both sexes, 1 to 3 y	1,908	15.34	3.16	5.20
Standard error		0.26	0.18	0.09
Both sexes, 4 to 8 y	1,711	15.52	4.50	6.75
Standard error		0.15	0.27	0.08
M 9 to 13 y	574	20.13	5.75	8.10
Standard error		0.36	0.34	0.19
M 14 to 18 y	474	24.76	6.59	8.61
Standard error		0.70	0.49	0.17
M 19 to 30 y	920	41.87	4.31	7.64
Standard error		1.48	0.32	0.18
M 31 to 50 y	1,805	36.58	5.36	8.74
Standard error		0.80	0.26	0.12
M 51 to 70 y	1,680	30.58	4.86	8.27
Standard error		0.66	0.30	0.12
M 71+ y	722	24.46	3.28	6.23
Standard error		0.74	0.40	0.17
F 9 to 13 y	586	16.57	4.68	6.52
Standard error		0.29	0.31	0.17
F 14 to 18 y	455	17.10	3.85	5.59
Standard error		0.40	0.35	0.20
F 19 to 30 y	880	21.43	3.85	6.07
Standard error		0.60	0.29	0.14
F 31 to 50 y	1,733	20.63	4.12	6.32
Standard error		0.33	0.25	0.09
F 51 to 70 y	1,605	19.25	3.43	6.09
Standard error		0.26	0.20	0.12
F 71+ y	669	18.04	2.92	5.73
Standard error		0.35	0.29	0.19
F Pregnant	81	22.26	4.61	7.68
Standard error		1.26	0.00	0.61
F Lactating	44	26.77	0.00	8.75
Standard error		1.80	0.00	0.45
All Individuals	15,941	23.92	3.52	6.35
Standard error		0.19	0.08	0.03
All Indiv (+P/L)	16,065	23.92	3.53	6.36
Standard error		0.19	0.08	0.03

[a] M = male, F = female, P/L = pregnant and lactating.
SOURCE: Health Technomics, Inc., 2000.

10th	25th	50th	75th	90th	95th	99th
4.16	19.00	34.59	44.47	77.45	133.32	182.03
0.34	0.47	0.24	0.29	0.88	0.67	2.49
6.50	10.64	28.82	40.95	65.89	114.13	151.76
0.36	0.34	0.43	0.30	0.91	1.17	1.85
6.64	8.69	11.60	15.44	20.37	25.92	34.80
0.06	0.05	0.05	0.05	0.08	0.12	0.27
8.06	10.00	12.76	16.38	20.76	25.04	30.59
0.07	0.05	0.05	0.05	0.07	0.11	0.19
10.09	12.89	16.54	21.24	26.81	33.08	40.27
0.14	0.11	0.09	0.11	0.15	0.26	0.38
10.93	14.06	19.37	25.58	33.02	41.43	55.10
0.15	0.14	0.13	0.13	0.19	0.34	0.62
10.61	14.93	22.53	34.98	62.77	105.67	165.58
0.13	0.11	0.11	0.15	0.30	0.49	0.78
11.94	16.10	22.86	32.84	52.44	80.41	122.98
0.10	0.08	0.07	0.09	0.17	0.27	0.55
11.07	14.82	20.70	28.71	40.99	60.48	96.85
0.09	0.08	0.07	0.08	0.13	0.29	0.54
9.26	12.56	17.85	24.79	33.00	43.08	62.36
0.15	0.11	0.10	0.12	0.16	0.29	0.67
8.33	10.74	13.81	17.39	22.33	36.34	32.69
0.15	0.10	0.08	0.09	0.14	0.17	0.37
7.57	10.16	13.59	18.27	23.18	28.50	35.84
0.18	0.10	0.11	0.12	0.15	0.26	0.45
7.79	10.54	14.72	20.65	29.63	40.63	61.02
0.11	0.09	0.09	0.10	0.16	0.28	0.63
8.36	10.92	15.18	21.11	28.49	36.65	51.17
0.08	0.06	0.06	0.07	0.10	0.16	0.38
8.50	11.27	15.07	20.41	26.30	32.65	41.12
0.09	0.06	0.06	0.07	0.09	0.14	0.26
7 71	10.39	14.07	19.38	25.27	30.65	39.73
0.12	0.10	0.09	0.10	0.13	0.22	0.39
8.93	11.64	17.45	23.85	32.86	38.96	45.60
0.08	0.40	0.31	0.31	0.56	0.56	1.53
11.30	15.66	21.92	28.51	37.01	50.20	56.93
0.75	0.64	0.46	0.50	0.63	0.21	0.53
8.44	11.15	15.53	22.08	31.98	46.27	79.63
0.03	0.02	0.02	0.02	0.04	0.07	0.17
8.45	11.15	15.55	22.11	32.01	46.21	79.28
0.03	0.02	0.02	0.02	0.04	0.07	0.17

TABLE E-9 Mean and Percentiles for Usual Intake of
Zinc (mg/day) from Food, Total Diet Study (1991–1997)

Sex/Age Category[a]	Number of Persons Examined	Mean	Percentile 1st	5th
Both sexes, 0 to 6 mo	204	6.00	0.00	0.10
Standard error		0.22	0.05	0.10
Both sexes, 7 to 12 mo	139	6.30	0.21	0.76
Standard error		0.22	0.00	0.26
Both sexes, 1 to 3 y	1,908	7.29	1.53	2.70
Standard error		0.08	0.18	0.07
Both sexes, 4 to 8 y	1,711	9.14	2.31	3.45
Standard error		0.10	0.14	0.07
M 9 to 13 y	574	12.46	3.22	4.80
Standard error		0.24	0.24	0.15
M 14 to 18 y	474	15.08	2.71	4.97
Standard error		0.38	0.44	0.18
M 19 to 30 y	920	14.64	2.18	4.09
Standard error		0.33	0.27	0.11
M 31 to 50 y	1,805	13.38	2.21	4.24
Standard error		0.16	0.23	0.08
M 51 to 70 y	1,680	11.78	1.53	3.60
Standard error		0.15	0.22	0.09
M 71+ y	722	9.56	1.45	2.79
Standard error		0.17	0.26	0.12
F 9 to 13 y	586	9.65	2.04	3.24
Standard error		0.19	0.19	0.14
F 14 to 18 y	455	9.47	1.33	2.58
Standard error		0.24	0.22	0.15
F 19 to 30 y	880	9.33	1.50	2.90
Standard error		0.17	0.24	0.11
F 31 to 50 y	1,733	8.51	1.24	2.49
Standard error		0.11	0.17	0.07
F 51 to 70 y	1,605	7.93	1.32	2.37
Standard error		0.10	0.15	0.08
F 71+ y	669	7.34	1.29	2.20
Standard error		0.15	0.21	0.10
F Pregnant	81	11.09	2.16	4.23
Standard error		0.52	0.00	0.61
F Lactating	44	12.79	0.00	4.59
Standard error		0.97	0.00	0.34
All Individuals	15,941	10.00	1.25	2.84
Standard error		0.05	0.06	0.03
All Indiv (+P/L)	16,065	10.01	1.26	2.85
Standard error		0.05	0.06	0.03

[a] M = male, F = female, P/L = pregnant and lactating.
SOURCE: Health Technomics, Inc., 2000.

10th	25th	50th	75th	90th	95th	99th
0.69	2.84	5.52	6.83	8.56	10.32	12.80
0.17	0.20	0.09	0.09	0.14	0.23	0.32
2.17	4.04	5.68	7.03	8.43	10.07	11.75
0.32	0.15	0.12	0.09	0.18	0.22	0.40
3.47	4.43	5.81	7.74	9.99	12.39	15.33
0.04	0.04	0.03	0.04	0.05	0.08	0.13
4.34	5.47	7.23	9.66	12.68	15.65	19.10
0.05	0.04	0.04	0.04	0.06	0.09	0.16
5.90	7.54	9.72	13.13	17.52	21.88	25.20
0.10	0.08	0.08	0.09	0.13	0.17	0.30
6.23	8.53	11.47	15.49	20.96	28.53	36.09
0.12	0.11	0.09	0.11	0.18	0.31	0.38
5.68	7.82	10.90	15.33	20.56	27.23	33.31
0.11	0.07	0.07	0.08	0.12	0.17	0.26
5.55	7.50	10.44	14.32	18.79	23.52	29.66
0.06	0.05	0.05	0.05	0.07	0.11	0.20
4.80	6.37	9.05	12.57	16.57	21.14	27.07
0.06	0.05	0.05	0.05	0.07	0.12	0.21
3.99	5.37	7.51	10.30	13.69	16.53	20.61
0.09	0.07	0.07	0.07	0.10	0.13	0.25
4.39	5.65	7.63	10.16	13.46	17.08	21.07
0.11	0.07	0.07	0.08	0.11	0.19	0.28
3.74	5.00	7.38	10.29	13.27	16.46	21.40
0.10	0.10	0.09	0.09	0.11	0.21	0.36
3.74	5.07	7.07	9.85	13.30	17.08	21.65
0.07	0.06	0.06	0.06	0.09	0.15	0.25
3.45	4.72	6.59	9.03	12.12	15.36	19.25
0.05	0.04	0.04	0.05	0.06	0.09	0.16
3.29	4.37	6.18	8.51	11.41	14.06	17.06
0.06	0.04	0.04	0.05	0.06	0.08	0.15
2.90	4.06	5.63	7.81	10.61	13.11	16.28
0.09	0.06	0.06	0.07	0.09	0.15	0.23
5.31	6.53	9.27	11.79	15.99	18.71	20.28
0.31	0.21	0.23	0.19	0.33	0.35	0.46
5.16	6.09	9.38	13.95	20.75	23.75	25.65
0.61	0.14	0.35	0.36	0.53	1.04	0.31
3.91	5.23	7.36	10.41	14.45	18.63	24.22
0.02	0.01	0.01	0.02	0.02	0.04	0.07
3.92	5.24	7.37	10.43	14.48	18.66	24.20
0.02	0.01	0.01	0.02	0.02	0.04	0.06

F

Canadian Dietary Intake Data, 1990

TABLE F-1 Mean and Percentiles for Intake of Vitamin A (µg/RE[a]/day) from Food, Nova Scotia and Québec, Canada (1990)

Sex/Age Category[b]	Number of Respondents	Mean	Percentile 5th
M 19–30 y	536	1,518	380
Standard error			37
M 31–50 y	724	1,281	417
Standard error			16
M 51–70 y	663	1,479	481
Standard error			43
M 71–74 y	149	2,093	464
Standard error			50
F 19–30 y	548	1,129	417
Standard error			17
F 31–50 y	826	1,137	401
Standard error			21
F 51–70 y	657	1,245	426
Standard error			24
F 71–74 y	148	1,298	431
Standard error			29

[a] RE = retinol equivalents. 1 RE = 6 µg β-carotene and 12 mg α-carotene or β-cryptoxanthin.
[b] M = male, F = female.
SOURCE: Nova Scotia Heart Health Program. 1993. *Report of the Nova Scotia Nutrition Survey*. Nova Scotia Department of Health, Health and Welfare Canada; Santé Québec.

10th	25th	50th	75th	90th	95th	99th
484	647	874	1,277	1,744	2,145	3,892
27	16	27	48	76	145	1,051
495	710	951	1,253	1,581	1,802	2,485
24	22	30	37	58	98	228
572	744	994	134	1,891	2,082	2,812
30	28	43	88	93	40	275
550	805	1,124	1,463	1,855	2,317	3,769
53	79	42	90	198	215	2,944
499	597	717	885	1,039	1,121	1,443
12	11	11	16	25	25	94
474	598	747	1,005	1,264	1,420	1,802
16	10	18	22	38	75	140
500	609	805	1,128	1,443	1,648	1,992
23	16	33	41	72	62	111
456	540	756	1,195	1,637	1,838	2,315
19	44	62	100	115	134	417

1995. *Les Québécoises et les Québécois Mangent-Ils Mieux? Rapport de l'Enquête Québécoise sur la Nutrition, 1990.* Montréal: Ministère de la Santé et des Services Sociaux, Gouvernement du Québec.

TABLE F-2 Mean and Percentiles for Intake of Iron (mg/day) from Food, Nova Scotia and Québec, Canada (1990)

Sex/Age Category[a]	Number of Respondents	Mean	Percentile 5th
M 19–30 y	536	17.9	10.3
Standard error			0.4
M 31–50 y	724	16.9	9.0
Standard error			0.4
M 51–70 y	663	15.1	8.2
Standard error			0.4
M 71–74 y	149	15.1	9.1
Standard error			0.8
F 19–30 y	548	11.8	6.2
Standard error			0.2
F 31–50 y	826	11.7	7.2
Standard error			0.2
F 51–70 y	657	11	7.0
Standard error			0.3
F 71–74 y	148	11	6.3
Standard error			0.3

[a] M = male, F = female.
SOURCE: Nova Scotia Heart Health Program. 1993. *Report of the Nova Scotia Nutrition Survey*. Nova Scotia Department of Health, Health and Welfare Canada; Santé Québec.

10th	25th	50th	75th	90th	95th	99th
11.2	13.7	16.1	19.2	22.4	23.9	31.6
0.3	0.2	0.2	0.4	0.3	1.0	2.2
10.2	12.6	15.7	18.7	21.9	24.7	31.6
0.4	0.3	0.3	0.3	0.6	1.2	2.2
9.0	11.2	14.5	17.8	20.4	22.2	29.5
0.5	0.3	0.4	0.4	0.7	0.8	2.4
10.0	11.4	13.6	16.8	20.4	21.6	31.6
0.3	0.4	0.7	1.0	1.1	2.6	5.2
7.1	8.6	10.9	13.4	15.9	17.5	20.8
0.2	0.2	0.2	0.3	0.4	0.4	0.9
8.2	9.6	10.8	12.1	13.7	14.8	17.8
0.2	0.1	0.1	0.2	0.2	0.4	0.5
7.8	9.0	10.5	11.8	13.3	14.0	17.3
0.2	0.2	0.2	0.2	0.3	0.2	1.1
6.6	8.0	9.7	11.9	13.7	17.2	24.9
0.4	0.3	0.4	0.4	1.4	3.2	4.6

1995. *Les Québécoises et les Québécois Mangent-Ils Mieux? Rapport de l'Enquête Québécoise sur la Nutrition, 1990.* Montréal: Ministère de la Santé et des Services Sociaux, Gouvernement du Québec.

TABLE F-3 Mean and Percentiles for Intake of Zinc (mg/day) from Food, Nova Scotia and Québec, Canada (1990)

Sex/Age Category[a]	Number of Respondents	Mean	Percentile 5th
M 19–30 y	536	15.9	11.2
Standard error			0.3
M 31–50 y	724	16.6	8.3
Standard error			0.3
M 51–70 y	663	12.6	7.4
Standard error			0.4
M 71–74 y	149	13.2	7.0
Standard error			0.6
F 19–30 y	548	9.9	5.9
Standard error			0.2
F 31–50 y	826	9.7	6.2
Standard error			0.2
F 51–70 y	657	8.8	4.0
Standard error			0.2
F 71–74 y	148	9.4	3.9
Standard error			0.3

[a] M = male, F = female.
SOURCE: Nova Scotia Heart Health Program. 1993. *Report of the Nova Scotia Nutrition Survey.* Nova Scotia Department of Health, Health and Welfare Canada; Santé Québec.

10th	25th	50th	75th	90th	95th	99th
12.0	13.0	14.0	14.9	15.8	16.5	20.2
0.1	0.1	0.08	0.1	0.1	0.4	1.4
9.4	11.2	13.1	14.9	16.6	18.2	21.9
0.3	0.3	0.2	0.2	0.3	0.6	1.0
8.5	9.7	11.3	13.2	15.8	18.0	20.1
0.2	0.2	0.3	0.3	0.7	0.8	0.6
8.0	8.9	11.0	13.3	15.1	16.2	21.9
0.4	0.3	0.5	0.5	0.7	1.4	2.5
6.6	7.6	8.8	10.1	11.3	12.1	14.1
0.1	0.09	0.1	0.1	0.1	0.2	0.8
6.7	7.5	8.5	9.7	10.8	11.6	13.9
0.09	0.1	0.1	0.1	0.2	0.2	0.6
5.8	6.8	8.2	9.3	10.6	11.5	13.2
0.2	0.1	0.2	0.2	0.2	0.4	1.1
4.2	6.2	7.4	9.0	12.0	13.0	20.7
0.5	0.4	0.2	0.8	0.8	2.8	4.1

1995. *Les Québécoises et les Québécois Mangent-Ils Mieux? Rapport de l'Enquête Québécoise sur la Nutrition, 1990.* Montréal: Ministère de la Santé et des Services Sociaux, Gouvernement du Québec.

G

Biochemical Indicators for Iron, Vitamin A, and Iodine from the Third National Health and Nutrition Examination Survey (NHANES III), 1988–1994

TABLE G-1 Mean and Percentiles for Hemoglobin (g/L), NHANES III (1988–1994)

Sex/Age Category[a]	n	Mean	SEM[b]	Percentile 5th	Percentile 10th
Both sexes, 1 to 3 y	2,389	120.9	0.2	108.0	110.8
Both sexes, 4 to 8 y	2,910	126.9	0.2	113.5	116.4
M 9 to 13 y	1,110	135.2	0.5	120.3	123.2
M 14 to 18 y	830	149.0	0.6	131.6	135.3
M 19 to 30 y	1,804	154.0	0.4	138.9	142.1
M 31 to 50 y	2,416	152.0	0.4	135.2	139.3
M 51 to 70 y	1,874	148.8	0.2	128.7	134.7
M 71+ y	1,189	143.7	0.6	117.6	125.1
F 9 to 13 y	1,090	131.8	0.5	117.9	121.3
F 14 to 18 y	883	132.4	0.5	116.8	120.3
F 19 to 30 y	1,809	132.8	0.3	115.8	119.8
F 31 to 50 y	2,805	132.2	0.3	112.9	118.3
F 51 to 70 y	1,976	135.1	0.3	117.4	121.7
F 71+ y	1,306	134.1	0.4	113.7	119.5
F Pregnant	317	121.0	1.0	105.1[c]	108.9
F Lactating	96	134.2	2.1	114.7[c]	117.6[c]
F P/L	408	123.9	1.0	106.7[c]	110.2
All Individuals	24,391	139.5	0.2	116.8	121.3
All Indiv (+P/L)	24,799	139.2	0.2	116.4	120.9

NOTE: Means, standard errors, and percentiles calculated with WesVar Complex Samples 3.0. Children fed human milk and females who had "blank but applicable" pregnancy and lactating status data or who responded "I don't know" to questions on pregnancy and lactating status were excluded from all analyses.

[a] M = male, F = female, P/L = pregnant and lactating.
[b] SEM = standard error of the mean.

25th	50th	75th	90th	95th	99th
115.7	120.4	125.7	130.5	133.3	138.3^c
121.1	127.2	132.1	136.4	139.2	145.1
128.3	134.6	141.2	146.3	150.1	161.9^c
141.5	149.4	156.1	161.0	164.2	169.7^c
147.1	153.7	160.1	164.9	168.5	177.7^c
145.6	152.2	158.2	164.5	167.8	174.6^c
141.7	149.1	155.7	162.2	166.6	174.5^c
135.8	144.2	152.6	159.7	164.3	173.2^c
126.3	130.6	136.5	143.1	146.2	154.6^c
125.9	132.5	138.8	143.8	147.3	153.0^c
126.3	133.0	139.2	144.8	147.7	154.6^c
126.0	132.5	139.1	145.2	149.5	156.9
128.3	135.0	141.7	147.8	151.6	158.6^c
127.4	134.1	141.3	147.7	152.4	160.9^c
114.5	120.7	126.2	136.1	137.9^c	148.8^c
128.7^c	134.4	140.2^c	146.9^c	150.7^c	151.9^c
115.7	122.4	131.1	138.9	145.4^c	151.3^c
129.1	138.8	149.7	158.1	162.7	170.9
128.8	138.5	149.5	158.0	162.6	170.8

^{c} These values are potentially unreliable in a statistical sense based on an insufficient sample size as indicated in statistical reporting standards (Life Sciences Research Office/ Federation of American Societies for Experimental Biology. 1995. *Third Report on Nutrition Monitoring in the United States*. Washington, DC: U.S. Government Printing Office). SOURCE: ENVIRON International Corporation, 2000.

TABLE G-2 Mean and Percentiles for Serum Transferrin Saturation (%), NHANES III (1988–1994)

Sex/Age Category[a]	n	Mean	SEM[b]	Percentile 5th	Percentile 10th
Both sexes, 1 to 3 y	1,935	18.6	0.3	5.6	7.6
Both sexes, 4 to 8 y	2,865	21.4	0.2	8.9	11.1
M 9 to 13 y	1,097	22.5	0.5	9.4	11.8
M 14 to 18 y	836	27.7	0.7	12.4	14.4
M 19 to 30 y	1,802	30.4	0.4	13.1	16.2
M 31 to 50 y	2,413	29.1	0.3	15.3	17.0
M 51 to 70 y	1,879	27.5	0.4	13.0	15.9
M 71+ y	1,188	27.1	0.4	12.2	14.5
F 9 to 13 y	1,087	22.6	0.6	8.8	10.7
F 14 to 18 y	884	23.4	0.5	7.3	10.0
F 19 to 30 y	1,795	25.4	0.5	8.5	11.3
F 31 to 50 y	2,802	23.4	0.4	7.3	9.9
F 51 to 70 y	1,980	23.6	0.3	11.1	13.0
F 71+ y	1,301	23.9	0.3	11.0	13.2
F Pregnant	318	22.8	1.0	9.3[c]	10.5
F Lactating	93	25.8[c]	1.9	10.1[c]	10.8[c]
F P/L	407	23.5	0.8	9.7[c]	10.6
All Individuals	23,864	25.5	0.1	9.6	12.6
All Indiv (+P/L)	24,271	25.5	0.1	9.6	12.5

NOTE: Means, standard errors, and percentiles calculated with WesVar Complex Samples 3.0. Females who had "blank but applicable" pregnancy and lactating status data or who responded "I don't know" to questions on pregnancy and lactating status were excluded from all analyses.

[a] M = male, F = female, P/L = pregnant and lactating.

[b] SEM = standard error of the mean.

25th	50th	75th	90th	95th	99th
11.4	17.6	24.6	29.8	35.3	44.9[c]
15.3	20.5	26.6	31.9	37.4	47.5
15.5	20.9	27.9	33.7	39.2	47.5[c]
19.2	25.1	34.8	44.2	49.7	63.6[c]
21.8	29.6	36.8	46.0	52.3	68.3[c]
21.5	27.5	34.9	43.0	48.9	64.0[c]
20.6	26.5	33.2	39.7	45.1	56.5[c]
19.6	25.9	33.2	39.9	45.9	65.7[c]
16.1	21.3	27.2	34.3	41.2	58.9[c]
15.9	22.0	29.5	36.0	44.1	59.6[c]
16.5	23.5	31.6	40.6	47.7	67.0[c]
15.0	21.4	29.8	39.0	45.1	57.4
17.0	22.4	28.6	35.2	41.3	54.2[c]
17.5	22.2	29.2	35.6	40.7	54.7[c]
14.0	21.4	28.5	38.2	43.8[c]	53.9[c]
15.3[c]	23.0[c]	33.6[c]	45.4[c]	46.6[c]	47.7[c]
14.5	22.0	29.5	40.7	46.2[c]	53.1[c]
17.6	24.0	31.5	39.8	46.0	59.7
17.5	24.0	31.4	39.8	46.0	59.6

[c] These values are potentially unreliable in a statistical sense based on an insufficient sample size as indicated in statistical reporting standards (Life Sciences Research Office/ Federation of American Societies for Experimental Biology. 1995. *Third Report on Nutrition Monitoring in the United States.* Washington, DC: U.S. Government Printing Office). SOURCE: ENVIRON International Corporation, 2000.

TABLE G-3 Mean and Percentiles for Serum Ferritin (µg/L), NHANES III (1988–1994)

Sex/Age Category[a]	n	Mean	Percentile 5th	Percentile 10th
Both sexes, 1–3 y	2,429	27.9	6.0	9.0
Both sexes, 4–8 y	2,906	34.1	14.3	17.0
Standard error		0.5	0.4	0.4
M 9–13 y	1,098	38.8	16.2	19.2
Standard error		1.1	0.7	1.3
M 14–18 y	837	56.6	20.0	24.0
Standard error		2.1	1.0	1.1
M 19–30 y	1,801	131.0	42.0	54.0
Standard error		2.5	3.2	6.0
M 31–50 y	2,418	189.4	41.0	60.0
Standard error		3.6	2.5	2.6
M 51–70 y	1,877	204.2	37.0	53.0
Standard error		6.8	2.5	3.1
M 71+ y	1,189	184.8	28.0	41.0
Standard error		6.4	1.7	1.9
F 9–13 y	1,092	36.4	12.3	16.0
Standard error		1.1	1.3	1.4
F 14–18 y	888	35.8	9.0	12.0
Standard error		2.9	1.0	1.0
F 19–30 years	1,797	47.8	9.0	13.0
Standard error		1.5	0.6	0.8
F 31–50 y	2,808	64.0	7.0	11.0
Standard error		3.1	0.4	0.6
F 51–70 years	1,980	120.1	19.0	28.0
Standard error		3.3	1.0	1.2
F 71+ y	1,300	135.1	21.0	30.0
Standard error		5.0	1.4	2.3
F Pregnant	320	37.6	12.0	15.0
Standard error		3.9	5.3	5.1
F Lactating	94	47.3	18.0	21.0
Standard error		6.1	5.6	6.1
F P/L	410	41.1	11.0	14.0
Standard error		3.3	1.7	2.1
All Individuals	24,420	104.3	12.0	18.0
Standard error		1.4	0.2	0.3
All Indiv (+P/L)	24,830	103.2	12.0	17.0
Standard error		1.4	0.2	0.3

NOTE: The intake distributions for 2–6 months, 7–11 months, and 1–3 years of age are unadjusted. Means and percentiles for these groups were computed using SAS PROC UNIVARIATE. For all other groups, data were adjusted using the Iowa State University method. Mean, standard errors, and percentiles were obtained using C-Side. Standard errors were estimated via jackknife replication. Each standard error has 49 degrees of freedom. Infants and children fed human milk and females who had "blank but applicable" pregnancy and lactating status data or who responded "I don't know" to ques-

25th	50th	75th	90th	95th
15.0	23.0	34.0	49.0	64.0
21.8	29.8	41.2	56.6	68.9
0.5	0.6	0.9	1.4	2.1
25.4	34.8	47.7	63.4	75.2
1.9	0.9	3.6	3.0	5.0
33.0	48.0	70.0	99.0	123.0
1.4	1.9	2.8	4.8	6.9
80.0	118.0	168.0	224.0	263.0
6.9	7.0	7.6	6.5	10.0
101.0	157.0	235.0	355.0	455.0
2.6	3.3	5.6	8.5	13.0
92.0	161.0	267.0	408.0	519.0
4.6	6.9	9.5	13.6	18.4
74.0	136.0	239.0	385.0	506.0
3.0	5.7	9.6	15.1	20.9
22.5	31.7	44.2	60.7	76.4
1.0	1.1	1.6	3.2	3.7
19.0	29.0	42.0	63.0	86.0
1.0	1.2	2.2	6.5	12.3
22.0	37.0	60.0	94.0	124.0
1.2	1.5	2.2	3.1	4.6
21.0	42.0	75.0	133.0	194.0
0.8	1.8	2.4	5.9	12.9
50.0	91.0	157.0	247.0	321.0
1.8	3.2	4.7	7.4	10.8
53.0	96.0	170.0	281.0	380.0
6.0	3.0	18.5	12.4	30.4
22.0	33.0	47.0	65.0	80.0
4.6	4.0	4.8	9.8	15.5
29.0	41.0	59.0	81.0	98.0
5.4	4.7	12.3	19.0	23.3
22.0	33.0	51.0	77.0	99.0
2.1	2.5	5.6	8.4	12.0
31.0	65.0	135.0	237.0	322.0
0.5	1.0	2.3	3.9	5.4
31.0	64.0	133.0	235.0	320.0
0.5	0.9	2.3	3.8	5.3

tions on pregnancy and lactating status were excluded from all analyses. Females who were both pregnant and lactating were included in both the Pregnant and Lactating categories. The sample sizes for the Pregnant and Lactating categories were very small so their estimates of usual serum ferritin distributions are not reliable.

[a] M = male, F = female, P/L = pregnant and lactating.

SOURCE: ENVIRON International Corporation and Iowa State University Department of Statistics, 2000.

TABLE G-4 Mean and Percentiles for Serum Vitamin A (Retinol) (μmol/L), NHANES III (1988–1994)

Sex/Age Category[a]	n	Mean	SEM[b]	Percentile	
				5th	10th
Both sexes, 4 to 8 y	2,704	1.22	0.01	0.84	0.91
M 9 to 13 y	1,076	1.43	0.01	0.99	1.06
M 14 to 18 y	823	1.76	0.02	1.22	1.31
M 19 to 30 y	1,784	2.01	0.02	1.38	1.50
M 31 to 50 y	2,397	2.22	0.01	1.43	1.59
M 51 to 70 y	1,870	2.27	0.02	1.48	1.65
M 71+ y	1,174	2.34	0.03	1.42	1.62
F 9 to 13 y	1,070	1.40	0.01	1.01	1.09
F 14 to 18 y	877	1.61	0.02	1.07	1.16
F 19 to 30 y	1,786	1.87	0.02	1.14	1.26
F 31 to 50 y	2,781	1.79	0.02	1.14	1.23
F 51 to 70 y	1,965	2.14	0.02	1.32	1.48
F 71+ y	1,282	2.24	0.02	1.32	1.49
F Pregnant	316	1.47	0.04	0.84[c]	0.99
F Lactating	94	1.82[c]	0.05	1.31[c]	1.39[c]
F P/L	406	1.55	0.03	0.88[c]	1.04
All Individuals	21,589	1.93	0.01	1.10	1.22
All Indiv (+P/L)	21,995	1.92	0.01	1.10	1.22

NOTE: Means, standard errors, and percentiles calculated with WesVar Complex Samples 3.0. Females who had "blank but applicable" pregnancy and lactating status data or who responded "I don't know" to questions on pregnancy and lactating status were excluded from all analyses.

[a] M = male, F = female, P/L = pregnant and lactating.
[b] SEM = standard error of the mean.

25th	50th	75th	90th	95th	99th
1.04	1.20	1.35	1.49	1.58	1.86
1.21	1.40	1.57	1.81	1.89	2.09^c
1.52	1.71	1.95	2.20	2.34	2.83^c
1.69	1.95	2.23	2.54	2.72	3.10^c
1.85	2.16	2.52	2.88	3.11	3.63^c
1.90	2.21	2.58	2.94	3.17	3.56^c
1.88	2.19	2.65	3.17	3.47	4.62^c
1.20	1.34	1.54	1.72	1.82	2.28^c
1.32	1.55	1.78	2.08	2.34	2.84^c
1.48	1.77	2.16	2.56	2.80	3.27^c
1.44	1.71	2.01	2.36	2.63	3.29
1.73	2.06	2.41	2.79	3.10	4.10^c
1.81	2.16	2.56	3.00	3.32	4.27^c
1.22	1.45	1.67	1.94	2.21^c	2.34^c
1.53^c	1.87^c	1.94^c	2.24^c	2.31^c	2.50^c
1.28	1.51	1.78	2.02	2.25^c	2.42^c
1.49	1.85	2.25	2.65	2.92	3.51
1.49	1.84	2.25	2.65	2.92	3.50

^{c} These values are potentially unreliable in a statistical sense based on an insufficient sample size as indicated in statistical reporting standards (Life Sciences Research Office/ Federation of American Societies for Experimental Biology. 1995. *Third Report on Nutrition Monitoring in the United States.* Washington, DC: U.S. Government Printing Office).
SOURCE: ENVIRON International Corporation, 2000.

TABLE G-5 Mean and Percentiles for Serum Retinyl Esters (μmol/L), NHANES III (1998–1994)

Sex/Age Category[a]	n	Mean	SEM[b]	Percentile 5th	Percentile 10th
Both sexes, 4 to 8 y	1,026	0.186	0.005	0.035	0.055
M 9 to 13 y	682	0.177	0.007	0.024	0.045
M 14 to 18 y	703	0.158	0.004	0.030	0.042
M 19 to 30 y	1,625	0.183	0.004	0.028	0.047
M 31 to 50 y	2,220	0.207	0.004	0.030	0.054
M 51 to 70 y	1,745	0.219	0.006	0.029	0.057
M 71+ y	1,090	0.196	0.007	0.018	0.038
F 9 to 13 y	651	0.171	0.005	0.032	0.054
F 14 to 18 y	770	0.154	0.004	0.024	0.039
F 19 to 30 y	1,669	0.174	0.004	0.017	0.039
F 31 to 50 y	2,625	0.187	0.003	0.028	0.049
F 51 to 70 y	1,809	0.247	0.016	0.038	0.062
F 71+ y	1,159	0.229	0.005	0.029	0.056
F Pregnant	268	0.221	0.010	0.048[c]	0.078
F Lactating	86	0.189[c]	0.017	0.031[c]	0.045[c]
F P/L	351	0.212	0.009	0.040[c]	0.068
All Individuals	17,774	0.198	0.003	0.028	0.049
All Indiv (+P/L)	18,125	0.198	0.003	0.028	0.049

NOTE: Means, standard errors, and percentiles calculated with WesVar Complex Samples 3.0. Females who had "blank but applicable" pregnancy and lactating status data or who responded "I don't know" to questions on pregnancy and lactating status were excluded from all analyses.

[a] M = male, F = female, P/L = pregnant and lactating.

[b] SEM = standard error of the mean.

25th	50th	75th	90th	95th	99th
0.097	0.146	0.220	0.295	0.379	0.517[c]
0.092	0.155	0.209	0.276	0.324	0.424[c]
0.082	0.135	0.192	0.238	0.278	0.355[c]
0.101	0.153	0.213	0.290	0.340	0.515[c]
0.110	0.173	0.239	0.340	0.400	0.629[c]
0.106	0.170	0.252	0.342	0.437	0.817[c]
0.081	0.148	0.237	0.331	0.410	0.781[c]
0.090	0.149	0.211	0.264	0.294	0.379[c]
0.073	0.128	0.184	0.249	0.294	0.407[c]
0.089	0.153	0.209	0.277	0.310	0.402[c]
0.092	0.156	0.225	0.302	0.352	0.490
0.120	0.191	0.274	0.379	0.451	0.868[c]
0.110	0.191	0.278	0.383	0.466	0.713[c]
0.142	0.194	0.256	0.330	0.385[c]	0.621[c]
0.103[c]	0.167[c]	0.235[c]	0.273[c]	0.327[c]	0.411[c]
0.129	0.189	0.249	0.306	0.369[c]	0.610[c]
0.097	0.161	0.231	0.310	0.377	0.597
0.097	0.161	0.231	0.310	0.376	0.598

[c] These values are potentially unreliable in a statistical sense based on an insufficient sample size as indicated in statistical reporting standards (Life Sciences Research Office/ Federation of American Societies for Experimental Biology. 1995. *Third Report on Nutrition Monitoring in the United States*. Washington, DC: U.S. Government Printing Office). SOURCE: ENVIRON International Corporation, 2000.

TABLE G-6 Mean and Percentiles for Urinary Iodine (µg/dL), NHANES III (1988–1994)

Sex/Age Category[a]	n	Mean	SEM[b]	Percentile 5th	10th
Both sexes, 6 to 8 y	1,369	30.0	1.7	6.0	9.2
M 9 to 13 y	1,184	96.1	73.7	7.0	9.0
M 14 to 18 y	876	26.0	1.4	6.0	8.4
M 19 to 30 y	1,852	21.3	0.9	3.8	5.7
M 31 to 50 y	2,481	18.2	0.7	2.9	4.6
M 51 to 70 y	1,896	29.7	6.2	3.6	4.6
M 71+ y	1,181	33.0	4.1	4.4	5.8
F 9 to 13 y	1,146	23.3	1.0	4.6	7.0
F 14 to 18 y	897	26.9	2.8	4.4	6.2
F 19 to 30 y	1,860	31.9	13.4	2.9	4.6
F 31 to 50 y	2,886	18.8	1.6	2.1	2.9
F 51 to 70 y	2,009	23.5	1.8	2.4	3.3
F 71+ y	1,228	39.7	11.5	3.5	4.4
F Pregnant	343	19.6	1.1	4.3[c]	5.8
F Lactating	95	16.1[c]	2.2	2.5[c]	2.9[c]
F P/L	433	18.7	1.0	3.7[c]	5.4
All Individuals	20,865	27.6	2.7	3.0	4.5
All Indiv (+P/L)	21,298	27.5	2.7	3.0	4.5

NOTE: Means, standard errors, and percentiles calculated with WesVar Complex Samples 3.0. Females who had "blank but applicable" pregnancy and lactating status data or who responded "I don't know" to questions on pregnancy and lactating status were excluded from all analyses.

[a] M = male, F = female, P/L = pregnant and lactating.
[b] SEM = standard error of the mean.

25th	50th	75th	90th	95th	99th
15.1	25.5	36.9	53.3	64.0	103.3[c]
14.3	23.7	39.6	57.6	70.5	138.8[c]
12.5	21.0	30.2	44.6	58.9	117.8[c]
10.0	15.3	23.9	38.3	52.7	123.0[c]
8.3	13.8	21.6	34.4	45.7	92.3[c]
8.0	14.1	23.2	37.7	50.0	114.4[c]
9.5	15.5	27.1	43.8	68.0	193.8[c]
11.4	17.9	26.5	42.3	52.2	140.3[c]
10.5	17.2	27.5	49.0	66.6	188.4[c]
7.8	12.9	19.9	29.4	41.2	98.4[c]
5.5	11.1	19.0	31.9	41.3	94.8
5.8	11.0	19.0	31.2	44.4	151.8[c]
6.8	12.6	21.4	36.1	50.3	131.5[c]
9.2	14.0	25.2	39.7	44.8[c]	72.7[c]
8.1[c]	10.9[c]	22.4[c]	32.3[c]	36.8[c]	59.3[c]
9.1	13.1	24.0	38.3	44.7[c]	72.4[c]
8.1	14.5	23.8	38.6	52.5	115.0
8.1	14.5	23.8	38.6	52.1	113.4

[c] These values are potentially unreliable in a statistical sense based on an insufficient sample size as indicated in statistical reporting standards (Life Sciences Research Office/ Federation of American Societies for Experimental Biology. 1995. *Third Report on Nutrition Monitoring in the United States*. Washington, DC: U.S. Government Printing Office).
SOURCE: ENVIRON International Corporation, 2000.

H

Comparison of Vitamin A and Iron Intake and Biochemical Indicators from the Third National Health and Nutrition Examination Survey (NHANES III), 1988–1994

TABLE H-1 Mean Serum Retinol Concentrations (µg/dl) by Quartile of Dietary Vitamin A Intake of Individuals Who Were Not Taking Supplements, NHANES III (1988–1994)

Sex/Age Category[a]	n	Quartile			
		1st	2nd	3rd	4th
M 4–8 y	950	35.6	34.5	35.2	34.4
M 9–13 y	885	39.5	40.5	41.8	39.4
M 14–18 y	698	47.8	49.7	49.9	51.4
M 19–30 y	1,210	54.0	58.2	56.1	56.8
M 31–50 y	1,520	60.7	62.6	62.5	61.7
M 51–70 y	1,035	62.6	59.7	64.2	65.4
M 71+ y	490	62.7	61.7	62.9	62.2
M Total	6,788	54.5	55.8	55.9	55.9
F 4–8 y	926	34.8	34.1	35.3	34.6
F 9–13 y	851	38.9	40.6	38.9	40.9
F 14–18 y	624	42.2	42.0	45.5	46.4
F 19–30 y	833	45.0	44.3	47.3	47.8
F 31–50 y	1,583	47.2	46.9	48.7	48.7
F 51–70 y	871	56.8	56.4	57.7	59.2
F 71+ y	524	58.4	61.5	60.0	59.6
F Total	6,212	46.9	46.9	48.3	48.9

[a] M = male, F = female.
SOURCE: C. Ballew and C. Gillespie, Division of Nutrition and Physical Activity, Centers for Disease Control and Prevention, unpublished data.

692

TABLE H-2 Mean Serum Retinol Concentrations (μg/dl) by Quartile of Total Vitamin A Intake of Individuals Who Were Taking Supplements, NHANES III (1988–1994)

Sex/Age Category[a]	n	Quartile			
		1st	2nd	3rd	4th
M 4–8 y	401	—[b]	33.0	35.6	35.2
M 9–13 y	159	—	33.0	45.0	41.6
M 14–18 y	71	—	52.0	53.0	53.8
M 19–30 y	227	—	—	64.0	60.5
M 31–50 y	360	—	—	63.3	68.4
M 51–70 y	295	—	—	59.4	68.6
M 71+ y	151	—	—	66.2	64.4
M Total	1,664	—	45.9	54.3	59.4
F 4–8 y	380	—	32.0	34.3	35.7
F 9–13 y	185	—	—	34.2	40.8
F 14–18 y	85	—	—	—	46.5
F 19–30 y	202	—	—	41.0	49.5
F 31–50 y	519	35.0	44.0	48.4	51.9
F 51–70 y	271	—	—	53.6	60.4
F 71+ y	194	—	—	59.6	63.0
F Total	1,836	35.0	36.9	44.2	51.2

[a] M = male, F = female.

[b] No value could be computed, primarily due to an empty data cell or the absence of sampling strata representation.

SOURCE: C. Ballew and C. Gillespie, Division of Nutrition and Physical Activity, Centers for Disease Control and Prevention, unpublished data.

TABLE H-3 Weighted Median Serum Ferritin by Body Mass Index (BMI) Quartiles, Adult Reference Sample, NHANES III (1988–1994)

	Men		Women	
	20–49 y	50+ y	20–49 y	50+ y
BMI Quartile[a]	Median	Median	Median	Median
Non-Hispanic White				
Quartile 1	118	138	39	77
Quartile 2	132	156	38	89
Quartile 3	132	165	48	92
Quartile 4	168	172	50	101
Regression Results, BMI (adjusted for age)				
Beta	4.007	3.619	1.434	2.358
p	0.0001	0.007	0.014	0.0017
Non-Hispanic Black				
Quartile 1	129	207	38	125
Quartile 2	143	146	51	120
Quartile 3	166	206	47	124
Quartile 4	186	191	59	150
Regression Results, BMI (adjusted for age)				
Beta	2.786	1.885	0.917	0.58
p	0.0048	NS[b]	0.03	NS
Mexican American				
Quartile 1	90	111	30	90
Quartile 2	128	160	34	87
Quartile 3	137	169	40	93
Quartile 4	178	174	65	112
Regression Results, BMI (adjusted for age)				
Beta	6.852	−0.6788	3.192	1.372
p	0	NS	0	0.019

NOTE: Excludes individuals with C-reactive protein levels > 1 and values indicative of iron deficiency for transferrin saturation, erythrocyte protoporphyrin, and mean corpuscular volume.

[a] BMI quartiles were defined using race/ethnicity-, age-, and sex-specific cutoffs.

[b] NS = not significant.

TABLE H-4 Lower and Upper Quartiles of Plasma Glucose (mmol/L) and Median Serum Ferritin Levels (µg/L), NHANES III (1988–1994)

Sex/Age Category[a]	Lower Quartile of Plasma Glucose		Upper Quartile of Plasma Glucose	
	Median Plasma Glucose (mmol/L)	Median Serum Ferritin (µg/L)	Median Plasma Glucose (mmol/L)	Median Serum Ferritin (µg/L)
M 20 to 30 y	4.66	108.4	5.57	116.2
M 31 to 50 y	4.77	147.5	5.82	177.8
M 51 to 70 y	4.87	131.2	6.57	188.6
M 71+ y	4.95	122.8	6.72	149.4
F 20 to 30 y	4.41	33.0	5.23	37.3
F 31 to 50 y	4.55	36.4	5.62	44.8
F 51 to 70 y	4.74	73.6	6.19	119.5
F 71+ y	4.90	87.8	6.37	120.0
F P/L	4.17	21.6	5.00	22.0

NOTE: The plasma glucose values used for constructing the lower and upper quartile populations were estimated using WestVarPC 2.12. Median serum ferritin values and plasma glucose values also were estimated with WestVarPC 2.12. Plasma glucose values were measured for individuals 20 years and older. Only individuals who reported fasting 4 or more hours prior to the blood draw and individuals not taking insulin were included in the analyses. Population groups included only those individuals for whom complete food intakes were reported. Females who had "blank but applicable" pregnancy and lactating status data or who responded "I don't know" to questions on pregnancy and lactating status were excluded from all analyses.

[a] M = male, F = female, P/L = pregnant and lactating.

SOURCE: ENVIRON International Corporation, 1999.

TABLE H-5 Lower and Upper Quartiles of Iron Intake from Food (mg/d) and Median Levels of Serum Ferritin (µg/L): Individuals Who Do Not Report Intake of Iron Supplements, NHANES III (1988–1994)

Sex/Age Category[a]	Lower Quartile of Iron Intake		Upper Quartile of Iron Intake	
	Median of Estimated Usual Iron Intake from Food	Median of Observed Serum Ferritin Levels	Median of Estimated Usual Iron Intake from Food	Median of Observed Serum Ferritin Levels
Both sexes, 1 to 3 y	4.6	21.0	16.3	23.5
Both sexes, 4 to 8 y	9.4	29.0	16.9	30.0
M 9 to 13 y	10.4	35.0	21.6	33.0
M 14 to 18 y	12.8	48.0	26.9	50.0
M 19 to 30 y	13.2	111.0	23.6	105.0
M 31 to 50 y	12.6	168.0	24.4	163.0
M 51 to 70 y	10.0	160.0	23.6	148.0
M 71+ y	8.3	148.0	25.1	134.0
F 9 to 13 y	10.5	29.0	16.4	31.0
F 14 to 18 y	7.8	28.0	16.5	25.0
F 19 to 30 y	9.9	33.0	15.4	31.0
F 31 to 50 y	8.4	43.0	16.9	40.0
F 51 to 70 y	7.3	102.0	17.0	93.5
F 71+ y	7.4	107.5	16.9	87.0
F P/L	10.8	32.0	21.1	28.5
All Individuals	9.2	51.0	19.6	49.0
All Individuals (+P/L)	9.2	51.0	19.6	49.0

NOTE: The iron intakes used for constructing the lower and upper quartiles were estimated using the Iowa State University method. Computations of the medians were completed with the C-SIDE program. Children fed human milk and females who had "blank but applicable" pregnancy and lactating status data or who responded "I don't know" to questions on pregnancy and lactating status were excluded from all analyses.
[a] M = male, F = female, P/L = pregnant and lactating.
SOURCE: ENVIRON International Corporation and Iowa State University Department of Statistics, 1999.

I

Iron Intakes and Estimated Percentiles of the Distribution of Iron Requirements from the Continuing Survey of Food Intakes by Individuals (CSFII), 1994–1996

TABLE I-1 Iron Content of Foods Consumed by Infants 7 to 12 Months of Age, CSFII (1994–1996)

Foods	Iron Content (mg/ 100 kcal)	Absorption (%)	Amount of Iron[a]	Estimate of Iron Absorbed (mg)	Weighted Mean Absorption (%)[b]
Human breast milk[c]	0.04	50	0.18	0.09	0.65
Meat and poultry	1.2	20	0.36	0.07	0.52
Fruits	0.4	5	0.27	0.13	0.10
Vegetables	1.2	5	0.56	0.03	0.20
Cereals[d]	8.75	6	12.1	0.73	5.24
Noodles	0.6	5	0.38	0.02	0.14
Total			13.85	1.07	6.85

[a] Based on a total daily energy intake of 845 kcal (Fomon SJ, Anderson TA. 1974. *Infant Nutrition*, 2nd ed. Philadelphia: WB Saunders. Pp. 104–111).

[b] Calculation based on the proportion of iron in each of the six food groups.

[c] Assumes an intake of 670 ml/day.

[d] Refers to iron-fortified infant cereals containing 35 mg iron/100 g of dry cereal.

TABLE I-2 Contribution of Iron from the 14 Food Groups for Children Aged 1 to 3 and 4 to 8 Years, CSFII (1994–1996)

Food Group	Iron Content (mg/100 kcal)[a]	Amount of Iron (mg), 1–3 y[b]	Amount of Iron (mg), 4–8 y[c]
Meat	1.19	1.57	2.17
Fruits	0.36	0.23	0.25
Vegetables	1.22	1.14	1.87
Cereals	2.65	8.64	11.98
Vegetables plus meat	0.7	0.17	0.18
Grain plus meat	0.78	1.12	1.53
Cheese	0.15	0.04	0.05
Eggs	0.9	0.22	0.19
Ice cream, yogurt, etc.	0.13	0.06	0.01
Fats, candy	0.05	0.03	0.05
Milk	0.08	0.18	0.15
Formula	1.8	0.18	0.00
Juices	0.44	0.34	0.22
Other beverages	0.11	0.07	0.12
Total		14.27	18.77

[a] Source: Whitney EN, Rolfes SR. 1996. *Understanding Nutrition,* 7th ed. St. Paul: West Publishing; Pennington JAT. 1998. *Bowes and Church's Food Values of Portions Commonly Used,* 17th ed. Philadelphia: Lippincott.

[b] The CSFII database provides total food energy (average of 2 days) and the proportion of energy from each of 14 food groups. The iron content of each food was determined from appropriate references (expressed as iron content per 100 kcal), thus the iron content of each food was calculated. The results are based on a total daily energy intake of 1,345 kcal (n = 1,868) as reported in CSFII.

[c] Calculated as shown above. Based on a total daily energy intake of 1,665 kcal (n = 1,711) as reported in CSFII. According to the Third National Health and Nutrition Examination Survey, the median intake of iron by infants is 15.5 mg/day; the iron mainly comes from fortified formulas and cereals, with smaller amounts from vegetables, pureed meats and poultry. It is estimated that the absorption of iron from fortified cereals is in the range of 6 percent, from breast milk 50 percent, and from meat, 20 percent.

TABLE I-3 Estimated Percentiles of the Distribution of Iron Requirements (mg/d) in Young Children and Adolescent and Adult Males, CSFII (1994–1996)

Estimated Percentiles of Requirements	Young Children, Both Sexes[a]			Male Adolescents and Adults		
	0.5–1 y[b]	1–3 y[c]	4–8 y[c]	9–13 y[c]	14–18 y[c]	Adult[c]
2.5	3.01	1.01	1.33	3.91	5.06	3.98
5	3.63	1.24	1.64	4.23	5.42	4.29
10	4.35	1.54	2.05	4.59	5.85	4.64
20	5.23	1.96	2.63	5.03	6.43	5.09
30	5.87	2.32	3.13	5.36	6.89	5.44
40	6.39	2.66	3.62	5.64	7.29	5.74
50[d]	6.90	3.01	4.11	5.89	7.69	6.03
60	7.41	3.39	4.65	6.15	8.08	6.32
70	7.93	3.82	5.27	6.43	8.51	6.65
80	8.57	4.39	6.08	6.76	9.03	7.04
90	9.44	5.26	7.31	7.21	9.74	7.69
95	10.15	6.06	8.45	7.58	10.32	8.06
97.5[e]	10.78	6.81	9.52	7.91	10.83	8.49

[a] Based on pooled estimates of requirement components (see Table 9-6); presented Estimated Average Requirement (EAR) and Recommended Dietary Allowance (RDA) based on the higher estimates obtained for males.
[b] Based on 10 percent bioavailability.
[c] Based on 18 percent bioavailability.
[d] Fiftieth percentile = EAR.
[e] Ninety-seven and one-half percentile = RDA.

TABLE I-4 Estimated Percentiles of the Distribution of Iron Requirements (mg/d) for Female Adolescents and Adults, CSFII (1994–1996)

	Group							
Estimated Percentile of Requirement	9–13 y	14–18 y	Oral Contraceptive User,[a] Adolescent	Mixed Adolescent Population[b]	Menstruating Adult	Oral Contraceptive User,[a] Adult	Mixed Adult Population[b]	Post Menopause
2.5	3.24	4.63	4.11	4.49	4.42	3.63	4.18	2.73
5	3.60	5.06	4.49	4.92	4.88	4.00	4.63	3.04
10	4.04	5.61	4.97	5.45	5.45	4.45	5.19	3.43
20	4.59	6.31	5.57	6.14	6.22	5.06	5.94	3.93
30	4.98	6.87	6.05	6.69	6.87	5.52	6.55	4.30
40	5.33	7.39	6.48	7.21	7.46	5.94	7.13	4.64
50[c]	5.66	7.91	6.89	7.71	8.07	6.35	7.73	4.97
60	6.00	8.43	7.34	8.25	8.76	6.79	8.39	5.30
70	6.36	9.15	7.84	8.92	9.63	7.27	9.21	5.68
80	6.78	10.03	8.47	9.77	10.82	7.91	10.36	6.14
90	7.38	11.54	9.47	11.21	13.05	8.91	12.49	6.80
95	7.88	13.08	10.42	12.74	15.49	9.90	14.85	7.36
97.5[d]	8.34	14.80	11.44	14.39	18.23	10.94	17.51	7.88

[a] Based on 60 percent reduction in menstrual blood loss.
[b] Mixed population assumes 17 percent oral contraceptive users, 83 percent nonusers, all menstruating.
[c] Fiftieth percentile = Estimated Average Requirement.
[d] Ninety-seven and one-half percentile = Recommended Dietary Allowance.

TABLE I-5 Probabilities of Inadequate Iron Intakes[a] and Associated Ranges of Usual Intake for Infants and Children 1 through 8 Years, CSFII (1994–1996)

Probability of Inadequacy	Associated Range of Usual Intakes (mg/d)		
	Infants 8–12 mo	Children 1–3 y	Children 4–8 y
1.0[b]	< 3.01	< 1.0	< 1.33
0.96	3.02–3.63	1.1–1.24	1.34–1.64
0.93	3.64–4.35	1.25–1.54	1.65–2.05
0.85	4.36–5.23	1.55–1.96	2.07–2.63
0.75	5.24–5.87	1.97–2.32	2.64–3.13
0.65	5.88–6.39	2.33–2.66	3.14–3.62
0.55	6.40–6.90	2.67–3.01	3.63–4.11
0.45	6.91–7.41	3.02–3.39	4.12–4.64
0.35	7.42–7.93	3.40–3.82	4.65–5.27
0.25	7.94–8.57	3.83–4.38	5.28–6.08
0.15	8.58–9.44	4.39–5.25	6.09–7.31
0.08	9.45–10.17	5.26–6.06	7.32–8.45
0.04	10.18–10.78	6.07–6.81	8.46–9.52
0[b]	> 10.78	> 6.81	> 9.52

[a] Probability of inadequate intake = probability that requirement is greater than the usual intake. Derived from Table I-3.

[b] For population assessment purposes, a probability of 1 has been assigned to all usual intakes falling below the two and one-half percentile of requirement and a probability of 0 has been assigned to all usual intakes falling above the ninety-seven and one-half percentile of requirement. This enables the assessment of population risk where precise estimates are impractical and effectively without impact.

TABLE I-6 Probabilities of Inadequate Iron Intakes[a] (mg/d) and Associated Ranges of Usual Intake in Adolescent Males and in Girls Using or Not Using Oral Contraceptives (OC), CSFII (1994–1996)

Probability of Inadequacy	9–13 y		14–18 y			
	Male	Female	Male	Female		
				Non-OC Users	OC Users[b]	Mixed Population[c]
1.0[d]	< 3.91	< 3.24	< 5.06	< 4.63	< 4.11	< 4.49
0.96	3.91–4.23	3.24–3.60	5.06–5.42	4.64–5.06	4.11–4.49	4.49–4.92
0.93	4.24–4.59	3.61–4.04	5.43–5.85	5.07–5.61	4.50–4.97	4.93–5.45
0.85	4.60–5.03	4.05–4.59	5.86–6.43	5.62–6.31	4.98–5.57	5.46–6.14
0.75	5.04–5.36	4.60–4.98	6.44–6.89	6.32–6.87	5.58–6.05	6.15–6.69
0.65	5.37–5.64	4.99–5.33	6.90–7.29	6.88–7.39	6.06–6.48	6.70–7.21
0.55	5.65–5.89	5.34–5.66	7.30–7.69	7.40–7.91	6.49–6.89	7.22–7.71
0.45	5.90–6.15	5.67–6.00	7.70–8.08	7.92–8.48	6.90–7.34	7.72–8.25
0.35	6.16–6.43	6.01–6.36	8.09–8.51	8.49–9.15	7.35–7.84	8.26–8.92
0.25	6.44–6.76	6.37–6.78	8.52–9.03	9.16–10.03	7.85–8.47	8.93–9.77
0.15	6.77–7.21	6.79–7.38	9.04–9.74	10.04–11.54	8.48–9.47	9.78–11.21
0.08	7.22–7.58	7.39–7.88	9.75–10.32	11.55–13.08	9.48–10.42	11.22–12.74
0.04	7.59–7.91	7.89–8.34	10.33–10.83	13.09–14.80	10.43–11.44	12.75–14.39
0[d]	> 7.91	> 8.34	> 10.83	> 14.80	> 11.44	> 14.39

[a] Probability of inadequate intake = probability that requirement is greater than the usual intake. May be used in simple computer programs to evaluate adjusted distributions of usual intakes. See Institute of Medicine. 2000. *Dietary Reference Intakes: Applications in Dietary Assessment.* Washington, DC: National Academy Press, for method of adjusting observed intake distributions. Not to be applied in the assessment of individuals. Derived from Tables I-3 and I-4.

[b] Assumes 60 percent reduction in menstrual iron loss.

[c] Mixed population represents 17 percent oral contraceptive users and 83 percent nonoral contraceptive users (Abma JC, Chandra A, Mosher WD, Peterson LS, Piccinino LJ. 1997. Fertility, family planning, and women's health: New data from the 1995 National Survey of Family Growth. *Vital Health Stat* 23:1–114).

[d] For population assessment purposes, a probability of 1 has been assigned to all usual intakes falling below the two and one-half percentile of requirement and a probability of 0 has been assigned to all usual intakes falling above the ninety-seven and one-half percentile of requirement. This enables the assessment of population risk where precise estimates are impractical and effectively without impact.

TABLE I-7 Probabilities of Inadequate Iron Intakes[a] (mg/d) and Associated Ranges of Usual Intake in Adult Men and Women Using and Not Using Oral Contraceptives (OC), CSFII (1994–1996)

Probability of Inadequacy	Adult Men	Menstruating Women			Postmenopausal Women
		Non-OC Users	OC Users[b]	Mixed Population[c]	
1.0[d]	< 3.98	< 4.42	< 3.63	< 4.18	< 2.73
0.96	3.98–4.29	4.42–4.88	3.63–4.00	4.18–4.63	2.73–3.04
0.93	4.30–4.64	4.89–5.45	4.01–4.45	4.64–5.19	3.05–3.43
0.85	4.65–5.09	5.46–6.22	4.46–5.06	5.20–5.94	3.44–3.93
0.75	5.10–5.44	6.23–6.87	5.07–5.52	5.95–6.55	3.94–4.30
0.65	5.45–5.74	6.88–7.46	5.53–5.94	6.56–7.13	4.31–4.64
0.55	5.75–6.03	7.47–8.07	5.95–6.35	7.14–7.73	4.65–4.97
0.45	6.04–6.32	8.08–8.76	6.36–6.79	7.74–8.39	4.98–5.30
0.35	6.33–6.65	8.77–9.63	6.80–7.27	8.40–9.21	5.31–5.68
0.25	6.66–7.04	9.64–10.82	7.28–7.91	9.22–10.36	5.69–6.14
0.15	7.05–7.69	10.83–13.05	7.92–8.91	10.37–12.49	6.15–6.80
0.08	7.70–8.06	13.06–15.49	8.92–9.90	12.50–14.85	6.81–7.36
0.04	8.07–8.49	15.50–18.23	9.91–10.94	14.86–17.51	7.37–7.88
0[d]	> 8.49	> 18.23	> 10.94	> 17.51	> 7.88

[a] Probability of inadequate intake = probability that requirement is greater than the usual intake. May be used in simple computer programs to evaluate adjusted distributions of usual intakes. See Institute of Medicine. 2000. *Dietary Reference Intakes: Applications in Dietary Assessment*. Washington, DC: National Academy Press, for method of adjusting observed intake distributions. Not to be applied in the assessment of individuals. Derived from Tables I-3 and I-4.

[b] Assumes 60 percent reduction in menstrual iron loss.

[c] Mixed population represents 17 percent oral contraceptive users and 83 percent nonoral contraceptive users (Abma JC, Chandra A, Mosher WD, Peterson LS, Piccinino LJ. 1997. Fertility, family planning, and women's health: New data from the 1995 National Survey of Family Growth. *Vital Health Stat* 23:1–114).

[d] For population assessment purposes, a probability of 1 has been assigned to all usual intakes falling below the two and one-half percentile of requirement and a probability of 0 has been assigned to all usual intakes falling above the ninety-seven and one-half percentile of requirement. This enables the assessment of population risk where precise estimates are impractical and effectively without impact.

J
Glossary and Acronyms

AAP	American Academy of Pediatrics
Action	Demonstrated effects in various biological systems that may or may not have physiological significance
Adverse effect	Any significant alteration in the structure or function of the human organism or any impairment of a physiologically important function that could lead to a health effect that is adverse
AI	Adequate Intake
AITD	Autoimmune thyroid disease
Association	Potential interactions derived from studies (e.g., epidemiological) of the relationship between specific nutrients and specific diseases
ASTDR	Agency for Toxic Substance and Diet Registry
Bioavailability	Accessibility of a nutrient to participate in unspecified metabolic and/or physiological processes
BMI	Body mass index: weight (kg)/height (cm)^2
CHD	Coronary heart disease
Cr	Elemental symbol for chromium

CRBP	Cellular retinol binding protein
CSFII	Continuing Survey of Food Intakes by Individuals; a survey conducted periodically by the Agricultural Research Service, U.S. Department of Agriculture
CV	Coefficient of variation: mean ÷ standard deviation
CVD	Cardiovascular disease
DNA	Deoxyribonucleic acid
Dose-response assessment	Second step in a risk assessment, in which the relationship between nutrient intake and an adverse effect (in terms of incidence or severity of the effect) is determined
DRI	Dietary Reference Intake
EAR	Estimated Average Requirement
EPA	U.S. Environmental Protection Agency
Erythrocyte	Red blood cell
FAO	Food and Agriculture Organization of the United Nations
FASEB	Federation of American Societies for Experimental Biology
FDA	Food and Drug Administration
Fe	Elemental symbol for iron
FNB	Food and Nutrition Board
Function	Role played by a nutrient in growth, development, and maturation
Gravid	Pregnant
Hazard identification	First step in a risk assessment, which is concerned with the collection, organization, and evaluation of all information pertaining to the toxic properties of a nutrient
HIV	Human immunodeficiency virus
HRT	Hormone replacement therapy

IAEA	International Atomic Energy Agency
IARC	International Agency for Research on Cancer
ICC	Indian childhood cirrhosis
ICCIDD	International Council for the Control of Iodine Deficiency Disorders
ICT	Idiopathic copper toxicosis
IM	Intramuscular
IOM	Institute of Medicine
IPCS	International Programme on Chemical Safety
IR	Insulin receptor
IRE	Iron response element
IRP	Iron response proteins
IU	International units
Lacto-ovo-vegetarian	Person who consumes milk (lacto), eggs (ovo), and plant foods and products, but no meat or fish
LDL	Low density lipoprotein
LMWCr	Low molecular weight chromium-binding substance
LOAEL	Lowest-observed-adverse-effect level: lowest intake (or experimental dose) of a nutrient at which an adverse effect has been identified
LSRO	Life Sciences Research Office
MCH	Mean corpuscular hemoglobin—the amount of hemoglobin in erythrocytes (red blood cells)
MCV	Mean corpuscular volume—the volume of the average erythrocyte
MI	Myocardial infarction
Mn	Elemental symbol for manganese
MnSOD	Manganese superoxide dismutase
MTF1	Metal response element transcription factor

NADH	Nicotinamide adenine dinuleotide hydride; a coenzyme
NHANES	National Health and Nutrition Examination Survey; a survey conducted periodically by the National Center for Health Statistics of the Centers for Disease Control and Prevention
NOAEL	No-observed-adverse-effect level; highest intake (or experimental dose) of a nutrient at which no adverse effect has been observed
NRC	National Research Council
OTA	Office of Technology Assessment
Phylloquinone	Plant form of vitamin K and a major form of this vitamin in the human diet
Provitamin A carotenoids	α-Carotene, β-carotenc, and β-cryptoxanthin
RAR	Retinoic acid receptor
RDA	Recommended Dietary Allowance
RE	Retinol equivalents
Risk assessment	Organized framework for evaluating scientific information, which has as its objective a characterization of the nature and likelihood of harm resulting from excess human exposure to an environmental agent (in this case, a nutrient); it includes the development of both qualitative and quantitative expressions of risk
Risk characterization	Final step in a risk assessment, which summarizes the conclusions from steps 1 through 3 of the risk assessment (hazard identification, dose response, and estimates of exposure) and evaluates the risk; this step also includes a characterization of the degree of scientific confidence that can be placed in the Tolerable Upper Intake Level
Risk management	Process by which risk assessment results are integrated with other information to make decisions about the need for, method of, and extent of risk reduction; in addition, risk management

considers such issues as the public health significance of the risk, the technical feasibility of
achieving various degrees of risk control, and
the economic and social costs of this control

RNA	Ribonucleic acid
RNI	Recommended Nutrient Intake
RXR	Retinoid X receptor
SD	Standard deviation
SE	Standard error
SEM	Standard error of the mean
SOD	Superoxide dismutase
sTfR	Soluble transferrin receptor
TDS	Total Diet Study; a study conducted by the Food and Drug Administration
TfR	Transferrin receptor
Tg	Thyroglobulin
Thyrotropin	Glycoprotein hormone that regulates thyroid function
TIBC	Total iron binding capacity
TPN	Total parenteral nutrition
TRH	Thyrotropin-releasing hormone
TSH	Thyroid stimulating hormone, also known as thyrotropin
UF	Uncertainty factor; number by which the NOAEL (or LOAEL) is divided to obtain the Tolerable Upper Intake Level (UL); the size of the UF varies depending on the confidence in the data and the nature of the adverse effect
UL	Tolerable Upper Intake Level
USDA	U.S. Department of Agriculture
VLDL	Very low density lipoprotein
WHO	World Health Organization

K

Conversion of Units

Nutrient	Système Internationale d'Unités (mole)	Conventional Unit (g)
Vitamin A (retinol)	1	286.5
Vitamin K	1	450.7
Arsenic	1	74.92
Boron	1	10.82
Chromium	1	52
Copper	1	63.54
Iodine	1	126.9
Iron	1	55.85
Manganese	1	54.94
Molybdenum	1	95.94
Nickel	1	58.71
Silicon	1	28.09
Vanadium	1	50.9
Zinc	1	65.4

L

Options for Dealing with Uncertainties

Methods for dealing with uncertainties in scientific data are generally understood by working scientists and require no special discussion here except to point out that such uncertainties should be explicitly acknowledged and taken into account whenever a risk assessment is undertaken. More subtle and difficult problems are created by uncertainties associated with some of the inferences that must be made in the absence of directly applicable data; much confusion and inconsistency can result if they are not recognized and dealt with in advance of undertaking a risk assessment.

The most significant inference uncertainties arise in risk assessments whenever attempts are made to answer the following questions (NRC, 1994):

- What set or sets of hazard and dose-response data (for a given substance) should be used to characterize risk in the population of interest?
- If animal data are to be used for risk characterization, which endpoints for adverse effects should be considered?
- If animal data are to be used for risk characterization, what measure of dose (e.g., dose per unit body weight, body surface, or dietary intake) should be used for scaling between animals and humans?
- What is the expected variability in dose-response between animals and humans?
- If human data are to be used for risk characterization, which adverse effects should be used?

710

• What is the expected variability in dose-response among members of the human population?

• How should data from subchronic exposure studies be used to estimate chronic effects?

• How should problems of differences in route of exposure within and between species be dealt with?

• How should the threshold dose be estimated for the human population?

• If a threshold in the dose-response relationship seems unlikely, how should a low-dose risk be modeled?

• What model should be chosen to represent the distribution of exposures in the population of interest when data relating to exposures are limited?

• When interspecies extrapolations are required, what should be assumed about relative rates of absorption from the gastrointestinal tract of animals and of humans?

• For which percentiles on the distribution of population exposures should risks be characterized?

At least partial, empirically based answers to some of these questions may be available for some of the nutrients under review, but in no case is scientific information likely to be sufficient to provide a highly certain answer; in many cases there will be no relevant data for the nutrient in question.

It should be recognized that for several of these questions, certain inferences have been widespread for long periods of time; thus, it may seem unnecessary to raise these uncertainties anew. When several sets of animal toxicology data are available, for example, and data are not sufficient for identifying the set (i.e., species, strain, and adverse effects endpoint) that best predicts human response, it has become traditional to select that set in which toxic responses occur at lowest dose (the most sensitive set). In the absence of definitive empirical data applicable to a specific case, it is generally assumed that there will not be more than a ten-fold variation in response among members of the human population. In the absence of absorption data, it is generally assumed that humans will absorb the chemical at the same rate as the animal species used to model human risk. In the absence of complete understanding of biological mechanisms, it is generally assumed that, except possibly for certain carcinogens, a threshold dose must be exceeded before toxicity is expressed. These types of long-standing assumptions, which are necessary to complete a risk assessment, are recognized by risk assessors as attempts to deal with uncertainties in knowledge (NRC, 1994).

A past National Research Council (NRC) report (1983) recommended adoption of the concepts and definitions that have been discussed in this report. The NRC committee recognized that throughout a risk assessment, data and basic knowledge will be lacking and risk assessors will be faced with several scientifically plausible options (called inference options by the NRC) for dealing with questions such as those presented above. For example, several scientifically supportable options for dose scaling across species and for high- to low-dose extrapolation will exist, but there will be no ready means to identify those that are clearly best supported. The NRC committee recommended that regulatory agencies in the United States identify the needed inference options in risk assessment and specify, through written risk assessment guidelines, the specific options that will be used for all assessments. Agencies in the United States have identified the specific models to be used to fill gaps in data and knowledge; these have come to be called *default options* (EPA, 1986).

The use of defaults to fill knowledge and data gaps in risk assessment has the advantage of ensuring consistency in approach (the same defaults are used for each assessment) and minimizing or eliminating case-by-case manipulations of the conduct of risk assessment to meet predetermined risk management objectives. The major disadvantage of the use of defaults is the potential for displacement of scientific judgment by excessively rigid guidelines. A remedy for this disadvantage was also suggested by the NRC committee: risk assessors should be allowed to replace defaults with alternative factors in specific cases of chemicals for which relevant scientific data are available to support alternatives. The risk assessors' obligation in such cases is to provide explicit justification for any such departure. Guidelines for risk assessment issued by the U.S. Environmental Protection Agency (EPA, 1986), for example, specifically allow for such departures.

The use of preselected defaults is not the only way to deal with model uncertainties. Another option is to allow risk assessors complete freedom to pursue whatever approaches they judge applicable in specific cases. Because many of the uncertainties cannot be resolved scientifically, case-by-case judgments without some guidance on how to deal with them will lead to difficulties in achieving scientific consensus, and the results of the assessment may not be credible.

Another option for dealing with uncertainties is to allow risk assessors to develop a range of estimates based on application of both defaults and alternative inferences that, in specific cases, have some degree of scientific support. Indeed, appropriate analysis of uncertainties seems to require such a presentation of risk results. Although presenting a number of plausible risk estimates has the advantage that it would seem to more faithfully reflect the true state of scientific understanding, there are no well-established criteria for using such complex results in risk management.

The various approaches to dealing with uncertainties inherent in risk assessment are summarized in Table L-1.

As can be seen in the nutrient chapters, specific default assumptions for assessing nutrient risks have not been recommended. Rather, the approach calls for case-by-case judgments, with the recommendation that the basis for the choices made be explicitly stated. Some general guidelines for making these choices are, however, offered.

TABLE L-1 Approaches for Dealing with Uncertainties in a Risk Assessment Program

Program Model	Advantages	Disadvantages
Case-by-case judgments by experts	Flexibility; high potential to maximize use of most relevant scientific information bearing on specific issues	Potential for inconsistent treatment of different issues; difficulty in achieving consensus; need to agree on defaults
Written guidelines specifying defaults for data and model uncertainties (with allowance for departures in specific cases)	Consistent treatment of different issues; maximization of transparency of process; resolution of scientific disagreements possible by resort to defaults	Possible difficulty in justifying departure or achieving consensus among scientists that departures are justified in specific cases; danger that uncertainties will be overlooked
Presentation of full array of estimates from all scientifically plausible models by assessors	Maximization of use of scientific information; reasonably reliable portrayal of true state of scientific understanding	Highly complex characterization of risk, with no easy way to discriminate among estimates; size of required effort may not be commensurate with utility of the outcome

REFERENCES

EPA (US Environmental Protection Agency). 1986. Proposed guidelines for carcinogen risk assessment; Notice. *Fed Regis* 61:17960–18011.

NRC (National Research Council). 1983. *Risk Assessment in the Federal Government: Managing the Process.* Washington, DC: National Academy Press.

NRC. 1994. *Science and Judgment in Risk Assessment.* Washington, DC: National Academy Press.

M
Biographical Sketches of Panel and Subcommittee Members

LENORE ARAB, Ph.D., is a professor of epidemiology and nutrition in the Departments of Epidemiology and Nutrition at the University of North Carolina at Chapel Hill, Schools of Medicine and Public Health. Dr. Arab's main research interests are anticarcinogens in foods, heterocyclic amines, breast cancer incidence and survival, the relationship of diet to athersclerosis, antioxidant nutrients in various diseases, iron nutriture, and multi-media approaches to dietary assessment. She has published over 140 original papers as well as numerous book chapters and monographs. Dr. Arab serves as a nutrition advisor to the World Health Organization (WHO) and is the founding director of the WHO Collaborating Center for Nutritional Epidemiology in Berlin. She is the North American editor of the journal *Public Health Nutrition* and sits on the editorial boards of the *European Journal of Clinical Nutrition, Journal of Clinical Epidemiology, Nutrition in Clinical Care,* and *Nutrition and Cancer: An International Journal.* She is the program director for nutritional epidemiology and leader of a training program and National Cancer Institute-sponsored training grant in that field. Dr. Arab received her M.Sc. from Harvard School of Public Health and her Ph.D. in nutrition from Justus Liebig University in Giessen, Germany.

SUSAN I. BARR, Ph.D., is a professor of nutrition at the University of British Columbia. She received a Ph.D. in human nutrition from the University of Minnesota and is a registered dietitian in Canada. Her research interests focus on the associations among nutrition, physical activity and bone health in women, and she has authored

Biology and the American Society for Nutritional Sciences, was an associate editor of the *Journal of Nutrition,* and is an associate editor of *Annual Review of Nutrition.* He has been a member of the Food and Nutrition Board since 1997, and the Standing Committee on the Scientific Evaluation of Dietary Reference Intakes since 1999. Dr. Cousins was elected to the National Academy of Sciences in 2000.

BARBARA L. DEVANEY, Ph.D., is a senior fellow at Mathematica Policy Research Inc. where she has specialized in designing and conducting program evaluations. She recently completed a study that produced a comprehensive and rigorous evaluation design for evaluating the impacts of a Universal-Free School Breakfast Program on dietary and educational outcomes of children. She currently is completing an evaluation of the effects of an infant mortality demonstration program, Healthy Start, and is involved in a study examining the impacts on health care utilization and costs of child participation in the Special Supplemental Nutrition Program for Women, Infants, and Children (WIC). She also is a co-investigator of a large national evaluation of abstinence education programs funded under the welfare reform legislation. Dr. Devaney was a member of the Institute of Medicine's Committee on Scientific Evaluation of WIC Nutrition Risk Criteria. She received her Ph.D. in economics from the University of Michigan.

JOHN T. DUNN, M.D., is a professor of internal medicine at the University of Virginia School of Medicine. He holds an M.D. from Duke University. Dr. Dunn's research interests include thyroid disease (goiter and cancer), iodine deficiency, and metabolism. Dr. Dunn is a member of the International Council for the Control of Iodine Deficiency Disorders. He has worked on various research and applied projects aimed at reducing iodine deficiency disorders in the developing world.

JOHANNA T. DWYER, D.Sc., R.D., is director of the Frances Stern Nutrition Center at New England Medical Center and professor in the Departments of Medicine and of Community Health at the Tufts Medical School and School of Nutrition Science and Policy in Boston. She is also senior scientist at the Jean Mayer U.S. Department of Agriculture Human Nutrition Research Center on Aging at Tufts University. Dr. Dwyer's work centers on life-cycle related concerns such as the prevention of diet-related disease in children and adolescents and maximization of quality of life and health in the elderly.

She also has a long-standing interest in vegetarian and other alternative lifestyles. Dr. Dwyer is currently the editor of *Nutrition Today* and on the editorial boards of *Family Economics* and *Nutrition Reviews*. She received her D.Sc. and M.Sc. from the Harvard School of Public Health, an M.S. from the University of Wisconsin, and completed her undergraduate degree with distinction from Cornell University. She is a member of the Food and Nutrition Board and the Standing Committee on the Scientific Evaluation of Dietary Reference Intakes, the Technical Advisory Committee of the Nutrition Screening Initiative, and past president of the American Society for Nutrition Sciences, past secretary of the American Society for Clinical Nutrition, and a past president of the Society for Nutrition Education.

GUYLAINE FERLAND, Ph.D., is associate professor of nutrition at the University of Montreal and director of Clinical Research at L'Institut Universitaire de Gériatrie de Montréal. She earned her B.Sc. from McGill University and received her M.Sc. and Ph.D. from the University of Montreal. Dr. Ferland did her postdoctoral research in human vitamin K metabolism at Tufts University and now heads a research program in vitamin K metabolism at the University of Montreal. Dr. Ferland served on the scientific consultative council for the Canadian National Institute of Nutrition and is a member of the External Advisory Panel, Government Working Group for the Review of Policies Concerning the Addition of Vitamins and Minerals to Foods.

JEAN-PIERRE HABICHT, M.D., Ph.D., is professor of nutritional epidemiology in the Division of Nutrition Sciences at Cornell University. His professional experience includes serving as special assistant to the director of the Division of Health Examination Statistics at the National Center for Health Statistics, World Health Organization (WHO) medical officer at the Instituto de Nutricion de Centro America y Panama, and professor of maternal and child health at the University of San Carlos in Guatemala. Currently, Dr. Habicht serves as an advisor to United Nations (UN) and government health and nutrition agencies. He is a member of the Expert Advisory Panel on Nutrition, WHO, and is past chairman of the UN Advisory Group on Nutrition. He has consulted to the UN's World Food Program and is involved in research with the UN High Commission for Refugees about the adequacy of food rations in refugee camps. Dr. Habicht has served on numerous Institute of Medicine Committees advising the U.S. Agency for International Development about issues in international nutrition. He served as a member of the Food and Nutrition Board (1981–1984) and as a member and past chair of the Committee on International Nutrition Programs. Dr. Habicht chaired the National Research Council's Coordinating Committee on Evaluation of Food Consumption Surveys, which produced the 1986 report, *Nutrient Adequacy: Assessment Using Food Consumption Surveys.*

K. MICHAEL HAMBIDGE, M.D., F.C.R.P., is professor emeritus of pediatrics and preventive medicine at the University of Colorado Medical Center. He received his B.A. and M.D. from Cambridge University. Dr. Hambidge has published numerous research articles on zinc metabolism and requirements during pregnancy and infancy. He received the American Institute of Nutrition Borden Award and the American Academy of Pediatrics Nutrition Award. He is a former member of the Food and Nutrition Board and served as liaison to the Committee on Scientific Evaluation of WIC Nutrition Risk Criteria.

RENATE D. KIMBROUGH, M.D., presently works as an independent consultant. From 1991 to 1999 she served as senior medical associate at the Institute for Evaluating Health Risks (IEHR). She earned her M.D. from the University of Goettingen in Germany. At IEHR, Dr. Kimbrough conducted several studies and consulted on a variety of matters involving environmental contamination and human health effects. Dr. Kimbrough has served previously as the Director for Health and Risk Capabilities and as Advisor on Medical Toxicology and Risk Evaluation for the U.S. Environmental Protection Agency's Office of the Administrator and as medical toxicologist for the Centers for Disease Control and Prevention. She has over 130 scientific publications in the fields of toxicology and risk assessment. Dr. Kimbrough is certified as a diplomate for the American Board of Toxicology and an honorary fellow of the American Academy of Pediatrics. In 1991, she received the American Conference on Governmental Industrial Hygienists' Herbert E. Stokinger Award for outstanding achievement in industrial toxicology. She also has served on the Scientific Advisory Board, United States Air Force, and the American Board of Toxicology.

HARRIET V. KUHNLEIN, Ph.D., R.D., is professor of human nutrition at McGill University and founding director of the Centre for Indigenous Peoples' Nutrition and Environment. She is a registered dietitian in Canada, and holds a Ph.D. in nutritional sciences from the University of California at Berkeley. The focus of Dr. Kuhnlein's research is on the nutrition, food patterns, and environment of indigenous peoples. Specifically, her work examines the traditional foods of indigenous peoples, nutrient and contaminant levels in indigenous food systems, and nutrition promotion programs for indigenous peoples. She has published numerous articles on these subjects. Dr. Kuhnlein is a member of both the American and Canadian Societies of Nutritional Sciences, the Society for International Nutrition Research, the Canadian Dietetic Association, and the Society for Nutrition Education. She serves on the Advisory Council of the Herb Research Foundation, and is a former co-chair of the committee on Nutrition and Anthropology of the International Union of Nutritional Sciences. Dr. Kuhnlein is a member of the editorial boards of *Ecology of Food and Nutrition, Journal of Food Composition and Analysis, International Journal of Circumpolar Health,* and *Journal of Ethnobiology.*

SEAN LYNCH, M.D., is a professor of medicine at the Eastern Virginia Medical School. Dr. Lynch received his M.D. from the University of Witwatersrand, South Africa. He has published numerous reviews and research articles in the area of iron metabolism, anemia, and iron overload. Dr. Lynch is a consultant to the International Nutritional Anemia Consultative Group.

RITA B. MESSING, Ph.D., received her Ph.D. in physiological psychology from Princeton University and did postdoctoral research in the Department of Nutrition and Food Science at Massachusetts Institute of Technology in the Laboratory of Neuroendocrine Regulation. Dr. Messing has been in the Department of Pharmacology, University of Minnesota Medical School since 1981, and is currently an associate professor. Since 1990 her primary employment has been at the Minnesota Department of Health in Environmental Toxicology, where she supervises the Site Assessment and Consultation Unit, which conducts public health activities at hazardous waste sites and other sources of uncontrolled toxic releases. Dr. Messing has 70 publications in toxicology and risk assessment, neuropharmacology, psychobiology, and experimental psychology. She has taught at Rutgers University, Northeastern University, University of California at Irvine, and University of Minnesota, and has had visiting appointments at Organon Pharmaceuticals in the Netherlands and the University of Paris.

SANFORD A. MILLER, Ph.D., is dean of the Graduate School of Biomedical Sciences and professor in the Departments of Biochemistry and Medicine at The University of Texas Health Science Center at San Antonio. He is the former director of the Center for Food Safety and Applied Nutrition at the Food and Drug Administration. Previously, he was professor of nutritional biochemistry at the Massachusetts Institute of Technology. Dr. Miller has served on many national and international government and professional society advisory committees, including the Federation of American Societies for Experimental Biology Expert Committee on GRAS Substances, the National Advisory Environmental Health Sciences Council of the National Institutes of Health, the Food and Nutrition Board and its Food Forum, the Joint World Health Organization/Food and Agriculture Organization of the United Nations (WHO/FAO) Expert Advisory Panel on Food Safety (chairman), and the Steering Committees of several WHO/FAO panels. He also served as chair of the Joint FAO/WHO Expert Consultation on the Application of Risk Analysis to Food Standards Issues. He is author or co-author of more than 200 original scientific publications. Dr. Miller received a B.S. in chemistry from the City College of New York, and an M.S. and Ph.D. from Rutgers University in physiology and biochemistry.

IAN C. MUNRO, Ph.D., is a consultant toxicologist and principal for CanTox, Inc. in Ontario, Canada. He is a leading authority on toxicology and has over 30 years experience in dealing with complex regulatory issues related to product safety. He has in excess of 150 scientific publications in the fields of toxicology and risk assessment. Dr. Munro formerly held senior positions at Health and Welfare Canada as director of the Bureau of Chemical Safety and director general of the Food Directorate, Health Protection Branch. He was responsible for research and standard setting activities related to microbial and chemical hazards in food and the nutritional quality of the Canadian food supply. He has contributed significantly to the development of risk assessment procedures in the field of public health, both nationally and internationally, through membership on various committees dealing with the regulatory aspects of risk assessment and risk management of public health hazards. Dr. Munro is a graduate of McGill University in biochemistry and nutrition and holds a Ph.D. from Queen's University in pharmacology and toxicology. He is a fellow of the Royal College of Pathologists, London, and a fellow of the Academy of Toxicological Sciences. He also was a former director of the Canadian Centre for Toxicology at Guelph, Ontario.

SUZANNE P. MURPHY, Ph.D., R.D., is a nutrition researcher (professor) at the Cancer Research Center of Hawaii at the University of

Hawaii, Honolulu. She received her B.S. in mathematics from Temple University and her Ph.D. in nutrition from the University of California at Berkeley. Dr. Murphy's research interests include dietary assessment methodology, development of food composition databases, and nutritional epidemiology. She is a member of the National Nutrition Monitoring Advisory Council and the Year 2000 Dietary Guidelines Advisory Committee, and serves on editorial boards for the *Journal of Nutrition, Journal of Food Composition and Analysis, Family Economics and Nutrition Review,* and *Nutrition Today.* Dr. Murphy is a member of numerous professional organizations including the American Dietetic Association, American Society for Nutritional Sciences, American Public Health Association, American Society for Clinical Nutrition, and Society for Nutrition Education. She has over 50 publications on dietary assessment methodology and has lectured nationally and internationally on this subject.

HARRIS PASTIDES, Ph.D., is dean of the University of South Carolina's School of Public Health and professor in the Department of Epidemiology and Biostatistics. Previously, he was chair and a professor of epidemiology in the Department of Biostatistics and Epidemiology at the School of Public Health and Health Sciences at the University of Massachusetts at Amherst. Dr. Pastides is a consultant to the World Health Organization's Program in Environmental Health and a fellow of the American College of Epidemiology. He has published widely and is the co-author of several books. He was a Fulbright Senior Research Fellow and visiting professor at the University of Athens Medical School in Greece from 1987 to 1988. Dr. Pastides earned his M.P.H. and Ph.D. from Yale University; he has been a principal investigator or co-investigator on over 30 externally-funded research grants, results of which have been published in numerous peer-reviewed journals. He previously served on the National Academy of Sciences' Committee on Pediatric Respiratory Infections in Developing Nations.

JAMES G. PENLAND, Ph.D., is a research psychologist at the U.S. Department of Agriculture, Agriculture Research Service, Grand Forks Human Nutrition Research Center and adjunct professor of psychology at the University of North Dakota. Since receiving his Ph.D. in experimental cognitive psychology from the University of North Dakota in 1984, Dr. Penland's research has focused on determining the role of mineral element nutrition in neuropsychological function and behavior throughout the lifespan. He has conducted numerous metabolic unit and community-based feeding and supplementation studies investigating a variety of minerals and functional outcomes, including zinc, iron, boron, and copper effects on cognitive performance; selenium effects on mood states; copper and iron effects on sleep behavior; and calcium and manganese effects on menstrual symptoms. He has also assessed the impact of boron, magnesium, zinc, copper and iron nutrition on brain electrophysiology. Computerized cognitive and psychomotor assessment methods developed by Dr. Penland have been used in collaborative nutrition studies with children and adults throughout the United States and in China, Guatemala, and New Zealand. Dr. Penland has served on several expert panels and scientific advisory groups, including the Food and Nutrition Board's Committee on Military Nutrition Research.

JOSEPH V. RODRICKS, Ph.D., is the managing director of The Life Sciences Consultancy LLC. He is one of the founding principals of the ENVIRON Corporation, with internationally recognized expertise in assessing the risks to human health of exposure to toxic substances. He received his B.S. from the Massachusetts Institute of Technology and his Ph.D. in biochemistry from the University of Maryland. Dr. Rodricks is certified as a diplomate of the American Board of Toxicology. Before working as a consultant, he spent 15 years at the Food and Drug Administration (FDA). In his final 3 years at FDA, he was Deputy Associate Commissioner for Science, with special responsibility for risk assessment. He was a member of the National Academy of Sciences (NAS) Board on Toxicology and Environmental Health Hazards, and has also served on or chaired ten other NAS committees. He has more than 100 scientific publications on food safety and risk assessment and has lectured nationally and internationally on these subjects. He is the author of *Calculated Risks,* a nontechnical introduction to toxicology and risk assessment.

IRWIN H. ROSENBERG, M.D., is an internationally recognized leader in nutrition science who serves as professor of physiology, medicine and nutrition at the School of Medicine and School of Nutrition, as well as director, Jean Mayer U.S. Department of Agriculture (USDA) Human Nutrition Research Center on Aging, and dean for nutrition sciences, all at Tufts University. He is the first holder of the Jean Mayer Chair in Nutrition at Tufts. Prior to joining Tufts, Dr. Rosenberg held faculty positions at the Harvard Medical School and University of Chicago where he served as the first director of the Clinical Nutrition Research Center. As a clinical nutrition investigator, he has helped develop a nutritional focus within the field of gastroenterology with his primary research interest being in the area of folate metabolism. His research for the past decade has focused on nutrition and the aging process. Among his many honors are the Josiah Macy Faculty Award, Grace Goldsmith Award of the American College of Nutrition, Robert H. Herman Memorial Award of the American Society of Clinical Nutrition, Jonathan B. Rhoads Award of the American Society for Parenteral and Enteral Nutrition, and 1994 W.O. Atwater Memorial Lectureship of the USDA. Dr. Rosenberg was elected to the Institute of Medicine in 1994 and in 1996 he received the Bristol Myers Squibb/ Mead Johnson Award for Distinguished Achievement in Nutrition Research.

A. CATHARINE ROSS, Ph.D., is professor of nutrition and Dorothy Foehr Huck Chair at the Pennsylvania State University. She earned her B.S. at the University California, Davis and received her Ph.D. from Cornell University. Dr. Ross has published numerous research articles in the area of vitamin A metabolism and immunity. Her research on infection and inflammation has included developing methods for assessing vitamin A status during infection in humans. Dr. Ross is a member of the Food and Nutrition Board and received the Mead Johnson Award of the American Society of Nutritional Sciences.

ROBERT M. RUSSELL, M.D., is professor of medicine and nutrition at Tufts University School of Medicine and associate director at the Jean Mayer U.S. Department of Agriculture (USDA) Human Nutrition Research Center on Aging. Dr. Russell served on the Panel on Folate and Other B Vitamins. He has a B.S. from Harvard University and an M.D. from Columbia University. His primary work involves studying the effects of aging on gastrointestinal absorption of micronutrients, including vitamin A. He has served on many national and international advisory panels, including chairman of the USDA Human Investigative Committee, U.S. Pharmacopeia Convention, Food and Drug Administration, National Digestive Diseases Advisory Board, American Board of Internal Medicine, and is currently a vice-chair on the Food and Nutrition Board. He has worked on international programs in several countries including Vietnam, Iran, Iraq, Guatemala, China, and the Philippines. Dr. Russell serves on the editorial boards of various professional journals. He is a staff gastroenterologist/nutritionist at the New England Medical Center Hospitals.

BARBARA J. STOECKER, Ph.D, R.D., is professor and head of nutritional sciences at Oklahoma State University. She received her B.S. at Kansas State University and holds a Ph.D. from Iowa State University. Her research interest is chromium metabolism and requirements. Specifically, she has investigated chromium absorption, impact on diabetes, and drug interactions. Dr. Stoecker is a member of the American Society for Nutritional Sciences, Institute of Food Technologists, and past chair of the Research Dietetic Practice Group of the American Dietetic Association.

JOHN W. SUTTIE, Ph.D., is the Katherine Berns Van Donk Steenbock Professor of in the Department of Biochemistry at the University of Wisconsin. He received his B.S., M.S., and Ph.D. from the University of Wisconsin. Dr. Suttie has published numerous research articles in the area of vitamin K action, metabolism, and nutritional importance. He is a member of the National Academy of Sciences, a member of the National Research Council's Board on Agriculture and Natural Resources, and is the editor of the *Journal of Nutrition*.

STEVE L. TAYLOR, Ph.D., serves as professor and head of the Department of Food Science and Technology and director of the Food Processing Center at the University of Nebraska. He also maintains an active research program in the area of food allergies through the Food Allergy Research and Resource Program at the University of Nebraska. He received his B.S. and M.S. in food science and technology from Oregon State University and his Ph.D. in biochemistry from the University of California at Davis. Dr. Taylor's primary research interests involve naturally occurring toxicants in foods, especially food allergens. His research involves the development of immunoassays for the detection of residues of allergenic foods contaminating other foods, the effect of processing on food allergens, and the assessment of the allergenicity of genetically engineered foods. Dr. Taylor has over 160 publications. He is a member of numerous professional associations including Institute of Food Technologists; American Chemical Society; American Academy of Allergy, Asthma, and Immunology; and Society of Toxicology.

JOHN A. THOMAS, Ph.D., received his undergraduate degree at the University of Wisconsin and his M.A. and Ph.D. at the University of Iowa. He has held professorships in departments of pharmacology and toxicology in several medical schools including Iowa, Virginia, and West Virginia. From 1973 to 1982 he served as associate dean of the School of Medicine at West Virginia University. In 1982

Dr. Thomas became Vice President for Corporate Research at Baxter Healthcare. Dr. Thomas served as vice president at the University of Texas Health Science Center at San Antonio from 1988 to 1998. He serves on several editorial boards of biomedical journals and serves as chairman of the Society of Toxicology Education Committee, chairman of the Expert Advisory Committee of the Canadian Network of Toxicology Centers, and vice president of the Academy of Toxicology. He is a diplomate, fellow, and member of the Board of Trustees in the Academy of Toxicological Sciences, and serves on many scientific boards and committees in the chemical and the pharmaceutical industry. He has received many awards, including the 1999 Distinguished Service Award from the American College of Toxicology, the Merit Award from the Society of Toxicology, Certificate of Scientific Service (U.S. Environmental Protection Agency), Distinguished Lecturer in Medical Sciences (American Medical Association), and the Distinguished Service Award from the Texas Society for Biomedical Research. He is an elected foreign member of the Russian Academy of Medical Sciences. Dr. Thomas is the author of over a dozen textbooks and research monographs and has published over 350 scientific articles.

JUDITH R. TURNLUND, Ph.D, R.D., is a research nutrition scientist at the U.S. Department of Agriculture Western Human Nutrition Research Center and an adjunct professor in the Department of Nutrition, University of California at Davis. She earned her B.S. at Gustavus Adolphus College and holds a Ph.D. from the University of California at Berkeley. Her research interests include human requirements for and bioavailability of trace elements (zinc, copper, molybdenum, and iron) and nutrition and aging. Dr. Turnlund received the American Institute of Nutrition Lederle Award for outstanding accomplishments in human nutrition.

KEITH P. WEST, Dr.P.H., R.D., is professor of human nutrition at the Johns Hopkins School of Hygiene and Public Health. He received his B.S. from Drexel University, earned his Dr.P.H. from the Johns Hopkins School of Hygiene and Public Health, and holds an R.D. from Walter Reed General Hospital. Dr. West recently headed two large community trials in Nepal to understand the impact of vitamin A interventions on the prevention of morbidity and mortality in women, children, and infants. In addition to vitamin A, Dr. West's research interests include nutritional epidemiology and dietary and anthropometric assessment. Dr. West is a member of the International Vitamin A Consultative Group.

GARY M. WILLIAMS, M.D., is a professor in the Department of Pathology and Director of Environmental Pathology and Toxicology at New York Medical College. He also serves as head of the Program on Medicine, Food and Chemical Safety. Previously, Dr. Williams served as director of the Naylor Dana Institute and chief of the Division of Pathology and Toxicology at the American Health Foundation. He earned his M.D. from the University of Pittsburgh. Dr. Williams has received numerous honors including the Arnold J. Lehman Award of the Society of Toxicology and the Sheard-Sandford Award of the American Society of Clinical Pathologists. He has served on the editorial boards for many scientific reports and journals. He is the author or co-author of over 430 scientific publications. He previously served on the Committee on Research Opportunities and Priorities for Environmental Protection Agency and the Committee on the carcinogenicity of Cyclamates for the National Academy of Sciences.

STANLEY H. ZLOTKIN, M.D., Ph.D., is a professor in the Departments of Pediatrics and Nutritional Sciences at the University of Toronto, senior scientist and medical director of nutrition support, and chief of the division of gastroenterology and nutrition at the Hospital for Sick Children. He received his Ph.D. from the University of Toronto, his M.D. from McMaster University, and his FRCP(C) from McGill University. His research interests include improved methods for assessing iron status and interventions to prevent iron deficiency anemia in infants and young children. Dr. Zlotkin has served as a consultant on nutrition issues to the Canadian Federal and Provincial Government and as past chairman of the Nutrition Committee of the Canadian Pediatric Society. Currently, he is the nutrition advisor for the International Life Sciences Institute's Food and Nutrition Safety Committee.

Index

A

Abortions, spontaneous, 248

Absorption of nutrients. *See also*
  Bioavailability of nutrients;
  Malabsorption syndromes;
  individual nutrients
  adults, 40, 86, 474, 479
  and adverse effects, 73
  aging and, 40, 86, 146, 474
  ascorbic acid interactions, 311-312, 521
  assessment methods, 445, 455, 472
  calcium interactions, 455-456
  carotenoids, 86-93, 107
  dietary fat and, 70, 106-107, 118, 121,
    163
  foods affecting, 521
  form of intake and, 267, 373, 395, 483
  form of nutrient and, 73 n 2, 87, 88-89,
    227-228, 455-456, 529
  fractional, 15, 447-448, 449, 450, 462,
    463, 464-465, 468, 469, 472, 473,
    474, 476, 478, 572
  gender and, 402
  human milk vs infant formula, 238, 404
  infections and, 107
  interaction of nutrients and, 70, 106-
    107, 118, 121, 163, 311-312, 455-
    456, 482-483
  interindividual variation in, 69, 397,
    402

intestinal environment and, 311-312,
    454-455
  lactation and, 244
  level of intakes and, 242, 399, 422, 115,
    473
  menaquinones, 164
  phytates and, 572, 576
  pregnancy and, 243
  processing of foods and, 107, 112, 146,
    174, 211
  solubility of compound and, 504
Aceruloplasminemia, 227, 377
Achlorhydria, 311
Achromotrichia, 435
Acid phosphatase activity, 529
Acrodermatitis enteropathica, 445, 477
Adenosine triphosphate (ATP), 225, 226
Adenosyl diphosphate, 357
S-Adenyl homocysteine, 509
S-Adenyl methionine, 509
Adequate intakes (AIs). *See also individual*
    nutrients
  appropriateness of intakes above,
    77
  criteria used to derive, 36, 37
  defined, 3, 6, 30, 34
  EAR distinguished from, 37
  extrapolation from other age groups,
    35, 51-52, 53, 111
  group applications, 554, 561, 564

729

C

M

X

Z

FOOD AND NUTRITION BOARD, INSTITUTE OF MEDICINE–NATIONAL ACADEMY OF SCIENCES
DIETARY REFERENCE INTAKES:
RECOMMENDED INTAKES FOR INDIVIDUALS, VITAMINS

Life Stage Group	Vitamin A (µg/d)[a]	Vitamin C (mg/d)	Vitamin D (µg/d)[b,c]	Vitamin E (mg/d)[d]	Vitamin K (µg/d)	Thiamin (mg/d)
Infants						
0–6 mo	400*	40*	5*	4*	2.0*	0.2*
7–12 mo	500*	50*	5*	5*	2.5*	0.3*
Children						
1–3 y	**300**	**15**	5*	**6**	30*	**0.5**
4–8 y	**400**	**25**	5*	**7**	55*	**0.6**
Males						
9–13 y	**600**	**45**	5*	**11**	60*	**0.9**
14–18 y	**900**	**75**	5*	**15**	75*	**1.2**
19–30 y	**900**	**90**	5*	**15**	120*	**1.2**
31–50 y	**900**	**90**	5*	**15**	120*	**1.2**
51–70 y	**900**	**90**	10*	**15**	120*	**1.2**
> 70 y	**900**	**90**	15*	**15**	120*	**1.2**
Females						
9–13 y	**600**	**45**	5*	**11**	60*	**0.9**
14–18 y	**700**	**65**	5*	**15**	75*	**1.0**
19–30 y	**700**	**75**	5*	**15**	90*	**1.1**
31–50 y	**700**	**75**	5*	**15**	90*	**1.1**
51–70 y	**700**	**75**	10*	**15**	90*	**1.1**
> 70 y	**700**	**75**	15*	**15**	90*	**1.1**
Pregnancy						
≤ 18 y	**750**	**80**	5*	**15**	75*	**1.4**
19–30 y	**770**	**85**	5*	**15**	90*	**1.4**
31–50 y	**770**	**85**	5*	**15**	90*	**1.4**
Lactation						
≤ 18 y	**1,200**	**115**	5*	**19**	75*	**1.4**
19–30 y	**1,300**	**120**	5*	**19**	90*	**1.4**
31–50 y	**1,300**	**120**	5*	**19**	90*	**1.4**

NOTE: This table (taken from the DRI reports, see www.nap.edu) presents Recommended Dietary Allowances (RDAs) in **bold type** and Adequate Intakes (AIs) in ordinary type followed by an asterisk (*). RDAs and AIs may both be used as goals for individual intake. RDAs are set to meet the needs of almost all (97 to 98 percent) individuals in a group. For healthy breastfed infants, the AI is the mean intake. The AI for other life stage and gender groups is believed to cover needs of all individuals in the group, but lack of data or uncertainty in the data prevent being able to specify with confidence the percentage of individuals covered by this intake.

[a] As retinol activity equivalents (RAEs). 1 RAE = 1 µg retinol, 12 µg β-carotene, 24 µg α-carotene, or 24 µg β-cryptoxanthin. To calculate RAEs from REs of provitamin A carotenoids in foods, divide the REs by 2. For preformed vitamin A in foods or supplements and for provitamin A carotenoids in supplements, 1 RE = 1 RAE.

Riboflavin (mg/d)	Niacin (mg/d)[e]	Vitamin B_6 (mg/d)	Folate (µg/d)[f]	Vitamin B_{12} (µg/d)	Pantothenic Acid (mg/d)	Biotin (µg/d)	Choline (mg/d)[g]
0.3*	2*	0.1*	65*	0.4*	1.7*	5*	125*
0.4*	4*	0.3*	80*	0.5*	1.8*	6*	150*
0.5	6	0.5	150	0.9	2*	8*	200*
0.6	8	0.6	200	1.2	3*	12*	250*
0.9	12	1.0	300	1.8	4*	20*	375*
1.3	16	1.3	400	2.4	5*	25*	550*
1.3	16	1.3	400	2.4	5*	30*	550*
1.3	16	1.3	400	2.4	5*	30*	550*
1.3	16	1.7	400	2.4[h]	5*	30*	550*
1.3	16	1.7	400	2.4[h]	5*	30*	550*
0.9	12	1.0	300	1.8	4*	20*	375*
1.0	14	1.2	400[i]	2.4	5*	25*	400*
1.1	14	1.3	400[i]	2.4	5*	30*	425*
1.1	14	1.3	400[i]	2.4	5*	30*	425*
1.1	14	1.5	400	2.4[h]	5*	30*	425*
1.1	14	1.5	400	2.4[h]	5*	30*	425*
1.4	18	1.9	600[j]	2.6	6*	30*	450*
1.4	18	1.9	600[j]	2.6	6*	30*	450*
1.4	18	1.9	600[j]	2.6	6*	30*	450*
1.6	17	2.0	500	2.8	7*	35*	550*
1.6	17	2.0	500	2.8	7*	35*	550*
1.6	17	2.0	500	2.8	7*	35*	550*

continued

[b] calciferol. 1 µg calciferol = 40 IU vitamin D.

[c] In the absence of adequate exposure to sunlight.

[d] As α-tocopherol. α-Tocopherol includes RRR-α-tocopherol, the only form of α-tocopherol that occurs naturally in foods, and the 2R-stereoisomeric forms of α-tocopherol (RRR-, RSR-, RRS-, and RSS-α-tocopherol) that occur in fortified foods and supplements. It does not include the 2S-stereoisomeric forms of α-tocopherol (SRR-, SSR-, SRS-, and SSS-α-tocopherol), also found in fortified foods and supplements.

[e] As niacin equivalents (NE). 1 mg of niacin = 60 mg of tryptophan; 0–6 months = preformed niacin (not NE).

[f] As dietary folate equivalents (DFE). 1 DFE = 1 µg food folate = 0.6 µg of folic acid from fortified food or as a supplement consumed with food = 0.5 µg of a supplement taken on an empty stomach.

[g] Although AIs have been set for choline, there are few data to assess whether a

Table Continued
FOOD AND NUTRITION BOARD, INSTITUTE OF MEDICINE–
NATIONAL ACADEMY OF SCIENCES
DIETARY REFERENCE INTAKES:
RECOMMENDED INTAKES FOR INDIVIDUALS, ELEMENTS

Life Stage Group	Calcium (mg/d)	Chromium (µg/d)	Copper (µg/d)	Fluoride (mg/d)	Iodine (µg/d)	Iron (mg/d)
Infants						
0–6 mo	210*	0.2*	200*	0.01*	110*	0.27*
7–12 mo	270*	5.5*	220*	0.5*	130*	11
Children						
1–3 y	500*	11*	340	0.7*	90	7
4–8 y	800*	15*	440	1*	90	10
Males						
9–13 y	1,300*	25*	700	2*	120	8
14–18 y	1,300*	35*	890	3*	150	11
19–30 y	1,000*	35*	900	4*	150	8
31–50 y	1,000*	35*	900	4*	150	8
51–70 y	1,200*	30*	900	4*	150	8
> 70 y	1,200*	30*	900	4*	150	8
Females						
9–13 y	1,300*	21*	700	2*	120	8
14–18 y	1,300*	24*	890	3*	150	15
19–30 y	1,000*	25*	900	3*	150	18
31–50 y	1,000*	25*	900	3*	150	18
51–70 y	1,200*	20*	900	3*	150	8
> 70 y	1,200*	20*	900	3*	150	8
Pregnancy						
≤ 18 y	1,300*	29*	1,000	3*	220	27
19–30 y	1,000*	30*	1,000	3*	220	27
31–50 y	1,000*	30*	1,000	3*	220	27
Lactation						
≤ 18 y	1,300*	44*	1,300	3*	290	10
19–30 y	1,000*	45*	1,300	3*	290	9
31–50 y	1,000*	45*	1,300	3*	290	9

continued

dietary supply of choline is needed at all stages of the life cycle, and it may be that the choline requirement can be met by endogenous synthesis at some of these stages.

[h] Because 10 to 30 percent of older people may malabsorb food-bound B_{12}, it is advisable for those older than 50 years to meet their RDA mainly by consuming foods fortified with B_{12} or a supplement containing B_{12}.

[i] In view of evidence linking folate intake with neural tube defects in the fetus, it is recommended that all women capable of becoming pregnant consume 400 µg from supplements or fortified foods in addition to intake of food folate from a varied diet.

Magnesium (mg/d)	Manganese (mg/d)	Molybdenum (µg/d)	Phosphorus (mg/d)	Selenium (µg/d)	Zinc (mg/d)
30*	0.003*	2*	100*	15*	2*
75*	0.6*	3*	275*	20*	3
80	1.2*	17	460	20	3
130	1.5*	22	500	30	5
240	1.9*	34	1,250	40	8
410	2.2*	43	1,250	55	11
400	2.3*	45	700	55	11
420	2.3*	45	700	55	11
420	2.3*	45	700	55	11
420	2.3*	45	700	55	11
240	1.6*	34	1,250	40	8
360	1.6*	43	1,250	55	9
310	1.8*	45	700	55	8
320	1.8*	45	700	55	8
320	1.8*	45	700	55	8
320	1.8*	45	700	55	8
400	2.0*	50	1,250	60	12
350	2.0*	50	700	60	11
360	2.0*	50	700	60	11
360	2.6*	50	1,250	70	13
310	2.6*	50	700	70	12
320	2.6*	50	700	70	12

^{j} It is assumed that women will continue consuming 400 µg from supplements or fortified food until their pregnancy is confirmed and they enter prenatal care, which ordinarily occurs after the end of the periconceptional period—the critical time for formation of the neural tube.

SOURCES: *Dietary Reference Intakes for Calcium, Phosphorus, Magnesium, Vitamin D, and Fluoride* (1997); *Dietary Reference Intakes for Thiamin, Riboflavin, Niacin, Vitamin B$_6$, Folate, Vitamin B$_{12}$, Pantothenic Acid, Biotin, and Choline* (1998); *Dietary Reference Intakes for Vitamin C, Vitamine E, Selenium, and Carotenoids* (2000); and *Dietary Reference Intakes for Vitamin A, Vitamin K, Arsenic, Boron, Chromium, Copper, Iodine, Iron, Manganese, Molybdenum, Nickel, Silicon, Vanadium, and Zinc* (2001). These reports may be accessed via www.nap.edu.